Terminology

for ALLIED HEALTH PROFESSIONALS

5TH EDITION

Carolee Sormunen, Ph.D.

Educational Consultant

Professor Emerita
Ball State University
Muncie, Indiana

Research and technical
assistance from
RONALD F. JONES

DELMAR
CENGAGE Learning™

Australia Canada Mexico Singapore Spain United Kingdom United States

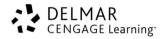
DELMAR
CENGAGE Learning

Terminology for
Allied Health Professionals
Fifth Edition
Carolee Sormunen

Executive Director,
Heath Care Business Unit:
William Brottmiller

Executive Editor:
Cathy L. Esperti

Acquisitions Editor:
Sherry Gomoll

Developmental Editor:
Deb Flis

Executive Marketing Manager:
Dawn F. Gerrain

Channel Manager:
Jennifer McAvey

Marketing Coordinator:
Mona Caron

Editorial Assistant:
Jennifer Conklin

Production Editor:
Mary Colleen Liburdi

Project Editor:
David Buddle

For product information and technology assistance, contact us at
Cengage Learning Customer & Sales Support, 1-800-354-9706

For permission to use material from this text or product,
submit all requests online at **cengage.com/permissions**
Further permissions questions can be emailed to
permissionrequest@cengage.com

ExamView® and ExamView Pro® are registered trademarks of FSCreations, Inc. Windows is a registered trademark of the Microsoft Corporation used herein under license. Macintosh and Power Macintosh are registered trademarks of Apple Computer, Inc. Used herein under license.

© 2007 Cengage Learning. All Rights Reserved. Cengage Learning WebTutor™ is a trademark of Cengage Learning.

Library of Congress Control Number: 2002073721

ISBN-13: 978-0-7668-6292-0

ISBN-10: 0-7668-6292-5

Delmar Cengage Learning
5 Maxwell Drive
Clifton Park, NY 12065-2919
USA

Cengage Learning products are represented in Canada by Nelson Education, Ltd.

For your lifelong learning solutions, visit **delmar.cengage.com**

Visit our corporate website at **www.cengage.com**

Notice to the Reader

Publisher does not warrant or guarantee any of the products described herein or perform any independent analysis in connection with any of the product information contained herein. Publisher does not assume, and expressly disclaims, any obligation to obtain and include information other than that provided to it by the manufacturer. The reader is expressly warned to consider and adopt all safety precautions that might be indicated by the activities described herein and to avoid all potential hazards. By following the instructions contained herein, the reader willingly assumes all risks in connection with such instructions. The publisher makes no representations or warranties of any kind, including but not limited to, the warranties of fitness for particular purpose or merchantability, nor are any such representations implied with respect to the material set forth herein, and the publisher takes no responsibility with respect to such material. The publisher shall not be liable for any special, consequential, or exemplary damages resulting, in whole or part, from the readers' use of, or reliance upon, this material.

Printed in China by CTPS
7 8 9 10 11 12 11 10 09 08

Contents

Preface

Terminology for Allied Health Professionals, fifth edition, is designed to integrate the entire spectrum of information needed by allied health professionals who must understand medical terminology.

PHILOSOPHY

Terminology for Allied Health Professionals, fifth edition, focuses on successful learning by applying information in the context in which it is used in the medical environment. A simple-to-complex instructional design begins with the basic structure of medical terms—including roots, prefixes, and suffixes—and an introduction to basic terms related to the human anatomy. Over 600 roots, prefixes, and suffixes are presented and defined in the specific chapter associated with a particular body system. A mix of anatomy, physiology, and pathophysiology is combined with information about the medical records in which these medical terms appear. Reinforcement activities are included that review each section of a chapter. Completion of these activities will provide an opportunity for you to highlight important information and focus review efforts in mastering content.

Anatomical medical illustrations are carefully designed to support explanations in the text. Each term in the text is numbered to coincide with a number in a related illustration. Whenever possible, these numbers move sequentially around the illustration to make it easier to locate a particular structure.

Medical history and physical examinations, surgical notes, radiology reports, discharge summaries, pathology reports, and autopsies are the basic six types of reports found in medical offices. In preparing these reports, the health care industry uses a variety of terms to describe patient health information: health record, medical record, clinical record, patient health record, and patient record. To avoid any confusion in discussions of the reports, the author has chosen to use the term "patient record" to identify all patient health information. Introduction of the various report types is not done until they have been discussed in the textual material. In other words, the history and physical report first appears as an example in Chapter 3, the surgical notes are not used as examples until Chapter 7, and so forth for the other four reports.

Every chapter related to body systems has a section called Working Practice that allows you to learn how the terms are used in the medical environment. Specialty chapters such as Pharmacology, Oncology, Radiology and Nuclear Medicine, and Mental Health add dimension and depth to your learning experience. Each chapter provides additional basic knowledge that helps increase your ability to secure employment.

The text and supporting materials encourage the development of critical thinking skills. Employers want individuals who can step beyond memorizing lists of words to use them confidently and to interact with the professionals who use them.

Dictionary Exercises are included in each chapter. Medical transcriptionists suggested many of the words used in these exercises, drawing on the terminology commonly found in dictation in their specialty offices. Medical reports have been provided from a variety of offices to give an in-depth exposure to the more common formats in a medical environment. These are included as Listening Exercises so that words can be heard in the context in which they are used. Reports have been dictated carefully for this initial exposure to hearing medical terminology. An audio CD containing the Listening Exercises is included in the back of the book. Listening to the correct pronunciation of the words and phrases as they are used in the context of a medical report provides "live" experience that will ease your move into the workplace.

CHANGES IN THE FIFTH EDITION

The fifth edition of *Terminology for Allied Health Professionals* retains its basic instructional design, but has been carefully reviewed by the author and panel of consulting physicians so that each chapter reflects the latest in medical developments.

Major revisions include the following elements:

1. New four-color anatomical medical illustrations and photos support text discussions.
2. Chapter 10, Oncology, has been substantially rewritten to reflect the continual expansion of knowledge in this area.
3. Chapter 16, The Female Reproductive System, is now a stand-alone chapter that includes the expanded section on pregnancy and childbirth.
4. Chapter 17, The Male Reproductive System, is now a stand-alone chapter that includes sexually transmitted diseases.
5. The diagnosis portion of the Working Practice sections has been reorganized for each specialty in a way that reflects the system. For example, in Chapter 8, The Cardiovascular System, the diagnoses have been grouped by diseases of the heart, heart valves, heart rate and rhythm, and arteries, veins, and circulation.
6. Frequently used terms that describe information pertinent to each system covering diagnostic procedures, diagnosis, treatment procedures, commonly used abbreviations, and medications were updated with cooperation from offices of the various medical specialties involved.
7. Activities were added to each chapter that introduce helpful and relevant Internet web sites.
8. Suggestions were added on how to proceed when you cannot find a term in your medical dictionary.
9. An audio CD containing listening exercises from the text provides real-world experience.

REFERENCES

Three primary sources were used in developing this instructional program. Pronunciations came from *Taber's Cyclopedic Medical Dictionary* and *Miller-*

Keane Encyclopedia and Dictionary of Medicine, Nursing, and Allied Health. For style, the reference was *Style Guide for Medical Transcription* by Tessier, American Association for Medical Transcription. In addition, extensive use was made of the Internet for research on various diseases, conditions, diagnostic and treatment procedures, medications, and other sources of information.

SPECIAL RESOURCES TO ACCOMPANY THIS TEXT

INSTRUCTOR'S MANUAL

A valuable resource, the Instructor's Manual (ISBN 0-7668-6293-3) includes

- Information on teaching and learning strategies, evaluations, and helpful suggestions based on the author's experience.
- A critical-thinking tip in each chapter designed to help students develop this highly desirable work skill.
- Medical illustrations ready to be reproduced or made into transparencies to be used for presentation, review, or evaluation activities.
- Word find and crossword puzzle activities that focus on words and definitions in specific chapters and add variety to repetitive drills.
- Lists of word elements in a larger, cleaner font to enhance reproduction on a transparency. These lists can be used for initial presentation, review, or evaluation activities.
- A test bank of objective questions. To assist you in a preparation of tests, the test bank includes nonrepetitious questions on the significant content of each chapter.
- Optional exercises such as charting exercises based on the listening exercises in Chapters 3, 7, 11, 14, and 18.
- Suggestions for assignments using the Internet to find chapter-related information.

WEBTUTOR™

Designed to complement the text, WebTutor™ is a content-rich, web-based teaching and learning aid that reinforces and clarifies complex concepts. The WebCT™ and Blackboard™ platforms also provide rich communication tools to instructors and students, including a course calendar, chat, e-mail, and threaded discussions.

WebTutor on WebCT™ (ISBN 0-7668-6294-1)
Text Bundled with WebTutor on WebCT™ (ISBN 1-4018-2100-6)
WebTutor on Blackboard™ (ISBN 0-768-6295-X)
Text Bundled with WebTutor on Blackboard™ (ISBN 1-4018-2099-9)

ADDITIONAL MULTIMEDIA RESOURCES

DELMAR'S MEDICAL TERMINOLOGY CD-ROM (INSTITUTIONAL VERSION)

This exciting interactive reference, practice, and assessment tool complements any medical terminology program. Features include the extensive use of multimedia—

animations, video, graphics, and activities—to present terms and word-building features. Difficult functions, processes, and procedures are included, so learners can more effectively learn from a textbook.

CD-ROM, Institutional Version, ISBN 0-7668-0979-X

DELMAR'S MEDICAL TERMINOLOGY VIDEO SERIES

This series of 14 medical terminology videotapes is designed for allied health and nursing students enrolled in medical terminology courses. The videos may be used in class to supplement a lecture or in a resource lab by users who want additional reinforcement. The series can also be used in distance learning programs as a telecourse. The videos simulate a typical medical terminology class and are organized by body system. The on-camera "instructor" leads students through various concepts, interspersing lectures with graphics, video clips, and illustrations to emphasize points. This comprehensive series is invaluable to students trying to master the complex world of medical terminology.

Complete Set of Videos, ISBN 0-7668-0976-5 (Videos can also be purchased individually.)

DELMAR'S MEDICAL TERMINOLOGY FLASH!: COMPUTERIZED FLASHCARDS

Learn and review over 1,500 medical terms using this unique electronic flashcard program. Flash! is a computerized flashcard-type question-and-answer program designed to help users learn correct spellings, definitions, and pronunciations. The use of graphics and audio clips makes it a fun and easy way for users to learn and test their knowledge of medical terminology.

CD-ROM, ISBN 0-7668-4320-3

ABOUT THE AUTHOR

The author brings a unique combination of experiences to the development of this edition of the textbook. As an instructional design and training specialist, the author applies her expertise to provide a solid instructional program for you. This expertise has been enhanced by her own experience in the medical environment, as well as her working relationship with individuals in a variety of positions in clinics, physician's offices, and hospitals. These experiences have resulted in a practical approach to preparing you for a variety of opportunities as an allied health professional.

ACKNOWLEDGMENTS

This text represents the efforts of many people. I am especially indebted to those who reviewed the manuscript drafts of the fifth edition and provided valuable suggestions.

Bradley S. Bowden, Ph.D.
Professor of Biology, Alfred University
Cheryl G. Davis, M.S., C.L.S. (N.C.A.)
Assistant Professor and Program Director, Medical Technology Program, Tuskegee University

Dr. Barbara A. Fortuna, R.H.I.A.
Professor and Program Coordinator, Miami-Dade Community College
Patsy Zink, B.S., M.S.
Business Technology Instructor, Oklahoma State University—Okmulgee

I also wish to acknowledge two individuals who provided invaluable help: Dr. Rosemary DeLoach, who spent many hours reading the original manuscript and providing constructive suggestions in the formative stage of this instruction program; and Marie Moisio, M.A., R.R.A., Northern Michigan University, who contributed significantly to the third edition by sharing her expertise. Both of these individuals have had a significant impact on the evolution of this textbook.

In addition to the medically related professional individuals and physicians identified on the following pages, I am indebted to staff members in the offices of the Marquette Medical Center and Marquette General Hospital, Marquette, Michigan, for their assistance.

Ronald F. Jones, my unofficial partner in this project, deserves special recognition for his valuable assistance with the revision of the text. He is a stalwart contributor who researched and verified portions of the text. His willingness to commit a significant amount of time, his technical writing skills, and his excellent editing skills added immeasurably to the creative process.

I especially appreciate the strong support I have had for this edition from Sherry Gomoll, acquisitions editor, and Deb Flis, developmental editor, at Delmar Learning.

Because a project of this nature is enriched by the efforts of each individual who assists in its completion, I wish to acknowledge the significant contributions all of you have made. Without that help, this book would not have been possible.

SPECIAL ACKNOWLEDGMENTS

I would like to thank the following contributors for their assistance in developing this text.

Cary Bjork, M.D., F.A.C.P.
American Board of Internal Medicine
Robert H. Blotter, M.D.
Fellow, American Academy of Orthopaedic Surgeons
Assistant Clinical Professor, Michigan State University College of Human Medicine, East Lansing, Michigan
Marquette General Hospital, Marquette, Michigan
Michael K. Conley, M.D.
Fellow, American College of Obstetricians and Gynecologists
Fellow, American College of Surgeons
Assistant Clinical Professor, Obstetrics and Gynecology, Michigan State University College of Human Medicine, East Lansing, Michigan
Randy Foker, M.D.
Board Certified Otolaryngologist
J. Marc Himes, M.D.
Assistant Clinical Professor of Internal Medicine, Michigan State University, College of Human Medicine, East Lansing, Michigan
Director of Hemodialysis Unit, Marquette General Hospital, Marquette, Michigan
James B. Keplinger, M.D.
American Board of Surgery

Ross G. Lane, Ph.D, H.S.P.P.

Ethelbert Lara, M.D.
Diagnostic Radiologist

Thomas D. LeGalley, M.D.
Board Certified in Cardiovascular Diseases
Fellow, American College of Cardiology
Fellow, American College of Chest Physicians

Vasilis Makris, M.D.
Fellow, American College of Surgeons

James H. Mering III, M.D.
Diplomate, American Board of Urology
Assistant Clinical Professor of Surgery, Michigan State University
College of Human Medicine, East Lansing, Michigan
Fellow, American College of Surgeons

Debra J. Morley, M.D., Ph.D.
Diplomate, American Board of Psychiatry and Neurology
Clinical Instructor, Michigan State University College of Human
Medicine, East Lansing, Michigan
Adjunct Faculty, Department of Biology, Northern Michigan University,
Marquette, Michigan

Reid Nishikawa, Pharm.D., B.C.N.S.P., F.L.S.H.P.
Director of Pharmacy and Coordinator, Clinical Services, Nutrishare,
Inc., Elk Grove, California
Clinical Associate Professor of Pharmacy, University of California—San
Francisco

Thomas F. Noren, M.D.
Associate, Upper Peninsula Digestive Disease Associates, Marquette,
Michigan

Aaron P. Scholnik, M.D.
American Subspecialty Board in Medical Oncology
American Subspecialty Board in Hematology
Associate Professor of Medicine—Hematology/Oncology, Michigan State
University College of Human Medicine, East Lansing, Michigan

Martha Short, M.D.
Clinical Associate Professor, Michigan State University College of
Human Medicine, East Lansing, Michigan

Milton D. Soderberg, M.D.
Diplomate, American Academy of Dermatology
Associate Clinical Professor, Michigan State University College of
Human Medicine, East Lansing, Michigan

Nicki Turner, M.D., F.A.C.P.
Division of Critical Care Medicine, Ball Memorial Hospital, Muncie,
Indiana

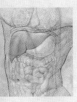

How to Use This Book

Terminology for Allied Health Professionals, fifth edition, focuses on successful learning by applying information in the context in which it is used in the medical environment. The following features are integrated throughout the text to assist you in learning and mastering medical terminology.

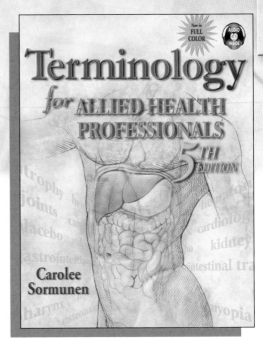

Chapter Quote

1 The quotation at the beginning of each chapter can be used to stimulate discussion and develop critical thinking. Reflect on the relevance of the quote in relation to the chapter material.

Objectives

2 Chapter objectives help you focus on key concepts presented in the chapter. The objectives are achieved through a combination of written and listening exercises, using a multisensory approach to learning.

Introduction

3 The introduction provides you with an overview of important concepts you will learn in the chapter.

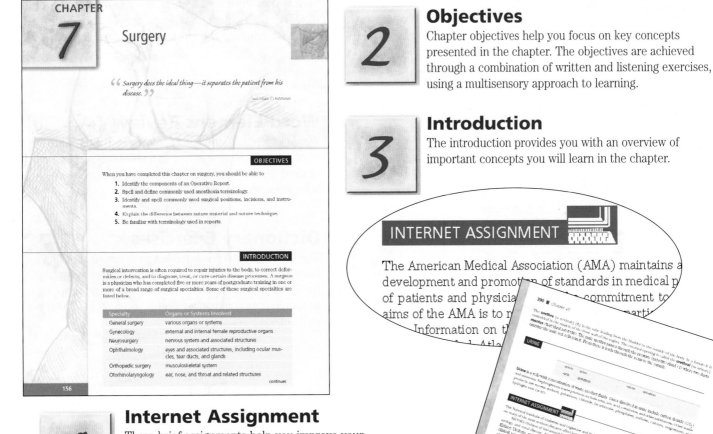

Internet Assignment

4 These brief assignments help you improve your research and Internet skills. Through the exploration of various web sites, you gain experience in locating chapter-related information.

Review

5 The review helps you assess your understanding of key facts presented in the chapter.

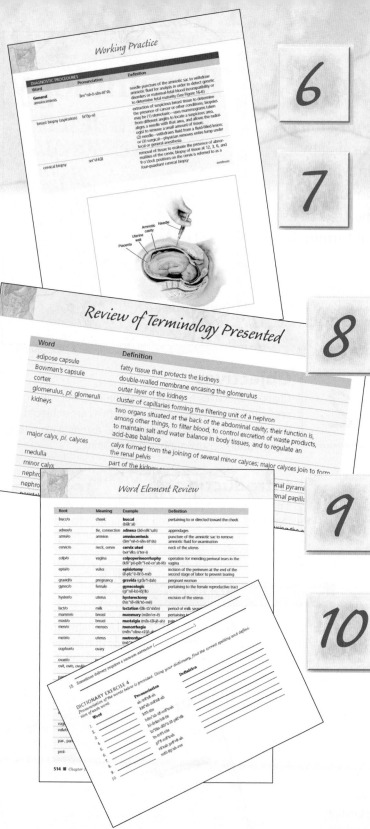

Working Practice

6 Every chapter related to body systems has a section called Working Practice that allows you to learn how the terms are used in medical environments. This section presents diagnostic and treatment procedures, diagnoses, abbreviations, and medications.

Full-color illustrations

7 **Full-color illustrations** of anatomical structures reinforce the terms used to describe them. Full-color illustrations in the Working Practice section reinforce diagnostic and treatment procedures.

Review of Terminology Presented

8 Key terms within chapters are **boldface**. The Review of Terminology Presented section serves as a chapter-level glossary of these important terms. Terminology Review Exercises reinforce the terms and their meanings.

Word Element Review

9 Word elements are integrated into each chapter. The Word Element Review serves as a chapter-level glossary of word elements. Word Element Review Exercises help you review roots, prefixes, and suffixes.

Dictionary Exercises

10 The Dictionary Exercises guide you in practicing using a medical dictionary effectively. Many of the words used in these exercises were identified by medical transcriptionists as terminology commonly found in dictation in their specialty offices.

Listening Exercises

11 The Listening Exercises, taken from actual medical documents, expose you to the most common formats in medical environments. The exercises allow you to *see* medical words in context. Listen to "real-life dictation" on the audio CD in the back of the book and *hear* words in the context in which they are used. Listening to the correct pronunciation of the words and phrases as they are used in the context of a medical report provides "live" experience that will ease your move into the workplace.

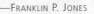
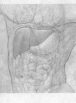

Building a Medical Vocabulary

Education isn't something you've had;
it's something you're always getting.

—FRANKLIN P. JONES

OBJECTIVES

When you have completed this chapter on building a medical vocabulary, you should be able to

1. Define medical terminology.
2. Define word elements, roots, prefixes, suffixes, combining vowels, and combining forms.
3. Create the adjective and noun forms of commonly used medical terms.
4. Create the singular and plural forms of commonly used medical terms.
5. Identify homonyms and eponyms used in medical reports.
6. Identify and spell the word elements and determine their meaning.
7. Use a medical dictionary effectively.

INTRODUCTION

Whether in a one-physician office, a major clinic, or a centralized laboratory, a behind-the-scenes health care team provides a variety of services. The list that follows provides a sampling of the positions that might comprise such a team.

Representative Health Care Positions

admissions clerk
coder-biller specialist
electrocardiogram technician
health information management
 technician
histologist
licensed practical nurse
medical transcriptionist
nurse practitioner
occupational therapist
office manager
paramedic

pharmacist
phlebotomist
physical therapist
physician's assistant
psychologist
radiologic technologist
radiology technician
registered nurse
respiratory therapy
 technician
ultrasound technician
unit clerk

The basic requirement for all members of a health care team is a working knowledge of medical terminology. It begins with a thorough understanding of roots, prefixes, and suffixes—referred to in this text as *word elements*—and how they can be combined in a variety of ways to create medical words. Chapter 1 introduces the rules for joining the word elements to form medical terms, along with information about adjective and noun forms, singular and plural forms, and homonyms and eponyms.

Because parts of the body are frequently referred to in the medical work environment, members of the health care team should be familiar with at least the more commonly used anatomical terms. Understanding how the systems of the body function helps to make sense of medical terms. Basic body structure is presented in Chapter 2; more detailed anatomy and associated terminology with each body system appear in subsequent chapters.

However, not all medical language is based on word elements, body structure, or anatomy. Some words are simply familiar words with a special medical meaning. For instance, a "thrill" appearing in a medical report is a vibration felt when the hand is placed on the body, whereas riding a roller coaster better fits your idea of a thrill. Similar frequently used words are integrated in the chapters and their listening activities.

Physicians also record or dictate the names and results of diagnostic procedures that they order. Therefore, the correct spelling of these procedures—as well as their resulting diagnoses, treatment procedures, and prescribed medications—is essential to the accurate recording of the physician's findings. In addition, it is also helpful to know metric measures (common in the medical field) and abbreviations. These terms will be introduced throughout the text as a part of their related body systems.

The knowledge you gain from this course of study will not only prepare you for a career in the allied health field but will also enable you to become an informed user of medical services, allowing you to make more intelligent choices about your personal health care.

WORD ELEMENTS

In this chapter, information about roots, prefixes, suffixes—the word elements—provides the foundation upon which a medical vocabulary is built. Many of these elements are derived from Greek and Latin. It is not necessary to know all of the word elements, but if you know those most commonly used, literally thousands of medical terms can be a part of your vocabulary.

However, it is often necessary to check the dictionary for an exact meaning. An example is *cardiectomy*. *Cardi-* means heart and *-ectomy* means surgical removal; thus, surgical removal of the heart would appear to be the correct meaning. Actually, the term *cardiectomy* means "surgical removal of the upper end of the stomach." *Check your dictionary frequently.*

Even if you knew every Greek and Latin root, prefix, and suffix, you would not know all medical terminology, because not all medical words are built from these word elements. They may come from a variety of sources.

Medical language is more extensive than many other specialized technical vocabularies. Progress in science and technology continually adds words to the language. Advances in the use of lasers, nuclear medicine, and computer technology, for example, have generated the addition of words that did not exist a few years ago. Even Greek and Latin word elements are sometimes combined in new ways to signify new meanings. Medical language, like all language, is constantly changing.

Nevertheless, the knowledge of roots, prefixes, and suffixes as well as the role of the combining vowels will provide the foundation for acquiring expertise with the language of medicine.

ROOTS

The foundation of a word is called the *root.* The root word in medical terminology usually indicates the part of the body under discussion and forms the main substance or meaning of the word. In the following terms, note that the root words are underlined.

EXAMPLES	gastric	cardiology
	gastr- means stomach	cardi- means heart

Gastr- and cardi-, then, are the root words that are the main elements of *gastric* and *cardiology*. A hyphen follows each root when it stands alone.

SUFFIXES

A *suffix* is added to the end of a word to further clarify the meaning of the root. Generally, when a suffix stands alone, a hyphen precedes it. For instance, use the root gastr-, which means stomach, and add the suffix -ectomy, which means removal of all or part of, as indicated below. The suffix in the example is underlined.

EXAMPLE	gastr- + -ectomy
	gastrectomy = removal of all or part of the stomach

Additionally, the suffix may indicate whether the word is a noun (name of a person, place, or thing) or an adjective (modifies a noun). Note the following example from the English language:

EXAMPLE	music	noun
	musical	adjective

In the language of medicine, the word ending also indicates whether the word is an adjective or noun, as in the following example:

EXAMPLE	tonsil	noun
	tonsillar	adjective

Some common adjective suffixes are as follows:

Adjective Suffixes	Meaning	Example
-ac, -iac	of, relating to	cardiac
-al	pertaining to	pleural
-ar	of, relating, resembling	tonsillar
-ary	pertaining to	pulmonary
-eal	pertaining to	peritoneal
-ic	having character of, producing	gastric
-ical	pertaining to	pathological
-oid	resembling	adenoid
-ose	pertaining to	adipose
-ous	full of, possessing qualities of	cancerous
-tic	pertaining to	narcotic

Common noun endings are *y, ia, um,* and *a.* Note the difference in the form of the following nouns and adjectives:

Noun Form	Adjective Form	Noun Form	Adjective Form
artery	arterial	pericarditis	pericarditic

continues

Noun Form	Adjective Form	Noun Form	Adjective Form
bacteria	bacterial	pericardium	pericardial
cell	cellular	spine	spinous
fascia	fascial	spleen	splenic
mania	manic	vein	venous

As a potential health professional, you will need to know whether words are nouns or adjectives. Using the correct form of a word is an important skill.

PREFIXES

A *prefix* is placed at the beginning of a word and modifies its meaning. In general use, when a prefix stands alone, a hyphen follows it. For example, take the word *gastrectomy* (meaning surgical removal of the stomach) and add the prefix *hemi-* (meaning half). The prefix is underlined in the following example:

> **EXAMPLE**
>
> hemi- + gastr- + -ectomy
> hemigastrectomy = surgical removal of half of the stomach

COMBINING FORMS

To facilitate the pronunciation of words made up of word elements, a vowel (usually *o*) is added to the root. This is referred to as a *combining vowel*. The root with the addition of the combining vowel is called a *combining form*. For instance, here is an example using the root *splen-* and the combining vowel *o*.

> **EXAMPLE**
>
> splen- (spleen) + o + -megaly (enlarged) = splenomegaly
> (Note the ease in saying the word with the addition of the *o*.)

However, if joining a combining form and suffix brings two vowels together, the combining vowel at the end of the root component is usually dropped.

> **EXAMPLE**
>
> gastr/o (stomach) + -itis (inflammation) = gastritis
> (Note that the *o* in *gastro-* is dropped.)

On the other hand, if two *roots* are joined bringing two vowels together, the combining vowel is retained.

> **EXAMPLE**
>
> gastr- (stomach) + o (combining vowel) + enter- (intestine) +
> -itis (inflammation) = gastroenteritis, *not* gastrenteritis

Identifying the meaning of words composed of roots, suffixes, and prefixes is an important skill to master.

SINGULAR AND PLURAL FORMS OF WORDS

To use medical terminology correctly, you must also understand the plural and singular forms of words. Plurals of medical words can be either in English or another language. For instance, the plural form of appendix becomes *appendixes* in English, but the foreign plural is *appendices*. The American Medical Association (AMA) suggests using the English plural whenever possible, but this practice varies widely.

The list that follows contains examples of some of the basic rules for forming the plurals of medical terms. Most are derived from the Latin or Greek languages.

If the word ends with		The plural form is	
a	(ampulla)	ae	(ampullae)
en	(lumen)	ina	(lumina)
is	(diagnosis)	es	(diagnoses)
ma	(stigma)	mata	(stigmata)
on	(criterion)	a	(criteria)
um	(bacterium)	a	(bacteria)
us	(bronchus)	i	(bronchi)

As in any language there are exceptions to the rules. For example, some words are always singular in usage (ascites, herpes), some are always plural (adnexa, genitalia), and some words retain the same form whether the usage is singular or plural (biceps, facies). Still other words are exceptions, such as

Singular	**Plural**
cornu	cornua
epididymis	epididymides
viscus	viscera

Always refer to a medical dictionary for proper guidance.

HOMONYMS AND OTHER WORDS THAT MAY CAUSE CONFUSION

The use of *homonyms* may cause confusion. Homonyms are words that have the same sound but different meanings. These are also words that resemble but are slightly different from others in sound or spelling.* In either case, careful discrimination is required. Examples of words that commonly cause confusion in medical records are the following.

Word	Definition
bare	naked
bear	to produce, give birth, sustain
breath	respiration
breathe	to inhale and exhale
cancer	malignant tumor
canker	an ulceration
chancre	primary lesion of syphilis
die	to cease to live
dye	to stain
facial	pertaining to the face
fascial	pertaining to fascia (connective tissue)

continues

---

*These words are also referred to as *homophones*.

Word	Definition
perineal	pertaining to the anatomical region between the thighs at the lower end of the trunk
peritoneal	pertaining to a membrane
peroneal	pertaining to the region of the fibula or outer side of the leg
sight	vision
site	place
cite	to quote
villous	shaggy with soft hair
villus	small vascular protrusion

EPONYMS

Eponyms are often used in medical reports. An eponym is the name given a medical disease, body part, or procedure derived from the name of the person who discovered or perfected it. This practice has existed for many years. Eponyms are the only medical terms that are capitalized, with the exception of trade names of drugs.

Some examples of eponyms with their comparable medical terms or definitions are as follows.

Eponym	Definition
Babinski's reflex	extension of the great toe with flexion of other toes on exciting the sole
Bell's palsy	peripheral facial paralysis
Dupuytren's contracture	flexion deformity of fingers
Graves' disease	exophthalmic (ek"sŏf-thal'mĭk) goiter
Hodgkin's disease	lymphogranulomatosis (lĭm"fō-grăn"ū-lō-mah-tō'sĭs)
Parkinson's disease	paralysis agitans (ăg'ĭ-tans)
Romberg's sign	swaying of the body and an inability to stand when the eyes are closed and the feet are placed together

Despite the AMA's recommendation that a comparable medical term be used rather than an eponym, eponyms do appear in all types of medical reports.

MEDICAL DICTIONARIES

A knowledge of word elements, the ability to form plurals correctly, the ability to provide noun or adjective word endings, and a knowledge of homonyms and eponyms will help you to learn medical terminology. However, there is one other skill you need to develop: how to use a medical dictionary.

A medical dictionary is a standard reference for a medical office because it includes terms from the basic sciences of anatomy, physiology, biochemistry, and pharmacology, as well as all the major specialties of clinical medicine and surgery.

To use a dictionary effectively, you should be familiar with its organization and the kinds of information it contains. In many medical dictionaries illustrations are placed within the text near the associated term. Some dictionaries include, as a separate section of the book, detailed anatomical plates (often in full color) that show the body in meaningful sections or by system. Other dictionaries have the plates integrated appropriately within the text.

When referencing a word or term, you will in most cases be able to quickly find it. However, sometimes—especially for phrases—you may need to determine the "key" word in the phrase in order to know where to look. For example, if you are looking for polycystic kidney disease, the key term is *disease* and is your starting point. Under *disease* there will be a list of phrases defining a specific disease where you should find *polycystic kidney d.* In some cases you may need to use your newfound word element knowledge to help in your search. Or you may need to reference a different dictionary, including a nonmedical dictionary or even the Internet.

Another important point about medical dictionaries is that most have a set of appendixes that provide additional useful information. It will be to your advantage to become familiar with the "extras" your dictionary provides.

Because many words sound different from their spelling, a variety of entries in the dictionary should be checked. Some examples follow.

Word Beginning	Sounds Like	Example
ch	(k)	chromatin
pn	(n)	pneumonia
ps	(s)	psychiatry
pt	(t)	ptosis
ae	(ay)	fasciae
i	(eye)	alveoli

Some word beginnings sound alike but are spelled differently. The following are commonly encountered.

EXAMPLES   dys, dis, des   sounds like dis   ker, cur   sounds like ker

cy, si, sy, psy   sounds like sy

The dictionary also includes pronunciation marks for medical words. Generally, pronunciation follows certain rules. These are

1. Words of two syllables are commonly accented on the first syllable.

EXAMPLES   renal (rē'năl)   ventral (vĕn'trăl)

ptosis (tō'sĭs)

2. In words of more than two syllables, the next to the last syllable is accented; the first syllable is rarely accented.

EXAMPLES   chromatic (krō-măt'ĭk)   orthoptic (or-thŏp'tĭk)

3. In the accented syllable, a vowel is short if it is followed by a consonant in the same syllable; if a vowel ends the accented syllable, it is long.

EXAMPLES   bronchoscopy (brong-kŏs'kō-pē)—accented syllable with short vowel

adrenal (ah-drē'năl)—accented syllable with long vowel

For the pronunciation of individual words, consult your medical dictionary. Read the notes or guidelines on the use of the dictionary that are usually found at the beginning of the reference source.

Practice in using the dictionary will build your skill in this area. Beginning with this chapter, exercises designed to acquaint you with the use of your dictionary are provided. Effective use of the dictionary will improve your production and effectiveness as an allied health professional.

INTERNET ASSIGNMENT

A wealth of medical information is available on the Internet. The challenge is knowing how and where to look for that one piece of information that fills your need, whether it be business or personal.

To give you some basic experience in finding "just the right" source, each chapter will introduce you to a web site and suggest an activity that will provide supplemental information about the topic of the chapter. For more practice, the Web Tutor Internet tool offers three additional web sites for each chapter.

An effort has been made to choose web sites that are well established and properly maintained and are likely to remain available for some time. However, over the life of this textbook, existing sites may be withdrawn—sometimes with little notice, other times with referrals to replacements—and new sites will be introduced. If an assigned web site is not available, your standing assignment is to find a suitable substitute.

Some web sites are limited in scope, often targeting a single topic. Others take a broad-brush approach, giving you overview information and then directing you to a wide range of specific subjects. This is the case with the site introduced in this chapter.

The National Institutes of Health (NIH) is one of the eight health agencies of the Public Health Services, which, in turn, is part of the U.S. Department of Health and Human Services. Its web site is located at **www.nih.gov**. The NIH has twenty-seven separate components, which are mainly research institutes and centers. The mission of the NIH is to uncover new knowledge that will lead to better health for everyone. Its goal is to help prevent, detect, diagnose, and treat disease and disability, from the rarest genetic disorder to the common cold. This valuable site has information about health conditions, research studies, drug information, health literature references, and special progams and provides links to other federal agencies.

By accessing each of these institutes and centers, you can obtain specific information that relates to the various topics covered in the textbook. These include cancer; the eye; heart, lung, and blood; alcohol abuse and alcoholism; allergy and infectious diseases; arthritis and musculoskeletal and skin diseases; biomedical imaging; child health and human development; deafness and other communication disorders; diabetes and digestive and kidney diseases; drug abuse; mental health; neurological disorders and stroke; and complementary and alternative medicine.

The NIH site is also home to the National Library of Medicine, which includes electronic data bases such as MEDLINE and MEDLINEplus, used extensively throughout the world by both professionals and the general public.

ACTIVITY

Access the National Health Institutes at **www.nih.gov**. Click on Health Information and explore the hyperlinks listed. Write a short summary of your findings with respect to the kinds of information and aids available on this site. Submit it to your instructor.

Review: Building a Medical Vocabulary

- To understand medical terminology requires knowledge of word elements, body structure, human anatomy, special medical meanings of otherwise familiar words, diagnostic and treatment procedures, medications, metric measures, and abbreviations.

- The language of medicine, derived primarily from Greek and Latin, is highly technical and extensive.

- The major word element is a root, which can be combined with a suffix, a prefix, or another root.

- The plural form of a word varies widely. The AMA suggests using the English plural, but foreign plurals are used as well.

- Adjective and noun suffixes must be used appropriately in reports.

- Homonyms (words that sound alike but differ in meaning) and words that are spelled similarly or sound similar require careful discrimination by medical office workers.

- Eponyms combine a person's name with a disease or part of the body.

- Effective use of a medical dictionary is essential; be familiar with its contents.

Terminology Review Exercises

Name: _____ Date: _____

COMPLETION*

Complete the following statements.

1. A large portion of the language of medicine comes from the _____ and _____ languages.

2. The major word element is called a _____.

3. An element placed at the end of a word that further defines the word is called a _____.

4. An element placed at the beginning of a word that modifies the meaning of the word is called a _____.

5. The root with the addition of the combining vowel is called a _____.

6. A word is a/an _____ when *-al, -ac, -ic, -ary, -eal,* or *-ous* is added as a suffix.

7. If two roots bring two vowels together, the combining vowel at the end of the first root is _____.

8. *Romberg's sign* is an example of a/an _____.

9. Words alike in sound but different in meaning are called _____.

10. If a combining form and suffix bring two vowels together, the combining vowel at the end of the root is usually _____.

11. Words of two syllables are commonly accented on the _____ syllable.

12. Place the accent on the correct syllable for these words: re-nal; chro-mat-ic.

PLURALS*

Form the plural of each of the singular words provided.

1. viscus _____

2. bacterium _____

3. epididymis _____

4. lumen _____

5. diagnosis _____

6. stigma _____

7. criterion _____

8. cornu _____

9. bronchus _____

10. ampulla _____

---

*Answers are in Appendix A.

CORRECT DEFINITION

Place a check next to the correct definition of the following words.

1. a place

   _____ site

   _____ sight

   _____ cite

2. an ulceration

   _____ cancer

   _____ canker

   _____ chancre

3. respiration

   _____ breath

   _____ breathe

4. pertaining to the face

   _____ facial

   _____ fascial

5. pertaining to a membrane

   _____ perineal

   _____ peritoneal

   _____ peroneal

NOUN/ADJECTIVE

Indicate whether the following words are nouns (N) or adjectives (A).

Word	N or A
1. adipose	_____
2. arterial	_____
3. bacteria	_____
4. cardiac	_____
5. cellular	_____
6. fascia	_____
7. mania	_____
8. narcotic	_____
9. pericarditis	_____
10. pericardium	_____
11. pleural	_____
12. pulmonary	_____
13. splenic	_____
14. vein	_____
15. venous	_____

Word Element Review

In each of the following chapters, you will learn some roots, prefixes, and suffixes. The roots will be shown with their combining vowel. Whenever possible, they are related to the subject matter of the text. Some of them, however, relate to many chapters.

Below are several basic prefixes and suffixes. A few root words with combining vowels are included to provide an opportunity for practice exercises.

Root	Meaning	Example	Definition
acr/o	extremity	**acrocyanosis** (ăk″rō-sī″ah-nō′sĭs)	bluish or reddish color in the fingers, wrists, and ankles
bas/o	base	**basic** (bā′sĭk)	pertaining to a base
cardi/o	heart	**cardiogenic** (kăr″dē-ō-jěn′ĭk)	originating in the heart
cyan/o	blue	**cyanophil** (sī-ăn′ō-fĭl)	cell easily stained with blue dyes
gastr/o	stomach	**gastrology** (găs-trŏl′ō-jē)	study of the stomach
pharmac/o	drug	**pharmacology** (fahr″mah-kŏl′ō-jē)	study of drugs
physi/o	nature	**physiology** (fiz″ē-ŏl′ō-jē)	study of the function of cells, tissues, and organs of living organisms
top/o	place	**topical** (tŏp′ě-kăl)	pertaining to place or surface

Prefix	Meaning	Example	Definition
a-, an-	without	**acardia** (ă-kăr′dē-ah)	congenital absence of the heart
gran-	grain	**granule** (grăn′ūl)	small grain

Suffix	Meaning	Example	Definition
-gen	originate, produce	**antigen** (ăn′tĭ-jěn)	any substance capable of inducing antibody formation
-gram	record, picture, tracing	**cardiogram** (kăr′dē-ō-grăm″)	picture of the heart
-(o)logist	specialist in the study of	**gastrologist** (găs-trŏl′ō-jĭst)	one who specializes in the study of the stomach
-(o)logy	study of	**cardiology** (kăr-dē-ŏl′ō-jē)	study of the heart
-osis	condition	**cyanosis** (sī″ah-nō′sĭs)	condition of blueness
-scopy	visual examination	**gastroscopy** (găs-trŏs′kō-pē)	visual examination of the stomach

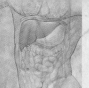

Word Element Review Exercises

Name: _____ Date: _____

ROOT, PREFIX, OR SUFFIX*

Circle the root and underline the prefix or suffix in the following words presented in the Word Element Review.

1. cardiology
2. gastrology
3. physiology
4. pharmacology
5. basic
6. cyanosis
7. antigen
8. topical
9. gastrologist
10. acardia
11. granule
12. acrocyanosis
13. cyanophil
14. cardiogenic
15. cardiogram
16. gastroscopy

WORD ENDING—NOUN OR ADJECTIVE*

Circle the word ending and specify whether the word is a noun (N) or an adjective (A).

	Word	N or A
1.	cardiac	_____
2.	basal	_____
3.	dermis	_____
4.	topical	_____
5.	gastroscopy	_____
6.	basic	_____
7.	endocardium	_____
8.	granule	_____

SPELLING

Rewrite the misspelled words.

1. cardiojenic   _____
2. granuell   _____
3. cyanosis   _____
4. antegen   _____
5. acrocyinosis   _____

---

*Answers are in Appendix A.

PRONUNCIATIONS AND DEFINITIONS
Provide the pronunciation and definition for each of the following terms.

1. physiology _____

_____

2. acardia _____

_____

3. basic _____

_____

4. granule _____

_____

5. cyanosis _____

_____

6. topical _____

_____

7. acrocyanosis _____

_____

8. cardiogram _____

_____

9. gastrology _____

_____

10. pharmacology _____

_____

WORD ELEMENT MEANINGS

Give the meaning of each word element. Then use your dictionary to find a new word that contains each of the word elements. Specify whether the new word is a noun or adjective by placing N or A in the last column.

Word Element	Meaning	Word	N or A
1. a-			
2. an-			
3. acr/o			
4. bas/o			
5. cardi/o			
6. cyan/o			
7. gastr/o			
8. -gen			
9. -gram			
10. gran-			
11. -(o)logist			
12. -(o)logy			
13. -osis			
14. pharmac/o			
15. physi/o			
16. -scopy			
17. top/o			

Dictionary Exercises

Name: _____ Date: _____

Each chapter contains exercises that will enable you to use your medical dictionary effectively. On occasion, you may have to use a regular dictionary, just as allied health professionals are required to do.

DICTIONARY EXERCISE 1*

Use your dictionary to find the definitions for the following homonyms and look-alike/sound-alike terms.

Word	Pronunciation	Definition
1. cord	_____	_____
chord	_____	_____
2. gait	_____	_____
gate	_____	_____
3. humerus	_____	_____
humorous	_____	_____
4. facet	_____	_____
faucet	_____	_____
5. colic	_____	_____
choleic	_____	_____
6. wen	_____	_____
when	_____	_____
7. acidic	_____	_____
acetic	_____	_____
acinic	_____	_____
8. form	_____	_____
forum	_____	_____
9. shocky	_____	_____
shotty	_____	_____
shoddy	_____	_____
10. radical	_____	_____
radicle	_____	_____
11. profusion	_____	_____
perfusion	_____	_____
12. casual	_____	_____
causal	_____	_____

---

*Answers are in Appendix A.

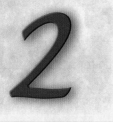

2

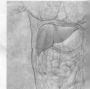

Introduction to Body Structure

> ❝ *You will have to learn many things . . . which you will forget the moment you have passed your final exam, but in anatomy it is better to have learned and lost than never to have learned at all.* ❞
>
> —W. SOMERSET MAUGHAM

OBJECTIVES

When you have completed this chapter on human anatomy, you should be able to

1. Spell and define the terms *cell, tissue, organ,* and *system* as they relate to the structure of living organisms.
2. Define the directions used in reference to the body structure.
3. Define the terms designated as planes of the body.
4. Define the cavities used to identify internal spaces of the body.
5. Name and define eleven systems of the body.
6. Identify the meanings of related word elements.

INTRODUCTION

Anatomy is defined as the science of the structure of living organisms. The study of human anatomy helps us to understand how our bodies work and is an important asset for anyone associated with the medical profession.

STRUCTURE OF THE BODY

Our bodies are marvelously intricate, delicate, and unique. Each part of the body has a purpose and function that fits into the total. Cells, tissues, organs, and systems are all part of the human anatomy.

CELLS

The smallest unit of life, the **cell**, is the basic structural unit of the body. Its contents are referred to collectively as **protoplasm** (prō'tō-plăzm). This thick, viscous colloidal material contains various organic and inorganic substances including, principally, the chemical elements oxygen, carbon, hydrogen, nitrogen, calcium, sulfur, and phosphorus.

Cells vary in size and purpose, as indicated in Figure 2-1. All have basic parts. The **cell membrane** is the outside covering. Next is the **cytoplasm** (si'tō-plăzm"), which carries on the work of the cell and contains water, food particles, and pigment. Finally comes the **nucleus** (nu'klē-ŭs), the controlling structure of the cell. It normally contains twenty-three pairs of **chromosomes** (krō'mō-sōmz), small, threadlike structures that transmit genetic information. These in turn contain **genes**, which control heredity.

In a more general sense, there are three types of cells present in the body: **differentiated cells** (static cells), **undifferentiated cells** (expanding cells), and **stem cells** (renewing cells that give rise to other kinds of cells). The key difference between differentiated and undifferentiated cells is that undifferentiated cells can grow again, but differentiated cells cannot. An example of differentiated, or static, cells is muscle cells. Examples of undifferentiated, or expanding, cells are those of the skin, lining of the gut, or bone marrow. Stem, or renewing, cells die regularly and are replaced at regular intervals, as in the case of hair or the lining of your intestinal tract. Stem cells obey signals to stop growth, whereas cancer cells lack a control mechanism to switch off growth.

TISSUES

Cells that are similar in nature group together to perform certain functions. Together they form **tissues**. These specialized cells make up four primary types of tissues: **epithelial** (ep"ĭ-thē'lē-ăl), **connective**, **muscular**, and **nervous**. Epithelial tissue forms glands, covers surfaces, and lines cavities. Connective tissue holds all parts of the body in place. Muscular tissue is comprised of fibers that contract and cause or allow movement. Nervous tissue conducts nerve impulses.

ORGANS

Two or more tissues combine to form an **organ**. Examples of cells and tissues grouped together to perform a certain function are the kidneys, heart, lungs, and liver. Internal organs are often referred to as **viscera** (vĭs'er-ah).

SYSTEMS

Organs do not function independently. They work in combinations to form a **system**, which performs a function or a related group of functions. Systems of the body may be identified in a variety of ways. We will study them in the following framework.

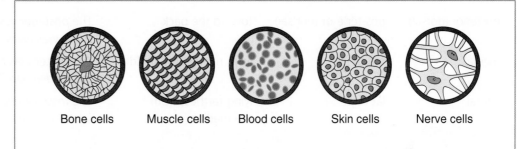

Bone cells   Muscle cells   Blood cells   Skin cells   Nerve cells

FIGURE 2-1
Types of Cells

System	Function
integumentary	The skin, hair, sweat, and sebaceous (sĕ-bā'shus) glands provide a covering and protection for the body.
musculoskeletal	Bones form the framework of the body, support organs, and provide a place to which muscles are attached; muscles permit motion and movement of the body.
blood and lymphatic	Blood carries oxygen and other substances to body parts; the lymph system furnishes protective mechanisms against infection.
cardiovascular	The heart pumps blood through the arteries and veins.
respiratory	The specialized organ group that transfers oxygen from air that is inhaled to the blood and transfers carbon dioxide from the blood to the air that is exhaled.
gastrointestinal	The alimentary canal transports and digests food, absorbs nutrients, and excretes waste products as necessary from the body.
urinary	The kidneys filter blood and excrete urine through the urinary tract.
reproductive	The function and composition of the male and female anatomies are designed for reproduction of the human race.
endocrine	The internal glands manufacture hormones.
nervous	The brain and nervous system integrate various intellectual and physical processes of the body.
sensory	The eyes, ears, nose, and throat provide information about the environment.

Each of these systems is presented later in this textbook.

BODY DIRECTION

Direction in the human body is identified in a specific way and is referred to as anatomical position (body upright, face forward, palms forward). Traditional indications of directions are not appropriate. (Have you ever heard of the eastern part of your body?) A number of terms have been devised to designate specific regions of the body. The following terms refer to the body when in the anatomical position.

Direction	Pronunciation	Meaning	Example
anterior (ventral)	ăn-tēr'ē-or	toward the front	Both *anterior* cerebral arteries filled from the right side.
posterior (dorsal)	pōs-tēr'ē-or (dor'sal)	toward the back	The *posterior* wall of the disc space was excised.
medial	mē'dē-ăl	lying nearest the middle	A catheter was placed beneath the *medial* skin flap.
lateral	lăt'er-ăl	lying farthest from the median	The mass extended to the left *lateral* wall of the pelvis.

continues

Direction	Pronunciation	Meaning	Example
superior	soo-pē'rē-or	referring to the upper or head end	An extension of the tumor was found in the *superior* portion of the breast.
inferior	ĭn-fēr'ē-or	referring to the lower, away-from-the-head end	The *inferior* rectus muscle was detached from its insertion.
proximal	prŏk'sĭ-măl	that part closest to the source	The muscles were resected and reflected *proximally*.
distal	dĭs'tăl	that part farthest from the source	The *distal* portion of the common duct was thoroughly irrigated.
apex	ā'pĕks	tip, summit	The uppermost part of the lung is the *apex* of the lung.
base	bās	bottom, lower part	The fracture was at the *base* of the skull.
supine	soo'pīn	lying face up	The patient was placed in the *supine* position.
prone	prōn	lying face down	The operation was done with the patient in the *prone* position.

BODY PLANES

Another way to identify structures and areas of the body is to refer to planes. As displayed in Figure 2-2, the **median** or **mid-sagittal plane** (1) passes through the center of the head, chest, and pelvis, dividing the body into two equal right and left portions. The **sagittal** (săj'ĭ-tăl) **plane** (2) is parallel to the median plane, can be in any location, and divides the body into any two right and left portions. The **vertical** or **frontal plane** (3) (also called the coronal plane) divides the body to create a posterior (back) and an anterior (front) portion. This line is at right angles to the median (center) plane. Finally, the **transverse** or **horizontal plane** (4) divides the body horizontally into an upper and a lower portion.

BODY CAVITIES

Sometimes the body is referred to in terms of a specific body cavity. Basically, as shown in Figure 2-3, there are two large internal spaces, which are called the **dorsal** (1) and **ventral** (8) **cavities**.

The two dorsal cavities are the **cranial cavity** (2), which contains the brain, and the **spinal cavity** (3), which encloses the spinal cord. Because they join, they are a continuous space.

The ventral cavities are much larger than the dorsal cavities and are not continuous. The **thoracic** (thō-răs'ĭk) **cavity** (4) is above and separated from the **abdominal cavity** (6) and the **pelvic cavity** (7) by a muscular membrane called the **diaphragm** (5). The thoracic cavity, shown in more detail in Figure 2-4, contains the heart, lungs, and large blood vessels. Included in this area are two smaller cavities, the **pleural** (ploo'răl) **cavity** and **mediastinum** (mē"dē-ah-stī'nŭm). The pleural cavity (one for each lung) is the space between the membranes that surround the lung, which is lined with a double-folded membrane called **pleura** (ploo'rah). The mediastinum is the area between the lungs that contains the heart and other organs. The abdominal cavity contains the stomach, intestines, kidney, liver, gallbladder, pancreas, and spleen. The pelvic cavity is joined with the abdominal cavity and contains the urinary bladder, rectum, and internal parts of the reproductive system.

Because the **abdominal cavity region** is so large, it is divided into nine sections, as shown in Figure 2-5. The three central regions are the epigastrium (ĕp"ĭ-găs'trē-ŭm) (1), umbilical (ŭm-bĭl'ĭ-kal) (2), and hypogastric (hī"pō-gas'trĭk) (3). At each side are the right and left hypochondrium (hī"pō-kon'drē-ŭm) regions (6), the right and left inguinal (ĭng'gwĭ-nal) (iliac [ĭl'ē-ak]) regions (4), and the right and left lumbar regions (5) near the waist. These directions allow a physician to identify specifically any area of the body.

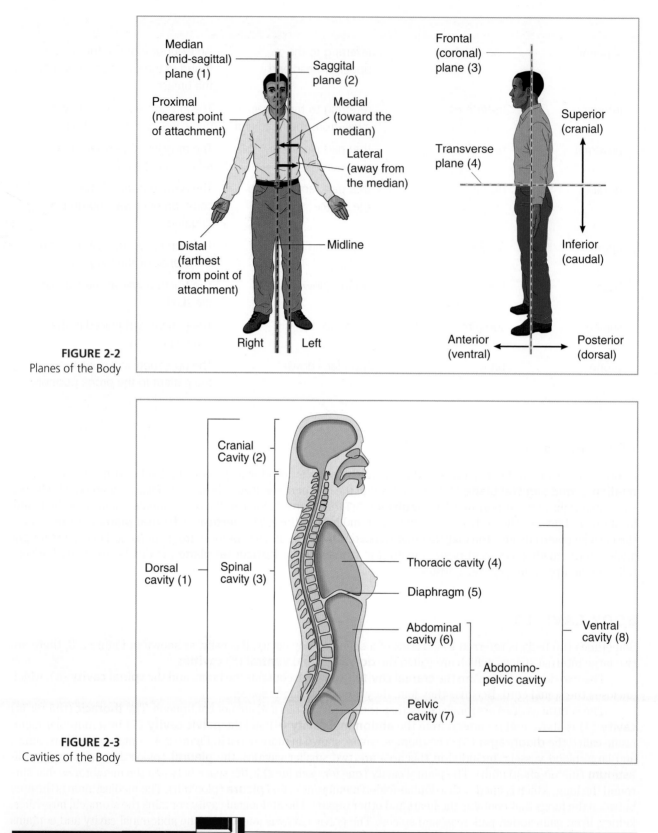

FIGURE 2-2
Planes of the Body

FIGURE 2-3
Cavities of the Body

Medical dictionaries are a source of a variety of information and often include anatomical drawings of body parts. No longer are health professionals limited to only hard copy versions of medical dictionaries. Several are available on the Internet, and most are free but may require registration.

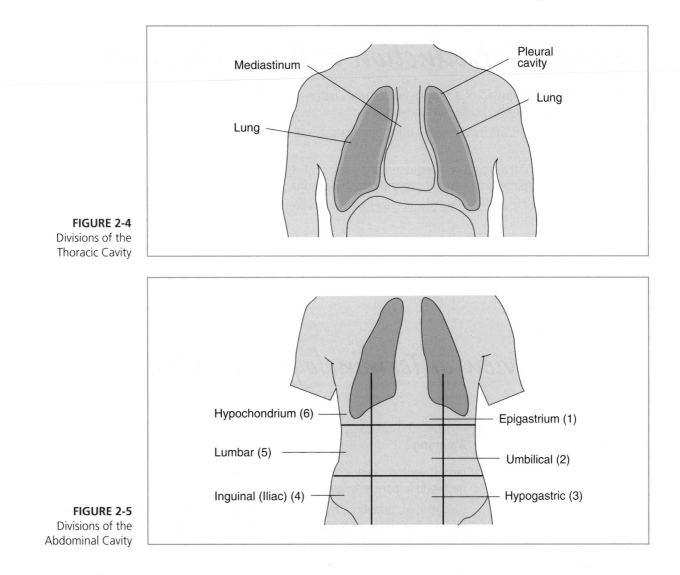

FIGURE 2-4
Divisions of the
Thoracic Cavity

FIGURE 2-5
Divisions of the
Abdominal Cavity

A list of free medical dictionaries online can be accessed at **www.online-dictionary.net**. Select Medical Dictionary. At the time of publication, the list included *Stedman's Medical Dictionary* (**www.pdr.net**; select Stedman's) and *Merriam-Webster's Medical Dictionary* (**www.intelihealth.com**; under Look It Up, select Medical Dictionary), and the *ADAM Medical Encyclopedia* (**my.webmd.com**; select Medical Library under Medical Info), which covers more than 4,000 topics including disease conditions, treatments, medical terms, procedures, and anatomy. (Some of these sources require registration, but it is free.) There are also some highly specialized sites such as the AIDS Medical Glossary (**www.critpath.org/research/gmhgloss.htm**) and the Alzheimer's Disease Medical Glossary (**www.alz.org**; select Glossary).

ACTIVITY

First, access **www.online-dictionary.net**. Then access *ADAM Medical Encyclopedia* to check out the anatomy available in it. Write a summary about the content. Next, access one of the other general medical dictionaries and summarize your investigation to the instructor. Finally, access one of the specialized dictionaries and report your findings to the instructor.

As an alternative assignment, use the keyword search function of your Internet service, your Internet browser, or search engine (**www.google.com** is a good one) to find a dictionary. Do this by keying a phrase such as "free online medical dictionaries" (the search argument) into the search window. Select three dictionaries and write a brief report to your instructor on their content and ease of use.

Review: Introduction to Body Structure

■ The body is composed of a progression of units beginning with a cell. Groups of specialized cells form tissues, which in turn form organs.

■ Although organs are independent units, they usually are part of a system that serves a particular function.

■ The systems of the body are integumentary, musculoskeletal, blood and lymphatic, cardiovascular, respiratory, gastrointestinal, urinary, reproductive, endocrine, nervous, and sensory.

■ Body direction is identified by planes: median (mid-sagittal), sagittal, frontal (vertical), and transverse (horizontal).

■ Two main body cavities are dorsal (containing the cranial and spinal cavities) and ventral (containing the abdominal, pelvic, and thoracic cavities).

Review of Terminology Presented

Word	Meaning
abdominal cavity	largest ventral cavity, containing the stomach, intestines, kidneys, liver, gallbladder, pancreas, and spleen
abdominal cavity regions	epigastrium, umbilical, hypogastric, right and left hypochondriac, right and left inguinal (iliac), and right and left lumbar regions
cell	smallest unit of life
cell membrane	outside covering of a cell
chromosome	threadlike structure that transmits genetic information; one of 23 pairs in a cell
connective tissue	groups of specialized cells that hold all parts of the body in place
cranial cavity	space that contains the brain; one of the dorsal cavities
cytoplasm	all substances of a cell other than the nucleus; carries on work of a cell
diaphragm	muscular membrane that separates ventral cavities
differentiated cells	static cells that cannot grow
dorsal cavity	large internal space containing cranial and spinal cavity
epithelial tissue	tissue that forms glands, covers surfaces, lines cavities
genes	blueprints that control heredity
median plane (mid-sagittal)	plane that passes through the center of the head, chest, and pelvis, dividing the body into two equal portions
mediastinum	middle portion of the thoracic cavity
muscular tissue	tissue comprised of fibers that contract and cause or allow movement
nervous tissue	tissue that conducts nerve impulses
nucleus	controlling structure of a cell

continues

Word	Meaning
organ	formed by two or more tissues working together to perform a certain function
pleura	double-folded membrane lining the pleural cavities
pleural cavities	right and left portions of the thoracic cavity; space between the membranes that surround each lung
protoplasm	collective name for the organic and inorganic substances that make up the contents of a cell
sagittal plane	plane that is parallel to the median plane in any location, dividing the body into any two portions, right and left
spinal cavity	dorsal cavity enclosing the spinal cord
stem cells	renewing cells that are replaced regularly
system	organs that combine to perform a function or related group of functions
thoracic cavity	uppermost section of the ventral cavity; contains heart, lungs, and large blood vessels as well as pleural cavities and mediastinum
tissues	groups of specialized cells that perform specific functions
transverse plane (horizontal)	plane that divides the body horizontally into two parts, upper and lower portions
undifferentiated cells	expanding cells that can grow again
ventral cavities	large cavities separated by the diaphragm
vertical plane (frontal)	plane that divides the body into a back and a front
viscera	name for internal organs

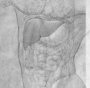

Terminology Review Exercises

Name: _____ Date: _____

CHOICES*

Circle the correct answer in each statement.

1. The (vertical, sagittal) plane divides the body into back and front portions.
2. The (vertical, transverse) plane divides the body horizontally into upper and lower portions.
3. The (sagittal, transverse) plane is parallel to the median plane, can be in any location, and divides the body into any two right and left portions.
4. The (median, sagittal) plane refers to a line from the center of the head through the center of the chest and pelvis and divides the body into two equal portions.
5. The tissues that form glands, cover surfaces, and line cavities are (epithelial, connective).
6. The tissue that holds body parts in place is (epithelial, connective).
7. Tissue that expands and contracts to allow movement is (connective, muscular).
8. The tissue that conducts nerve impulses is (nervous, epithelial).

COMPLETION*

Complete the following statements.

1. The three ventral cavities are the _____, _____, and _____.
2. Cells and tissues grouped together to perform certain functions are called _____.
3. Internal organs are often referred to as the _____.
4. The cavity that contains the urinary bladder, rectum, and internal parts of the reproductive system is called the _____ cavity.
5. A continuous space that contains the cranial and spinal cavities is called the _____ cavity.
6. The muscular membrane separating the thoracic cavity from the abdominal and pelvic cavities is the _____.
7. The thoracic cavity has two smaller cavities: the _____ and the _____.
8. The abdominal cavity is divided into _____ regions.
9. The central regions of the abdominal cavity are called _____, _____, and _____ regions.
10. The right and left regions next to the three central regions are _____, _____, and _____.
11. The difference between differentiated and undifferentiated cells is _____.
12. Cells that are replaced on a regular basis are _____ cells.

DEFINITIONS*

Define the following body directions.

1. distal _____
2. proximal _____
3. inferior _____
4. lateral _____
5. anterior _____

---

*Answers are in Appendix A.

MATCHING
Match the systems to their functions.

1. _____ manufactures hormones
2. _____ filters blood and excretes urine
3. _____ covers and protects the body
4. _____ forms the framework of the body; permits motion and movement of the body
5. _____ handles the integration of intellectual and physical processes
6. _____ transfers oxygen from the air we inhale to the blood and transfers carbon dioxide from the blood to the air we exhale
7. _____ transports blood throughout the body through veins and arteries
8. _____ transports and digests food, absorbs nutrients, and excretes waste products
9. _____ provides for perpetuation of the human species
10. _____ carries oxygen and other materials to body parts; furnishes protection against infection
11. _____ provides the body with information about the environment

a. cardiovascular
b. endocrine
c. gastrointestinal
d. urinary
e. integumentary
f. blood, lymphatic
g. musculoskeletal
h. nervous
i. respiratory
j. reproductive
k. sensory

IDENTIFICATION
Identify the direction intended in the following phrases.

1. anterior cerebral artery _____
2. medial skin flap _____
3. superior portion of the breast _____
4. distal portion of the common duct _____
5. supine position _____
6. in the prone position _____
7. base of the organ _____
8. apex of the organ _____

DESCRIPTIONS
Describe each of the terms that are associated with a cell.

1. cell _____
2. protoplasm _____
3. cell membrane _____
4. cytoplasm _____
5. nucleus _____
6. chromosomes _____
7. genes _____

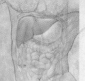

Word Element Review

Root	Meaning	Example	Definition
cyt/o	cell	**cytogenous** (sī-tŏj'ĕ-nŭs)	producing cells
		cytology (sī-tŏl'ō-jē)	study of cells
dors/o	back	**dorsal** (dor'săl)	pertaining to the back
end/o	inside	**endocardium** (ĕn"dō-kar'dē-ŭm)	innermost lining membrane of the heart
later/o	side	**lateral** (lăt"er-ăl)	pertaining to a side
somat/o	body	**somatic** (sō-măt'ĭk)	pertaining to the body
viscer/o	internal organ	**visceral** (vĭs'er-ăl)	pertaining to the organs of the body

Prefix	Meaning	Example	Definition
contra-	against	**contraindicated** (kŏn"trah-ĭn'dĭ-kā"tĕd)	not advisable; not recommended
		contralateral (kŏn-trah-lăt'er-ăl)	pertaining to the opposite side
ex-	out, away from	**excise** (ĕk-sīz')	to remove by cutting
		excrete (ĕks-krēt')	to throw off or eliminate
inter-	between	**intermuscular** (ĭn"ter-mŭs'kū-lăr)	between muscles
intra-	within	**intra-abdominal*** (ĭn"trah-ăb-dŏm'ĭ-năl)	within the abdomen
		intramuscular (ĭn"trah-mŭs'kū-lăr)	within the muscle
peri-	about, around, surrounding	**pericardium** (pĕr"ĭ-kăr'dē-ŭm)	fibrous sac enclosing the heart
retro-	backward	**retroversion** (rĕt"rō-ver'zhŭn)	turning backward of an organ
		retrograde (rĕt'rō-grād)	moving backward; degenerating to a worsened state
sub-	under, below	**subconscious** (sŭb-kŏn'shŭs)	below the level of conscious perception
		subnormal	below normal
trans-	through, across	**transplant** **transport**	to graft tissue from one place to another movement of materials in biological systems

---

*Note an exception to the rule: The *a* is not dropped; instead it is hyphenated.

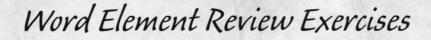

Word Element Review Exercises

Name: _____ Date: _____

ROOT OR COMBINING FORM*
Circle the root or combining form in the following words.

1. dorsolateral
2. cytology
3. lateral
4. somatic
5. visceral
6. endocardium

PREFIX*
Circle the prefix in the following words.

1. retrograde
2. transport
3. intermuscular
4. contralateral
5. subconscious
6. excrete
7. pericardium
8. intra-abdominal

WORD ENDINGS—NOUN OR ADJECTIVE*
Circle the word ending and specify whether the word is a noun (N) or an adjective (A).

1. visceral   _____
2. somatic   _____
3. cytogenous   _____
4. lateral   _____
5. dorsal   _____
6. pericardium   _____

COMPLETION
Complete the following statements.

1. To graft tissue from one place to another is to _____.
2. The study of cells is called _____.
3. To remove by cutting is to _____.
4. _____ means pertaining to the side of the body.
5. The fibrous sac that surrounds the heart is the _____.
6. _____ means pertaining to the body.

_____

*Answers are in Appendix A.

7. _____ means pertaining to the back.

8. In medical usage, _____ means that something is not recommended.

9. _____ means pertaining to the organs of the body.

10. _____ means between muscles.

11. The innermost lining membrane of the heart is the _____.

12. Below normal is called _____.

MEANINGS

Give the meaning of the underscored words.

1. The <u>dorsal</u> lobes of the brain are the occipital lobes.

   _____

2. The little toes are <u>lateral</u> to the big toes.

   _____

3. Administering antibiotics is <u>contraindicated</u> at this time.

   _____

4. An <u>intramuscular</u> injection was given.

   _____

5. The uterus was in a <u>retroverted</u> position.

   _____

WORD ELEMENT MEANINGS

Give the meaning of each word element. Then use your dictionary to find a new word that contains each of the word elements. Specify whether the new word is a noun or adjective by placing N or A in the last column.

Word Element	Meaning	Word	N or A
1. contra-	_____	_____	_____
2. cyt/o	_____	_____	_____
3. dors/o	_____	_____	_____
4. end/o	_____	_____	_____
5. ex-	_____	_____	_____
6. inter-	_____	_____	_____
7. intra-	_____	_____	_____
8. later/o	_____	_____	_____
9. peri-	_____	_____	_____
10. retro-	_____	_____	_____
11. somat/o	_____	_____	_____
12. sub-	_____	_____	_____
13. trans-	_____	_____	_____
14. viscer/o	_____	_____	_____

Dictionary Exercises

Name: _____ Date: _____

DICTIONARY EXERCISE 1

Use your dictionary to find the pronunciation and definition of the following words.

	Word	Pronunciation	Definition
1.	metabolism	_____	_____
2.	histologist	_____	_____
3.	endogenus	_____	_____
4.	peritoneum	_____	_____
5.	quadrant	_____	_____
6.	superficial	_____	_____
7.	catabolism	_____	_____
8.	hypochondriac	_____	_____
9.	megakaryocyte	_____	_____
10.	mitochondria	_____	_____
11.	viscera	_____	_____
12.	retroflexion	_____	_____

DICTIONARY EXERCISE 2*

Pronunciation of the words below is provided. Using your dictionary, find the correct spelling and definition of each word.

	Word	Pronunciation	Definition
1.	_____	en"dō-kăr-dī'tĭs	_____
2.	_____	lăt"ĕr-ō-vĕr'shŭn	_____
3.	_____	trăns"thō-răs'ĭk	_____
4.	_____	rĕt"rō-ăk'shŭn	_____
5.	_____	sŭb-frĕn'ĭk	_____
6.	_____	vĭs"ĕr-ō-jĕn'ĭk	_____
7.	_____	si"tō-păth-ŏl'ō-jē	_____
8.	_____	dor"sō-vĕn'trăl	_____
9.	_____	sō"măt-ō-jĕn'ĭk	_____
10.	_____	ĭn"tĕr-mē'dē-ār-ē	_____
11.	_____	ĭn-tră-vē'nŭs	_____
12.	_____	ĕks-prĕs'	_____

---

*Answers are in Appendix A.

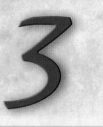

The Medical History and Physical Examination

" *The doctor may also learn more about the illness from the way the patient tells the story than from the story itself.* *"*

—JAMES HERRICK

When you have completed this study of the medical history and physical examination, you should be able to

1. Identify and define the components of such reports.
2. Spell and abbreviate the names of frequently used diagnostic tests.
3. Describe other reports based on the medical history and physical examination.
4. Compare and define the source oriented and problem oriented medical record.
5. Identify and spell commonly used abbreviations.

INTRODUCTION

The Medical History and Physical Examination report is a key document associated with patient care. Often called the History and Physical (H&P), the document records baseline information and an overall evaluation of the patient's state of health. This can be done as part of an office visit or in preparation for a hospital-based episode of care. The patient's physician usually does the History and Physical Examination, but it may be done by a nurse practitioner or a physician assistant.

A complete medical record has several important purposes. It is the foundation on which planning and evaluating patient care and ongoing treatment is based. The course of the patient's medical evaluation, treatment, and change in condition is documented in the medical record. It also provides evidence of communication between the physician and any other health professionals assisting in the patient's care. The medical record protects both the patient and physician and helps to establish a factual database for use in continuing education and research so vital to the medical profession and, ultimately, patient care.

The Medical History and Physical Examination contains both subjective and objective information. Symptoms and feelings that the patient describes to the physician are categorized as *subjective*. What the examiner can see, hear, or touch provides *objective* information. Test results are also considered objective information. For example, a young child may pull at his ear and say his head hurts. This is subjective information. When the physician looks into the ear canal and sees an inflamed, bulging eardrum, an ear infection can be objectively identified.

While a health practitioner may complete the History and Physical Examination and dictate the information to be included, members of another allied health profession will be responsible for producing the printed report. Understanding the document requires familiarity with the components of a history and physical examination report and the associated terminology.

The basic content of a History and Physical Examination report is determined by convention. Various regulatory and statuary agencies require certain components, as do such groups as health insurance companies and health maintenance organizations (HMO). But because no one format is exactly right for every physician, every patient, or every situation, medical facilities often develop their own format and expect it to be used. For example, abbreviations indicated for each report component are acceptable in some offices and hospitals while others do not allow their use.

On the occasion that an error is noted in a completed medical report, there is a proper procedure to correct it to maintain the report's integrity. The person finding the error should draw a single line through the incorrect data, indicate what the error is, provide the corrected information, and then initial and date the notation.

CONFIDENTIALITY OF MEDICAL RECORDS

Confidentiality is a very important factor when working in the medical environment. Both the information the patient shares with the physician and the physician's observations during the course of consultation or treatment are considered privileged communication. It may be given to other members of the health care team if it pertains directly to the course of treatment, but to no one else without the express authorization of the patient.

This authorization may be made on a preprinted form (the AMA offers several variations) or as a simple letter. However, it must include certain specific items. For example, the release must specify exactly what information is to be disclosed, to whom it is to be disclosed, and the reason for the disclosure. It must also be signed and dated by the patient. The signed release form is kept in the patient's file.

There are a few exceptions to the physician-patient privileged communication. These primarily relate to court-ordered or other limited legal situations, which vary from state to state.

The need for confidentiality extends beyond the clinical staff, who deal directly with a patient, to include the support staff, who are privy to patient information. These employees are bound by the same moral and legal restrictions as a physician. Should a physician's employee repeat confidential information, not only the employee, but the physician, too, becomes liable for legal action by the patient. If for no other reason than this single example, *confidentiality is absolutely essential and must be maintained at all times.*

COMPONENTS OF THE MEDICAL HISTORY AND PHYSICAL EXAMINATION

The history and physical report is usually treated as one document with two distinct parts—the Medical History and the Physical Examination. Although it is possible and acceptable to generate this report as two separate documents, the components remain the same. There is a signature block at the end of the Physical Examination. There may also be one at the end of the Medical History section. In this textbook the History and Physical report will be treated as one document with two distinct parts.

HISTORY

The first section of the Medical History and Physical Examination is the patient's **history**. The section contains several headings: Chief Complaint, Present Illness, Past History, Family History, Social History, and Review of Systems. Each will be identified and defined.

Chief Complaint (CC)

The **Chief Complaint** is a subjective description of the **symptom** or symptoms that caused the patient to seek medical attention. These symptoms may be indications of disease as reported by the patient. Symptoms are further identified as **primary symptoms**, which are directly related to a disease, and **secondary symptoms**, which are the results or consequences of the disease process. The information can be recorded as a series of words or as a phrase.

EXAMPLES	
	CHIEF COMPLAINT: Tiredness, headaches, increased thirst and hunger, frequency of urination, general **malaise*** (măl-āz').
	CHIEF COMPLAINT: Severe pain of approximately eight hours' duration radiating into the groin from the right side.

Present Illness (PI)

Present Illness can also be called *History of Present Illness (HPI)*. The patient gives detailed information as to when the symptoms were first noticed, their extent and intensity, and the patient's opinion as to what caused the symptoms. To gather additional relevant information the physician may prompt the patient by asking questions about the symptoms. Any medications the patient is taking to relieve the symptoms, whether home remedy, over the counter, or prescription, should be listed.

EXAMPLE	
	PRESENT ILLNESS: This is the first admission for this 70-year-old white male, a retired dockhand, who enters with the chief complaint of gradual loss of clear sight in his right eye over a period of four months. The left eye presents no problem. The patient describes his sight like "looking through a frosted window." He denies eye pain or discomfort, change in appearance, **diplopia** (dĭ-plō'pē-ah), discharge, or change in **lacrimation** (lăk"rĭ-mā'shŭn).

Past History (PH)

The **Past History** may also be called the *Past Medical History (PMH)*. The past history includes any childhood or adult diseases, surgical procedures, accidents, pregnancies, deliveries, and allergies to medications or other items. The past medical history can be especially important for identification of allergies or patterns of disease.

EXAMPLE	
	PAST HISTORY: Patient had an appendectomy in 1959. No other history of surgery, disease, or accident. She does not take any medication and claims to have no allergies.

Family History (FH)

The **Family History** should include relevant medical information about family members. Many diseases are hereditary; others can be found in families. A family history of breast cancer would be very significant for a female patient. A significant family history of diabetes or heart disease may alert the physician and the patient to begin preventive measures. The patient's marital status is sometimes included in this section.

EXAMPLE	
	FAMILY HISTORY: Father died at age 50 of prostate cancer; mother died as a result of heart disease. The patient has been married for 25 years. There are three children.

---

*Words appearing in boldface in the examples are defined in the Review of Terminology Presented section of this chapter.

Social History (SH)

The purpose of the **Social History** is to summarize the patient's lifestyle and environment and determine whether something about the environment may be contributing to the disease. The use of alcohol, tobacco, and drugs is of particular interest because these can be factors affecting a person's health. The patient's occupation should be included, especially in those cases where occupational hazards may occur.

EXAMPLE	SOCIAL HISTORY: The patient reports occasional use of alcohol, no more than three times per week. Consumes six to twelve cups of coffee per day. She has worked for an asbestos removal company for the past ten years. Quit smoking approximately two years ago. Denies any drug use.

Review of Systems (ROS)

The **Review of Systems** is an exchange between the physician and the patient. The physician will ask specific questions and record significant responses. At this time, the presence or absence of signs and symptoms can be identified. A **sign** is an objective, observable or measurable manifestation of a disease as noted or observed by the physician or health care practitioner. Signs are often accompanied by symptoms.

The order of the review usually starts with the patient's head and continues down to the fingers and toes. The length and detail of this section will vary according to the patient's physical condition.

Several headings pertain to the names of body systems, which were discussed in Chapter 2. These headings, with representative narratives, are presented below. Some agencies allow the use of abbreviations to identify the headings. Those most commonly used are shown. HEENT is frequently used for the heading Head, Eyes, Ears, Nose, and Throat.

EXAMPLE	**REVIEW OF SYSTEMS:**
	HEENT: Postnasal drip. Occasional sinus trouble. Migraine headaches about twice a month. No change in vision or hearing.
	CARDIOVASCULAR: Denies prior history of chest pain, **murmurs**, or arrhythmias.
	RESPIRATORY: No pneumonia, tuberculosis, pleurisy or **hemoptysis** (hē-mŏp'tĭ-sĭs). Has a dry cough occasionally productive of clear **sputum** (spū'tŭm).
	GASTROINTESTINAL (GI): Mild, recurrent heartburn. Denies food intolerance or vomiting.
	GENITOURINARY (GU): Recent urinary tract infection (UTI). Menstrual history is unremarkable.
	MUSCULOSKELETAL: No complaints at this time.
	NEUROLOGICAL: Denies **vertigo** (ver'tĭ-gō), weakness, or problems with coordination.

PHYSICAL EXAMINATION (PX, PE)

The **Physical Examination** is usually completed at the same time as the medical history, especially when the Medical History and Physical Examination report is generated as a single document with two distinct parts.

The Physical Examination is the objective assessment of the patient. It is most often completed by the patient's physician. The physician uses general observation techniques as well as special or unique evaluation methods. These methods are defined in the following list.

Auscultation (aws"kŭl-tā'shŭn)
Listening for sounds within the body chiefly to determine the condition of thoracic or abdominal organs. Using a stethoscope achieves the best results with this technique.

Palpation (păl-pā'shŭn)
Feeling with fingers or hands to determine the physical characteristics of organs or tissues.

Percussion (per-kŭsh'ŭn)
Using the fingertips to tap the surface area of the body to produce sound, as shown in Figure 3-1. Solid and hollow areas will produce different tones. This information helps the physician determine size, position, and density of body organs and cavities.

Visualization or inspection
Using both observation and inspection to assess parts of the body that can be evaluated by sight alone.

General

The first part of the Physical Examination section is a general description of the patient. The description is based on the physician's observation and information that can be supported in an objective manner. The patient's vital signs can be included under the general heading or may be documented as a separate heading.

EXAMPLE

GENERAL: This 40-year-old black female appears to be in no acute distress. **Vital signs** include oral temperature, 98.6°F; pulse rate, 80 beats per minute; blood pressure, 180/100; weight, 180 lb.; height, 5'6".

The physical examination continues with an objective assessment of each area or body system. As with the review of systems, the physician begins with the head and neck and proceeds all the way to the extremities. Although other headings may be included, the example presented here represents those most frequently employed. Formats will vary depending on patient need, physician training, and the documentation policies of the specific health care setting.

EXAMPLE

HEAD AND NECK: Eyes: Pupils are equal, round, and react to light and accommodation. Normal **extraocular** (ĕks"trah-ŏk'ū-lar) movements. **Fundi** (fŭn'dĭ) are normal. Ears: External auditory canals are clear. **Tympanic** (tĭm-păn'ĭk) **membranes** are clear. Nose: Normal nasal mucosa. No **septal** (sĕp'tăl) deviation. Mouth and throat: No pathological findings. Neck: Supple. **Trachea** (trā'kē-ah) in midline. Thyroid gland not palpably enlarged. **Carotid** (kah-rŏt'ĭd) pulses are equal.

CHEST: Normal expansion. Breasts: No masses palpable. Heart: Not enlarged; no **thrills**; heart tones good; regular rhythm; no murmurs or **rubs**. Lungs: Clear to percussion and auscultation.

ABDOMEN: Soft, nontender; no rebound tenderness; no masses palpable. Bowel sounds are present. No **hepatosplenomegaly** (hĕp"ah-tō-splē"nō-mĕg'ah-lē). No inguinal hernia. **Femoral** (fĕm'or-ăl) pulses are equal.

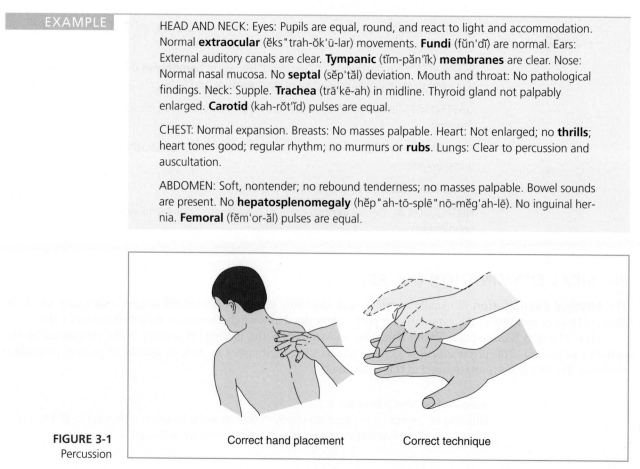

FIGURE 3-1
Percussion

Correct hand placement   Correct technique

EXTREMITIES: Symmetrical. No **edema** (ĕ-dē'mah). No varicose veins. No limitation of motion.

NEUROLOGICAL: Cranial nerves intact. Normal deep tendon reflexes. No Babinski's reflex. Romberg's sign negative.

Impressions/Diagnoses

Once the physical examination has been completed, the physician will state diagnostic conclusions in a section called **Impressions/Diagnoses**. A **diagnosis** is the identification of a disease or condition by a scientific evaluation of physical signs, symptoms, history, laboratory tests, and procedures. There are four types of diagnoses.

Clinical diagnosis
A diagnosis made on the basis of the knowledge obtained from the medical history and physical examination without the benefit of laboratory tests or x-ray films.

Differential diagnosis
A diagnosis that distinguishes between two or more diseases with similar symptoms by systematically comparing their signs and symptoms.

Laboratory diagnosis
A diagnosis derived from the results of laboratory tests.

Physical diagnosis
A diagnosis supported by both the clinical diagnosis and the laboratory diagnosis.

This section may also be called *Impression, Diagnosis, Diagnostic Impression,* or *Findings*. The conclusions can be written in paragraph form or listed and enumerated.

EXAMPLE

IMPRESSION: Hypertension. Obesity. Rule out **atherosclerosis** (ăth"er-ō-sklĕ-rō'sĭs).

DIAGNOSES:
1. Hypertension
2. Obesity
3. Rule out atherosclerosis

Plan

Accrediting and regulatory agencies require the inclusion of a treatment plan that relates to the impressions or diagnoses. The **Plan** may include specific laboratory and diagnostic tests, referrals to specialists, specific instructions to the patient, and/or follow-up appointments as needed. The Plan may be written as a paragraph or in a list format.

EXAMPLE

PLAN: Consultation with the dietitian for a 1,500 calorie, low salt, reducing diet. Monitor blood pressure, weekly. Complete Blood Count (CBC) with **lipid** (lĭ'pĭd) profile.

Refer to the listening exercise at the end of this chapter to examine a complete History and Physical report.

DIAGNOSTIC TESTS

Diagnostic tests help the physician to clarify or rule out suspected or provisional diagnoses. In the past, a physician ordered routine tests such as a complete blood count (CBC), urinalysis (UA), chest x-ray, and other blood chemistry tests so that the results would be available at the time of the annual physical examination. Today cost-containment regulations limit this practice. This may require the physician to order only those tests that specifically relate to the diagnostic findings documented in the physical examination.

If the physical examination is done in preparation for a surgical or diagnostic procedure, the tests ordered would relate to both the diagnosis and procedure. Laboratory and diagnostic test terminology is included in each chapter of this text. Some of the more frequently used tests are identified and defined below.

COMPLETE BLOOD COUNT (CBC)

The complete blood count is one of the most frequently ordered blood tests. The CBC provides valuable information about the patient's state of health; it measures and evaluates the cellular component of blood. Some of the tests included in the CBC are

Red blood cell (RBC) count
Determines the number of red blood cells found in a cubic millimeter of blood.

Hemoglobin (Hgb)
A component of red blood cells necessary for transporting oxygen throughout the body. The CBC measures the amount of hemoglobin in the blood.

Hematocrit (Hct)
Determines the percentage of red blood cells contained in a volume of blood. Literally translated, it means to separate blood.

Red blood cell indices
A collective name for three separate diagnostic test results. The results are calculated by a mathematical formula using the hemoglobin, hematocrit, and red blood cell count. The tests are the mean corpuscular volume (MCV), mean corpuscular hemoglobin (MCH), and mean corpuscular hemoglobin concentration (MCHC). The purpose of these tests is to define the size and hemoglobin concentration of the red blood cell.

White blood cell (WBC) count
Determines the number of white blood cells found in a cubic millimeter of blood.

Differential white blood cell count (diff)
Determines the number of different types of circulating white blood cells. The test is often called the differential count.

Blood smear
Examines peripheral blood to determine variations and abnormalities in RBCs, WBCs, and platelets.

Platelet count
Measures the number of platelets per cubic milliliter of blood.

NOTE: A more complete presentation on blood cell terminology is found in Chapter 9.

BLOOD CHEMISTRY PROFILE

A **blood chemistry profile** is an analysis of the chemical components of the patient's blood. This type of test is often ordered as part of the physical assessment of the patient. This profile might include an analysis of electrolytes (sodium, potassium, chloride, and carbon dioxide) and glucose (blood sugar); a series of liver tests; and tests for uric acid, creatinine (a kidney function test), and albumin (a major protein in the blood). Different combinations may be used in different institutions. The abbreviation and unit of measure for some of the more common tests are as follows:

Element	Abbreviation	Unit of Measure
calcium	Ca	milligrams% (mg%)
		continues

Element	Abbreviation	Unit of Measure
cholesterol	Chol*	milligrams% (mg%)
creatinine	creat*	milligrams% (mg%)
glucose	glu*	milligrams% (mg%)
phosphorus	phos*	milligrams% (mg%)
total bilirubin	T bili*	milligrams% (mg%)
uric acid		milligrams% (mg%)
albumin	alb*	grams% (gm%)
total protein	TP*	grams% (gm%)
alkaline phosphatase	alk phos	IU/L (international units per liter)
lactic dehydrogenase	LDH	IU/L
aspartate aminotransferase	AST	IU/L

MISCELLANEOUS BLOOD TESTS

Other blood tests taken may include sedimentation rate and coagulation prothrombin time. The **erythrocyte sedimentation rate** (ESR) is the rate at which red blood cells settle in a tube within a given amount of time to determine the degree of inflammation in the body. The **coagulation prothrombin time** measures the effectiveness of several blood-clotting factors. If there is insufficient quantity of any of these factors, prothrombin time is prolonged.

For those individuals with high cholesterol, a lipid profile measures **cholesterol** (kō-lĕs'tĕr-ōl), **triglycerides** (trī-glĭs'ĕr-īdz), low-density **lipoprotein** (lĭp"ō-prō'tēn) (LDL), and high-density lipoprotein (HDL) in the blood. These tests help to assess the risk of coronary artery disease, stroke, and myocardial infarction.

URINALYSIS

A routine urinalysis (UA) is often ordered in preparation for a diagnostic or surgical procedure or as a screening test for a physical examination. The test identifies various physical properties and chemical components of the patient's urine. On occasion, a twenty-four hour urine specimen may be called for. Color, specific gravity, and clarity may be indicators of problems, but microscopic laboratory examination will provide definitive analysis.

ELECTROCARDIOGRAM

An electrocardiogram (ECG, EKG) is a graphic recording of the electrical activity of the heart. A highly sensitive machine that uses electrodes is attached to the body to record the heart's electrical activity. The activity is recorded as tracings and can indicate cardiac abnormalities and changes in the heartbeat.

STOOL SPECIMEN

Blood in the stool (occult blood) can be an indicator of serious problems. Hemoccult Sensa is the trademark for a guaiac reagent strip that indicates the presence of blood and, consequently, the need for additional testing to determine the source of the blood. This test is given routinely to patients over 40 and for those who have a personal history of inflammatory bowel disease.

---

*These abbreviations will appear only on preprinted lab requisition slips or on automated lab report printouts. They are not used in written or dictated medical reports.

REPORTS BASED ON THE HISTORY AND PHYSICAL EXAMINATION

There are several other types of reports based on the History and Physical Examination. They are Interval History and Physical Examination, Short-Stay History and Physical Examination, Consultations, and Progress Notes. Each is used in specific circumstances, as discussed in the following sections.

INTERVAL HISTORY AND PHYSICAL EXAMINATION

When a patient is repeatedly hospitalized for the same condition, the physician may complete an **Interval History and Physical Examination** report. The use of this abbreviated format is governed by accrediting and regulatory standards, quality care issues, and physician training and preference. (Check with local agencies to determine the appropriate use of this format.) The Interval History and Physical Examination report must include a summary of what has happened to the patient since last being examined. Any changes in the patient's physical status must be thoroughly documented. Figure 3-2 is an example of the Interval History and Physical Examination.

SHORT-STAY HISTORY AND PHYSICAL EXAMINATION

With the explosion of ambulatory, same-day, and short-stay surgical interventions, there may be a limited amount of time to do a thorough history and physical examination during the hospitalization. In these situations, the History and Physical Examination may be completed in the physician's office, with a copy provided for the hospital record, or the physician may complete a shortened form of the History and Physical Examination called a **Short-Stay History and Physical Examination**. Figure 3-3 is an example of this abbreviated format.

CONSULTATIONS

There are situations when the patient's primary physician sometimes requests input from another physician. The most common situation is when a specialist is asked to evaluate a specific problem or condition or give a second opinion. Documentation of such a request is called a **Consultation** report. The Consultation report format varies from physician to physician. When the consultation occurs between physician offices, a letter format is used. If the consultation is part of a hospitalization, the hospital usually has a format that must be followed.

The consulting physician conducts an evaluation of the patient and records the results. Particular attention is given to the consultant's area of specialization. Impressions or diagnoses with treatment plans must be included in the report.

PROGRESS NOTES

After the initial physical examination, the physician generates brief notes about the patient's progress or lack of progress. The physician's **Progress Notes** will include updated information based on implementation of the treatment plan. The physician may also use the Progress Notes to change the course of treatment.

Although physician Progress Notes are often handwritten, the physician may dictate Progress Notes in some settings, including the physician's office progress note, nursing facility (long-term care) progress notes, and emergency department progress notes.

EXAMPLE

PROGRESS NOTE: March 5, 20—. Doing well. No further episodes of chest pain. Has not taken any nitroglycerin. Continue with digoxin 0.25 mg daily. Physical exam today reveals blood pressure of 150/88. Pulse is 72 and regular. No neck vein distention. Lungs are clear to percussion and auscultation. Heart perhaps slightly enlarged to the left, although this is equivocal. Heart tones are somewhat distant and of poor to fair quality. No murmurs heard. PLAN: Continue as stated. Return in three months. (Signature.)

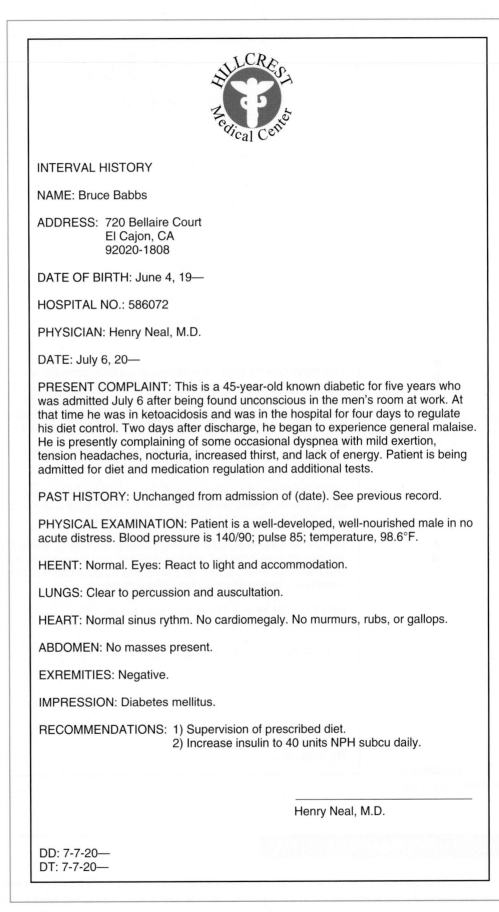

INTERVAL HISTORY

NAME: Bruce Babbs

ADDRESS: 720 Bellaire Court
El Cajon, CA
92020-1808

DATE OF BIRTH: June 4, 19—

HOSPITAL NO.: 586072

PHYSICIAN: Henry Neal, M.D.

DATE: July 6, 20—

PRESENT COMPLAINT: This is a 45-year-old known diabetic for five years who was admitted July 6 after being found unconscious in the men's room at work. At that time he was in ketoacidosis and was in the hospital for four days to regulate his diet control. Two days after discharge, he began to experience general malaise. He is presently complaining of some occasional dyspnea with mild exertion, tension headaches, nocturia, increased thirst, and lack of energy. Patient is being admitted for diet and medication regulation and additional tests.

PAST HISTORY: Unchanged from admission of (date). See previous record.

PHYSICAL EXAMINATION: Patient is a well-developed, well-nourished male in no acute distress. Blood pressure is 140/90; pulse 85; temperature, 98.6°F.

HEENT: Normal. Eyes: React to light and accommodation.

LUNGS: Clear to percussion and auscultation.

HEART: Normal sinus rythm. No cardiomegaly. No murmurs, rubs, or gallops.

ABDOMEN: No masses present.

EXREMITIES: Negative.

IMPRESSION: Diabetes mellitus.

RECOMMENDATIONS: 1) Supervision of prescribed diet.
2) Increase insulin to 40 units NPH subcu daily.

_____
Henry Neal, M.D.

DD: 7-7-20—
DT: 7-7-20—

FIGURE 3-2
An Interval History

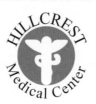

SHORT-STAY HISTORY

NAME: Jamie Holtz

ADDRESS: 363 Poe Drive
          Winter Haven, FL
          33880-1225

DATE OF BIRTH: August 29, 20—

HOSPITAL NO.: 383490

PHYSICIAN: Clara Stewart, M.D.

DATE: February 25, 20—

PRESENT COMPLAINT: This 10-month-old child comes in with a history of ear infections occurring about every three weeks since she was born. She has been on multiple antibiotics and decongestants and is just finishing a course of Ceclor. Examination in the office has revealed bilateral serous otitis media. With a history of recurrent infection, she is now admitted for bilateral myringotomy.

REVIEW OF SYSTEMS: Unremarkable. No respiratory, cardiovascular, GI or GU problems.

PAST HISTORY: Operations: None. Allergies: None. Medications: She is finishing up her Ceclor. Illness: No other serious. Family history is unremarkable. No history of bleeding tendencies or anesthetic problems.

PHYSICAL EXAMINATION: Shows a healthy-appearing, young child in no acute distress. Both ears are dull red and retracted with serous fluid. Nose is unremarkable. Mouth shows no oral lesions. Neck is normal and lungs are clear. Heart has a regular sinus rhythm without murmurs.

IMPRESSION: History of recurrent otitis media.
            Serous otitis.

RECOMMENDATIONS: Myringotomy and tubes.

_____
Clara Stewart, M.D.

DD: 2-26-20—
DT: 2-26-20—

FIGURE 3-3
A Short-Stay History

HEALTH INFORMATION SYSTEMS

Patient medical and health information must be maintained and stored for a variety of clinical and legal reasons. There are several record management systems available to physicians and other health care providers. The two most commonly used systems are described in this chapter.

SOURCE ORIENTED RECORD (SOR)

The **Source Oriented Record** (SOR) is a traditional way to organize patient records according to the source of the documents involved. Each patient record is subdivided into sections that describe the source of the document or information. In a hospital or large clinic, the record (also called the patient's chart) has dividers labeled "physician," "nursing," "lab and x-ray," "social services," and so forth. As various reports are generated, they are placed behind the appropriate divider. This method is easy to use and requires little training for clerical or support staff. Simply note who signed the report and place it behind the appropriate divider.

For example, behind the *physician divider* you may find the History and Physical Examination, physician orders, physician progress notes, or any other report or document generated or signed by a physician. Following the *nursing divider* would be the nurse's progress notes, nursing assessments, nursing care plans, or other documents that a nurse generated or signed.

Record holders and dividers are available from various record management companies. Commercially prepared divider sets may have dividers that are not necessary in your office or hospital.

PROBLEM ORIENTED (MEDICAL) RECORD (POR, POMR)

In the 1960s Dr. Lawrence Weed presented a new method for organizing patient medical or health information. The problem oriented record was considered to be a major departure from the traditional source oriented record. The **Problem Oriented Record** (POR) integrates information from all health care practitioners. The organizing factor of this system is the patient's problems or diagnoses. The patient's record is generated in the same manner that care is delivered. For example, the patient is evaluated, problems or diagnoses are identified, a plan for each problem is developed, and progress or lack of progress is recorded. The patient's record is set up to reflect that process. Each patient's record is divided into four basic sections, described below.

Data Base

The first section of a Problem Oriented Record is the **Data Base**, including a record divider labeled as such. The Data Base would include patient profile, chief complaint, and all patient evaluations, such as the History and Physical Examination, Nursing Assessment, Dietitian Assessment, Social Services Evaluation, and other documents evaluating the patient's state of health.

Problem List

Once the patient has been evaluated, problems or diagnoses are entered on a master **Problem List**. Each problem is given a title and number that stays with that problem during the entire episode of care. Problems can be identified as active or inactive. Active problems are expected to be addressed in the treatment plan.

Plan

The Plan section of the POR must address *each* active problem. All plans for a single problem should be identified by the problem's name and number. Plans can be written on physician order forms, nursing care plans, or other types of patient record forms. Subjective impression, objective clinical evidence, and assessment or diagnosis for each problem are included.

Progress Notes

The **Progress Notes** section of the POR includes both narrative and flow sheet documentation. A narrative progress note can be written by anyone who provides care to the patient. Progress notes are numbered and titled to relate to a specific problem. Whenever possible, the notes address **s**ubjective information, **o**bjective results, **a**ssessment of both the subjective and objective data, and a comment about the need to update or change the treatment **p**lan. Narrative notes written in this format are often called SOAP notes.

Flow sheets include various documents that carry only a check mark or the initials of the person providing patient care. One example of a flow sheet is the medication record. There is little, if any, narrative documentation on a flow sheet.

The POR requires training for all users, including clerical and support staff. This system is well suited to the physician's office and long-term care settings. Many acute care settings, such as hospitals, have modified the POR to fit the agency's needs. Supplies necessary to set up a POR are readily available from many commercial vendors.

ABBREVIATIONS

The following abbreviations are commonly found in medical History and Physical Examination reports, as well as other patient records. (Note that abbreviations may vary slightly from institution to institution.)

A&P, P&A	auscultation and percussion
AMA	American Medical Association
BP	blood pressure
BUN	blood urea nitrogen
CBC	complete blood count
CC	Chief Complaint
diff	differential white blood cell count
DX, Dx	diagnosis
ECG, EKG	electrocardiogram
ESR	erythrocyte sedimentation rate
FH	family history
GI	gastrointestinal
GU	genitourinary
H&P	history and physical
Hct	hematocrit
HDL	high-density lipoprotein
HEENT	head, eyes, ears, nose, throat
Hgb	hemoglobin
HMO	health maintenance organization
HPI	History of Present Illness
LDL	low-density lipoprotein
MCH	mean corpuscular hemoglobin
MCHC	mean corpuscular hemoglobin concentration
MCV	mean corpuscular volume
PERRLA	pupils are equal, round, react to light and accommodation
PH	Past History
PI	Present Illness
PMH	Past Medical History
POR (POMR)	Problem Oriented (Medical) Record
Pt	patient

continues

PX, PE	Physical Examination
RBC	red blood cell count
ROS	Review of Systems
RX, Rx	treatment, prescription
SH	Social History
SOAP	subjective, objective, assessment, plan
SOR	Source Oriented Record
TPR	temperature, pulse, respirations
UA	urinalysis
UTI	urinary tract infection
W/D	well developed
W/N	well nourished
WBC	white blood cell count

ABBREVIATIONS USED WITH LAB RESULTS

cm	centimeters
gm%	grams percent
HPF	high-power field
IU/L	international units per liter
L	liter
LPF	low-power field
mEq	milliequivalent
mEq/L	milliequivalent per liter
mg	milligram
mg%	milligrams percent
mm/Hg	millimeters of mercury
mm^3	millimeters cubed

INTERNET ASSIGNMENT

The American Health Information Management Association (AHIMA) is the professional association that represents specially educated health information management professionals who work to manage, analyze, and utilize data vital for patient care. Their goal is to make this information accessible to health care providers when it is needed to enhance individual care. They also work to safeguard the confidentiality and privacy of an individual's medical records.

ACTIVITY

Visit the AHIMA's site at **www.ahima.org** and click on About AHIMA in the heading banner to acquaint yourself with this organization. Check its history, mission, and code of ethics. Then provide your instructor with a written response to this question: What role has the AHIMA played in safeguarding the confidentiality of information in the medical record?

Review: The Medical History and Physical Examination

■ The Medical History and Physical Examination includes the Chief Complaint, Present Illness, Past History, Family History, Social History, Review of Systems, and Diagnostic Impressions and Treatment Plans.

■ The Medical History and Physical Examination can be completed by a physician, nurse practitioner, or physician assistant and must satisfy clinical, legal, and regulatory requirements.

■ The report may include the names of various diagnostic tests related to blood count, blood chemistry, and lipid profiles; x-rays and other tests may be ordered as patient need indicates.

■ There are specific situations when an abbreviated medical history and physical examination format may be used, such as a Short-Stay History and Physical, Interval History and Physical, Consultation, or physician Progress Notes.

■ The two most commonly used health information systems are the Problem Oriented Record (POR), which uses the patient's problems as the organizing factor, and the Source Oriented Record (SOR), which is organized by the source of the report or document.

Review of Terminology Presented

In each chapter beginning with this one, words printed in boldface in the text are considered important to your learning process. These words are summarized in the Review of Terminology Presented for easy reference and use in the practice exercises that follow.

Word	Meaning
atherosclerosis	hardening of arterial walls due to deposits of cholesterol or fats
auscultation	act of listening for sounds within the body
blood chemistry profile	analysis of chemical components of the patient's blood
carotid	principal artery in the neck
chief complaint (CC)	subjective description of the symptoms that caused the patient to seek medical attention
cholesterol	fat-soluble, crystalline, steroid alcohol found in animal fat

continues

Word	Meaning
clinical diagnosis	diagnosis made on the basis of knowledge obtained from the medical history and physical examination
coagulation prothrombin time	measurement of the effectiveness of several blood-clotting factors to adjust prothrombin time
Consultation	report written by consulting physician on the request of a patient's primary physician
data base	first section of a problem oriented record, including all patient evaluations such as the History and Physical Examination, Nursing Assessment, Dietitian Assessment, Social Services Evaluation, and other documents that evaluate the patient's state of health
diagnosis	identification of a disease or condition by a scientific evaluation of physical signs, symptoms, laboratory tests, and procedures
differential diagnosis	distinguishing between two or more diseases with similar symptoms by comparing their signs and symptoms
diplopia	perception of two images of a single object; double vision
edema	abnormal accumulation of fluid in intercellular spaces; swelling
erythrocyte sedimentation rate (ESR)	rate at which red blood cells settle in a tube within a given amount of time to determine the degree of inflammation in the body
extraocular	outside of the eye
family history (FH)	relevant medical information about the patient's family members
femoral (pulse)	pulse of the femoral artery felt in the groin
fundi	back portion of the interior of the eyeball
hemoptysis	spitting up of blood or blood-tinged sputum
hepatosplenomegaly	enlargement of liver and spleen
history	section of the physical and history that contains information to document patient care, justify physician's actions, and secure payment for services rendered
impressions/diagnoses	section of the report in which the physician indicates diagnostic conclusions
interval history and physical examination	abbreviated format sometimes used when a patient is repeatedly hospitalized for the same condition
laboratory diagnosis	diagnosis arrived at after the study of laboratory findings
lacrimation	secretion and discharge of tears
lipid	fat or fatlike substance
lipoprotein	combination of a lipid and a protein having the general properties of proteins
malaise	vague feeling of bodily discomfort
murmur	auscultatory sound, particularly a periodic, short-duration sound of cardiac or vascular origin
palpation	feeling with fingers or hands to determine the physical characteristics of organs or tissues
past history (PH)	information that includes any childhood or adult diseases, surgical procedures, accidents, pregnancies, deliveries, and allergies to medications or other items

continues

Word	Meaning
percussion	using fingertips to tap the surface area of the body in order to produce sound
physical diagnosis	diagnosis supported by both the clinical diagnosis and the laboratory diagnosis
physical examination (PX, PE)	physician's objective assessment of the patient, using auscultation, palpation, percussion, and visualization
plan	section of the report that includes specific laboratory and diagnostic tests, referrals to specialists, specific instructions to the patient, and/or follow-up appointments as needed
present illness (PI)	information provided by patient as to when the symptoms were first noticed, the extent and intensity, and the patient's opinion about what caused the symptoms
primary symptoms	symptoms directly related to a disease
Problem List	section of the problem oriented patient record that identifies each problem of a patient (active and inactive)
problem oriented record (POR)	organizes information in a patient's record by problems or diagnoses
progress notes	brief notes from a physician documenting a patient's progress
review of systems (ROS)	exchange between doctor and patient to determine presence or absence of signs and symptoms
rubs	scraping or grating noise
secondary symptoms	symptoms that are the result of a disease process
septal	pertaining to a septum
short-stay history and physical examination	abbreviated form of a history and physical often used for ambulatory, same-day, or short-stay surgical interventions
sign	objective, observable, or measurable manifestation of a disease
social history (SH)	information summarizing the patient's lifestyle and environment to determine whether something about these factors is contributing to the problem
source oriented record (SOR)	record organized according to the source of the documents included
sputum	matter ejected from the trachea, bronchi, and lungs via the mouth
symptom	subjective indication of disease as reported by the patient
thrills	vibrations felt by way of palpation
trachea	windpipe
triglyceride	neutral fat that is the usual storage form of lipids
tympanic membrane	eardrum
vertigo	sensation as if the patient or the environment is revolving; dizziness
visualization	observation and inspection to assess various body parts by simple use of sight
vital signs	measurement of pulse rate, respiration rate, and body temperature; can also include blood pressure

Terminology Review Exercises

Name: __Kerivanveghel__ Date: __1/20/09__

DEFINITIONS*

Give the medical term for the following.

1. Listening to sounds in the body — __auscultation__
2. Feeling with fingers or hands to determine the physical characteristics of organs or tissues — __palpation__
3. Observation and inspection by the use of sight — __visualization__
4. Tapping surface area of body with fingertips — __percussion__
5. Measurement of temperature, pulse, and respiration — __vital signs__
6. Scraping or grating noise — __rubs__
7. A vibration felt by way of palpation — __thrills__
8. Abnormal accumulation of fluid — __edema__
9. Enlargement of liver and spleen — __hepatosplenomegaly__
10. Eardrum — __tympanic eardrum__
11. First section of the history and physical — __history__

SHORT ANSWER*

From the Review of Terminology Presented, identify and define the terms that relate to the eye.

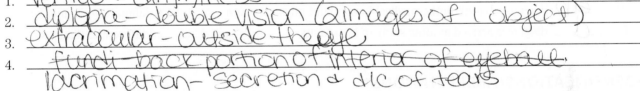

1. vertigo – dimminess
2. diplopia – double vision (2 images of 1 object)
3. extraocular – outside the eye
4. fundi – back portion of interior of eyeball.
   lacrimation – secretion & d/c of tears

SIGN, SYMPTOM, OR DIAGNOSIS*

Identify each of the following terms as a sign, symptom, or diagnosis. (Review the definition of sign, symptom, and diagnosis.)

1. atherosclerosis — diagnosis
2. edema — sign
3. malaise — symptom
4. thrills — sign
5. diplopia — symptom
6. hemoptysis — sign
7. rubs — sign
8. hepatosplenomegaly — diagnosis

---

*Answers are in Appendix A.

SPELLING*

Rewrite the misspelled words.

1. coratid — carotid
2. lipid
3. femural — femoral
4. vertigo
5. triglyceride
6. sputum
7. trachia — trachea
8. lipoprotein
9. cholesterol
10. murmer — murmur
11. septol — septal

MATCHING*

Match the type of diagnosis with its definition.

1. __c__ supported by both the clinical and laboratory diagnosis
2. __a__ identification of diseases by scientific evaluation
3. __e__ distinguishing between two or more diseases
4. __ab__ diagnosis based on the medical history and physical exam
5. __d__ diagnosis arrived at after study of lab results

a. diagnosis
b. clinical diagnosis
c. physical diagnosis
d. laboratory diagnosis
e. differential diagnosis

IDENTIFICATIONS/ABBREVIATIONS*

List the headings of a Medical History and Physical Examination in the order in which they appear in a report. Then provide the abbreviation (if any) for each heading.

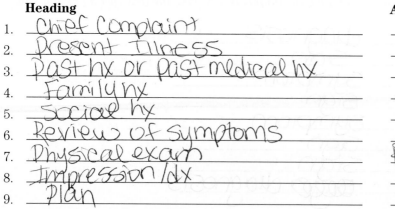

Heading	Abbreviation
1. Chief Complaint	CC
2. Present Illness	PI
3. Past hx or past medical hx	PH PMH
4. Family hx	FH
5. Social hx	SH
6. Review of symptoms	ROS
7. Physical exam	PX (PE)
8. Impression /dx	
9. Plan	

IDENTIFICATIONS

Write out the words for the following abbreviations. Identify the section of the Medical History and Physical Examination in which each would most likely be found.

1. BP — blood pressure
2. DX — diagnosis
3. PERRLA — pupils re equal round reactive to light & accomodation
4. RX — reaction
5. TPR — temperature, pulse, respiration
6. W/D — well developed
7. W/N — well nourished
8. A&P — assessment & auscultation & persussion
9. UTI — urinary tract infection
10. HEENT — head eye ear neck throat

Write out the words for the following abbreviations of laboratory and diagnostic tests.

11. BUN — blood urea nitrogen
12. ECG — electrocardiogram
13. UA — urinalysis
14. HDL — high density lipoproteins
15. LDL — low density lipoproteins

Write out the words for the following abbreviations.

16. POR (POMR) — problem oriented record
17. SOR — source oriented record
18. SOAP — subjective objective assessment physical
19. Pt — patient
20. H&P — history & physical

ABBREVIATIONS/IDENTIFICATIONS

Identify the tests included in a complete blood count (CBC). Give the abbreviation and write out the test name.

	Abbreviation	Name of Test
1.	WBC	
2.	RBC	
3.	Hg	
4.	Hct	
5.	RBC indices	
6.	diff	
7.	blood smear	
8.	platelets	

MATCHING

Match the abbreviations to their meanings.

1. __D__ millimeters cubed
2. __F__ milligram
3. __E__ grams percent
4. __K__ low-power field
5. __H__ milliequivalent
6. __D__ millimeters of mercury
7. __L__ milligrams percent
8. __A__ centimeters
9. __G__ international units per liter
10. __C__ high-power field
11. __B__ liter
12. __I__ milliequivalent per liter

a. cm
b. L
c. HPF
d. mm^3
e. gm%
f. mg
g. IU/L
h. mEq
i. mEq/L
j. mm/Hg
k. LPF
l. mg%

SHORT ANSWER

1. Name the four components of the Problem Oriented (Medical) Record.

_____

_____

_____

2. How is the Source Oriented Record organized?

_____

_____

3. Differentiate between symptom, sign, and diagnosis.

_____

_____

4. Briefly describe the following terms:

a. Interval History and Physical Examination

_____

_____

b. Short-Stay History and Physical Examination

_____

_____

c. Consultation

_____

_____

d. Progress Notes

_____

_____

Word Element Review

Root	Meaning	Example	Definition
path/o	disease	**cardiopathy** (kar"dē-ŏp'ah-thē)	any disease of the heart

Prefix	Meaning	Example	Definition
dys-	bad, labored	**dyspnea** (dĭsp'nē-ah)	labored breathing
ect-	out, outside	**ectopic** (ĕk-tŏp'ĭk)	situated outside of the usual location
epi-	above, upon	**epigastric** (ĕp"ĭ-gă-s'trĭk)	above the stomach
hemi-	half	**hemiplegia** (hĕm"ē'plē'jē-ah)	paralysis of one side of the body
in-	not, into	**incurable** (ĭn-kū'rah-b'l)	not able to cure
infra-	beneath	**infra-axillary** (ĭn"frah-ak'sĭ-lār-ē)	below the axilla
para-	beside	**paraneural** (păr"ah-nū'răl)	alongside a nerve
super-	above, in the upper part of	**superior** (soo-pē'rē-or)	situated above
supra-	above, over	**suprapelvic** (soo"prah-pĕl'vĭk)	above the pelvis

Suffix	Meaning	Example	Definition
-algia	pain	**arthralgia** (ar-thrăl'jē-ah)	pain in a joint
-emesis	vomiting	**hematemesis** (hēm"ah-tĕm'ĕ-sĭs)	vomiting of blood
-ia, -iasis	condition, formation	**lithiasis** (lĭ-thī'ah-sĭs)	condition marked by the formation of stones
-itis	inflammation	**gastritis** (găs-trī'tĭs)	inflammation of the stomach
-malacia	softening	**cardiomalacia** (kăr"dē-ō-mah-lā'shē-ah)	softening of the muscular tissue of the heart
-osis	condition	**fibrosis** (fī-brō'sĭs)	condition of forming fibrous tissue
-ptosis	prolapse, downward	**nephroptosis** (nĕf"rŏp-tō'sĭs)	downward displacement of the kidney
-rrhage, -rrhagia	bursting forth, excessive flow	**hemorrhage** (hĕm'ōr-ĭj)	excessive flow of blood
-trophy	development, growth	**atrophy** (ăt'rō-fē)	wasting away; without growth

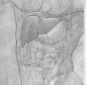

Word Element Review Exercises

Name: _____ Date: _____

MATCHING
Match the word elements to their meanings.

1. __G B F__ above, over   a. ect-
2. __E__ beside   b. epi-
3. __G F__ above, in the upper part of   c. hemi-
4. __A__ out, outside   d. infra-
5. __B__ above, upon   e. para-
6. __C__ half   f. super-
7. __H__ prolapse, downward   g. supra-
8. __D__ beneath   h. -ptosis
9. __I__ not, into   i. in-

MEANINGS*
In the underlined words below, circle the word element presented in this chapter. Provide the meaning of the word.

1. The patient complains of <u>dyspnea</u>.

   _____

2. The condition, unfortunately, is <u>incurable</u> at the present time.

   _____

3. <u>Cardiopathy</u> of undetermined origin was listed as the final diagnosis.

   _____

4. The patient presented with <u>arthralgia</u>.

   _____

5. As a result of the wound, the patient began to <u>hemorrhage</u>.

   _____

6. Her deteriorating condition was marked by <u>cardiomalacia</u>.

   _____

7. <u>Gastritis</u> can be caused by any number of factors.

   _____

8. Her last pregnancy was an <u>ectopic</u> pregnancy.

   _____

9. His aches and pains were attributed to <u>fibrosis</u>.

   _____

10. <u>Epigastric</u> discomfort led her physician to order a series of GI tests.

    _____

*Answers are in Appendix A.

11. <u>Hematemesis</u> is a sign of a critical illness.

   _____

12. Gallstones and kidney stones are evidence of <u>lithiasis</u>.

   _____

13. The urologist was concerned about the patient's <u>nephroptosis</u>.

   _____

14. The <u>infra-axillary</u> area was tender to palpation.

   _____

15. Disuse <u>atrophy</u> can be caused by long periods of inactivity.

   _____

WORD ELEMENT MEANINGS

Give the meaning of each word element. Then use your dictionary to find a new word that contains each of the word elements. Specify whether the new word is a noun or an adjective by placing N or A in the last column.

Word Element	Meaning	Word	N or A
1. -algia			
2. dys-			
3. ect-			
4. -emesis			
5. dermat/o			
6. hemi-			
7. -ia, -iasis			
8. in-			
9. infra-			
10. -itis			
11. -malacia			
12. -osis			
13. para-			
14. path/o			
15. -ptosis			
16. -rrhage, -rrhagia			
17. super-			
18. supra-			
19. -trophy			

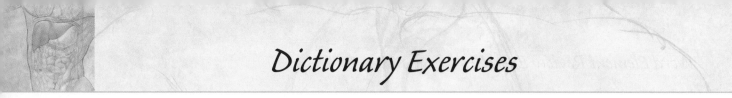

Name: _____ Date: _____

DICTIONARY EXERCISE 1

Use your dictionary to find the pronunciation and definition of the following words.

	Word	Pronunciation	Definition
1.	adnexa	_____	_____
2.	afebrile	_____	_____
3.	atresia	_____	_____
4.	bruit	_____	_____
5.	cachexia	_____	_____
6.	emaciation	_____	_____
7.	hypertrophy	_____	_____
8.	lesion	_____	_____
9.	rebound pain	_____	_____
10.	rupture	_____	_____

DICTIONARY EXERCISE 2*

Pronunciation of the words below is provided. Using your dictionary, find the correct spelling and definition of each word.

	Word	Pronunciation	Definition
1.	atypical	ā-tĭp'ĭ-kal	_____
2.	bilateral	bī-lăt'er-al	_____
3.	congestion	kŏn-jĕst'shŭn	_____
4.	dehydration	dē"hī-drā'shŭn	_____
5.	inflammation	ĭn"flah-mā'shŭn	_____
6.	insomnia	ĭn-sŏm'nē-ah	_____
7.	migraine	mī'grān	_____
8.	obstruction	ŏb-strŭk'shŭn	_____
9.	supple	sŭp'l	_____
10.	unilateral	ū"nĭ-lăt'er-al	_____
11.	arrhythmia	ă-rĭth'mē-ă	_____
12.	serous	sēr'ŭs	_____
13.	accumulation	ă-kŏm"ō-elā'shŭn	_____

DICTIONARY EXERCISE 3

Look up the meaning of each italicized word. Place the pronunciation in the space provided. Then rewrite the sentence in your own words.

1. Even though the child was *asymptomatic* (_____), she had an ear infection.

   _____

2. Abdominal *distention* (_____) hampered the physical examination.

   _____

3.   Once the nerve was severed, *flaccid* (_____) paralysis resulted.

   _____

4.   *Gait* (_____) disturbances can be caused by many different factors.

   _____

5.   A *gallop* (_____) rhythm may signal the need for further cardiac assessment.

   _____

6.   *Pallor* (_____) is a symptom and does not identify a specific disease.

   _____

7.   Dry and moist *rales* (_____) must be identified by location.

   _____

8.   The *residual* (_____) effects of a stroke can be as devastating as the disease itself.

   _____

9.   On physical examination, a strident *rhonchus* (_____) was identified.

   _____

10.   No *cardiomegaly* (_____), no murmurs, rubs, or gallops were identified.

   _____

11.   The patient was in *ketoacidosis* (_____) at the time of admission to the hospital.

   _____

12.   With a history of recurrent infection, the patient is admitted for bilateral *myringotomy*
   (_____).

   _____

13.   The little girl had a history of recurrent *otitis media* (_____).

   _____

Listening Exercise

Name	Date

INSTRUCTIONS

All the listening exercises in this text are actual medical documents. The words provided in the preview section should be reviewed and practiced before listening to the tape. The words appear in the preview in the same order in which they are used to fill in the blanks in the listening activity.

1. Review the spelling, pronunciation, and meaning of the words provided in the preview.
2. Listen to the audio CD and fill in the blank as the word is dictated.
3. At the end of the exercise, check your spelling against the preview words. They appear in the preview in the order in which they are encountered in the exercise.
4. Review and practice the words you missed.
5. Look up words that are not familiar.

PREVIEW OF WORDS FOR LISTENING EXERCISE 3-1

Word	Pronunciation	Definition
hemicolectomy	hĕm"ē-kō-lĕk'tō-mē	excision of approximately half of the colon
hematuria	hē"māh-tū'rē-ă	presence of blood in the urine
cataract	kăt'ă-răkt	clouding of the lenses of the eye
ptosis	tō'sĭs	drooping or downward placement
varicosities	văr"ĭ-kŏs'ĭ-tees	enlarged veins
hepatosplenomegaly	hĕp"ă-tō-splē"nō-mĕg'ă-lē	enlargement of liver and spleen

History and Physical

HISTORY

This 63-year-old male is admitted for a planned right _____ for a recently discovered cecal carcinoma. The patient denies any history of rectal bleeding, _____, change in bowel habits, bloating, cramping, or any history of colorectal disorder.

No family history of colon cancer.

PAST MEDICAL HISTORY

No previous medical or surgical hospitalization. Had outpatient removal of a _____ with lens implant. Hemorrhoidectomy recently accomplished.

PHYSICAL EXAMINATION

Blood pressure is 145/100. Pulse is 88 and regular. Respirations are 16. Temperature is 98.6°F. The patient is sedated, pleasant, and in no acute distress.

HEENT: Wears glasses. Has _____ of right upper eyelid. Teeth are in good repair. Tympanic membranes are clear. Neck is supple. No evidence of thyroid enlargement or cervical lymphadenopathy.

EXTREMITIES: Femoral and popliteal pulses intact. Minor _____ in the right lower leg.

NEUROMUSCULAR: Within normal limits.

ABDOMEN: Soft and nontender; no rebound tenderness. No masses are palpable. Blower sounds are present. There is no _____or inguinal hernia. Femoral pulsations are equal.

Rectal not done at this time.

IMPRESSION

1. Cecal carcinoma in a mildly hypertensive man.

PLAN: As noted above.

CHAPTER

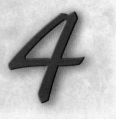

4

Pharmacology

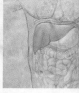

> *There are no really "safe" biologically active drugs. There are only "safe" physicians.*
>
> —HAROLD KAMINETZKY

OBJECTIVES

When you have completed this chapter on pharmacology, you should be able to

1. Identify significant legislation designed to protect consumers.
2. Distinguish among types of drug names.
3. Name and define drug classifications and abbreviations.
4. Explain various effects of drugs and drug actions.
5. Identify and define methods of drug administration.
6. Identify commonly used drug references.

INTRODUCTION

A natural or synthetic chemical substance that affects body function is referred to as a **drug**. These substances may come from plants, minerals, or animals, or they may be synthetic sources manufactured in laboratories (Figure 4-1). **Pharmacology** (fahr"mah-kŏl'ō-jē), the study of chemical substances, is an important specialty area addressing the following topics.

1. The production of new drugs
2. The use of drugs in treating disease
3. How drugs exert their effects on the body and interact with cells
4. The absorption, distribution, elimination, and duration of effectiveness of drugs
5. The study of drugs as they interact with other drugs or foods
6. The study of drugs as they interact with enzyme systems
7. The study of drugs and their harmful effects, including contraindications

The registered **pharmacist** (R.Ph. or Pharm.D.) dispenses medications ordered by the physician and is the professional who has the ultimate responsibility for the accuracy and appropriateness of those medications. A patient should get the right medication, in the right amount, at the right time, by the right route of

58

Source	Example	Drug name	Classification
Plants	cinchona bark	quinidine	antiarrhythmic
	purple foxglove	digitalis	cardiotonic
Minerals	magnesium	Milk of Magnesia	antacid, laxative
	gold	Solganal; auranofin	anti-inflammatory used to treat rheumatoid arthritis
Animals	pancreas of cow, hog	insulin	antidiabetic hormone
	thyroid gland of animals	thyroid, USP	hormone
Synthetic	meperidine	Demerol	analgesic
	diphenoxylate	Lomotil	antidiarrheal

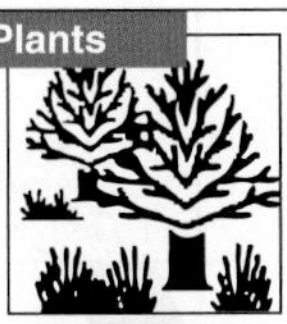

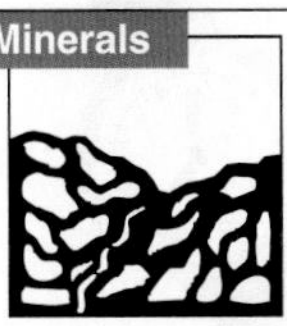

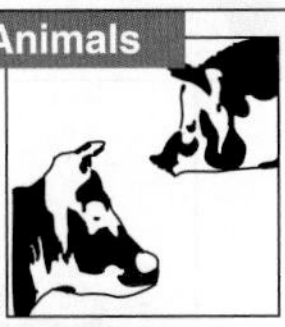

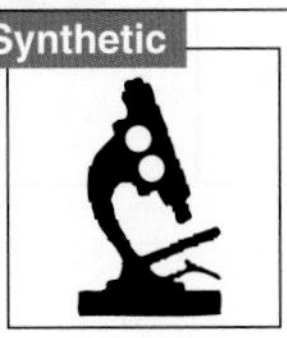

FIGURE 4-1
Sources of Drugs

administration. These *rights of medication administration* are illustrated in Figure 4-2.

Recognizing these rights, recent federal requirements mandate that a pharmacist shall provide patient counseling concerning drug effects, dosage and form, medication and food compatibility, and dose scheduling. This is very important to the patient because the interaction a medication has with other drugs or foods may determine the potential for an adverse reaction and may alter its effectiveness.

This is where the work of a **toxicologist** (tŏk"sĭ-kŏl'ō-jĭst) becomes significant. This pharmacology specialist studies harmful chemicals and their effects on the body and seeks antidotes for drugs that have toxic effects.

Pharmacy and toxicology are but two of the many specialties within the field of pharmacology. Others include medicinal chemistry, nuclear pharmacology, pharmacodynamics, pharmacokinetics, and molecular pharmacology. As modern medicine evolves, new areas continue to open.

CONSUMER SAFETY

In the early 1900s, the first of three laws was passed regulating the dispensing of drugs. The Pure Food and Drug Act, enacted in 1906, required all drugs marketed in the United States to meet minimal standards of strength, purity, and quality. It also established the two references of officially approved drugs: the *United States Pharmacopoeia* (USP) and the *National Formulary* (NF). These two books were later combined into one book, referred to as the USP/NF.

The second law, passed in 1938, was the federal Food, Drug, and Cosmetic Act (with amendments in 1951 and 1965). This legislation provided for more specific regulation of the industry and established the Food and Drug Administration (FDA) as the enforcement agency.

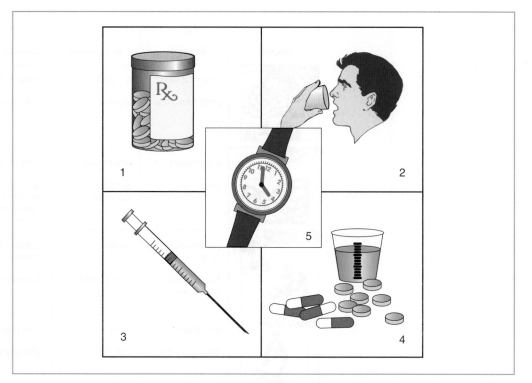

FIGURE 4-2
Five Rights of
Medication
Administration:
(1) right medication,
(2) right patient,
(3) right route,
(4) right amount,
(5) right time

The third law, the Controlled Substances Act, which passed in 1970, established the Drug Enforcement Administration (DEA). The law set much tighter controls on drugs that are depressants, stimulants, psychedelics, and narcotics. One significant part of this act established five levels or schedules into which all drugs are classified. As shown below, the levels—C-I through C-V—are determined by the degree of danger the drug presents. The first three levels all lead to some form of addiction or dependency.

As a result of these three laws, health care workers often are required to keep records according to specific regulations. For example, because prescription pads have the physician's DEA registration number, all pads should be in a secure location.

Class	Description of the Drug	Examples
I	not considered for legitimate use; high risk for addiction	LSD, heroin
II	accepted medical use; high risk for addiction	morphine, codeine, Demerol
III	strict limitation on quantity and length of time; moderate potential for addiction	Butisol
IV	strict limitation on quantity and length of time; less potential for addiction than Class III	Librium, Valium, Darvon, Equanil
V	no limits on prescription; low potential for addiction	Robitussin A-C, Lomotil

DRUG NAMES

Drugs can have four names—a generic name (which any drug manufacturer may use); an official name; a trade, private, or brand name; and a chemical name.

The **generic name** is the common or nonproprietary name by which a medication is known and assigned by the United States Adopted Names (USAN) Council. The name can be used by any manufacturer.

The **official name** is the name of the medication as it appears in the official reference, the USP/NF. Generally, it is the same as the generic name.

The **trade**, **private**, or **brand name** indicates ownership by a manufacturer and usually bears a superscript ® or ™ to the right of the name. The ® indicates registry with the United States Patent and Trademark Office, and ™ indicates a trademark but no federal registration.

The **chemical name** indicates the chemical content of the medication. The chemical name is not commonly used in a physician's practice.

The following is an example of one drug's brand, chemical, and generic names: Sinemet, (-)-3-(3,4-dihydroxyphenyl)-L-alanine, levodopa.

Sometimes a number is a part of the trade name. The purpose of this number is to differentiate it from a product that is almost identical. The number often refers to the *amount* of one of the components of the medication (e.g., 650 mg), but may simply indicate a difference in delivery medium (e.g., liquid vs. tablet) or dosage level (e.g., Tylenol #1, #2, #3, #4). The referenced component of the medication may also be a controlled substance. As a rule, the higher the number, the more of a given substance is present.

A physician may order medications using either the trade or generic name. A list of the fifty most prescribed medications and their generic names follows.

The Fifty Most Prescribed Medications by Number of Prescriptions Dispensed*

Brand Name	Generic Name
Accupril	quinapril
Allegra	fexofenadine hydrochloride
Ambien	zolpidem tartrate
Anexsia, Bancap-HC, Vicodin, Lorcet	hydrocodone with acetaminophen
Ativan	lorazepam
Augmentin	amoxicillin and potassium clavulanate
Bactrim, Septra	trimethoprim/sulfamethoxazole
Cefzil	cefprozil monohydrate
Celebrex	celecoxib
Cipro	ciprofloxacin
Claritin	loratadine
Coumadin	warfarin sodium
Darvon	propoxyphene
Deltasone	prednisone
Dyazide	triamterene/HCTz
Elavil	amitiriptyline hydrochloride
Esidrix, HydroDIURIL	hydrochlorothiazide
Excedrin	acetaminophen, APAP, and caffeine
Flexeril	cyclobenzaprine hydrochloride
Glucophage	metformin
Keflex	cephalexin
Lanoxin	digoxin

continues

Classification	Effect on Body	Example
• *cholesterol-reducing agents*	decreases the breakdown of body fats	Questran (cholestyramine), Mevacor (lovastatin), Lopid (gemfibrozil)
• *diuretics*	lowers blood pressure by promoting kidneys to excrete urine	Lasix (furosemide)
• *vasodilator*	stimulates arteries of the heart to enlarge	Capoten (captopril)
endocrine medications	acts in the same manner as naturally occurring hormones	
• *androgens*	hormones that stimulate the production of male sexual characteristics	Halotestin (fluoxymesterone), Virilon (methyltestosterone)
• *estrogens*	hormones used to treat menopause, prevent osteoporosis, used in oral contraceptives and to treat some types of cancer	Premarin, estradiol, Nolvadex (tamoxifen)
• *progestin*	medications that treat abnormal uterine bleeding	Provera (medroxy-progesterone acetate), Megace (megestrol acetate)
gastrointestinal medications	treats gastrointestinal diseases	
• *antacids*	neutralizes acid in stomach	Rolaids (calcium carbonate and magnesia)
• *antiulcer*	blocks secretion of acid in the stomach	Tagamet (cimetidine), Zantac (ranitidine)
• *cathartics*	treats constipation	Peri-Colace (casanthranol and docusate sodium)
• *antinauseants/ antiemetics*	treats nausea and vomiting	Antivert (meclizine), Compazine (prochlorperazine maleate), Zofran (ondanse-tron hydrochloride), Reglan (metoclopramide)
• *antidiarrheal*	decreases rapid movement of walls of colon	Lomotil (diphenoxylate and atropine), Imodium (loperamide)
• *proton pump inhibitors*	inhibits acid secretion	Prilosec (omeprazole), Prevacid (lansoprazole), Protonix (pantoprazole)
respiratory medications	treats emphysema, asthma, and respiratory infections	Proventil (albuterol), Theo-Dur (theophylline), Vanceril (beclomethasone)
sedatives–hypnotics	induces a state of drowsiness to relax and calm nervousness	Halcion (triazolam), Seconal (secobarbital)

continues

Classification	Effect on Body	Example
stimulants	acts on the brain to speed up vital processes	caffeine, Dexedrine (dextroamphetamine sulfate)
tranquilizers	treats stress and anxiety	Xanax (alprazolam), Thorazine (chlorpromazine)

EFFECTS OF MEDICATIONS

Effects of medications are categorized as being either systemic or local. Any substance that has the ability to be absorbed and distributed throughout the body has a **systemic** (sĭs-tĕm′ĭk) **effect**. However, when the effect is limited to the area of the body where it is administered, it has a **local effect**.

Once the chemical substance is in the body, it is absorbed, distributed, metabolized, and finally, excreted. **Absorption** (ab-sŏrp′shun) is the process of getting a chemical substance into the bloodstream. This process is affected by the medication's degree of acidity and lipid (fat) solubility, as well as whether there is food in the stomach. That is why some prescriptions are labeled "Give before meals" or "Take with food." Another factor that may either impair or enhance the absorption process is whether other prescription drugs might be present in the system. Only when the physician is aware of all medications being taken by the patient can the proper prescription be written.

The specific composition of the chemical substance will determine its **distribution**—that is, the process of moving from the bloodstream into the tissues and fluids of the body. Some chemical substances are attracted to specific organs or cells, whereas others may or may not be able to cross a lipid membrane.

The chemical substance undergoes physical and chemical alterations in the body. This process is referred to as **metabolism** (mĕ-tăb′ō-lĭzm). Most chemical substances are transformed in the liver to more water-soluble by-products that can be easily excreted by the kidneys. Some drugs may be eliminated through perspiration, feces, bile, or breast milk, as well as through the kidneys.

Excretion (eks-krē′shun) is the process of eliminating substances such as the waste products of drug metabolism from the body. If not excreted properly, some chemicals may accumulate and may cause **toxicity** (tŏk-sĭs′ĭ-tē)—a poisonous and potentially dangerous situation for the patient. This occurs often during renal insufficiency. These toxic effects must be monitored carefully when certain medications are prescribed. Toxic and other unintended effects that may occur with some medications are called **side effects**. For individual patients, the use of a particular drug may have harmful effects. **Contraindications** (kŏn-trah-ĭn″dĭ-kā′shuns) are the specific conditions that preclude the use of a drug or greatly increase the risk of adverse drug reactions or interactions that the physician considers in selecting medications for an individual patient.

Other factors that affect the pharmacologic response to drugs include age, weight, gender, psychological state, other medications and food interacting with one another, dosage, drug resistance or tolerance, genetic factors, allergies, and method of administration.

Use of a plant's seeds, berries, roots, leaves, bark, or flowers can be traced back centuries to the people of Egypt, Greece, India, and Asia. Currently, at least one-third of Americans use herbs and have spent billions of dollars yearly on these substances, despite the fact that no organization or government body regulates their manufacture or certifies the labeling of herbal preparations. Unfortunately, individuals taking these substances often do not tell their physicians of their use. This omission can lead to unwanted or unexpected results should a physician prescribe a medication or suggest an OTC product that reacts adversely with the chemical combinations found in herbal medicines.

Because there is little clinical evidence associated with specific herbal agents, claims of effectiveness or safety may not be adequately substantiated. Drug interactions can be significant and may lead to morbidity. Some herbal products can cause allergic reactions and others act like a diuretic or a hormone. Still others can effect heart rate, blood pressure, or clotting factors. For example, patients facing surgery are advised to stop taking St. John's wort and ginkgo biloba to avoid bleeding problems or other complications associated with anesthesia. Coumadin's blood-thinning effect is enhanced by Dong Quai root, a popular menopause remedy. Feverfew, sometimes used to prevent migraines, should not be used with nonsteroidal anti-inflammatories such as Advil, Motrin, and Aleve; anti-clotting drugs such as warfarin; or blood thinners such as aspirin.

Herbs come in different forms: teas, syrups, oils, liquid extracts, tincture, and dry extracts (pills and capsules). Because of the lack of industry regulation, there is no guarantee that the herb content of any given bottle or package or even from dose to dose is the same. Therefore, it is essential that the physician is consulted before herbal medicines are added to one's diet. In addition, infants and pregnant women should not take any herbal remedies.

A list of some of the herbs and their medicinal claims include those in the following chart.

Representative Herbal Medicines and Their Medicinal Claims	
Herbal Medicine	Medicinal Claim
aloe	heals
astragalus	enhances energy reserves
barberry	treats bad breath
bilberry leaf	increases night vision
black cohosh	relieves menstrual cramps
burdock leaf, root	treats severe skin problems, cases of arthritis
calendula flower	mends cuts
celery leaf, seed	treats incontinence
chamomile flower	relieves nervous stomach
cranberry	treats, prevents bladder, kidney infections
dandelion leaf	detoxifies poison in liver
Don Quai root	prevents, treats menstrual problems
echinacea root	treats strep throat, lymph glands
feverfew herb	treats migraines
garlic capsules	"nature's antibiotic"
ginger root	treats sore throat
ginkgo biloba	improves blood flow to brain; memory enhancer
ginseng root	slows aging; relieves stress
goldenseal	treats bladder infection, cancers, mouth sores, ulcers
gata kola	improves memory, "memory herb"
hawthorn	strengthens, regulates heart
horsetail	develops strong fingernails, hair
kava kava	induces sleep, calms nervousness
licorice	treats constipation
marshmallow leaf	treats inflammation
pau d'arco	protects immune system
St. John's wort	treats mood disorders
skullcap	sedates nerves
uva-ursi leaf	stimulates digestion
wild yam	helps expel gas
yarrow root	treats flu, fever

Vitamins are not commonly regarded as drugs, but actually are because their administration is associated with a pharmacologic response. They are natural or synthetic substances that have a positive or negative effect on the body. Water-soluble vitamins (vitamins B and C) must be replaced on a regular basis. On the other hand, vitamins A,

D, E, and K are fat-soluble vitamins whose effects are cumulative. Therefore, if excessive amounts of vitamin A, D, and K are consumed, whether in foods or in natural or synthetic forms, they may increase the risk of toxicity. Vitamin E, however, is not toxic in adults and older children except in extremely rare cases.

ADMINISTRATION OF MEDICATIONS

GASTROINTESTINAL (GI) TRACT ROUTES

Medications can be administered in a variety of ways to achieve a desired pharmacologic effect. The most common route of administration is via the **gastrointestinal** (găs″trō-ĭn-tĕs′tĭ-năl) **tract** (GIT). The gastrointestinal tract includes oral (p.o.), nasogastric (NG), and the rectal route of administration.

The oral route of administration is the most frequent route utilized, but the effects of the medications are delayed 30–60 minutes as adequate absorption must occur from the GIT. These medications may be represented by tablets, capsules, or various forms of liquids (solutions, suspensions, or elixirs). Oral medications may also be administered through a nasogastric tube (NGT) as shown in Figure 4-3. The NGT is generally not inserted for the sole purpose of administering these types of medications, but it may be used when the tube is placed for other reasons.

When drugs are administered rectally, they may be in the form of suppositories or enemas. Actual absorption of a drug given this way may vary depending on its characteristics and therefore influence the therapeutic effect.

PARENTERAL ROUTES

Administration of medications by other than the gastrointestinal tract is referred to as **parenteral** (păr-ĕn′tĕr-ăl). Most frequently they are introduced into the system by *intramuscular* (IM), *subcutaneous* (SC), *intravenous* (IV), or *intradermal* (ID) routes (each illustrated in Figure 4-4). Infusion of medications through an IV may be done continuously or by injection with a syringe as shown in Figure 4-5. This method, which generally requires prior placement of an indwelling catheter, provides an almost immediate effect from the drug because it is being introduced directly into the bloodstream.

Medications may also be administered several other ways, one of which is into the ear for direct absorption. Some additional methods are

intra-articular (into a joint space)
epidural (into the epidural space)
intra-ocular (into the eye)
intracardiac (into the heart)
buccal (between the gum and cheek)
sublingual (under the tongue)

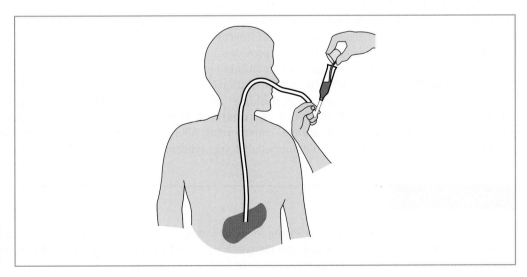

FIGURE 4-3
Medication Delivered
Through a
Nasogastric Tube

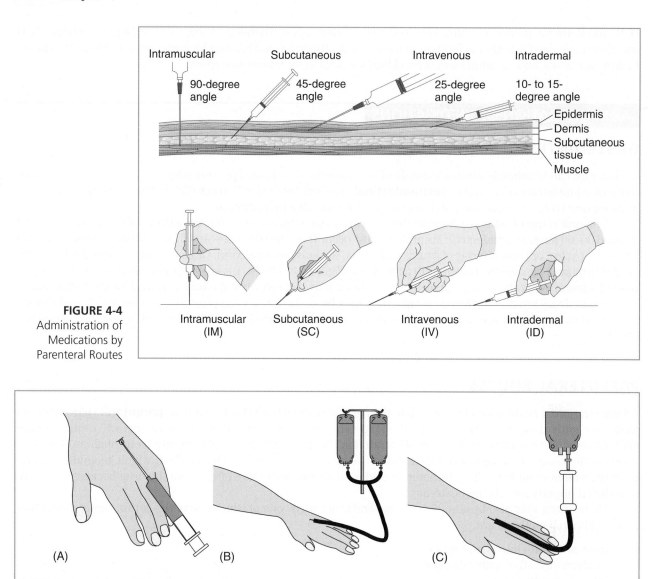

FIGURE 4-4
Administration of
Medications by
Parenteral Routes

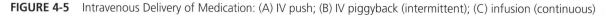

FIGURE 4-5   Intravenous Delivery of Medication: (A) IV push; (B) IV piggyback (intermittent); (C) infusion (continuous)

Topical administration of a drug refers to the application of a cream, ointment, lotion, or solution where its active ingredient is absorbed through the skin. These medications include vaginal creams, hemorrhoidal preparations, suppositories, oral analgesic creams, and topical steroids. Another example of the topical route is the use of a **transdermal** (trăns-dĕr'măl) **patch**, which provides a sustained delivery of a drug, shown in Figure 4-6. Examples include a synthetic narcotic (fentanyl) and an antimotion sickness medication (transdermal scopolamine).

The **inhalation** route includes the administration of drugs from an especially designed device through the nose or mouth. The device may contain a spray, mist, gas, powder that is delivered through a special apparatus such as an inhaler, vaporizer, nebulizer (Figure 4-7), respirator, atomizer, or intermittent positive pressure machine. Examples include medications for asthma, osteoporosis, allergic rhinitis, chronic obstructive pulmonary disease (COPD), cystic fibrosis, and acquired immunodeficiency syndrome (AIDS).

DRUG ACTIONS

Drug action has several meanings. For example, drug action can refer to the action the drug has on specific cells, tissues, organs, or systems. Drug action can also refer to the effect the drug has on a disease or disease symptoms. The following words refer to the latter usage of the term *drug action.*

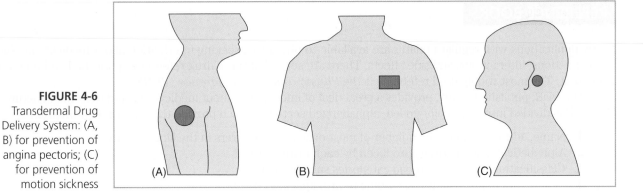

FIGURE 4-6
Transdermal Drug Delivery System: (A, B) for prevention of angina pectoris; (C) for prevention of motion sickness

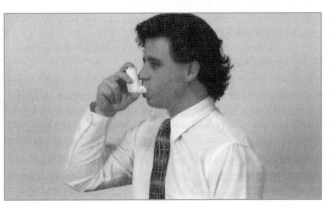

FIGURE 4-7
Nebulizer: medication by inhalation

PALLIATIVE

A drug is said to have a **palliative** (păl'ē-ă"tĭv) effect when it relieves the symptoms of the disease but does not cure the disease. A common example is the use of Tylenol to reduce a fever: The medication relieves the symptom (fever) but does not cure or combat the underlying cause of the fever.

PLACEBO

A **placebo** (plah-sē'bō) contains an inert substance lacking any pharmacologic effect. The layman's term for a placebo is sugar pill. Currently, placebos are most commonly used in controlled studies to help determine how well a tested medication works. In the past, however, patients who insisted on medication they did not need were given a placebo—an inactive substance or preparation to satisfy their psychological need.

PROPHYLACTIC

Medications can have a **prophylactic** (prō"fĭ-lăk'tĭk) effect when used to ward off or prevent disease. Immunizations using vaccines are prime examples of prophylactic medications. Antibiotics are often given prophylactically to prevent infection.

THERAPEUTIC

A medication used to cure or treat the disease or disease process is defined as **therapeutic** (ther"-ah-pū'tĭk). Many of the antibiotics are therapeutic medications in that they actually produce a cure.

REFERENCE BOOKS

Yearly publications with regular updates are available to physicians seeking information about medications, such as their actions, interactions, and side effects. There are several of these drug references published and they vary in content. The most widely used reference is the *Physicians' Desk Reference* (PDR).

The PDR, published yearly, provides a great deal of information about medications and their manufacturers. The PDR is divided into eight color-coded, alphabetized sections, which provide the following information.

1. Name, address, and phone number of most drug manufacturers in the United States
2. Alphabetical index of drugs produced by each manufacturer
3. Classification of drugs by broad categories such as laxatives
4. Generic or chemical names according to principal ingredients
5. Drug identification by means of color pictures of medications
6. List of drugs with use, dosage, composition, action, and side effects
7. An index of diagnostic products
8. A guide to management of drug overdose

The PDR is distributed to practicing physicians in a single hardcover volume; several supplements are published throughout the year.

Although the PDR is widely available, there are several other pharmaceutical reference guides. The two most frequently found in pharmacies are *Facts and Comparisons* (updated monthly) and, from The American Hospital Formulary Service, *Drug Information* (released annually and updated quarterly). Both serve as excellent sources of drug information. Pharmacies and other medical facilities often maintain many other drug-related books containing a variety of material about drugs including:

administration	drug comparisons	pharmacology
adverse reactions	drug interactions	precautions
available products	indications	relative costs
cautions	investigational drugs	stability
chemistry	overdosage	uses
contraindications	patient information	
dosage	pharmacokinetics	

Depending on the medical environment, you may find one or more of these references available. Examine the introductory section and learn to use its features.

ABBREVIATIONS

According to the American Association for Medical Transcription (AAMT) guidelines, periods are not used with short forms of words, such as caps for capsule, or with metric abbreviations. However, time and frequency abbreviations should have periods, as listed in the following tables. The AAMT guide also states that periods for English units of measure should be used as convention dictates and to avoid confusion.

Medication Forms

Medication	Forms
aloe	heals
cap	capsule
inj	injection
ung.	ointment
sol, soln	solution
supp	suppository

continues

Medication Forms *(continued)*

Medication	Forms
susp	suspension
syr	syrup
tabs	tablets
tinct, tr	tincture

Time and Frequency of Administration

Abbreviation	Latin Phrase	Meaning
a.c.	*ante cibum*	before meals
ad lib	*ad libitum*	at pleasure
b.i.d.	*bis in die*	twice a day
h.s.	*hora somni*	at bedtime
noc., noct.	*nocte*	night
p.c.	*post cibum*	after meals
p.r.n., PRN	*pro re nata*	as required, as necessary
q.d.	*quaque die*	every day
q.h.	*quaque hora*	every hour
q.4h.	*quaque quarta hora*	every 4 hours
q.i.d.	*quater in die*	4 times/day
q.n., q.noc.	*quaque nocte*	every night
q.o.d.		every other day
stat., STAT	*statim*	immediately
t.i.d.	*ter in die*	3 times/day

Dosages and Measurements

Abbreviation	Meaning
cc	cubic centimeter
dr.	dram
fl. oz.	fluid ounce
fl. dr.	fluid dram
gr.	grain
g, gm	gram
gt., gtt.	gutta (drop), guttae (drops)
mEq	milliequivalent
mg	milligram
ml, mL	milliliter
mMol, mMole	millimole
oz.	ounce

Site of Administration

Abbreviation	Latin Phrase	Meaning
AD	*auris dextra*	right ear

continues

Site of Administration *(continued)*

Abbreviation	Latin Phrase	Meaning
AS	*auris sinistra*	left ear
AU	*aures unitas*	both ears
ID		intradermal
IM		intramuscularly
IV		intravenously
OD	*oculus dexter*	right eye
OS	*oculus sinister*	left eye
OU	*oculus unitas*	both eyes
p.o.	*per os*	orally
PR		rectally
SL		sublingually
SQ, SC, subq, subQ		subcutaneously
vag.		vaginally

Other Abbreviations

Abbreviation	Meaning
c̄	with
disp	dispense
FDA	Food and Drug Administration
NPO	nothing by mouth
OTC	over the counter
pt.	patient
s̄	without
sig., Sig.	let it be labeled
×	times, multiplied by

See Appendix D for additional abbreviations.

INTERNET ASSIGNMENT

The U.S. Food and Drug Administration (FDA) is an agency within the U.S. Department of Health and Human Services. Its mission is to review clinical research and take action on the marketing of regulated products and to protect the public health by ensuring product safety and effectiveness. The Center for Drug Evaluation and Research (CDER) is part of the U.S. Food and Drug Administration. One of its best-known activities is the evaluation of new drugs prior to their being made available to the public. Its web site is located at **www.fda.gov/cder**. Clicking the Drug Information button will bring up a list of general and specific drug topics that include

New Prescription Drug Approvals
Prescription Drug Information
Major Drug Information Pages
Consumer Drug Information
Over-the-Counter Drug Information
Drug Safety and Side Effects

Clinical Trials Information
Public Health Alerts and Warning Letters
Reports and Publications
Special Projects and Programs

Selecting any of these topics will lead you to detailed articles and lists concerning drugs. For example, under New Prescription Drug Approvals, information is provided about New and Generic Drug Approvals (an alphabetical list updated daily), FDA Drug Approvals List (a reverse chronological list updated weekly), and New Drugs Approved for Cancer Indications (a current listing of new cancer drugs).

ACTIVITY

Visit the CDER site and select an article of interest from the Consumer Drug Information selection. Summarize what you have read in a brief memo to your instructor.

Review: Pharmacology

- Any chemical substance that affects body function is a drug.
- Three major legislative acts standardize the strength, purity, and quality of drugs, and control dangerous, addictive drugs.
- Drugs have four different names: generic, trade, chemical, and official.
- Drugs have either a local or systemic effect and are absorbed, distributed, metabolized, and excreted by the body and/or organ systems.
- Drugs may be administered through the GI tract or parenterally.
- The most widely used drug reference is the *Physicians' Desk Reference* (PDR).

Review of Terminology Presented

Word	Definition
absorption	process of getting a chemical substance into the bloodstream
chemical name	name that indicates chemical content of a drug
contraindications	patient factors that make use of a drug inadvisable
controlled substances	medications or drugs that may become addictive
distribution	process of drug movement from the bloodstream into body tissues and fluids
drug	chemical substance that affects body function
excretion	process of eliminating from the body substances such as the waste products or drugs metabolites
gastrointestinal tract (GIT)	most common drug administration route; includes oral, nasogastric, intramuscular, subc taneous, and rectal routes

continues

FILL IN THE BLANK*

Complete the following statements.

1. The common name by which a drug is known, assigned by the United States Adopted Names Council, is the _____ name.

2. The name that indicates the chemical content of the drug is _____.

3. The study of chemical substances is called _____.

4. The pharmacology specialist who studies the effect of harmful chemicals in the body is a _____.

5. The drug reference distributed by the American Hospital Formulary Service is _____.

6. _____ is the cumulative effect of drugs that may be harmful.

7. _____ is the external application of a drug using a cream, ointment, spray, or transdermal patch.

8. The two main categories for administering drugs are _____ and _____.

9. Drugs that are not safe to take without a doctor's guidance are _____ drugs.

10. A chemical substance that affects body function is a _____.

11. The most common route of medication administration is via the _____.

12. A drug that relieves the symptoms, but does not cure the disease, is a _____ medication.

13. The medical term for a sugar pill is _____.

14. Medications that ward off or prevent disease are _____ medications.

15. A medication used to treat and cure a disease process is _____.

16. A nebulizer is used when the route of administration is _____.

MATCHING

Match the abbreviations to their meanings.

1.	_____ three times a day		a.	cap
2.	_____ ointment		b.	syr
3.	_____ capsule		c.	IV
4.	_____ intravenously		d.	p.r.n.
5.	_____ syrup		e.	q.i.d.
6.	_____ four times a day		f.	p.o.
7.	_____ when requested		g.	susp
8.	_____ suspension		h.	SL
9.	_____ sublingually		i.	tab
10.	_____ orally		j.	t.i.d.
			k.	ung.

_____

*Answers are in Appendix A

Word Element Review

Root	Meaning	Example	Definition
bucc/o	cheek	**buccal** (bŭk'al)	pertaining to or directed toward the cheek
chem/o	chemical	**chemoreceptor** (kē"mō-rē-sĕp'tor)	receptor sensitive to stimulation by chemical substances
cutane/o, cut/o	skin	**cutaneous** (kū-tā'nē-us)	pertaining to the skin
derm/o	skin	**dermatologic** (der"mah-tō-lŏj'ik)	pertaining to or affecting the skin
hypn/o	sleep	**hypnotic** (hĭp-not'ik)	inducing sleep
lingu/o	tongue	**lingual** (lĭng'gwal)	pertaining to the tongue
narc/o	stupor	**narcosis** (nar-kō'sĭs)	stuporous state induced by a drug
pharmac/o	drug	**pharmaceutical** (fahr"mah-sū'tĭ-kal)	pertaining to pharmacy or drugs
tox/o	poison	**toxic** (tŏk'sik)	poisonous
toxic/o	poison	**toxicant** (tŏk'sĭ-kănt)	poison; poisonous

Prefix	Meaning	Example	Definition
anti-	against	**antispasmodic** (an"tĭ-spăz-mŏd'ik)	prevents or relieves spasms
contra-	against, opposite	**contraindication** (kon"tră-ĭn"dĭ-kā'shun)	any condition that renders a particular line of treatment improper or undesirable
intra-	within	**intravenous** (in"tră-vē'nŭs)	within a vein
par-	other than	**parenteral** (pah-ren'tĕr-al)	not through the alimentary canal, but by another route
sub-	under, below	**subliminal** (sŭb-lĭm'ĭ-nal)	below the threshold of sensation or conscious awareness
syn-	together, with	**synergy** (sĭn'er-jē)	cooperation of two drugs
trans-	through, across	**transdermal** (trăns-dĕr'măl)	through the skin

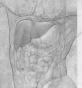

Word Element Review Exercises

Name: _____ Date: _____

CIRCLE AND DEFINE*

Circle and define the combining form in the following words.

1. pharmaceutical _____
2. toxicant _____
3. cutaneous _____
4. narcosis _____
5. buccal _____
6. chemoreceptor _____
7. dermatologic _____
8. hypnotic _____
9. toxic _____
10. lingual _____

Circle and define the prefix in the following words.

1. transdermal _____
2. synergy _____
3. parenteral _____
4. intravenous _____
5. subliminal _____
6. antispasmodic _____
7. contraindication _____

COMPLETION*

Provide the correct word element to complete the following words.

1. receptor sensitive to stimulation by chemical substances _____ receptor
2. stuporous state induced by a drug _____ sis
3. any condition that renders a particular line of treatment improper _____ indication
4. poison _____ ant
5. prevents or relieves spasms _____ spasmodic
6. below the threshold of sensation or conscious awareness _____ liminal
7. pertaining to or directed toward the cheek _____ al
8. poisonous _____ ic

_____

*Answers are in Appendix A

MATCHING
Match the terms to their meanings.

1. _____ not through the alimentary canal, but by another route
2. _____ poisonous
3. _____ pertaining to the skin
4. _____ affecting the skin
5. _____ inducing sleep
6. _____ poison
7. _____ cooperation of two drugs
8. _____ pertaining to the tongue
9. _____ injected into the vein
10. _____ through the skin

a. cutaneous
b. dermatologic
c. hypnotic
d. lingual
e. toxic
f. toxicant
g. intravenous
h. parenteral
i. synergy
j. transdermal

WORD ELEMENT MEANINGS
Give the meaning of each word element. Then use your dictionary to find a new word that contains each of the word elements. Specify whether the new word is a noun or an adjective by placing N or A in the last column.

Word Element	Meaning	Word	N or A
1. anti-	_____	_____	_____
2. bucc/o	_____	_____	_____
3. chem/o	_____	_____	_____
4. contra-	_____	_____	_____
5. cutane/o, cut/o	_____	_____	_____
6. derm/o	_____	_____	_____
7. hypn/o	_____	_____	_____
8. intra-	_____	_____	_____
9. lingu/o	_____	_____	_____
10. narc/o	_____	_____	_____
11. par-	_____	_____	_____
12. pharmac/o	_____	_____	_____
13. sub-	_____	_____	_____
14. syn-	_____	_____	_____
15. tox/o	_____	_____	_____
16. toxic/o	_____	_____	_____
17. trans-	_____	_____	_____

Dictionary Exercises

DRUG-RELATED WORDS

Below are drug-related words that have particular meanings for pharmacists and other allied health specialists. After reviewing them, complete the dictionary exercises that follow.

Word	Pronunciation	Definition
allergy		adverse response to a foreign chemical resulting from a previous exposure to that substance
amphetamine	ăm-fĕt'ă-mēn	stimulant for the central nervous system
analgesic	ăn"ăl-jē'zĭk	drug that relieves pain
anaphylactic reaction	ăn"ăh-fĭ-lăk'tĭk	severe allergic response (possibly fatal)
antagonism		interaction created when drugs work against each other
anesthetic	ăn"ĕs-thĕt'ĭk	drug agent that reduces or eliminates sensation
anthelmintic	ănt"hĕl-mĭn'tĭk	antiparasitic drug that destroys worms
antiasthmatic	ănt"ăz-măt'ĭk	agent that prevents or relieves an asthma attack
antibiotic		drug that slows down or stops the growth of bacteria, fungi, or parasites
anticoagulant	ăn"tĭ-kō-āg'ū-lănt	drug that prevents clotting or coagulation of blood
anticonvulsant	ăn"tĭ-kŏn-vŭl'sănt	drug that prevents or reduces the severity of seizure disorders
antidepressant	ăn"tĭ-dē-prĕs'ănt	drug that elevates moods and treats symptoms of depression
antidiabetic	ăn"tĭ-dī"ah-bĕt'ĭk	drug that treats Type I and Type II diabetes mellitus
antiemetic	ăn'tĭ-ĕ-mĕt'ĭk	agent that prevents or relieves nausea or vomiting
antihistamine	ăn"tĭ-hĭs'tah-mēn	drug that blocks the action of histamine, a substance that causes allergic reactions
anti-inflammatory	ăn"tĭ-ĭn-flăm'ă-tō-rē	agent that counteracts inflammation
barbiturate	bar-bĭch'oo-rĭt	drug with sedative properties
beta-blockers		drugs that block beta adrenergic receptors used as antiarrhythmics, antianginals, and antihypertensives
cardiovascular drug	kăr"dē-ō-văs'kū-lăr	drug that acts on the heart and/or blood vessels
dependence		situation where removal or withholding of a drug may cause psychological and/or physical symptoms
diuretic	dī"ū-rĕt'ĭk	drug that increases volume of urine excreted
emetic	ĕ-mĕt'ĭk	drug that induces vomiting
endocrine drug	ĕn'dō-krīn	drug that simulates naturally occurring hormones such as androgens, estrogens, progestins, thyroid, or glucocorticoids
gastrointestinal drug	găs"trō-ĭn-tĕs'tĭ-nal	drug, such as an antacid, antiulcer, antidiarrheal, antinauseant, cathartic, or laxative, which acts on various areas of the gastrointestinal tract
hypersensitivity	hī"pĕr-sĕn"sĭ-tĭv'ĭ-tē	immune response (allergy to a drug)

continues

Word	Pronunciation	Definition
idiosyncrasy	ĭd"ē-ō-sĭn'krah-sē	unusual response to a drug that is peculiar to the individual
isotonic	ī"sō-tŏn'ĭk	pertaining to solutions that possess the same osmotic pressure
lipid		family of compounds soluble in organic solvents but not in water (e.g., triglycerides, phospholipids, and steroids)
narcotic		drug having both an analgesic and a sedative action; can include substances with morphine-like activity (e.g., meperidine, hydrocodone codeine)
OTC		over the counter
placebo	plă-sē'bō	substance that resembles a medication but lacks pharmacologic effect
placebo effect		perceived pharmacologic effect from the administration of a placebo
potentiation	pō-tĕn"shē-ā'shŭn	interaction of two drugs such that one prolongs or multiplies the effect of the other
resistance		decrease in the response to a drug by various factors (e.g., bacteria) or other drugs
sedative		drug that quiets the central nervous system
stimulant		drug that excites or arouses vital processes such as heart rate, respiration, central nervous system activity, or blood flow
synergism	sĭn'ĕr-jĭzm	combining of two or more drugs that work together to produce a greater effect than either produces separately
teratogenic effect	tĕr"ah-tō-jĕn'ĭk	effect of a drug taken by a pregnant woman that may cause physical defects in a fetus
tincture	tĭnk'tūr	alcoholic or hydroalcoholic solution
tolerance		decrease in the response to a drug due to its continued use
tranquilizer		drug used to control anxiety
uricosuric agent	ū"rĭ-kō-sū'rĭk	drug that increases the excretion of uric acid in the urine

Name: _____ Date: _____

DICTIONARY EXERCISE 1
Select the correct meaning of each word.

1. Potentiation is
   a. an unusual response to a drug.
   b. interaction of two drugs so that one prolongs or multiplies the effect of the other.
   c. a drug that promotes vomiting.

2. Synergism is
   a. repeated doses that decrease the response to the drug.
   b. an unusual response to a drug.
   c. when drugs work together.

3. A beta-blocker is
   a. a drug that blocks beta adrenergic receptors.
   b. a drug that speeds up vital processes such as heart and respiration.
   c. a drug that reduces or eliminates sensation.

4. An amphetamine is
   a. a drug that sedates a person.
   b. a drug used to control anxiety.
   c. a stimulant for the central nervous system.

5. Drugs that mimic naturally occurring hormones such as androgens, estrogens, progestins, and thyroid are
   a. endocrine drugs.
   b. anticonvulsant drugs.
   c. antidiabetic drugs.

6. Drugs such as antacids, antiulcer, anti-diarrheal, antinauseants, cathartics, or laxatives are
   a. endocrine drugs.
   b. gastrointestinal drugs.
   c. antihistamines.

7. An interaction created when one drug cancels or decreases the effect of another is referred to as
   a. synergism.
   b. antagonism.
   c. potentiation.

8. A drug agent that reduces or eliminates sensation is
   a. an anticonvulsant.
   b. an analgesic.
   c. an anesthetic.

9. Drugs that block the action of histamine, a substance that causes allergic reactions, are
   a. anticonvulsants.
   b. antidepressants.
   c. antihistamines.

10. A reduced pharmacologic response to a drug after multiple doses is known as
    a. tolerance.
    b. antagonism.
    c. synergism.

11. Drugs used to control anxiety are
    a. stimulants.
    b. analgesics.
    c. tranquilizers.

12. Drugs that relax an individual by depressing the central nervous system are referred to as
    a. sedatives.
    b. stimulants.
    c. anticonvulsants.

13. Drugs that arouse or excite vital processes such as heart rate and respiration are
    a. sedatives.
    b. stimulants.
    c. amphetamines.

14. An unusual response to a drug is referred to as
    a. an idiosyncrasy.
    b. a teratogenic effect.
    c. an anaphylactic reaction.

15. If a drug produces symptoms of withdrawal, the patient is experiencing
    a. drug dependence.
    b. placebo effect.
    c. anaphylactic reaction.

16. If solutions have the same osmotic pressure, they are referred to as
    a. isotonic.
    b. teratogenic.
    c. anaphylactic.

17. An adverse reaction to a substance is
    a. an antidepressant.
    b. an allergy.
    c. a placebo effect.

18. A drug that treats Types 1 and 2 diabetes mellitus is an
    a. antibiotic.
    b. amphetamine.
    c. antidiabetic.

DICTIONARY EXERCISE 2*

Rewrite the following sentences in your own words. Provide the spelling for the underlined pronunciation in the space provided.

1. In the emergency department, the physician ordered an ĕ-mĕt'ĭk (_____) for the child.

_____

2. The control group took a plah-sē'bō (_____) for the entire year.

_____

3. The patient has been taking an ăn"tĭ-kō-ag'ū-lănt (_____).

_____

4. The infant exhibited hĭ"pĕr-sĕn"sĭ-tĭv'ĭ-tē (_____) to penicillin.

_____

5. It was apparent the patient was having an ăn"ah-fĭ-lăk'tĭk (_____) reaction.

_____

6. The drug was identified as having a tĕr"ah-tō-jĕn'ĭk (_____) effect.

_____

7. She was taking a bar-bĭch'oo-rĭt (_____).

_____

8. The results may be explained by the plah-sē'bō (_____) effect.

_____

9. He asked the physician to prescribe an ăn"ăl-jē'zĭk (_____).

_____

10. Her recovery was assisted by the ăn"tĭ-bī-ŏt'ĭk (_____) prescribed.

_____

11. The ah-lĕr'jĭk (_____) reaction to the drug was severe.

_____

12. The drug was classified as ănt"hĕl-mĭn'tĭk (_____).

_____

13. Because the drug was a dī"ū-rĕt'ĭk (_____), she experienced some minor inconvenience.

_____

---

*Answers are in Appendix A

14. The substance was classified as a lĭp'ĭd (_____).

_____

15. The physician indicated that use of năr-kŏt'ĭks (_____) was a primary factor in this situation.

_____

16. The pneumonia demonstrated rē-zĭs'tăns (_____) to antibiotic therapy.

_____

17. The physician prescribed tĭnk'tūr (_____) of opium.

_____

18. The physician prescribed a ū"rĭ-kō-sū'rĭk (_____) agent.

_____

19. The physician prescribed an ăn"tĭ-kŏn-vŭl'sănt (_____).

_____

20. An ăn"tĭ-dē-prĕs'sănt (_____) was prescribed for several weeks.

_____

Listening Exercise

History and Physical

Name	Date

INSTRUCTIONS

1. Review the spelling, pronunciation, and meaning of the words provided in the preview.

2. Listen to the audio CD and fill in the blank as the word is dictated.

3. At the end of the exercise, check your spelling against the preview words. They appear in the preview in the order in which they are encountered in the exercise.

4. Review and practice the words you missed.

5. Look up words that are not familiar.

PREVIEW OF WORDS FOR LISTENING EXERCISE 4-1

Word	Pronunciation	Definition
Elavil		an antidepressant
pharmaceutical	fahr"mah-sū'tĭ-kal	a medicinal drug
Isordil		coronary vasodilator
h.s.		at bedtime (hour of sleep)
conjunctiva	kŏn"jŭnk-tī' vă	delicate membrane lining the eyelid and covering the eyeball
antidepressant	ăn"tĭ-dē-prĕs'sănt	drugs that prevent or relieve depression

History and Physical

History

CHIEF COMPLAINT: This 53-year-old female presents with vague symptoms of dizziness and nausea.

PRESENT ILLNESS: The patient felt quite well until last Wednesday when she experienced a gradual onset of the above-mentioned symptoms. She had been started on _____ and it was felt that the symptoms could be related to a reaction to her medication. The patient was seen in the office today to assess her _____ regimen.

PAST MEDICAL HISTORY: Past medical history is significant as the patient takes a wide variety of prescription medications. They include Synthroid 0.25 mg per day, _____ 20 mg b.i.d., Capoten 50 mg t.i.d., Zantac 150 mg b.i.d., Reglan 10 mg _____, prednisone 25 mg q.i.d., Lopid 600 mg daily in divided doses. The patient denies the use of any OTC drugs.

SOCIAL AND FAMILY HISTORY: Noncontributory.

REVIEW OF SYSTEMS: No significant change from recent examination done on Wednesday, with the exception of the symptoms described above.

Physical Examination

GENERAL: The patient is a well-developed, well-nourished female who expresses concern over the recent onset of nausea and dizziness.

VITAL SIGNS: Wt. 178 lb., BP 150/88. P is 72 and regular; T 98.6°F. RR 20 and labored.

HEENT: Pupils are equal and reactive, and _____ are clear. Neck pulses are clear. No bruit.

HEART: No evidence of enlargement or murmurs.

LUNGS: Although respirations are labored, lungs are clear and resonant.

ABDOMEN: No tenderness or guarding. Bowel sounds are present and normal.

GENITALIA: External genitalia is normal female. Vaginal exam not done.

NEUROLOGICAL: Cranial nerves are intact. No evidence of pathology. Remainder of the examination is noncontributory.

IMPRESSION: Current symptoms appear to be related to a reaction to the recently prescribed _____.

PLAN: The patient was advised to discontinue Elavil for two days; and if symptoms subside, we will try another antidepressant.

The Integumentary System

> " A mole on the neck
> You shall have money by the peck. "
>
> —Old English rhyme

OBJECTIVES

When you have completed this study of the integumentary system, you should be able to

1. Spell and define major system components and explain how they operate.
2. Identify the meanings of word elements.
3. Spell and define diagnostic procedures, diagnoses, treatment procedures, and abbreviations.
4. Spell the names of commonly used medications.
5. Be familiar with terminology used in reports.

INTRODUCTION

The average adult has approximately 7 pounds of skin, which amounts to about 20 square feet of tissue—literally all the general public ever sees. As an organ system of the body, the skin, or **integument** (ĭn-tĕg'ū-mĕnt), is considered to be one of the most important systems. The integumentary system includes not only the skin but the hair, nails, and sweat and oil glands. Although the breast is considered an appendage of the skin, its discussion has been deferred to Chapter 16, The Female Reproductive System.

SKIN

Dermatology (dĕr"mă-tŏl'ō-gē) is the branch of medicine concerned with the diagnosis, interpretation, and treatment of diseases of the skin. The physician who specializes in the study of the skin is called a **dermatologist** (dĕr"mă-tŏl'ō-jĭst).

FUNCTIONS OF THE SKIN

The skin is an organ containing millions of cells and other biological components that protect the inner vital organs. This remarkable organ, the body's first line of defense, serves many functions, but the most important of these are as follows:

1. To protect deeper tissues against drying and being invaded by organisms and many chemicals.
2. To regulate body temperature. Blood vessels in the skin contract when we are cold but dilate when we are warm to dissipate heat. When we are very warm, we perspire and are cooled by the evaporation of the sweat.
3. To sense information about the environment and our position in it.
4. To lubricate the body surface to keep it soft and pliable.

In addition, because of the skin's visibility, it provides valuable information about an individual's general health.

In each chapter that pertains to organ systems of the body and oncology, the roots, prefixes, and suffixes that pertain to a particular part of the system are identified and defined. Thus, in this chapter the word elements that refer to the skin, hair, and nails are listed and defined.

STRUCTURE OF THE SKIN

| adip/o | fat | dermat/o, derm/o | skin |
| cutane/o, cut/o | skin | | |

The surface of the body is covered by three layers of tissue, each different in structure and function. As shown in Figure 5-1, the **epidermis** (ĕp"ĭ-dĕr'mĭs) (6) is the outermost layer. The **dermis** (dĕr'mĭs) (5) is the second layer and contains a framework of connective tissue. These first two layers are referred to as the skin. The third layer is referred to as the **subcutaneous** (sŭb"kū-tā'nē-ŭs) tissue (4) and is composed of deposits of fat in modified connective tissue (**adipose** [ăd'ĭ-pōs] tissue). This layer of fat is sometimes referred to as the panniculus adiposus.

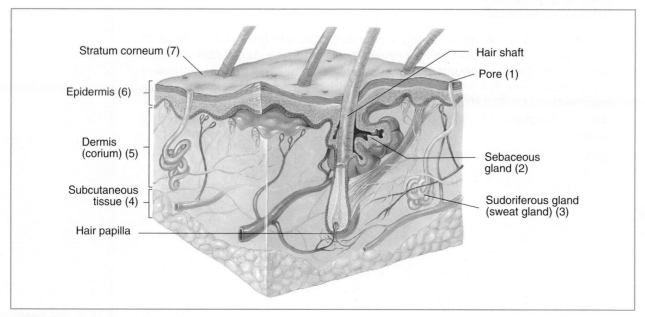

Stratum corneum (7)
Hair shaft
Pore (1)
Epidermis (6)
Dermis (corium) (5)
Sebaceous gland (2)
Subcutaneous tissue (4)
Sudoriferous gland (sweat gland) (3)
Hair papilla

FIGURE 5-1 Structures of the Skin

Epidermis

corne/o	horny		melan/o	black
kerat/o	horny			

The epidermis itself has several layers. The outermost layer (**stratum corneum** [strā'tŭm kor'nē-ŭm]) (7) is composed of flat, horny cells. These cells—which are dead by the time they reach this layer—have become filled with a dense, fibrous protein material called **keratin** (kĕr'ah-tĭn). The dead cells are shed constantly and replaced by new cells pushed outward from deeper layers of the epidermis.

Color in the epidermis is the result of pigment granules called **melanin** (mĕl'ah-nĭn) granules. This pigmentation protects the body from injurious ultraviolet light rays and also accounts for color differences among the races. When unbroken, the epidermis can prevent most disease germs from entering the body. Ridges in the epidermis can be seen most easily in fingerprints.

Dermis (Corium)

hidr/o	sweat		sud/o, sudor/o	sweat
seb/o	sebum			

The second layer, the dermis, is also called the **corium** (kō'rē-ŭm) (5). It has a framework of elastic, fibrous connective tissues and contains blood vessels and lymphatics, as well as sweat glands, sebaceous glands, and nerves. Involuntary muscle fibers are also found in the dermis, especially near hairs. Some areas of the dermis are thicker than others, for example, the soles of the feet compared with the eyelids.

There are primarily two types of glands located in the dermis—sweat or **sudoriferous** (sū"dō-rĭf'ĕr-ŭs) **glands** (2) and oil or **sebaceous** (sĕ-bā'shŭs) **glands** (2). The oily secretion of the sebaceous gland is called **sebum** (sē'bŭm).

The body has some 2 million sweat glands. There are two kinds of sweat glands. The **apocrine** (ăp'ō-krĭn) glands, which are found in the pubic, anal, and mammary regions, open into hair follicles. **Eccrine** (ĕk'rĭn) glands are present almost everywhere and help the body to dissipate excessive heat. These coiled, tubelike structures have an excretory tube that leads to the surface and to a pore (1). Sweat glands can produce two quarts or more of sweat per day under extreme conditions.

There are about as many oil-secreting glands as there are sweat glands. The sebaceous glands have ducts around the hair follicles. Oil secretions prevent the hair from becoming brittle, thus helping the hair remain vital. A certain amount of natural skin oil is also necessary to keep the skin soft and pliable. The largest number of these glands are found in regions of the scalp, face, neck, and upper trunk, which are the areas commonly involved with acne.

A pilosebaceous unit consists of a sebaceous gland opening into the hair canal, the hair apparatus, the arrector pili (smooth muscle attached to the hair follicle wall), and the apocrine gland (in areas where there are apocrine sweat glands). The smooth muscle may contract when the body is chilled, causing piloerection or visible "gooseflesh."

Subcutaneous Layer (Hypodermis)

fasci/o	sheet, band

The dermis is connected to the underlying fascia of the muscles by the subcutaneous layer, also called the hypodermis. The hypodermis is made up of connective tissue, which specializes in the formation of fat. This subcutaneous layer protects deeper tissues and acts as a heat insulator. Some areas of the body, such as the abdomen and buttocks, have characteristically larger accumulations of fat.

HAIR AND NAILS

onych/o	nail
pil/o	hair
trich/o	hair

Although the epidermis, dermis, and subcutaneous layers are associated with the skin, one does not normally think of the hair and nails as skin. In fact, hair, fingernails, and toenails are simply modified forms of skin cells.

The major structural material of the hair and nails is keratin. Keratin is produced by the same process that changes living cells into dead, horny cells in the epidermis. A **papilla** (pah-pĭl'ah) is a tiny, cone-shaped structure located at the bottom of a hair follicle, as shown in Figure 5-2. It is here that the root cells grow. Most hair tips project from the skin at a slant.

Oil from the sebaceous gland provides gloss. The hair follicle itself gets its nourishment through tiny capillaries that bring it minerals, proteins, vitamins, fats, and carbohydrates. Like the skin, scalp hair can provide protection and is a visible indicator of age and sometimes general health.

Nails have essentially the same structure as hair, except that nails are flat, hard plates. The living part of a nail (1) lies in the matrix (2), shown in Figure 5-3, which is comprised of modified epidermal cells that produce the hard keratin of the nail.

The matrix lies under the skin fold (3) nearest to the nail and is partially evident under the base of the nail. This is referred to as the **lunula** (loo'nū-lah) (4) or white crescent. As long as the matrix remains intact, new nail will grow. Changes in the appearance of your nails can be a first signal of illness.

INTERNET ASSIGNMENT

The United States National Library of Medicine (**www.nlm.nih.gov**), the world's largest medical library, provides information through several venues. Its goal is to offer reference and customer service to those in need of biomedical information. The site is divided into five sections: Health Information, Library Services, Research Programs, News and Noteworthy, and General Information.

Each of these sections offers a wide range of topics that can be accessed by clicking the name of the listed sections or through the site index in the page header. To illustrate, Health Information leads you to MEDLINEplus,

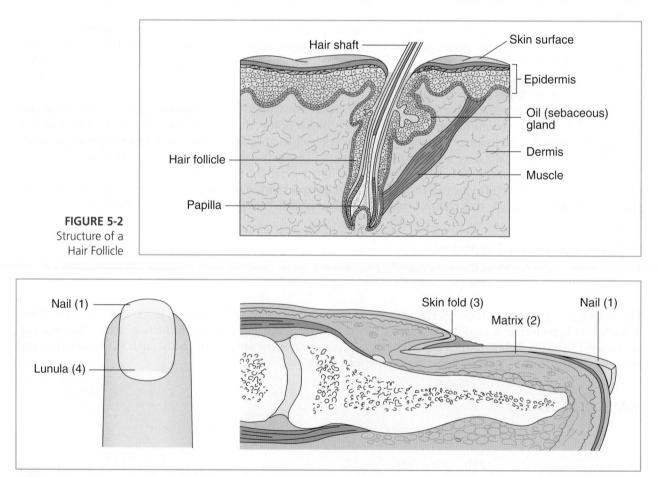

FIGURE 5-2
Structure of a
Hair Follicle

FIGURE 5-3 Structure of the Fingernail

MEDLINE/PubMed, DIRLINE, LOCATORplus, NLM Gateway, TOXNET, and several other sites. MEDLINEplus provides links to dictionaries, drug information, and more.

ACTIVITY

Sign on to the U.S. National Library of Medicine site and select DIRLINE. Enter "skin" in the search window and get a list of associations interested in the skin. The list is presented in order of relevancy with respect to the inquiry topic (skin). Scroll down the list until you find the American Academy of Dermatology. Connect to it by clicking its name (it is in hyperlink format). Select Patient Information. Then scroll to Patient Education and click it. Links are displayed for information about thirty-five different conditions. Click on one of the links and summarize your findings for your instructor.

Review: The Integumentary System

- The skin protects the body, regulates body temperature, and secretes oil to maintain its softness and pliability.
- The first layer of skin, the epidermis, protects the body from injurious light rays or pathogens.
- The second layer, the dermis, contains a network of blood vessels, lymphatics, connective tissue, glands, and nerves.
- The third or subcutaneous layer acts as a heat insulator and protects deeper tissue.
- Hair and nails are modified forms of skin cells and can be indicators of general health.

Review of Terminology Presented

Word	Meaning
adipose tissue	fat
apocrine glands	sweat glands found in the pubic, anal, and mammary regions and which open into hair follicles
corium	dermis
dermatologist	physician who specializes in the study of the skin
dermatology	branch of medicine concerned with the diagnosis, interpretation, and treatment of diseases of the skin
dermis	second layer of skin; also called the corium
eccrine glands	sweat glands that help dissipate excessive heat
epidermis	outermost layer of skin
integument	skin
keratin	major structural material of hair, fingernails, and toenails; a dense, fibrous protein material
lunula	portion of the nail-forming matrix evident at the base of the nail as a white crescent
melanin	pigment granules that give color to the skin and protect the body from injurious ultraviolet light rays
papilla	small cone-shaped prominence located at the bottom of a hair follicle
sebaceous glands	oil glands located in the dermis
sebum	oily secretion of the sebaceous gland
stratum corneum	outermost layer of the epidermis
subcutaneous tissue	third layer of tissue covering the body; also called the hypodermis
sudoriferous glands	sweat glands

Terminology Review Exercises

Name: _____ Date: _____

DEFINITIONS*
Define the following terms.

1. adipose tissue _____

2. sebaceous glands _____

3. stratum corneum _____

4. corium _____

5. lunula _____

6. sudoriferous glands _____

7. sebum _____

COMPLETION*
Complete the following statements.

1. Color pigmentation in the skin is created by _____.

2. There are approximately _____ sweat glands in the body.

3. Sweat glands are of two types; they are the _____ and _____.

4. A tiny, cone-shaped structure at the bottom of the hair follicle is called a _____.

5. A physician who specializes in the study of the skin is called a _____.

6. The three layers of tissue covering the body are the _____, _____, and _____.

7. The major structural material of hair and nails is _____.

8. Integument means _____.

9. Outermost layer of the epidermis is the _____.

10. The subcutaneous layer of skin is composed of deposits of _____.

SHORT ANSWERS
Supply a short answer to the following.

1. Why are hair and nails considered part of the skin system?

    _____

    _____

2. List the four functions of the skin.

    _____

    _____

    _____

    _____

    _____

---

*Answers are in Appendix A.

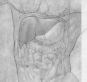

Working Practice

The information pertaining to each of the body systems about the type of work done in that specialty is entitled "Working Practice." These sections will vary considerably among specialties. For example, some practices include a great deal of surgery, whereas others have very little or none.

The diagnostic procedures may include radiologic procedures, laboratory tests of blood and other body products, and examinations with instruments. Treatment procedures are indicated for the specific practices they apply to. However, there will be some overlap because certain procedures are pertinent to more than one body system. Common diagnoses for the practices are included, as are abbreviations used and drugs prescribed.

The information presented with each body system is considered sufficient for job-entry qualification. By no means is it intended to be a comprehensive summary of the entire specialty dealing with that body system. You will continue to learn as you begin your career in the allied health field.

DIAGNOSTIC PROCEDURES

Word	Pronunciation	Definition
General		
fungal, bacterial, viral cultures	fŭng'găl	tissue scrapings, purulent (pus-filled) material, exudate (accumulated) fluid, or normal body fluids sent to a lab for identification of pathogenic organisms present
immunofluorescent studies for epidermal autoantibodies	ĭm"ū-nō-floo"ō-rĕs'ĕnt ĕp"ĭ-der'măl aw"tō-ăn'tĭ-bŏd"ēz	fluorescent studies of skin or blood serum under a microscope to identify the specific, abnormal antibody proteins of some cutaneous diseases
KOH smears		skin scrapings from suspect fungal lesions immersed in twenty percent aqueous potassium hydroxide and examined under the microscope for hypha (mold) or spores
skin biopsy	bī'ŏp-sē	removal of lesions for pathological examination, usually microscopic; a *punch or incisional biopsy* is done when it is not possible to remove the entire section of tissue involved
skin tests for allergy or disease		three types of test procedures where the site becomes red and swollen when the results are positive after the indicated period of time; tests reveal multinucleated giant cells (e.g., herpes virus infection)
• *patch test*		small piece of gauze or filter paper treated with a suspected allergy-causing substance is placed on the skin; reaction occurs after 48 hours
• *scratch test*		small scratches are made in the skin and minute amounts of suspected material are applied; results are examined after 20–60 minutes and again after 24 hours
• *intradermal test*		reactive substances are injected between the dermis and epidermis; results are examined after 20–60 minutes and again after 24 hours
Tzanck smear	tsănk	test of fluid from base of a vesicle; fluid is applied to a glass slide, stained, and examined under microscope
Wood's light examination		examination to detect fluorescent characteristic of certain skin infections (usually fungal) in which skin is viewed in a darkened room under ultraviolet light filtered through Wood's glass

continues

DIAGNOSTIC PROCEDURES

Word	Pronunciation	Definition
Blood		
antibody titer for viral, bacterial, fungal illness	tī'tĕr	blood test used to determine whether the patient has or has had an infection
antinuclear antibody titer (ANA)	ăn"tī-nū'klē-ăr	blood test used to screen for cutaneous lupus erythematosus and similar diseases of the connective tissues
enzyme-linked immunosorbent assay (ELISA)		blood-screening test for certain bacterial antigens and antibodies; one of the primary tests for several infectious diseases, in particular HIV
T3, T4, T7, TSH		blood tests to determine thyroid function

DIAGNOSES

Word	Pronunciation	Definition
Infectious Diseases Caused by Virus, Bacteria, Fungus, and Parasites		
abscess, furuncle, carbuncle	fū'rŭng-k`l, kăr'bŭng"k`l	localized collection of pus occurring in any body tissue including the skin; a *furuncle* generally occurs around a hair follicle; *carbuncles* are larger abscesses and involve several interconnected furuncles
candidiasis	kăn"dĭ-dī'ă-sĭs	yeast-type fungal infection caused by the yeast *candida*, often affecting individuals with chronic diseases
cellulitis	sĕl-ū-lī'tĭs	diffuse or spreading inflammation of the skin usually caused by *Staphylococcus*.
cheilitis	kī-lī'tĭs	lip inflammation
exanthem	ĕg-zăn'thĕm	measleslike eruption or rash that may be due to a virus, bacterial toxin, or allergic reaction to a drug
herpes	hĕr'pēz	family of viruses characterized by skin inflammation and the eruption of groups of small vesicles along the course of affected cutaneous nerves; associated with neuralgic pain, especially in the elderly
• *simplex type 1*		commonly called fever blisters and cold sores; usually around lips and nose
• *genitalis (simplex type 2)*	gĕn-ĭ-tăl'ĭs	commonly called genital herpes; highly contagious disease that may be sexually transmitted, but not exclusively so
• *varicella*	văr'ĭ-sĕl'ah	highly contagious childhood disease, commonly called chickenpox; virus becomes dormant after the infection clears
• *zoster*	zŏs'tĕr	reactivation of the varicella virus in adults; appears as blisters grouped along cutaneous nerves; commonly called shingles
impetigo	ĭm-pĕ-tī'gō	bacterial, inflammatory skin disease caused by *Staphylococci* and *Streptococci* characterized by vesicles, pustules, and crusted lesions (See Figure 5-4)

continues

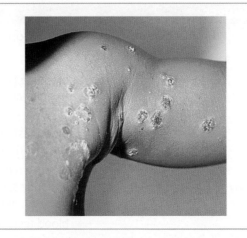

FIGURE 5-4
Impetigo (Courtesy of Robert A. Silverman, M.D., Pediatric Dermatology, Georgetown University)

DIAGNOSES

Word	Pronunciation	Definition
Infectious Diseases Caused by Virus, Bacteria, Fungus, and Parasites *(continued)*		
Lyme disease	līm	multisystem infection caused by the lyme spirochetes or Brorrelia burgdorferi, a bacterium; transmitted to humans by the bite of a deer tick
measles		highly communicable disease caused by the rubeola virus, marked by fever and rash; also known as rubeola
pediculosis	pĕ-dĭk"ū-lō'sĭs	condition of being infested with lice, either in the head, body, or pubic area (crabs)
pityriasis rosea	pĭt"ĭ-rī'ă-sĭs	benign rash characterized by scaling, rose-colored spots
scabies	skă'bēz	contagious, parasitic infection of the skin causing intense itching
tinea	tĭn'ē-ă	skin disease caused by fungus; ringworm; the term usually includes the name of the body part affected: may be *corporis* (body), *pedis* (foot), *unguium* (nails), *cruris* (genital area), *faciei* (face), or *capitis* (scalp) (See Figure 5-5)
tinea versicolor	tĭn'ē-ă vĕr'sĭ-kŏl"or	type of superficial fungal infection on the trunk and arms caused by the overgrowth of a saprophytic yeast normally present (*pityrosporum*)
verruca	vĕ-roo'kah	wart; type of common viral skin infection (See Figure 5-6)
Metabolic, Hypersensitivity, Immune, or Idiopathic Disease		
acne vulgaris	ăk'nē vŭl-ga'rĭs	inflammatory disease characterized by oil plugs and inflammation in and around the sebaceous glands; characterized by formation of *comedones*, either whiteheads or blackheads, pustules and in severe cases deep, inflammatory nodules
contact dermatitis	dĕr"mă-tī'tĭs	acute or chronic allergic reaction affecting the skin

continues

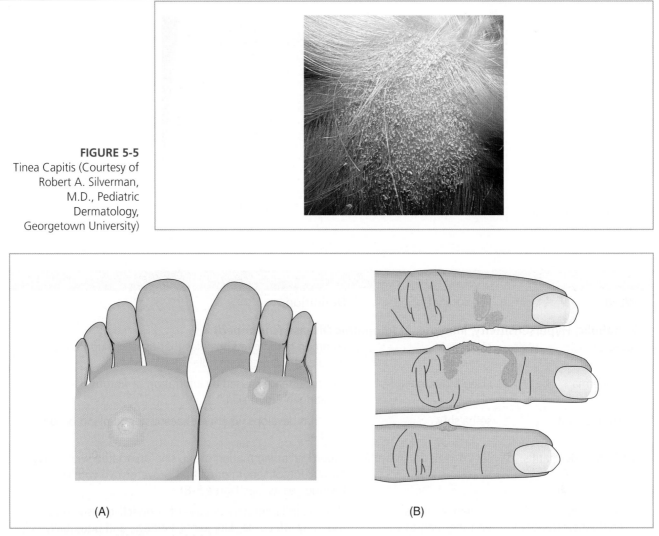

FIGURE 5-5
Tinea Capitis (Courtesy of Robert A. Silverman, M.D., Pediatric Dermatology, Georgetown University)

(A)   (B)

FIGURE 5-6   Warts: (A) Plantar and (B) Verruca

DIAGNOSES		
Word	Pronunciation	Definition
Metabolic, Hypersensitivity, Immune, or Idiopathic Disease *(continued)*		
eczema	ĕk'zĕ-mă	inflammation of the skin characterized by itching, redness, and vesicles; causes skin thickening in acute stages or dry lichenifications in chronic stages; *atopic dermatitis* is a chronic type of eczema often in families with a history of allergies and asthma; onset is usually two months after birth (See Figure 5-7)
lichen planus	lī'kĕn plā'nŭs	recurrent, itchy, inflammatory skin eruption often accompanied by oral lesions
psoriasis	sō-rī'ah-sĭs	chronic skin disease of unknown cause characterized by red, raised plaques with distinct borders and silvery scales

continues

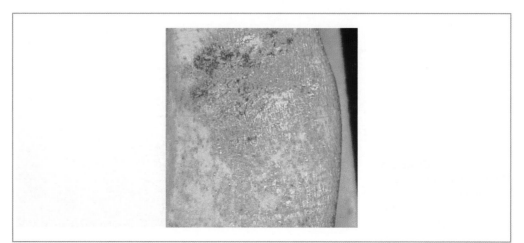

FIGURE 5-7
Eczema (Courtesy of the Centers for Disease Control and Prevention)

DIAGNOSES		
Word	Pronunciation	Definition
Metabolic, Hypersensitivity, Immune, or Idiopathic Disease *(continued)*		
rosacea	rō-zā'sē-ă	common chronic red pustules that usually erupt in the middle of the face in middle-aged individuals
scleroderma	sklĕr"ă-dĕr'mah	chronic disease caused by infiltration of fibrous tissue resulting in "hard skin"
sebaceous cyst	sē-bā'shŭs	cyst that develops when a sebaceous or oil gland becomes blocked
seborrheic dermatitis	sĕb"ō-rē'ĭk dĕr"mă-tī'tĭs	superficial inflammation of the skin associated with heavy production of sebum or oil that is overgrown with oil-bearing yeasts (See Figure 5-8)
systemic lupus erythematosus (SLE)	sĭs-tĕm'ĭk lū'pŭs ĕr"ĭ-thē-mah-tō'sŭs	chronic, inflammatory disease of connective tissue that that may affect the skin, joints, kidneys, and potentially any organ of the body

continues

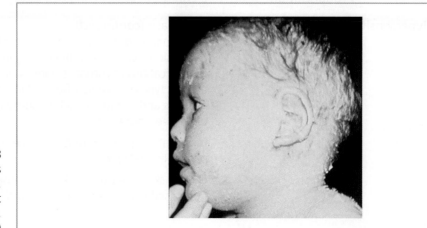

FIGURE 5-8
Seborrheic Dermatitis (Courtesy of Robert A. Silverman, M.D., Pediatric Dermatology, Georgetown University)

DIAGNOSES

Word	Pronunciation	Definition
Metabolic, Hypersensitivity, Immune, or Idiopathic Disease (continued)		
urticaria	ŭr-tĭ-kā'rē-ă	skin condition that may be a reaction to internal or external allergens and often remains of unknown cause; characterized by wheals or hives and local skin swelling; often itchy due to fluids leaking from blood vessels; individual lesions clear within 4 hours, but others appear; hives
Benign, Premalignant, and Malignant Tumors and Abnormal Pigmented Lesions		
actinic keratosis	ăk-tĭn'ĭk kĕr-ă-tō'sēs	premalignant condition characterized by growth of wart-like lesions on sun-exposed areas of skin
albinism	ăl'bĭn-ĭzm	genetic total or partial absence of pigment in skin, eyes, and hair
basal cell carcinoma	bā'săl kăr"sĭ-nō'mah	malignant tumor of the basal cell layer of the epidermis
ephelis, *pl.* ephelides	ĕf-ē'lĭs, ĕf-ĕl-ī'dēs	freckle
hemangioma	hĕ-măn"jē-ō'mah	benign tumor made up of newly formed blood vessels
Kaposi sarcoma	kăp'ō-sē săr-kō'mah	malignant vascular skin tumor; usually not highly malignant except in the case of AIDS
keloid	kē'loid	abnormally large, thickened scar
lentigo, *pl.* lentigines	lĕn-tī'gō, lĕn-tīj"ĭ-nēz"	larger, brown patches in the skin
leukoplakia	loo"kō-plā'kē-ah	white, thickened patches on the mucous membrane tissue of the tongue, cheek, or female external genitalia
malignant melanoma	mĕl"ah-nō'mah	malignant, pigmented mole or tumor of the melanocytes that may metastasize (spread) widely
melasma	mĕl-ăz'mah	condition characterized by dark patches of skin on the face; commonly called mask of pregnancy
nevus, *pl.* nevi	nē'vŭs, nē'vī	mole, birthmark (See Figure 5-9)

continues

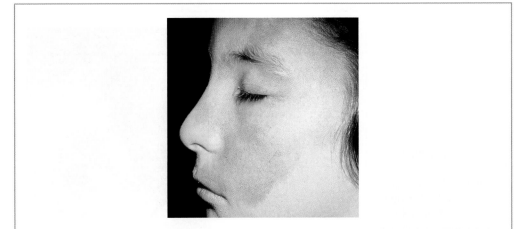

FIGURE 5-9
Nevus Flammeus
(Courtesy of Robert
A. Silverman, M.D.,
Pediatric Dermatology,
Georgetown University)

DIAGNOSES

Word	Pronunciation	Definition
Benign, Premalignant, and Malignant Tumors and Abnormal Pigmented Lesions *(continued)*		
seborrheic keratosis	sĕb"ō-rē'ĭk kĕr-ă-tō'sĭs	benign overgrowth of epithelial cells into brown warty lumps in older individuals
squamous cell carcinoma	skwā'mŭs kăr"sĭ-nō'mah	malignant tumor of the squamous epithelial cells of the epidermis
vitiligo	vĭt-ĭl-ī'gō	condition characterized by destruction of melanocytes in patches of skin and are seen as abnormally white patches in the skin
Diseases of Nail and Hair		
alopecia	ăl"ō-pē'shē-ah	partial or complete hair loss (See Figure 5-10)
folliculitis	fō-lĭk"ū-lī'tĭs	inflammation and infection of the hair follicle
hirsutism	hŭr'sūt-ĭzm	excessive growth of hair
paronychia	păr-ō-nĭk'ē-ah	infection of the skin around the nail
Trauma, Mechanical, Thermal, Electrical, Radiation, and Pressure		
abrasion	ă-brā'zhŭn	scrape, commonly called friction burns or rug burns
avulsion	ă-vŭl'shŭn	trauma caused when a portion of skin or appendage is pulled or torn away
burns		damage to the skin by fire, sun, chemicals, heated objects or fluids, electricity, or other means ranging from minor incidents to life-threatening emergencies; burns are described using four classifications: (1) superficial, or first-degree burns, which affect only the epidermis; (2) partial thickness, or second-degree burns, which affect the epidermis and dermis; (3) full thickness, or third-degree burns, which affect all dermal structures; and (4) deep full thickness, or fourth-degree burns, which extend to the underlying muscles and bones (See Figure 5-11)

continues

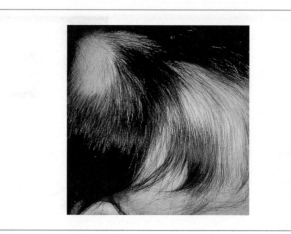

FIGURE 5-10
Alopecia Areata (Courtesy of Robert A. Silverman, M.D., Pediatric Dermatology, Georgetown University)

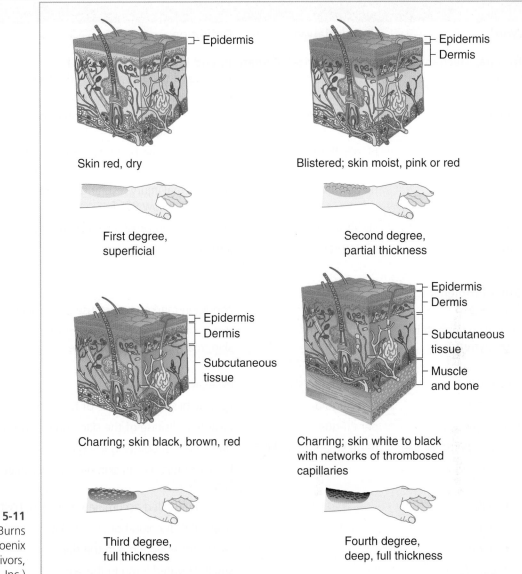

Skin red, dry

First degree,
superficial

Blistered; skin moist, pink or red

Second degree,
partial thickness

Charring; skin black, brown, red

Third degree,
full thickness

Charring; skin white to black
with networks of thrombosed
capillaries

Fourth degree,
deep, full thickness

FIGURE 5-11
Four Stages of Burns
(Courtesy of The Phoenix
Society for Burn Survivors,
Inc.)

DIAGNOSES		
Word	Pronunciation	Definition
Trauma, Mechanical, Thermal, Electrical, Radiation, and Pressure (*continued*)		
callus	kăl'ŭs	localized thickening of the horny layer of the epidermis due to pressure or friction; usually on the palms of the hands or on the feet
contusion	kŏn-too'zhŭn	bruise
corns		local thickening of tissue, usually on the feet, often painful to pressure and walking
decubitus ulcer	dē-kū'bĭ-tŭs	pressure sore
excoriation	ĕks-kō"rē-ā'shŭn	scratch

continues

DIAGNOSES		
Word	Pronunciation	Definition

Trauma, Mechanical, Thermal, Electrical, Radiation, and Pressure (*continued*)

frostbite		freezing of tissue, usually on the face, fingers, toes, and ears
hematoma	hē"mah-tō'mah	blood accumulation in the skin or other tissues resulting from bleeding
hyperthermia	hī"pĕr-thĕr'mē-ah	occurs when the body is overheated due to excessive exposure to the sun or a hot environment
hypothermia	hī"pō-thĕr'mē-ah	cold thermal injury resulting when the body's core temperature falls below 95° F
laceration	lăs"ĕr-ā'shŭn	cut in the skin caused by a sharp object
purpura	pŭr'pū-rah	large bruises in the skin

Other Problems

diaphoresis	dī"ă-fō-rē'sĭs	condition marked by profuse perspiration
exfoliative dermatitis or erythroderm	eks-fō'lē-ă-tĭv dĕr"mă-tī'tĭs, ĕ-rĭth"rō-dĕr'mah	generalized scaling eruption of the skin; many causes are possible
hyperhidrosis	hī"pĕr-hī-drō'sĭs	excessive perspiration
pemphigoid	pĕm'fĭ-goid	specific blistering disease of the skin
pemphigus	pĕm'fĭ-gŭs	blistering disease of the skin and mucous membrane
petechia, *pl.* petechiae	pĕ-tē'kē-ah, pĕ-tē'kē-ē	fine bleeding points in the skin
primary lesions		basic irregularities in skin disease identified as follows (See Figure 5-12)
• *bulla*		large, fluid-filled accumulation in skin; blister
• *macule*		small, flat discoloration in the skin
• *nodule*		larger, rounded lump in the skin
• *papule*		small, elevated lump in the skin
• *patch*		larger, flat discoloration in the skin
• *plaque*		wider elevation in the skin
• *pustule*		pus-filled swelling in the skin
• *vesicle*		small, clear, liquid accumulation in the skin
• *wheal*		hive; transient swelling in the skin
pruritus	proo-rī'tŭs	itch
secondary lesions		lesions that arise from primary lesions; scales, crusts (scabs), erosions, ulcers, scars, atrophy, excoriations, and lichenification (thickening of skin)
xanthoma	zăn-thō'mah	distinct yellow growth caused by deposits of fat in the skin; usually reflects increased fatty materials in the bloodstream

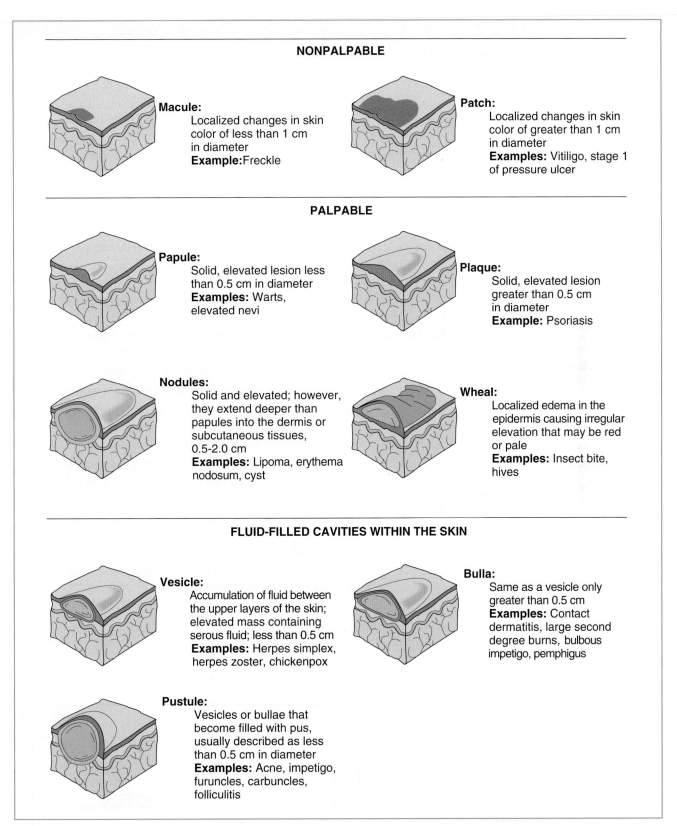

NONPALPABLE

Macule:
Localized changes in skin color of less than 1 cm in diameter
Example: Freckle

Patch:
Localized changes in skin color of greater than 1 cm in diameter
Examples: Vitiligo, stage 1 of pressure ulcer

PALPABLE

Papule:
Solid, elevated lesion less than 0.5 cm in diameter
Examples: Warts, elevated nevi

Plaque:
Solid, elevated lesion greater than 0.5 cm in diameter
Example: Psoriasis

Nodules:
Solid and elevated; however, they extend deeper than papules into the dermis or subcutaneous tissues, 0.5-2.0 cm
Examples: Lipoma, erythema nodosum, cyst

Wheal:
Localized edema in the epidermis causing irregular elevation that may be red or pale
Examples: Insect bite, hives

FLUID-FILLED CAVITIES WITHIN THE SKIN

Vesicle:
Accumulation of fluid between the upper layers of the skin; elevated mass containing serous fluid; less than 0.5 cm
Examples: Herpes simplex, herpes zoster, chickenpox

Bulla:
Same as a vesicle only greater than 0.5 cm
Examples: Contact dermatitis, large second degree burns, bulbous impetigo, pemphigus

Pustule:
Vesicles or bullae that become filled with pus, usually described as less than 0.5 cm in diameter
Examples: Acne, impetigo, furuncles, carbuncles, folliculitis

FIGURE 5-12   Primary Lesions

TREATMENT PROCEDURES

Word	Pronunciation	Definition
allergy immunotherapy		treatment of an allergy by using desensitizing injections of allergy serum for specific allergens
cryosurgery	krī"ō-sŭr'jer-ē	use of extreme cold in a localized part of the body to freeze and destroy unwanted tissues
curettage	kū"rĕ-tahzh'	destruction and removal of the surface of the skin or the covering of an organ by scraping with a spoon-shaped, sharp instrument
débridement	dā-brēd-mŏn'	removal of debris, foreign objects, or damaged tissue from a wound to prevent infection
dermabrasion	dĕr"mah-brā'shun	removal of facial scars, keratose, or nevi by use of mechanical or chemical abrasives
electrocoagulation	ē-lĕk"trō-kō-ăg"ū-lā'shŭn	solidification of tissue by means of a high-frequency electric current concentrated at one point as it passes through tissue (See Figure 5-13)
electrodesiccation	ēlĕk"trō-dĕs"ĭ-kā'shŭn	destruction of warts, growths, or unwanted areas of tissue with a diathermy (electric current) instrument by drying tissue with a hot, electric spark (See Figure 5-13)
escharotomy	ĕs-kăr-ŏt'ō-mē	incision into necrotic tissue resulting from a severe burn
fulguration	fŭl"gū-rā'shŭn	destruction of tissue by electric sparks; uses the same electrode tip as desiccation, but the needle tip is not inserted into the tissue (See Figure 5-13)
laser therapy		destruction of various skin lesions with the use of certain types of lasers, intense monochromatic light that is known to be absorbed by certain skin lesions
Mohs' surgery	mōz	technique for removal of a malignant growth in mapped layers with rapid microscopic evaluation of frozen sections of each layer
photochemotherapy		use of oral or topical psoralen medications followed by exposure to light bulbs emitting light in the long wavelength, ultraviolet light spectrum for treatment of psoriasis

continues

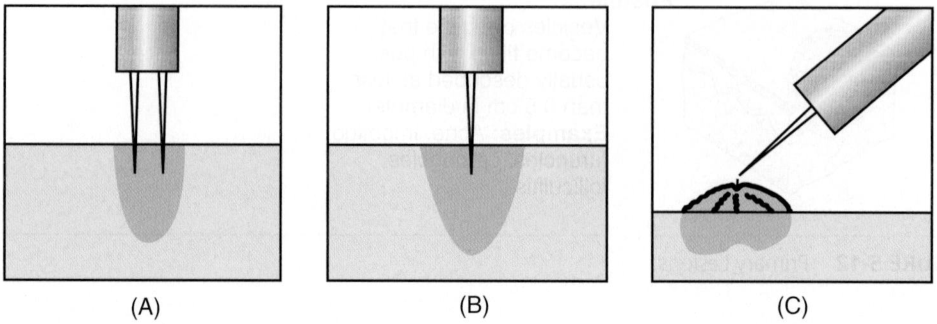

FIGURE 5-13
(A) Electrocoagulation;
(B) Electrodesiccation;
(C) Fulguration

TREATMENT PROCEDURES

Word	Pronunciation	Definition
skin grafts		procedure to cover a burn wound to promote healing; may be autograft (from patient), homograft (from another individual), heterograft (from an animal), or synthetic substitutes
UVB		exposure to ultraviolet B light (sunburn spectrum) for treatment of psoriasis

MEDICATIONS PRESCRIBED

Trade Name	Generic Name
Anti-acnes	
Accutane	isotretinoin
Azelex	azelek acid
Cleocin	clindamycin
Differin	adapalene
Emgel, T-Stat, A/T/S, Deramycin	topical erythromycin
Retin A, Avita, Renova	tretinoin
Antifungals	
Diflucan	fluconazole
Exelderm	sulconazole nitrate
Fulvicin P/C, Grifulvin V, Grisactin	griseofulvin
Lamisil	terbinfine
Loprox	ciclopirox topical
Lotrimin, Mycelex	clotrimazole topical
Lotrisone	betamethasone and clotrimazole
Monistat, Mitrazol, Monistat-Derm	miconazole
Naftin	naftifine topical
Nizoral	ketoconazole
Oxistat	oxiconazole topical
Spectazole	econazole topical
Sporanox	itraconazole
Antihistamines	
Atarax, Rezine, Vistaril	hydroxyzine
Benadryl, Banophen	diphenhydramine

continues

MEDICATIONS PRESCRIBED

Trade Name	Generic Name
Anti-infectives	
Bactroban	mupirocin topical
Bio-Statin, Nilstat, Mycostatin	nystatin
E-Mycin, E.E.S., Robimycin	erythromycin
Keflex, Keftab, Zatran	cephalexin
Antivirals	
Valtrex	valacyclovir
Zovirax	acyclovir
Bath Dermatologics	
Alpha Keri	
Aveeno Bath	
Balnetar oil	
Lubath	
Zetar	
Burn Treatments	
Baciguent	bacitracin
Betadine	povidone-iodine
Furacen	nitrofurazone
Garamycin	gentamicin sulfate
Myciguent	neomycin sulfate
Silvadene	silver sulfadiazine
Sulfamylon	mafenide acetate
Psoriasis Medications	
Dovonex	calcipotriene
Mexate	methotrexate
Oxsoralen	methoxsalen
Tegison	etretinate
Scabicides	
Elamite, Acticin	permathrin
Eurax	crotimaton
—	lindane topical

continues

MEDICATIONS PRESCRIBED

Trade Name	Generic Name
Topical Steroids	
Aristocort Topical, Kenalog	triamcinolone acetonide
Cordran	flurandrenolide topical
Cort-Dome, Hytone, Nutracort, Cortaid, A-Hydrocort, Westcort	hydrocortisone topical
Cutivate	fluticasone propionate
Dermatop	prednicarbate topical
Lidex, Dermacin, Fluex, Flurosyn	fluocinonide topical
Medrol	methylprednisolone
Synalar, Fluonid	fluocinolone acetonide
Temovate, Ciobrevate, Cormax	clobetasol topical
Topicort	desoximetasone topical
Ultravate	halobetasol propionate
Valisone, Diprosone, Maxivate, Betaderm, Diprolene	betamethasone

ABBREVIATIONS*

ANA	antinuclear antibody
bx	biopsy
decub	decubitus ulcer (bed sore)
derm	dermatology
ELISA	enzyme-linked immunosorbent assay
FANA	fluorescent antinuclear antibody
FS	frozen section
I&D	incision and drainage
ID	intradermal
KOH	potassium hydroxide
PUVA	psorafen ultraviolet A-range
SLE	systemic lupus erythematosus
subcu, subq, SC, SQ	subcutaneous
TENS	transcutaneous electrical nerve stimulation
ung, unst	ointment
UV	ultraviolet

*See Appendix D for additional abbreviations.

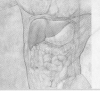

Word Element Review Exercises

Name: _____ Date: _____

COMPLETION*
Complete the following statements.

1. Three word elements that mean sweat are _____, _____, and
   _____.

2. Two word elements that mean skin are _____ and _____.

3. Two word elements that refer to the hair are _____ and _____.

IDENTIFY*
Provide the word that fits the following definitions.

1. banding together   _____
2. hornlike   _____
3. pertaining to the skin   _____
4. scaly   _____
5. sweaty hands or feet   _____
6. oily, fatty matter secreted by sebaceous glands   _____
7. discolored spot on the skin   _____
8. inflammation of the nail bed   _____
9. horny growth   _____
10. inflammation of the skin   _____
11. producing sweat   _____
12. hairy   _____

REWRITE
Rewrite the misspelled words.

1. cornious   _____
2. melinoderma   _____
3. triciasis   _____
4. fasicular   _____
5. miycosis   _____
6. pillose   _____
7. suderiferous   _____
8. adiposele   _____

---

*Answers are in Appendix A.

WORD ELEMENT MEANINGS

Give the meaning of each word element. Then use your dictionary to find a new word that contains each of the word elements. Specify whether the new word is a noun or an adjective by placing N or A in the last column.

Word Element	Meaning	Word	N or A
1. adip/o			
2. corne/o			
3. cutane/o			
4. cut/o			
5. dermat/o			
6. derm/o			
7. fasci/o			
8. hidr/o			
9. kerat/o			
10. macul/o			
11. melan/o			
12. myc/o			
13. onych/o			
14. pil/o			
15. seb/o			
16. squam/o			
17. sud/o			
18. sudor/o			
19. trich/o			

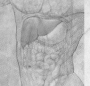

Dictionary Exercises

Name: _____ Date: _____

Additional words commonly used by physicians specializing in the system are included at the end of each chapter. They are presented in the form of exercises that will assist you in learning how to use the medical dictionary.

DICTIONARY EXERCISE 1*

Use your dictionary to find the pronunciation and definition of the following words.

	Word	**Pronunciation**	**Definition**
1.	acrochordon	_____	_____
2.	bulla	_____	_____
3.	melanoderma	_____	_____
4.	collagen	_____	_____
5.	balanitis xerotica obliterans	_____	_____
6.	strawberry hemangioma	_____	_____
7.	dermatitis herpetiformis	_____	_____
8.	Candida	_____	_____
9.	dermographism	_____	_____
10.	photosensitivity	_____	_____
11.	neurodermatitis	_____	_____
12.	mycosis fungoides	_____	_____

DICTIONARY EXERCISE 2*

Pronunciation of the words below is provided. Using your dictionary, find the correct spelling and definition for each word.

	Word	**Pronunciation**	**Definition**
1.	_____	sĭk-ā'trĭks	_____
2.	_____	ĕks-kō-"rē-ā'shŭn	_____
3.	_____	pū'roo-lĕnt	_____
4.	_____	tĭn'ē-ă pĕd'ĭs	_____
5.	_____	kŏn"dĭ-lō'mah	_____
6.	_____	kŏm'ē-dō	_____
7.	_____	sĭl'ē-ah	_____
8.	_____	mŏ-lŭs'kŭm	_____
9.	_____	stē"ah-tō'mah	_____
10.	_____	tĕl'ō-jĕn ĕf-floo'vē-ŭm	_____
11.	_____	pĭt"ĭ-rī'ă-sĭs rō'zē-ah	_____

---

*Answers are in Appendix A.

DICTIONARY EXERCISE 3

Rewrite the following sentences in your own words. Provide pronunciation marks for each italicized word.

1. The baby's past medical history included urticaria and *varicella* (_____).

   _____

2. The skin of the feet was characterized by *xerosis* (_____), *pruritus* (_____), and *melasma* (_____), with a *clavus* (_____) on the left toe.

   _____

3. The rash was diagnosed as *erysipelas* (_____).

   _____

4. There was no evidence of *dermatosis* (_____).

   _____

5. The *eruption* (_____) looked like *pityriasis rosea* (_____).

   _____

6. The baby was born with a strawberry *hemangioma* (_____) near the knee.

   _____

7. The final diagnosis was *elephantiasis* (_____).

   _____

8. The *verrucous* (_____) area is located near the *dermatofibroma* (_____).

   _____

9. Psoriasis is an *idiopathic* (_____) disease.

   _____

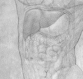

Listening Exercise

Name	Date

INSTRUCTIONS

1. Review the spelling, pronunciation, and meaning of the words provided in the preview.

2. Listen to the audio CD and fill in the blank as the word is dictated.

3. At the end of the exercise, check your spelling against the preview words. They appear in the preview in the order in which they are encountered in the exercise.

4. Review and practice the words you missed.

5. Look up words that are not familiar.

PREVIEW OF WORDS FOR LISTENING EXERCISE 5-1

Word	Pronunciation	Definition
malar	mā'lăr	relating to the cheekbone or the cheek; cheekbone
dermatoses	dĕr"mă-tō'sēs	skin disorders not characterized by inflammation
verrucous	vĕr-rŏo'kŭs	pertaining to wartlike elevations
papules	păp'ūlz	small, superficial, solid elevations of the skin
actinic	ăk-tĭn'ĭk	producing chemical action
keratoses	kĕr-ă-tō'sēs	horny growths such as warts or callosities

Listening Exercise 5-1

Letter of Consultation

Dear Dr. Ober:

I examined our mutual patient, Brian Westerhoff, on 8/7/20—. Thank you for sending your clinic notes. As you mentioned, he has had an irregularity on his lip present for several months. This has somewhat diminished since he began using Chapstick with an SPF of 30. In addition, he had a patch on his right _____ area that was treated in the last six months with applications of Aclovate cream, that did not clear. The patient is an outdoors person and has had much sun exposure over the years. There is no family history of _____ or allergies.

On examination, he exhibited a fine 6 mm irregular scaling patch on his right lower lip centrally. There was also a fine scaling patch on his right malar area. There were tan _____ _____ on his upper chest, and there were several on his back.

It was my impression he exhibited several _____ _____, as well as multiple seborrheic keratoses. I discussed these with him and proceeded to treat the two actinic keratoses with application of liquid nitrogen.

I did suggest he return for follow-up in several months.

Thank you for this consultation.

Sincerely yours,

George Quackenbush, MD

The Musculoskeletal System

> *Those who think they have no time for bodily exercise will sooner or later have to find time for illness.*
>
> —EDWARD STANLEY

When you have completed this study of the musculoskeletal system, you should be able to

1. Spell and define major system components and explain how they operate.
2. Identify the meanings of related word elements.
3. Spell and define diagnostic procedures, diagnoses, treatment procedures, and abbreviations.
4. Spell the names of commonly used medications.
5. Be familiar with terminology used in reports.

INTRODUCTION

The musculoskeletal system is composed of bones, muscles, tendons, ligaments, and joints. This system involves the specialties of orthopedic surgery, physical medicine, rheumatology, and sports medicine. **Orthopedic** (or"thō-pē'dĭk) **surgery** is the surgical correction of deformities, traumas, and chronic diseases of bones and joints. **Physical medicine** is the treatment of illnesses by clinical use of physical agents such as heat, water, electricity, ultraviolet radiation, massage, and exercise. **Rheumatology** (roo"mă-tŏl'ō-jē) is the study of diseases of the joints. **Sports medicine** and **exercise science** are committed to the diagnosis, treatment, and prevention of sports-related injuries. Basic to all of these specialties are the various components of the musculoskeletal system: bones, joints, and muscles.

BONES

oste/o	bone

There are 206 bones in the human body. Each bone is an organ with its own system of blood and lymphatic vessels and nerves. Bones are divided into four classes according to their shape—long, short, flat, and irregular.

COMPOSITION OF BONES

Bones are living **osseous** (ŏs'ē-ŭs) tissue, one of the hardest materials in the body. Note in Figure 6-1 that almost all bones are covered on the outside by a membrane called **periosteum** (pĕr"ē-ŏs'tē-ŭm) (1), which contains many nerve fibers and lymphatics. The hard material forming the exterior of the bone is called **compact** or **cortical** (kor'tĭ-kăl) **bone** (2). **Cancellous** or **spongy bone** (3) is found in the interior. Spaces within the cancellous bone contain two kinds of marrow, red and yellow bone marrow (4). **Red bone marrow** is found in certain parts of all bones and manufactures most of the blood cells. **Yellow bone marrow** is found primarily in the central cavities of the long bones and is composed chiefly of fat cells.

PROCESSES AND DEPRESSIONS

The contour of bones has many projections. Often there are places for muscle attachments. To identify these areas the term **process** is used. Some of the common bony processes are as follows.

Process	Pronunciation	Meaning
condyle	kŏn'dīl	rounded portion of bone that joins with another
epicondyle	ĕp"ĭ-kŏn'dīl	small projection located on or above a condyle

continues

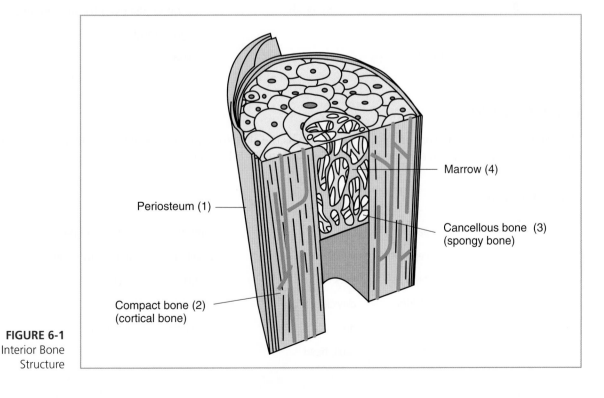

Periosteum (1)

Marrow (4)

Cancellous bone (3) (spongy bone)

Compact bone (2) (cortical bone)

FIGURE 6-1
Interior Bone
Structure

Process	Pronunciation	Meaning
head		larger end of a long bone, often set off from the shaft of the bone by a neck
trochanter	trō-kăn'ter	large, somewhat blunt process on the femur that serves as a site for attachment
tubercle	too'ber-k'l	nodule or small, rounded process that serves as the site for tendon or muscle attachment
tuberosity	too"bĕ-rŏs'ĭ-tē	broad process, larger than a tubercle

Openings or hollow regions that help to join one bone to another are **depressions**. The following are some of the common bony depressions.

Depression	Pronunciation	Meaning
fissure	fĭs'sur	narrow, deep, slitlike opening
foramen	fō-rā'mĕn	hole for blood vessels and nerves
fossa	fŏs'ah	depression or cavity in a bone, for articulation or muscle attachment
sinus	sī'nŭs	air cavity within a bone
sulcus	sŭl'kŭs	groove

Other descriptive structural terms include the following:

Term	Pronunciation	Meaning
crest		sharp, prominent, bony ridge
facet	făs'ĕt	small, flat-surfaced area on a bone
fovea	fō'vē-ah	pit generally used for attachment
line		slight, bony ridge
meatus	mē-ā'tŭs	canal

THE SKELETON

The complete bony framework of the body is known as the skeleton. It is divided into two main groups of bones—the axial (ăk'sē-ăl) skeleton and the appendicular (ăp"ĕn-dĭk'ū-lar) skeleton.

Axial Skeleton

caud/o	tail		lumb/o	loin, lower back
cephal/o	head		maxill/o	upper jaw bone
cervic/o	neck		sacr/o	sacrum
cleid/o	clavicle		spondyl/o	vertebra
cost/o	rib		vertebr/o	vertebra
crani/o	skull, head			

The **axial skeleton** includes the bony framework of the head and trunk.

Head. The framework of the head is called the **skull**; it is subdivided into two parts, called the cranium and the facial bones. Figure 6-2 illustrates the cranium bones: frontal (1), parietal (pah-rī'ĕ-tăl) (2), temporal (3), ethmoid (ĕth'moid) (10), sphenoid (sfē'noid) (11), and occipital (ŏk-sĭp'ĭ-tăl) (4). The facial bones shown in Figure 6-2 are the mandible (măn'dĭ-bl) (7), maxillary (măk'sĭ-lĕr"ē) (8), zygomatic (zī"gō-măt'ĭk) (6), and smaller bones, including the nasal (9) and lacrimal (lăk'rĭ-măl) (5).

Trunk. The framework of the trunk includes the vertebral column and rib cage. The **spinal column** is divided into five regions, shown in Figure 6-3. These spinal column regions are the cervical (1), thoracic (2), lumbar (3), sacral (să'krăl) (4), and coccygeal (kŏk-sĭj'ē-ăl) (5). These bones protect the spinal cord and enable a human to stand in an upright position. A physician records or identifies each by indicating region and number; for example, the twelfth thoracic vertebra is T12.

The **rib cage** has twelve pairs of ribs attached to the vertebral column at the back. Ten of these pairs are also attached directly or indirectly to the breastbone or **sternum** (ster'nŭm) in the front. The remaining two pairs, referred to as floating ribs, are attached only to the vertebral column. The rib cage serves to support the chest and protect the heart, lungs, and other organs.

Appendicular Skeleton

carp/o	wrist	ili/o	ilium
cheir/o, chir/o	hand	ischi/o	hip
dactyl/o	finger, toe	ped/o, pod/o	foot
digit/o	finger, toe	tars/o	of or pertaining to the edge of the foot

The **appendicular skeleton** is usually referred to as the extremities and includes both upper and lower extremities.

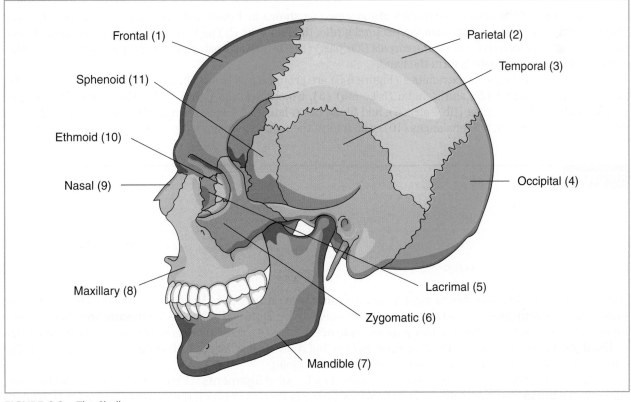

FIGURE 6-2 The Skull

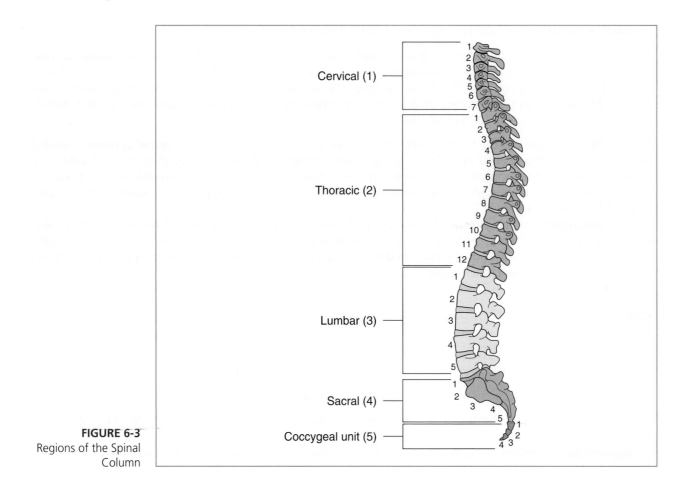

FIGURE 6-3
Regions of the Spinal
Column

The bones of the upper extremities are grouped as shown in Figure 6-4: the clavicle (klăv'ĭ-kl) (1) and scapula (skăp'ū-lah) (2), which form the pectoral girdle; the humerus (hū'mer-ŭs) (3); the ulna (ul'nah) (4) and radius (5), which form the forearm; the carpals (kăr'păls) (6), the metacarpals (mĕt"ah-kăr'păls) (8), and the phalanges (fah-lăn'jēz) (7), which form the hand.

The bones of the lower extremities (Figure 6-5) are grouped in a similar fashion, as follows: the ilium (ĭl'ē-ŭm) (1), pubis (pū'bĭs) (2), and ischium (ĭs'kē-ŭm) (3), which form the pelvic girdle; the femur (fē'mur) (4), patella (pah-tĕl'ah) (5), tibia (tĭb'ē-ah) (6), and fibula (fĭb'ū-lah) (7), which form the leg; the tarsals (tahr'săls) (8), the metatarsals (9), and phalanges (10), which form the foot. The femur is the strongest bone in the body.

JOINTS

arthr/o	joint	ligament/o	ligament
articu/o	joint	synov/o	synovial membrane
burs/o	sac		

A region where two or more bones meet is called a **joint** or an articulation. Most are classified as freely movable joints, called **diarthroses** (dī"ăr-thrō'sēz), and are lined with a **synovial** (sĭ-nō'vē-ăl) **membrane** that secretes lubricating synovial fluid. The shoulder is an example of this type of joint. Others are classified as slightly movable or **fixed joints**, which occasionally allow slight motion, but these do not have a distinct cavity containing fluid. The suture joints of the skull are considered examples of a fixed joint.

Stability is added to joints by connective tissue bands called **ligaments**. Certain joints have a saclike structure called a **bursa** (bĕr'sah) surrounding them that prevents friction between the moving parts, such as tendons and bones. Common bursal locations are at the elbow, knee, and shoulder joints.

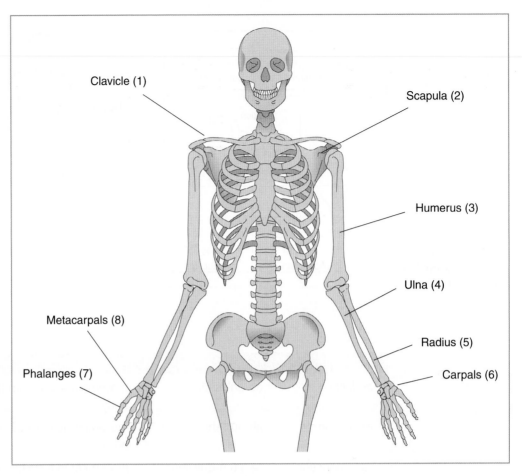

FIGURE 6-4
Bones of the Upper
Extremities

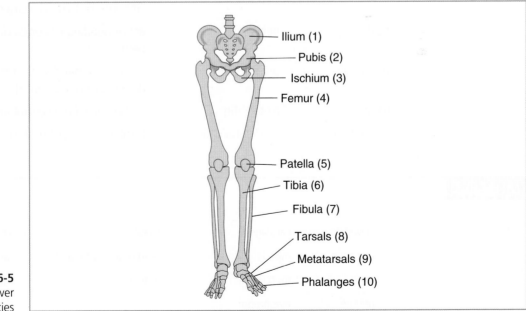

FIGURE 6-5
Bones of the Lower
Extremities

The chief function of the freely movable joints is to allow changes of position and to provide for motion. Some of these movements are identified and illustrated in Figure 6-6.

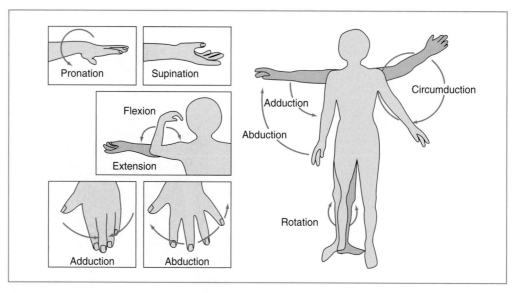

FIGURE 6-6
Movement of Joints

Movement	Pronunciation	Meaning
abduction	ăb-dŭk'shŭn	movement away from the midline of the body
adduction	ah-dŭk'shŭn	movement toward the midline of the body
circumduction	ser'kŭm-dŭk'shŭn	movement in a circular direction
extension	ĕk-stĕn'shŭn	movement that brings the members of a limb into or toward a straight condition
flexion	flĕk'shŭn	act of bending or condition of being bent
pronation	prō-nā'shŭn	turning the hand so that the palm faces downward or backward
rotation	rō-tā'shŭn	motion around a central axis
supination	soo"pĭ-nā'shŭn	turning of the palm or foot upward

MUSCLES

chondr/o	cartilage	spas/o	draw, pull
muscul/o	muscle	tend/o, ten/o, tendin/o	tendon
my/o	muscle	tens/o	stretch
phren/o	diaphragm		

The three kinds of basic muscle tissue—skeletal, smooth, and cardiac—are illustrated in Figure 6-7. Skeletal (or striated) muscles may be regarded as organs because they are made of a combination of muscle and connective tissue. These muscles give form and shape to the body and are referred to as **voluntary muscles** because they operate at will. Enveloping and separating the skeletal muscles is a fibrous tissue called **fascia** (fāsh'ē-ah). It contains the blood, nerves, and other supplies for muscles. Smooth and cardiac muscles are considered **involuntary muscles** because

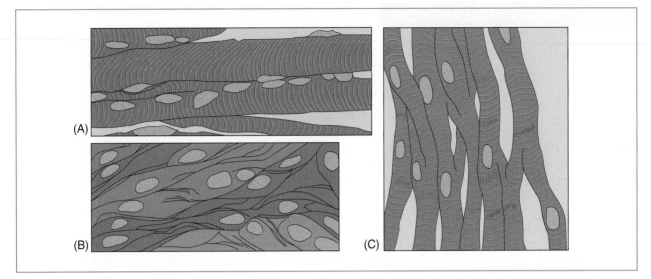

FIGURE 6-7 Kinds of Muscle Tissue: (A) skeletal (voluntary); (B) smooth (involuntary); (C) cardiac (involuntary)

they generally function without direction from an individual. Examples of involuntary muscles are the muscles that control the digestive tract, blood vessels, and heart.

Most muscles have two or more attachments to the skeleton. The method of attachment varies. In some cases, the connective tissue within the muscle is attached directly to the periosteum of the bone. These attachments are called **tendons**. If these connective tissues are broad and sheetlike and attached to bone or to other tissue, they are referred to as **aponeurosis** (ăp"ō-nū-rō'sĭs).

Muscle may in some instances attach to **cartilage**. Cartilage, a specialized type of dense connective tissue, appears in the adult body in several regions, including the nasal septum, external ear, lining of the eustachian tube, larynx, trachea, bronchi, between bodies of the vertebrae, and on the surfaces of movable joints. Cartilage can withstand a great deal of stress; however, interference with this surface of the bone may result in arthritis.

The human body contains more than 400 skeletal muscles, making up about forty to fifty percent of body weight. The one muscle or set of muscles that initiates movement is called the **prime mover**. When an opposite movement is to be made, another set of muscles known as the **antagonist** takes over. In this way, body movements are coordinated, and a large number of complicated movements are carried out without the necessity of planning in advance how to perform them. All muscular activity occurs as a result of messages transmitted from the brain through the central nervous system to the muscles.

Following are some of the most commonly referred to muscles in the body. For a more comprehensive list, consult *A Syllabus for the Surgeon's Secretary, Gray's Anatomy,* or a medical dictionary.

Muscles of the shoulder and upper extremities
biceps, triceps, deltoid (injection site), pectoralis major

Muscles of the chest and back
pectoralis major and minor, serratus anterior, intercostal muscles, latissimus dorsi

Muscles of the lower extremities
gluteus maximus (injection site), gluteus medius and minimus, iliopsoas, quadriceps femoris, hamstring group, gastrocnemius, soleus, tibialis anterior and posterior, peroneus brevis and longus

Muscles of the abdomen
external and internal oblique, transversus and rectus abdominis

Diaphragm
The diaphragm is an important muscle that divides the thoracic cavity from the abdominal cavity. It has three major openings for the esophagus, aorta, and inferior vena cava, as well as several smaller structures.

When muscles do not function as they should, a disability occurs and a physiatrist may become involved.

THE ROLE OF PHYSICAL MEDICINE

dynam/o	power		therm/o	heat
-plegia	paralysis		traumat/o	wound, injury
therap/o	treatment, therapy			

A **physiatrist** (fĭz"ē-ăt'rĭst) is a physician who specializes in physical medicine and rehabilitation. Skill in applying physical agents is combined with evaluating the patient's mental, social, and vocational problems. Rehabilitation helps a person reach maximum potential for normal living. This practice recognizes that diagnosing the problem is not enough. The critical issue is finding a solution that best benefits the patient.

Disabilities occur because of trauma, such as an accident, a birth defect, a disease, or a cerebrovascular or cerebrocardiovascular accident. Three sources account for most cerebrovascular accidents: thrombosis, embolism, and hemorrhage. Diseases may be of the connective tissue or the nervous system. Trauma may affect the brain or spinal cord, as do several congenital diseases. Sports medicine, a field that deals with injuries related to sports, has evolved from the treatment of trauma and accidents.

Regardless of the type of trauma, a variety of evaluative methods are used to diagnose the nature and degree of disability. Taking the patient's history and examining him or her physically are the first steps.

HISTORY

The physiatrist takes a patient's history using a format similar to that identified in Chapter 3; however, the focus is somewhat different. The first step involves determining the chief complaint. The diseases most likely to produce the complaints a physiatrist addresses usually involve the musculoskeletal, neurological, or cardiovascular system.

Present illness will specify what effect the illness has on self-care activities. The physiatrist wants to know how much the patient depends on others to perform activities of daily living, such as walking, transfer activities, dressing activities, eating skills, and personal hygiene.

Social and vocational history evaluates the patient's environment and provides insight into the patient's psychological makeup.

Review of systems and past medical history contribute to the assessment of residual capacity. Essentially, the physician is looking for the following cardinal signs in each of these systems.

System	Pronunciation	Cardinal Signs
cardiovascular	kăr"dē-ō-văs'kū-lăr	dyspnea (dĭsp'nē-ah) or orthopnea (or"thŏp-nē'ă) (types of labored breathing), chest pain, limb claudication (klaw"dĭ-kā'shŭn) (pain from exercise resulting in limping), palpitations
musculoskeletal	mŭs"kū-lō-skĕl'ĕ-tăl	pain, deformity, weakness, limitation of movement, stiffness
nervous		numbness, weakness, fainting, loss of consciousness, dizziness, pain, headache, defective memory or thinking
respiratory	rĕ-spĭ'rah-tō"rē	cough, sputum, hemoptysis (hē-mŏp'tĭ-sĭs) (spitting up blood), chest pain, dyspnea

Past medical history attempts to identify residual effects of prior disease or trauma.

PHYSICAL EXAMINATION

A physical examination serves three functions: It searches for deviations from normal, tries to identify secondary problems, and attempts to assess residual strengths. All areas of a traditional examination are covered, with emphasis on the neurological and musculoskeletal areas.

An essential step in the evaluation of function in a patient is measuring joint movement or motion, or **goniometry** (gō-"nē-ŏm'ĕ-trē). Methods for recording measurements vary. In addition to the planes and directions indicated in Chapter 2 and the movements illustrated in Figure 6-6, the following directions are used.

Direction	Pronunciation	Meaning
dorsiflexion	dor"sǐ-flĕk'shŭn	backward bending of the hand or foot
opposition		moving the thumb into contact with the pads of the other digits
plantar flexion	plăn'tăr flĕk'shŭn	bending the foot toward the ground

The rehabilitative process includes assessment of speech and language disorders, psychological assessment and management, psychosocial diagnoses, vocational assessment and management, and electrodiagnosis. All help determine realistic goals and the types of therapeutic techniques necessary to achieve those goals. Therapeutic techniques include heat and cold treatment (local), **diathermy** (dī'ah-ther"mē) (deep heating), hydrotherapy, ultraviolet therapy, electrical stimulation, **iontophoresis** (ī-ŏn"tō-fō-rē'sǐs), and exercise.

Physical medicine is a creative practice that utilizes the expertise of people trained in occupational therapy, physical therapy, and speech therapy. A team approach is most effective in providing the various types of therapeutic treatments that will enable an individual to regain as much normalcy as possible.

MASSAGE THERAPY

Massage therapy—the systematic manual treatment of disease—and physical exercise are techniques that have a curative effective on the human condition. The modern day version of these techniques was first used as far back as 3000 B.C. by the Chinese, Hindu, Egyptian, Japanese, Persian, and Turkish cultures. They claim massage therapy can relieve stress and anxiety, increase the blood supply to tissues, hasten the elimination of waste stored in muscles, improve energy level, aid recovery from damaged muscles and ligaments, and relieve certain repetitive motion injuries related to job activities. In the broad perspective, it may provide anything from soothing relaxation to deeper therapy for specific physical problems as well as compensate for the lack of physical activity when an individual must remain sedentary.

The medical profession views massage therapy as an addition or possible alternative to regular medical treatment. Research confirms its benefits. Recent publications such as the *International Journal of Neuroscience* and the *Professional Nurse* have reported the use of compression to treat lymphoedema in breast cancer patients and the enhancement of the immune system's cytotoxic capacity in treating cancer or human immunodeficiency virus (HIV) positive patients.

Integrated approaches such as prenatal therapy, infant therapy, and geriatric therapy have become part of certain practices. But perhaps one of the most widely accepted and utilized approaches is in sports massage.

Sports massage is based on **osteology** (ŏs-tē-ŏl'ō-jē), the study of the skeleton, and **myology** (mī-ŏl'ō-jē), the study of muscles, their attachments, and the actions they perform. Deep and repetitive compressions of fiber-spreading techniques produce a hyperemia (dilation of the total range of blood vessels). These treatments bring blood and oxygen to the muscles and result in an increase in free motion.

The American Massage Therapy Association has spearheaded a national certification process, and some states have already begun to license massage therapists. Some of the techniques used are listed below.

Technique	Pronunciation	Meaning
compression		use of pressure on the body to spread tissue against underlying structures; may be pinpoint compression (direct pressure) or ischemic pressure (applied at acupressure points)

continues

Technique	Pronunciation	Meaning
effleurage	ĕf-loor-ăzh'	use of gliding strokes applied horizontally in relation to tissue masses
friction		use of small deep movements, either circular or transverse, performed on a local area; movements focus directly on underlying tissue
petrissage	pā"trē-săzh'	use of kneading-like action where soft tissue is lifted, rolled, wrung, and squeezed
rocking		use of rhythmic motion applied with a deliberate full-body movement
shaking		use of quick, loose movements to a body area to relax muscle groups or an entire limb
tapotement (percussion)	tă-pōt-mŏn'	use of springy blows to the body at a fast rate to create rhythmical compression
vibration		use of compression first and then a trembling action; transmits to surrounding tissue to create reflexive response

Other professions that use manipulation techniques described above are chiropractic and osteopathy.

Chiropractic treats disease by manipulating the vertebral column based on the assumption that all diseases are caused by pressure on the nerves. This pressure is the result of faulty alignment of the bones.

Osteopathy is founded on the theory that the body is a single organism made up of interrelated systems dependent upon one another for good health. Practitioners are called Doctors of Osteopathic Medicine (D.O.s) or osteopaths. They treat specific illnesses in the context of the whole person by utilizing generally accepted physical, medicinal, and surgical methods of diagnosis and therapy. The emphasis of this treatment is on the importance of normal body mechanics and manipulative methods to detect and correct faulty structure.

Massage therapy, chiropractic, and osteopathy practitioners each use their knowledge of the musculoskeletal system to help their patients remain healthy and pain free.

INTERNET ASSIGNMENT

The American Academy of Orthopaedic Surgeons (AAOS) is a not-for-profit organization that advocates for improved patient care and informs the public about the science of orthopedics. Members of the Academy are concerned with the diagnosis, care, and treatment of musculoskeletal disorders. The orthopedist's scope of practice includes disorders of the body's bones, joints, ligaments, muscles, and tendons. AAOS's web site is **www.aaos.org**.

On the home page clicking the Patient/Public Information button in the header brings up a picture representation of each component of the musculoskeletal system. A list of links to fact sheets about each system component is presented by clicking on the appropriate picture. For more information, make a selection from the list. The patient information has been reviewed by surgeons to ensure accuracy. Other features of the site are free access to abstracts of the professional journals sponsored by AAOS (complete articles require a fee), news releases, and a surgeon locator. Some information is available to members only.

ACTIVITY

Access the AAOS at **www.aaos.org**. On the home page, click Patient/Public Information and then one of the pictures. From the hyperlinks provided, select one that interests you. Summarize your findings in a short report for your instructor, focusing on new information that you learned.

Review: The Musculoskeletal System

■ Bones are made up of one of the hardest materials in the body. They are long, short, flat, or irregular in shape; covered by periosteum; and filled with red and/or yellow marrow.

■ The skeleton consists of the axial skeleton (head and trunk) and appendicular skeleton (upper and lower extremities).

■ Contours on the bones, called processes and depressions, provide places for muscle attachments that join one bone to another.

■ A joint, or articulation, is where two or more bones join. Some joints are movable; others are not.

■ Skeletal muscles are voluntary muscles. They give shape to the body and are regarded as organs.

■ Smooth and cardiac muscles are involuntary muscles and function without direction from the individual.

■ Muscles are attached to the bone with tendons or connective tissue called aponeurosis.

■ The physiatrist, a physician specializing in physical medicine, diagnoses problems with special attention to the residual effects on the mental, social, and vocational aspects of a patient's life.

■ Massage therapists, chiropractors, and osteopaths are some of the professionals who use knowledge of the musculoskeletal system in helping individuals to be healthy and pain free.

Review of Terminology Presented

Word	Definition
antagonist	muscle that opposes movement initiated by a prime mover muscle
aponeurosis	broad, sheetlike connective tissue that attaches muscles to bone or other tissue
appendicular skeleton	bony framework of the extremities
axial skeleton	bony framework of the head and trunk
bursa	saclike structure surrounding certain bony processes to prevent friction
cancellous (spongy) bone	soft, spongy material found in the interior of bone
cartilage	specialized type of dense connective tissue
chiropractic	system of treating disease by manipulating the vertebral column
compact (cortical) bone	hard material forming the exterior of bone
depressions	openings or hollow regions that help to join one bone to another
diarthroses	freely movable joints lined with a synovial membrane that secretes synovial fluid
diathermy	deep heating
fascia	fibrous tissue separating and enveloping muscles

continues

Word	Definition
fixed joints	joints that have little or no movement
goniometry	measurement of joint movement
involuntary muscles	smooth and cardiac muscles that move without conscious thought
iontophoresis	process of transferring ions of the body by an electromotive force
joint	region where two or more bones join
ligaments	connective tissue bands that add stability to joints
massage therapy	systematic, therapeutic manual treatment of disease
myology	study of the muscles and their parts
orthopedic surgery	surgical correction of deformities, traumas, and chronic diseases of bones and joints
osseous	referring to bone; bony
osteology	study of the structure and function of bones
osteopathy	treatment based on the importance of normal body mechanics and manipulative methods to detect and correct faulty structure
periosteum	membrane covering the outside of most bones
physiatrist	physician specializing in physical medicine and rehabilitation
physical medicine	treatment of illnesses by clinical use of physical agents such as heat and water
prime mover	muscle that initiates a movement
process	projection on bones for muscle attachments
red bone marrow	soft, organic material found in spaces within the spongy bone; source of red blood cells
rheumatology	study of diseases of the joints
rib cage	24 bones attached to the vertebral column and sternum; supports chest and protects heart, lungs, and other organs
skull	framework of the head
spinal column	structure that protects spinal cord and allows humans to stand upright
sports medicine and exercise science	diagnosis, treatment, and prevention of sports-related injuries
sternum	breastbone
synovial membrane	inner layer of a movable joint that secretes lubricating synovial fluid
tendons	connective tissues within muscles that attach directly to the periosteum of bones
voluntary muscles	skeletal (or striated) muscles; operate at will
yellow bone marrow	soft organic material found in central cavities of long bones; composed chiefly of fat cells

Terminology Review Exercises

Name: _____ Date: _____

COMPLETION*

Complete the following statements.

1. The systematic therapeutic manual treatment of disease is referred to as _____ _____.

2. Projections of the bones that often serve as places for muscle attachment are called _____.

3. Bones are made of _____ tissue.

4. The two kinds of bone are _____ and _____.

5. Most bones are covered by a membrane called _____.

6. A physician would identify the fifth lumbar vertebra as _____.

7. A physician who specializes in physical rehabilitation is a _____.

8. The five regions of the spinal column are the _____, _____, _____, _____, and _____.

9. Muscles make up from _____ to _____ percent of body weight.

10. The measurement of joint function is _____.

CHOICES

Circle the correct answer in each statement.

1. (Red marrow/yellow marrow) is composed chiefly of fat cells.

2. The (axial skeleton/appendicular skeleton) is composed of the extremities.

3. A (joint/bursa) is the region where two or more bones come together.

4. A (tendon/ligament) is connective tissue within a muscle that attaches directly to the periosteum of the bone.

5. (Synovial membrane/bursa) is the lining that secretes lubrication for movable joints.

6. (Cartilage/ligaments) are connective tissue bands that add stability to joints.

MATCHING

Match the terms to their meanings.

1. _____ motion around a central axis
2. _____ motion away from the body
3. _____ motion toward the body
4. _____ straightening or stretching
5. _____ bending motion
6. _____ backward bending of the hand or foot
7. _____ moving the thumb toward the digit pads
8. _____ bending the foot toward the ground

a. rotation
b. extension
c. flexion
d. abduction
e. adduction
f. plantar flexion
g. dorsiflexion
h. opposition

_____

*Answers are in Appendix A.

DIAGNOSES

Word	Pronunciation	Definition
Diseases of Bone (continued)		
myeloma	mī-ě-lō'mah	tumor originating in the bone marrow
osteomalacia	ŏs"tē-ō-mah-lā'shē-ah	condition marked by softening of the bones as a result of calcium loss from the bones
osteomylitis	ŏs"tē-ō-mī"ě-lī'tǐs	inflammation of bone and bone marrow due to infection
osteoporosis	ŏs"tē-ō-pō-rō'sǐs	condition caused by decrease in bone mass resulting in thinning and weakening of bone (See Figure 6-9)
osteosarcoma	ŏs"tē-ō-sǎr-kō'mah	malignant cancer of the bone
Paget's disease	pǎj'ět	chronic metabolic bone disease that affects bone formation
scoliosis	skō"lē-ō'sǐs	abnormal rotational and lateral curvature of the spine (See Figure 6-8D)
spondylosis	spŏn"dǐ-lō'sǐs	disorder in which the spine becomes stiff and loses flexibility over time
talipes	tǎl'ǐ-pēz	congenital deformity of the foot; clubfoot

Diseases of Joints, Muscles, and Connective Tissue

Word	Pronunciation	Definition
arthritis	ǎr-thrī'tǐs	inflammation of bone joints; *atrophic* (rheumatoid) and *hypertrophic* (osteoarthritis) are the two most common forms; may also be infectious; caused by bacteria, virus, or fungus (See Figure 6-10)

continues

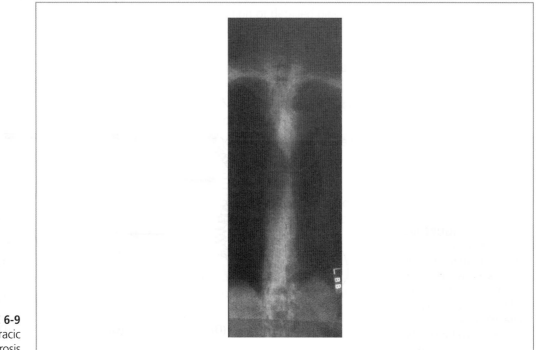

FIGURE 6-9
Fracture of the Thoracic
Spine Due to Osteoporosis

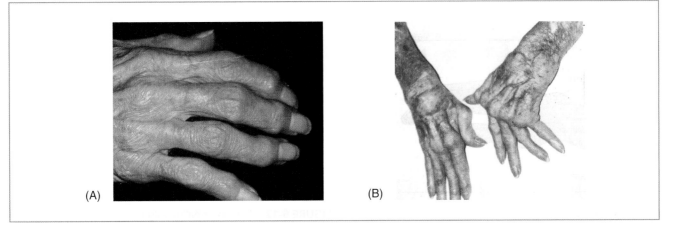

FIGURE 6-10 Comparison of (A) Osteoarthritis and (B) Rheumatoid Arthritis: hands and joints

DIAGNOSES

Word	Pronunciation	Definition
Diseases of Joints, Muscles, and Connective Tissue (*continued*)		
Dupuytren's contracture	dū-pwē-trănz' kŏn-trăk'chūr	disorder characterized by a hardening of the lining of tissue beneath skin of the palm of the hand
fibromyalgia	fī''brō-mī-ă'jē-ah	chronic disorder characterized by aches, pain, and stiffness in joints and muscles
ganglion cyst	găng'glē-ŏn	cystic lump on the wrist and other areas (See Figure 6-11)
gout	gowt	inflammation of joints caused by excessive uric acid in the body
hallux valgus	hăl'ŭks văl'gŭs	bunion; thickening and inflammation of the bursa of the great toe (See Figure 6-12)
muscular dystrophy (MD)	dĭs'tro-fē	inherited disease characterized by a progressive weakness of muscle fibers
myasthenia gravis	mī"ăs-thē'nē-ah grăv'ĭs	disorder marked by lack of muscle strength and by paralysis
osteoarthritis	ŏs"tē-ō-ăr-thrī'tĭs	chronic, noninflammatory, degenerative disease of bones and joints due to degenerative changes in cartilage
rheumatoid arthritis	roo'mah-toyd ăr-thrī'tĭs	condition marked by inflammation of a joint as well as stiffness
systemic lupus erythematosus (SLE)	sĭs tĕm'ĭk lū'pŭs ĕr"ĭ-thĕm"ah-tō'sŭs	chronic, inflammatory disease involving the joints, skin, kidneys, nervous system, heart, and lungs
temporomandibular joint (TMJ) syndrome	tĕm"pō-rō-măn-dĭb'ū-lăr	condition characterized by severe headaches and pain in the jaw joint with decreased ability to open the mouth
tetanus	tĕt'ă-nŭs	acute infectious, life-threatening disease characterized by painful, uncontrolled contractions of skeletal muscle; lockjaw

continues

DIAGNOSES		
Word	**Pronunciation**	**Definition**
Trauma (continued)		
plantar fasciitis	plăn'tăr făs"ē-ī'tĭs	inflammation of the thick connective tissue and the sole of the foot
shin splint		overuse injury to the periosteum and extensor muscles of the lower leg
sprains		traumatic injury to a joint with partial or complete tearing of ligaments
strains		overstretching injury of a muscle leading to tenderness, soreness, and pain
subluxation	sŭb"lŭks-ā'shŭn	a partial separation of a bone from its normal position in a joint (See Figure 6-13)
tendonitis	tĕn"dah-nī'tĭs	inflammation of a tendon, often in the shoulder
torn rotator cuff		injury to the tendonous portion of a group of muscles that hold the head of the humerus in the shoulder socket area
torn meniscus	mĕn-ĭs'kŭs	injury to cartilage pads that are in the knee

TREATMENT PROCEDURES		
Word	**Pronunciation**	**Definition**
anterior cruciate ligament (ACL) reconstruction	ăn-tēr'ē-or kroo'shē-āt	replacement of a torn ACL with a biological or synthetic graft; usually done by arthroscopic surgery
arthrodesis	ăr"thrō-dē'sĭs	stiffening or fusion of a joint to provide stability; sometimes done for pain from arthritis
arthroplasty	ăr'thrō-plăs"tē	surgical reconstruction of a joint
arthroscopy	ăr'thrŏ-skō"pē	surgical procedures performed on joints with an arthroscope (a fiber-optic camera) (See Figure 6-16)
arthrotomy	ăr-thrŏt'ŏ-mē	surgical opening of a joint
bunionectomy	bŭn-yŭn-ĕk'tō-mē	removal of the bursa and bone of the great toe
capsulorrhaphy	kăp"sū-lor'ah-fē	suture of a tear in any joint capsule
carpal tunnel release	kăr'păl	cutting the wrist ligament to relieve nerve pressure (See Figure 6-17)
chondroplasty	kŏn'drō-plăs"tē	shaving or smoothing of rough or fragmented articular cartilage; done by arthroscopic surgery
fasciectomy	făs"ē-ĕk'tō-mē	surgical removal of fascia
laminectomy	lăm"ĭ-nĕk'tō-mē	removal of a portion of a vertebra in order to remove disc tissue
meniscectomy	mĕn"ĭ-sĕk'tō-mē	removal of knee cartilage (meniscus)
microdiskectomy	mī"krō-dĭs-kĕk'tŏ-mē	removal of ruptured disc or disc fragments using small incisions and minimal approach

continues

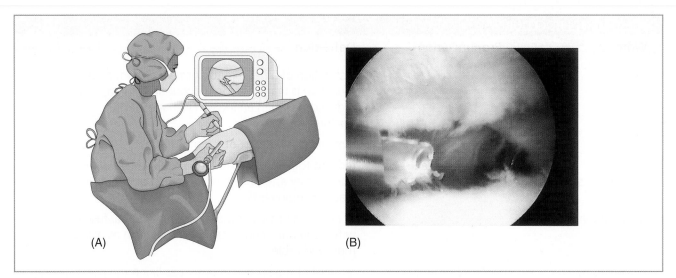

FIGURE 6-16   Arthroscopy of the Knee: (A) arthroscope in use; (B) internal view of the knee during arthroscopy

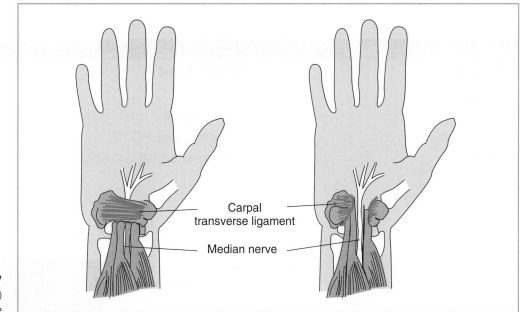

FIGURE 6-17
Carpal Tunnel Release: (A)
before; (B) after procedure

Carpal
transverse ligament

Median nerve

TREATMENT PROCEDURES

Word	Pronunciation	Definition
microvascular anastomosis	mī"krō-văs'kū-lăr ah-năs"tō-mō'sĭs	use of an operating microscope to repair minute blood vessels and nerves
neurolysis	nū-rōl'ĭ-sĭs	freeing the nerve of surrounding scar tissue; may be median, ulnar, or radial
ostectomy	ŏs-tĕk'tō-mē	correction of a bone deformity by cutting and repositioning the bone

continues

TREATMENT PROCEDURES

Word	Pronunciation	Definition
reduction		restoration of a fracture to normal position; *closed reduction* is manipulation without an incision; *open reduction* is when an incision is made into the fracture site
resection		removal of all or part of a bone
revision arthroplasty	ăr'thrō-plăs"tē	redoing total hip arthroplasty or total knee arthroplasty after failure or loosening of originally placed components
spinal fusion		bony union of two or more vertebrae; spinal fusion with bone graft and internal fixatives such as plates, rods, and cables
synovectomy	sĭn"ō-věk'tō-mē	removal of the synovium or tissues lining the joints
total hip replacement		surgical reconstruction by implanting a prosthetic hip joint (See Figure 6-18)

MEDICATIONS PRESCRIBED

Trade Name	Generic Name
Analgesics	
Darvon	propoxyphene
Flexeril, Cycloflex	cyclobenzaprine HCl
Fioricet	caffeine, butalbital, and APAP

continues

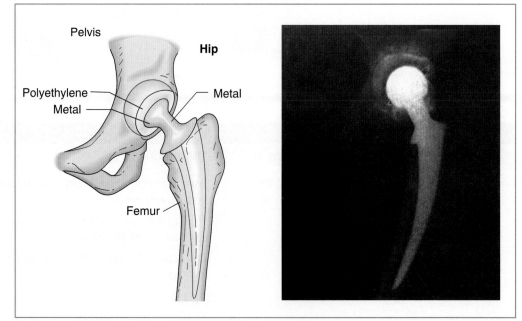

FIGURE 6-18
Total Hip Replacement: implanted artificial joint

MEDICATIONS PRESCRIBED

Trade Name	Generic Name
Analgesics (continued)	
Fiorinal	caffeine, butalbital, and ASA
Lortab, Lorcet, Vicodin, Dolacet, Hydrocet	hydrocodone and acetaminophen
OxyContin	oxycodone
Robaxin	methocarbamol
Soma	carisoprodol
Tylenol, Panadol, Excedrin, Anacin	acetaminophen and APAP
Ultram	tramadol HCl
Antibiotics	
Cipro	ciprofloxacin
Keflex	cephalexin
Mandol	cefamandole
Muscle Relaxants	
Flexeril, Cycloflex	cyclobenzaprine HCl
Robaxin	methocarbamol
Soma	carisoprodol
Valium	diazepam
Disease-Modifying Antirheumatic Drugs (DMARDs)	
Azulfidine	sulfasalazine
Cytoxan	cyclophosphamide
Imuran	azathioprine
Minocin	minocycline
Neoral, Sandimmune	cyclosporine
Rheumatrex, Trexall	methotrexate
Osteoporosis Treatment	
Actonel	risedronate sodium
Calcimar, Miacalcin	calcitonin
Didronel	etidronate
Menest	esterified estrogen
Evista	raloxifene hydrochloride
Fosomax	alendronate
Rocaltrol	calcitriol

continues

MEDICATIONS PRESCRIBED

Trade Name	Generic Name
Nonsteroidal Anti-Inflammatory Drugs (NSAIDs)	
Advil, Motrin, Midol, Rufen	ibuprofen
Anaprox, Naprosyn	naproxen sodium
Ansaid	flurbiprofen
Celebrex	celecoxib
Clinoril	sulindac
Daypro	oxaprozin
Feldene	piroxicam
Indocin	indomethacin
Lodine	etodolac
Nalfon	fenoprofen calcium
Orudis, Oruvail	ketoprofen
Relafen	nabumetone
Tolectin	tolmetin sodium
Vioxx	rofecoxib
Voltaren	diclofenac sodium ophthalmic
Gout	
—	colchicine
Anturane	sulfinpyrazone
Benemid, Probalan	probenecid
Lopurin, Zyloprim	allopurinol
Glucocorticoids	
Artisocort	triamcinolone acetonide
Cortone	cortisone
Cortef, Hydrocortone	hydrocortisone
Decadron, Hexadrol	dexamethasone
Deltasone, Orasone	prednisone
Medrol	methylprednisolone
Prelone	prednisolone
Biological Response Modifiers	
Enbrel	etanercept
Remicade	infliximab

ABBREVIATIONS

ACL	anterior cruciate ligament
ANA	antinuclear antibody
C1, C2, etc.	cervical vertebrae
Ca	calcium
CK	creatine kinase
CPK	creatine phosphokinase
CTS	carpal tunnel syndrome
DEXA	dual-energy x-ray absorptiometry
DTR	deep tendon reflex
EMG	electromyography
ESR	erythrocyte sedimentation rate
Ga	gallium
IM	intramuscular
L1, L2, etc.	lumbar vertebrae
LE	lower extremity
LE cell	lupus erythematosus cell
ortho	orthopedics
phos, P	phosphorus
RA	rheumatoid arthritis
RF	rheumatoid factor
ROM	range of motion
SLE	systemic lupus erythematosus
T1, T2, etc.	thoracic vertebrae
TMJ	temporomandibular joint
UE	upper extremity

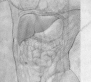

Working Practice Review Exercises

Name: _____ Date: _____

SPELLING*

Rewrite the misspelled words.

1. capsuloraphy   _____
2. fascectomy   _____
3. lupis erythematosis   _____
4. arthrotomy   _____
5. menisectomy   _____

DEFINITIONS*

Define the following diagnostic procedures.

1. arthroscopy

   _____

2. arthrography

   _____

3. synovial fluid studies

   _____

4. latex fixation or rheumatoid factor

   _____

5. electromyography

   _____

6. skeletal survey

   _____

7. C-reactive protein

   _____

8. magnetic resonance imaging

   _____

9. serum creatine kinase

   _____

10. erythrocyte sedimentation rate

    _____

11. gallium scan

    _____

12. myelography

    _____

*Answers are in Appendix A.

IDENTIFICATION
Name the following treatment procedures.

1. removal of knee cartilage _____

2. removal of the bursa and bone of the great toe _____

3. incision made into a fracture site to return bone to its normal position _____

4. cutting the wrist ligament to relieve nerve pressure _____

5. surgical opening of a joint _____

6. surgical implantation of a prosthetic hip joint _____

7. union of two or more vertebrae _____

8. surgical procedures performed on joints with an arthroscope _____

9. surgical reconstruction of a joint _____

10. restoration of a fracture to normal position _____

DEFINITIONS
Define the underscored diagnoses.

1. The patient was seen today because of suspected atrophic arthritis.

   _____

2. The injury to the leg was a greenstick fracture.

   _____

3. He complained of gout for years.

   _____

4. The patient has myasthenia gravis.

   _____

5. The diagnosis in her case is osteomyelitis.

   _____

6. The dentist was suffering from carpal tunnel syndrome.

   _____

7. The doctor suspected he suffered from Paget's disease.

   _____

8. The patient complained of discomfort related to a ganglion cyst.

   _____

9. The doctor indicated that scoliosis was causing her symptoms.

   _____

10. James has a torn meniscus as a result of his participation in the football game.

   _____

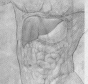

Word Element Review

Root	Meaning	Example	Definition
arthr/o	joint	**arthrocentesis** (ăr"thrō-sĕn-tē'sĭs)	puncture of a joint with a needle to remove fluid
articul/o	joint	**articular** (ăr-tĭk'ū-lăr)	pertaining to a joint
burs/o	sac	**bursitis** (bĕr-sī'tĭs)	inflammation of a bursa (fluid-filled sac)
carp/o	wrist	**carpal** (kăr'păl)	pertaining to the wrist
caud/o	tail	**caudal** (kaw'dăl)	pertaining to a tail-like structure; inferior position
cephal/o	head	**cephalic** (sĕ-făl'ĭk)	pertaining to the head
cervic/o	neck	**cervical** (sĕr'vĭ-kĭl)	pertaining to the neck
cheir/o, chir/o	hand	**cheirospasm** (kī'rō-spăsm)	spasm of the muscles of the hand; writer's cramp
		chirospasm (kī'rō-spăzm)	writer's cramp (Note the similar pronunciation and meaning of these two terms but the different spellings.)
chondr/o	cartilage	**chondrocostal** (kŏn'drō-kŏs'tăl)	pertaining to the ribs and costal cartilages
cleid/o	clavicle	**sternocleidomastoid** (ster"nō-klī"dō-măs'toid)	one of two muscles arising from the sternum and inner part of the clavicle
cost/o	rib	**intercostal** (ĭn"ter-kŏs'tăl)	between the ribs
crani/o	skull, head	**cranial** (krā'nē-ăl)	pertaining to the skull and head
dactyl/o	finger, toe	**dactylitis** (dăk"tĭ-lī'tis)	inflammation of a finger or toe in very young children
digit/o	finger, toe	**digital** (dĭj'ĭ-tăl)	pertaining to or resembling a finger or toe
ili/o	ilium	**iliac** (ĭl'ē-ăk)	referring to the ilium
ischi/o	hip	**ischium** (ĭs'kē-ŭm)	lower portion of the hip bone
ligament/o	ligament	**ligamentous** (lĭg"-ah-men'tăs)	pertaining to or of the nature of a ligament
lumb/o	loin, lower back	**lumbago** (lŭm-bā'gō)	nonspecific term for a dull, aching pain in the lumbar region of the back
maxill/o	upper jaw bone	**maxilla** (măk-sĭl'ah)	upper jaw bone

continues

Root	Meaning	Example	Definition
muscul/o	muscle	**musculoskeletal** (mŭs'kū-lō-skĕl'ĕ-tăl)	pertaining to the muscles and skeleton
my/o	muscle	**myocarditis** (mī"ō-kăr-dī'tĭs)	inflammation of the middle layer of the heart wall
oste/o	bone	**osteoarthritis** (ŏs"tē-ō-ăr-thrī'tĭs)	chronic disease involving the joints
ped/o, pod/o	foot	**podiatry** (pŏ-dī'ah-trē)	specialized field dealing with the study and care of the foot
phren/o	diaphragm	**phrenic nerve** (frĕn'ik)	nerve to the diaphragm
sacr/o	sacrum	**sacroiliac** (sā"krō-ĭl'ē-ăk)	pertaining to the sacrum and ilium
spas/o	draw, pull	**spasticity** (spăs-tĭs'ĭ-tē)	state of increased muscle tone over the normal
spondyl/o	vertebra	**spondylolysis** (spŏn"dĭ-lŏl'ĭ-sĭs)	degenerative changes in the spine
synov/o	synovial membrane	**synovitis** (sĭn-ō-vī'tĭs)	inflammation of the synovial membrane, especially that of a joint
tars/o	foot	**tarsus** (tahr'sŭs)	ankle
tend/o, ten/o, tendin/o	tendon	**tendinitis** (tĕn"dĭ-nī'tŭs) (preferred spelling) **tendonitis** (tĕn"dō-nī'tĭs) **tenorrhaphy** (tĕn-or'ah-fē)	inflammation of a tendon suturing of a tendon
tens/o	stretch	**tensor** (tĕn'sor)	any muscle that makes a body part tense
vertebr/o	vertebra	**vertebral column** (ver'tē-brăl)	spinal column

Physical Medicine

Root	Meaning	Example	Definition
dynam/o	power	**dynamometer** (dī"nah-mŏm'ĕ-ter)	an instrument for measuring muscular strength
therap/o	treatment, therapy	**physical therapist** (thĕr'a-pĭst)	a person skilled in the treatment of diseases or disorders using physical agents such as massage, heat, hydrotherapy (water), radiation, electricity, and exercise
therm/o	heat	**thermotherapy** (ther"mō-thĕr'ah-pē)	therapeutic application of heat
traumat/o	wound, injury	**traumatic** (traw-măt'ĭk)	pertaining to or resulting from a wound or an injury (trauma)

continues

Suffix	Meaning	Example	Definition
-plegia	paralysis	**paraplegia** (păr"ah-plē'jē-ah)	paralysis of the lower part of the body
		quadriplegia (kwŏd"rĭ-plē'jē-ah)	paralysis of all four limbs

Word Element Review Exercises

Name: _____ Date: _____

WORD ELEMENTS*
Name the word elements that refer to the following parts.

1. head _____
2. hand _____
3. foot _____
4. back _____

MATCHING*
Match the word elements to their meanings.

1. _____ clavicle
2. _____ muscle
3. _____ sac
4. _____ ilium
5. _____ diaphragm
6. _____ bone
7. _____ rib
8. _____ joint
9. _____ hip
10. _____ upper jawbone

a. arthr/o

b. burs/o

c. cleid/o

d. cost/o

e. ili/o

f. ischi/o

g. maxill/o

h. muscul/o, my/o

i. oste/o

j. phren/o

PRONUNCIATION AND DEFINITION*
Provide the pronunciation and definition for the following terms.

1. intercostal _____

_____

2. arthrocentesis _____

_____

3. bursitis _____

_____

4. myocarditis _____

_____

5. osteoarthritis _____

_____

6. spondylolysis _____

_____

7. tensor _____

_____

_____

*Answers are in Appendix A.

MATCHING

Match the terms to their meanings.

1. _____ paralysis of the lower limbs
2. _____ person skilled in the treatment of diseases and disorders either with or using physical agents
3. _____ instrument for measuring muscular strength
4. _____ pertaining to the wrist
5. _____ upper jaw bone
6. _____ pertaining to or resulting from a wound or injury
7. _____ any muscle that makes a body part tense
8. _____ specialized field studying the foot
9. _____ pertaining to a ligament
10. _____ pertaining to a joint
11. _____ pertaining to the neck
12. _____ state of increased muscle tone over the normal
13. _____ therapeutic application of heat
14. _____ writer's cramp
15. _____ pertaining to ribs and costal cartilages

a. articular
b. carpal
c. cervical
d. chirospasm
e. chondrocostal
f. dynamometer
g. ligamentous
h. maxilla
i. paraplegia
j. physical therapist
k. podiatry
l. spasticity
m. tensor
n. thermotherapy
o. traumatic

WORD ELEMENT MEANINGS

Give the meaning of each word element. Then use your dictionary to find a new word that contains each of the word elements. Specify whether the new word is a noun or an adjective by placing N or A in the last column.

Word Element	Meaning	Word	N or A
1. arthr/o			
2. articul/o			
3. burs/o			
4. carp/o			
5. caud/o			
6. cephal/o			
7. cervic/o			
8. cheir/o			
9. chir/o			
10. chondr/o			
11. cleid/o			
12. cost/o			

Word Element	Meaning	Word	N or A
13. crani/o			
14. dactyl/o			
15. digit/o			
16. dynam/o			
17. ili/o			
18. ischi/o			
19. ligament/o			
20. lumb/o			
21. maxill/o			
22. muscul/o			
23. my/o			
24. oste/o			
25. ped/o			
26. phren/o			
27. -plegia			
28. pod/o			
29. sacr/o			
30. spas/o			
31. spondyl/o			
32. synov/o			
33. tars/o			
34. tend/o			
35. ten/o			
36. tendin/o			
37. tens/o			
38. therap/o			
39. therm/o			
40. traumat/o			
41. vertebr/o			

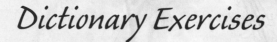

Dictionary Exercises

Name: _____ Date: _____

DICTIONARY EXERCISE 1*

Use your dictionary to find the pronunciation and definition of the following words.

	Word	**Pronunciation**	**Definition**
1.	anomaly	_____	_____
2.	calcific	_____	_____
3.	collateral ligaments	_____	_____
4.	costochondral	_____	_____
5.	coxa	_____	_____
6.	de Quervain's disease	_____	_____
7.	flail joint	_____	_____
8.	genu	_____	_____
9.	Legg-Calvé-Perthes disease	_____	_____
10.	pes planus	_____	_____
11.	osteoplasty	_____	_____
12.	ossification	_____	_____
13.	intertrochanteric	_____	_____
14.	osteoclast	_____	_____

DICTIONARY EXERCISE 2*

Select the correct meaning and provide the pronunciation of each term.

1. capitulum (_____)
   a. small, rounded end of a bone
   b. the shaft of a long bone

2. diaphysis (_____)
   a. resembling a pit or socket
   b. the shaft of a long bone

3. giant cell tumor (_____)
   a. bony outgrowth, usually branched in shape
   b. arises from the marrow of a long bone or from a tendon sheath

4. glenoid (_____)
   a. resembling a pit or socket
   b. the bony process of the ulna at the elbow

5. glenoid cavity (_____)
   a. removal of tissue to form a shallow depression
   b. hollow socket in the head of the shoulder blade that receives the head of the humerus

6. hemarthrosis (_____)
   a. passage of blood into the cavity of a bony joint
   b. spotty osteoporosis of bone in post-traumatic states

7. lamina (_____)
   a. bony outgrowth, usually branched in shape
   b. a thin, flat layer

8. metaphysis (_____)
   a. fusing together of two or more toes or fingers
   b. growth zone of a long bone between the epiphysis and diaphysis

9. nucleus pulposus (_____)
   a. semi-fluid cushion in the center of an intervertebral disk
   b. bonelike structure that develops on a bone or occasionally at another site

---

*Answers are in Appendix A.

10. olecranon (_____)
   a. free-floating bone that resembles a grain of sesame in size and shape
   b. bony process of the ulna at the elbow

11. ostectomy (_____)
   a. surgical removal of dead bone
   b. excision or resection of bone

12. osteoma (_____)
   a. arises from the marrow of a long bone or from a tendon sheath
   b. bonelike structure that develops on a bone or occasionally at another site

13. osteophyte (_____)
   a. a bony outgrowth, usually branched in shape
   b. resembling a pit or socket

14. rheumatologist (_____)
   a. physician who treats joint diseases
   b. physician who manipulates the spinal column

15. polymyositis (_____)
   a. inflammatory condition of muscular tissue in which an area of abnormal bone formation occurs
   b. inflammation of uncertain origin of several muscles at once

16. saucerization (_____)
   a. removal of tissue to form a shallow depression
   b. surgical removal of dead bone

17. sequestrectomy (_____)
   a. surgical removal of dead bone
   b. removal of synovial membrane lining a joint capsule

18. sesamoid (_____)
   a. free-floating bone that resembles a grain of sesame in size and shape
   b. resembling a pit or socket

19. Sudeck's atrophy (_____)
   a. complete or incomplete separation of a portion of joint cartilage from underlying bone
   b. spotty osteoporosis of bone in post-traumatic states

20. syndactylism (_____)
   a. hollow back; convexity of spine
   b. fusing together of two or more toes or fingers

DICTIONARY EXERCISE 3

Pronunciation of the words below is provided. Using your dictionary, find the correct spelling and the definition of the word.

	Word	**Pronunciation**	**Definition**
1.	_____	ăs"ĕ-tăb'ū-lŭm	_____
2.	_____	mī"ĕ-lō'mah	_____
3.	_____	ŏs"tē-ō-kŏn-drī'tĭs	_____
4.	_____	dĭs'ĕ-kănz sŭb"lŭk-sā'shŭn	_____
5.	_____	zĭf'oid prŏs'ĕs	_____
6.	_____	krĕp"ĭ-tā'shŭn	_____
7.	_____	făs"ē-ī'tĭs	_____
8.	_____	dĭs-plā'sē-ah	_____
9.	_____	kŏn"drō-mah-lā'shē-ah	_____
10.	_____	ăng"kĭ-lō'sĭs	_____
11.	_____	ŏs"ĭ-fĭ-kā'shŭn	_____
12.	_____	lah-săgz' sign	_____
13.	_____	mĕ-nĭs'kŭs	_____
14.	_____	mī"ō-sī'tĭs ŏ-sĭf'ĭ-kănz	_____
15.	_____	spŏn"dĭ-lō-lĭs'thē-sĭs	_____
16.	_____	ō-lĕk'răn-ŏn	_____
17.	_____	tor"tĭ-kŏl'ĭs	_____

DICTIONARY EXERCISE 4

Look up the definition of each of the italicized words. Write the pronunciation in the space provided. Then rewrite the sentence in your own words.

1. The patient was placed in a *Denis Browne* splint.

_____

2. *Ortolani's* (_____) sign was evident.

_____

3. She was scheduled for a *patellectomy* (_____) on Thursday.

_____

4. There was evidence of *spondylolysis* (_____), as well as *myositis* (_____).

_____

5. During the procedure *tenodesis* (_____) was achieved.

_____

6. A *tenoplasty* (_____) was performed two years ago.

_____

7. On examination, a *trigger finger* was noted on the right hand.

_____

8. Both a *tenosynovectomy* (_____) and *tenotomy* (_____) were required.

_____

9. The pathology report indicated an *osteochondroma* (_____).

_____

10. On physical examination, the patient presented with a *metatarsus varus* (_____).

_____

11. There was a *contracture* (_____) present, as well as *lordosis* (_____).

_____

12. The problem was diagnosed as *Baker's cyst.*

_____

13. Patient is suffering from *Paget's* (_____) *disease.*

_____

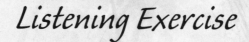

Listening Exercise

Name	Date

INSTRUCTIONS

1. Review the spelling, pronunciation, and meaning of the words provided in the preview.

2. Listen to the audio CD and fill in the blank as the word is dictated.

3. At the end of the exercise, check your spelling against the preview words. They appear in the preview in the order in which they are encountered in the exercise.

4. Review and practice the words you missed.

5. Look up words that are not familiar.

PREVIEW OF WORDS FOR LISTENING EXERCISE 6-1

Word	Pronunciation	Definition
crepitus	krĕp'ĭ-tŭs	dry, crackling sound or sensation, as in the grating of the ends of a fractured bone
effusion	ĕ-fū'zhŭn	escape of fluid into a part
varus gait	vā'rŭs gāt	style of walking characterized by an inward bend toward the midline of the body
medially	mē'dĕ-ăl-lē	toward the midline of the body
patellofemoral	pă-tĕl"ō-fĕm'ō-răl	pertaining to the patella (kneecap) and femur (thigh bone)
arthroplasty	ăr'thrō-plăs"tē	surgical reconstruction of a joint

Letter of Consultation

Dear Dr. Zemstov:

I had the pleasure of seeing your patient, Mr. Roger Petrov, who is a 75-year-old very active gentleman who has had a long history of increasing pain associated with his right knee. He states his problem began when he sustained trauma to his knee while playing high school football. Although he got better originally, over the last few years he has experienced increasing discomfort within his knee with activities. In addition, he has noted a deformity, specifically a genu varum or bow-leggedness, that has gotten worse. He finds that on occasion he will sense catching and locking. He has noted considerable amounts of _____ along with periodic episodes of _____.

You have maintained him so appropriately over these last few years with anti-inflammatory medication, the use of cold therapy, and some physical therapy with reasonable success. However, his symptoms now have worsened to the point where his daily living activities have become more difficult, including such simple things as walking to the mailbox, cutting the grass and doing minimal manual tasks around his house, or going shopping.

On physical examination he is a healthy appearing, very pleasant man complaining of right knee pain. He walks with a limp with an obvious _____. Closer examination reveals no limb-length discrepancy. He does carry about a half inch of atrophy of his thigh. There is relative instability _____ with a 2+ effusion. Considerable crepitus is noted throughout his knee. There is discomfort along the medial side during the course of the exam as well. He has no edema, has full pulses, and no other lower extremity joint problems.

We have obtained standing x-rays, in addition to the usual lateral and Merchant views. The films show end-stage degenerative arthritis involving primarily the medial compartment of his knee with lesser involvement of the _____ compartment. He is bone on bone medially.

I think this man has exhausted all forms of conservative measures for his condition of degenerative arthritis. He is an excellent candidate for a total knee _____ in an effort to improve his pain and reduce his other symptoms, as well as to alter his alignment. He is interested in pursuing a corrective course and arrangements will be made for this to be done sometime within the next few weeks.

Thank you for this referral. I will keep you informed as to his progress, both in the hospital and postoperatively.

Sincerely yours,

Juanita Montoya, MD

Surgery

> 66 *Surgery does the ideal thing—it separates the patient from his disease.* 99
>
> —Logan Clendening

When you have completed this chapter on surgery, you should be able to

1. Identify the components of an Operative Report.
2. Spell and define commonly used anesthesia terminology.
3. Identify and spell commonly used surgical positions, incisions, and instruments.
4. Explain the difference between suture material and suture technique.
5. Be familiar with terminology used in reports.

INTRODUCTION

Surgical intervention is often required to repair injuries to the body, to correct deformities or defects, and to diagnose, treat, or cure certain disease processes. A surgeon is a physician who has completed five or more years of postgraduate training in one or more of a broad range of surgical specialties. Some of these surgical specialties are listed below.

Specialty	Organs or Systems Involved
General surgery	various organs or systems
Gynecology	external and internal female reproductive organs
Neurosurgery	nervous system and associated structures
Ophthalmology	eyes and associated structures, including ocular muscles, tear ducts, and glands
Orthopedic surgery	musculoskeletal system
Otorhinolaryngology	ear, nose, and throat and related structures

continues

Specialty	Organs or Systems Involved
Plastic surgery	repair and reconstruction of various body structures
Thoracic surgery	thorax (chest) and diseases related to the bronchi, lungs, and mediastinum
Urology	male and female urinary tract, male reproductive organs
Vascular and cardiac surgery	heart, blood vessels, and lymphatic vessels

The terminology associated with surgery and surgical reports is highly specialized as well. Surgical terminology includes terms related to anesthesia; names of surgical positions, instruments, and incisions; and suture techniques and materials. The surgical report contains a detailed technical description of how the procedure was done.

Although the surgeon is responsible for providing the information for the report, support staff may be responsible for processing or producing it. Therefore, it is important to recognize the required components of the report, know basic information about anesthetics, and become familiar with other surgical terminology.

COMPONENTS OF THE OPERATIVE REPORT

A written report is required for every surgical procedure. The report may be called an operative note, an operative report, a surgical note, or a surgical report. The term **Operative Report** will be used throughout this chapter.

The Operative Report is used to assist in further patient care, to secure payment for services provided, and as a legal document to support the surgeon's actions. There are required components of the Operative Report mandated by various state and federal laws and by other regulatory agencies. Each report must contain a preoperative and postoperative diagnosis, the name of the operation or procedure, indications for the procedure, and a description of findings and techniques.

In addition, the Operative Report will include the patient's name, date of the procedure, and the surgeon's name. These items may be listed at the beginning of the report under appropriate headings. Some agencies include the case number, patient room number, and the names of any assisting surgeons or physicians.

PREOPERATIVE DIAGNOSIS

All regulatory and accrediting agencies require a **Preoperative Diagnosis**, which helps explain why the operation or procedure is necessary. The diagnosis can be stated as a specific disease. When the diagnosis is not clearly evident, the Preoperative Diagnosis is stated as a "rule out" or "suspected" diagnosis, or in other general terms.

EXAMPLES

Patient A has been diagnosed with acute appendicitis. An appendectomy is performed. In this case the Preoperative Diagnosis will be appendicitis.

Patient B may have several symptoms of appendicitis, but the physician cannot make a clear-cut diagnosis. In this case the Preoperative Diagnosis could be suspected appendicitis, rule out appendicitis, or it could be severe abdominal pain with high fever, with an unknown reason or cause.

In any case the Preoperative Diagnosis *must* be present and *must* be related to the procedure performed.

> **LAYMAN'S INTERPRETATION:** The patient was brought to the operating room. The table was raised so he was sitting up. The glands at the back and sides of the throat were given a shot of a medicine to make them numb. When the glands were completely numb, a curved clamp was used to grab them. Two kinds of cutting methods (blunt and sharp) were used. The tonsils were trapped in the clamp and removed.

Closure

The final paragraphs of the Findings and Technique section describe how the incision was closed, state that all surgical tools have been accounted for, and may include information about blood loss.

The surgeon describes how each layer of skin and tissue was sutured, the type of suture material and techniques used, and the condition of the incisional wound. There are many types of suture materials and techniques, which are discussed later in this chapter.

An important part of the Findings and Techniques section is the sponge count. Every Operative Report must state that the surgeon can account for all surgical tools. Prior to every procedure, a member of the surgical team counts items like sponges, needles, and instruments. After the procedure, these items are counted again to ensure that nothing was left inside the patient. The Operative Report *must* have a statement that the count was done.

> EXAMPLE
>
> The sponge, needle, and instrument counts were correct.

You *must not* include a sponge count statement if the surgeon does not include one. You should, however, alert the surgeon of this omission, because it is the surgeon's responsibility to authorize the inclusion of this information.

If the patient received blood during the procedure, information about blood loss and blood replacement may appear in this section. This information may be included as a separate heading of the Operative Report.

> EXAMPLE
>
> Due to excessive blood loss, the patient received 2 units of whole blood.

Patient Condition

The final statement in the Operative Report concerns the condition of the patient and is usually one or two sentences in length.

> EXAMPLE
>
> The patient was sent to the recovery room in stable condition.

If there is some question about the patient's ability to survive the operation, the statement could read:

> EXAMPLE
>
> The patient was sent to the recovery room in poor condition. Prognosis is poor.

In the case of a poor **prognosis** (prŏg-nō'sĭs) (probable outcome), a reason will be given.

SIGNATURE BLOCK

The surgeon must sign the Operative Report. It is important to *carefully proofread* the completed report before you submit it for signature. A standard signature block format is acceptable. It contains the name of the surgeon followed by the initials of the individual who transcribed or typed the report. If the report was dictated and transcribed, a notation beneath the signature block indicates the date dictated and the date transcribed.

Figure 7-1 is an example of a completed Operative Report.

ANESTHESIA TERMINOLOGY

Anesthesiology (ăn"ĕs-thē"zē-ŏl'ŏ-jē), a specialty that developed as a result of Joseph Priestley's discovery of nitrous oxide in 1772, is the study of anesthesia and anesthetic agents. An **anesthesiologist** (ăn"ĕs-thē"zē-ŏl'ō-jĭst)

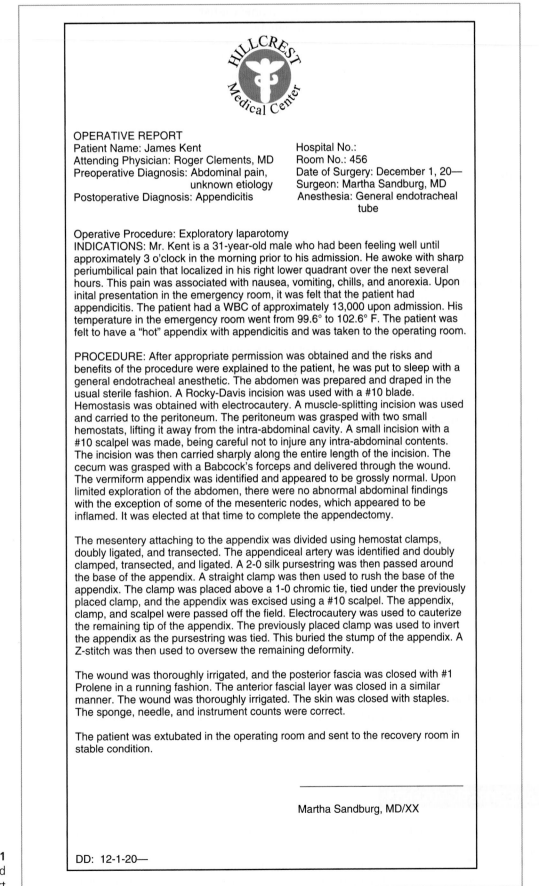

OPERATIVE REPORT

Patient Name: James Kent
Attending Physician: Roger Clements, MD
Preoperative Diagnosis: Abdominal pain,
                         unknown etiology
Postoperative Diagnosis: Appendicitis

Hospital No.:
Room No.: 456
Date of Surgery: December 1, 20—
Surgeon: Martha Sandburg, MD
Anesthesia: General endotracheal
                         tube

Operative Procedure: Exploratory laparotomy

INDICATIONS: Mr. Kent is a 31-year-old male who had been feeling well until approximately 3 o'clock in the morning prior to his admission. He awoke with sharp periumbilical pain that localized in his right lower quadrant over the next several hours. This pain was associated with nausea, vomiting, chills, and anorexia. Upon inital presentation in the emergency room, it was felt that the patient had appendicitis. The patient had a WBC of approximately 13,000 upon admission. His temperature in the emergency room went from 99.6° to 102.6° F. The patient was felt to have a "hot" appendix with appendicitis and was taken to the operating room.

PROCEDURE: After appropriate permission was obtained and the risks and benefits of the procedure were explained to the patient, he was put to sleep with a general endotracheal anesthetic. The abdomen was prepared and draped in the usual sterile fashion. A Rocky-Davis incision was used with a #10 blade. Hemostasis was obtained with electrocautery. A muscle-splitting incision was used and carried to the peritoneum. The peritoneum was grasped with two small hemostats, lifting it away from the intra-abdominal cavity. A small incision with a #10 scalpel was made, being careful not to injure any intra-abdominal contents. The incision was then carried sharply along the entire length of the incision. The cecum was grasped with a Babcock's forceps and delivered through the wound. The vermiform appendix was identified and appeared to be grossly normal. Upon limited exploration of the abdomen, there were no abnormal abdominal findings with the exception of some of the mesenteric nodes, which appeared to be inflamed. It was elected at that time to complete the appendectomy.

The mesentery attaching to the appendix was divided using hemostat clamps, doubly ligated, and transected. The appendiceal artery was identified and doubly clamped, transected, and ligated. A 2-0 silk pursestring was then passed around the base of the appendix. A straight clamp was then used to rush the base of the appendix. The clamp was placed above a 1-0 chromic tie, tied under the previously placed clamp, and the appendix was excised using a #10 scalpel. The appendix, clamp, and scalpel were passed off the field. Electrocautery was used to cauterize the remaining tip of the appendix. The previously placed clamp was used to invert the appendix as the pursestring was tied. This buried the stump of the appendix. A Z-stitch was then used to oversew the remaining deformity.

The wound was thoroughly irrigated, and the posterior fascia was closed with #1 Prolene in a running fashion. The anterior fascial layer was closed in a similar manner. The wound was thoroughly irrigated. The skin was closed with staples. The sponge, needle, and instrument counts were correct.

The patient was extubated in the operating room and sent to the recovery room in stable condition.

Martha Sandburg, MD/XX

DD: 12-1-20—

FIGURE 7-1
Completed
Operative Report

Block

Block is a generic term that means the anesthetic agent is injected near or along a nerve path in order to stop nerve impulses to the area supplied by the nerve. The block method is also called nerve block and can include the name of the nerve or nerve group to be anesthetized. Block modes of induction are associated with regional anesthetics. Some of the more frequently used block methods are presented here.

Epidural (ĕp"ĭ-dū'ral) **block**
An anesthetic injected into the epidural space of the spinal column to anesthetize the pelvic, abdominal, or genital area.

Intercostal (ĭn"ter-kŏs'tal) **block**
An anesthetic injected into the intercostal nerves to prevent the conduction of nerve impulses. Intercostal nerves are located near or along the rib cage.

Saddle block
A local anesthetic injected into the area of the spine that affects the buttocks, perineum, and inner aspects of the thighs. The **perineum** (per"ĭ-nē'ŭm) is the area between the anus and genitalia. This type of anesthesia is frequently associated with childbirth.

Spinal block
A local anesthetic injected into the **subarachnoid** (sŭb"ah-răk'noid) **space** around the spinal cord. The area below the injection site is affected.

Endobronchial

The **endobronchial** (ĕn"dō-brong'kē-al) mode of induction is the administration of a gaseous mixture through a tube placed in a large bronchus. The **bronchus** (brŏng'kŭs) is one of two larger air passages to the lung beyond or below the trachea. The endobronchial mode is associated with general anesthesia.

Endotracheal

The **endotracheal** (ĕn"dō-trā'kē-al) method is the administration of a gaseous mixture through a tube placed in the **trachea** (trā'kē-ah), or windpipe. This method produces a general anesthetic condition.

Infiltration

Infiltration is the injection of anesthetic agent into tissues. This is a common way to administer a local anesthetic.

Inhalation

Inhalation is when the patient breathes in or inhales a gaseous anesthetic agent. This method is used most often with general anesthetics.

Insufflation

Insufflation (ĭn"sŭ-flā'shŭn) is the introduction of a gaseous anesthetic agent into the respiratory tract through a slender tube. It is another method of general anesthesia.

Intravenous

The **intravenous** method is the administration of an anesthetic agent into a vein by injection. This method usually indicates a general anesthesia.

Topical

The **topical** mode of induction is the application of an anesthetic agent directly to the surface of the area involved in the procedure. Topical induction does not compromise the integrity of the skin or membrane involved.

OTHER SURGICAL AND OPERATIVE TERMINOLOGY

There are several other categories of specialized surgical and operative terminology. These categories include the names of surgical positions, instruments, and incisions, as well as suture materials and techniques.

POSITION

Surgical position describes how the patient is placed on the operative or examination table. The surgeon chooses the position best suited for the procedure to be performed. The Operative Report includes the surgical position. The names of several surgical positions and when they are used are identified below. The more commonly used surgical positions are illustrated in Figure 7-2.

Position	Description
decubitus (right, left, lateral)	lying on the right or left side; position for urological procedures
dorsal (supine)	flat on back with legs extended; position for abdominal surgery
dorsal recumbent	flat on back with knees drawn up and thighs turned outward; position for vaginal procedures
Fowler	trunk raised to form a 45-degree angle, thighs also raised, pelvis at bottom of "V"
Kraske	prone on abdomen with head and foot of table dropped, buttocks raised; position for rectal surgery
lateral decubitus	on side, body elevator raised under patient, head and foot lower; position for kidney procedure
lithotomy	on back with legs in stirrups; position for obstetrics and gynecology
prone	flat on abdomen; position for back surgery
Sims'	on left side with left arm in back, resting on chest, right knee drawn up; position for rectal procedures
Trendelenburg	on back with table tilted 45 degrees toward head, bent at knees; stirrups may be used; position for pelvic surgery

INSTRUMENTS

A wide variety of instruments are used to perform surgical procedures. They are classified according to their function: cutting, grasping/holding, clamping, retracting, probing, dilating, suturing, or suctioning. Specific examples are shown in the list of Commonly Used Surgical Instruments below. Other instruments that do not fit into these classifications are referred to as accessory instruments.

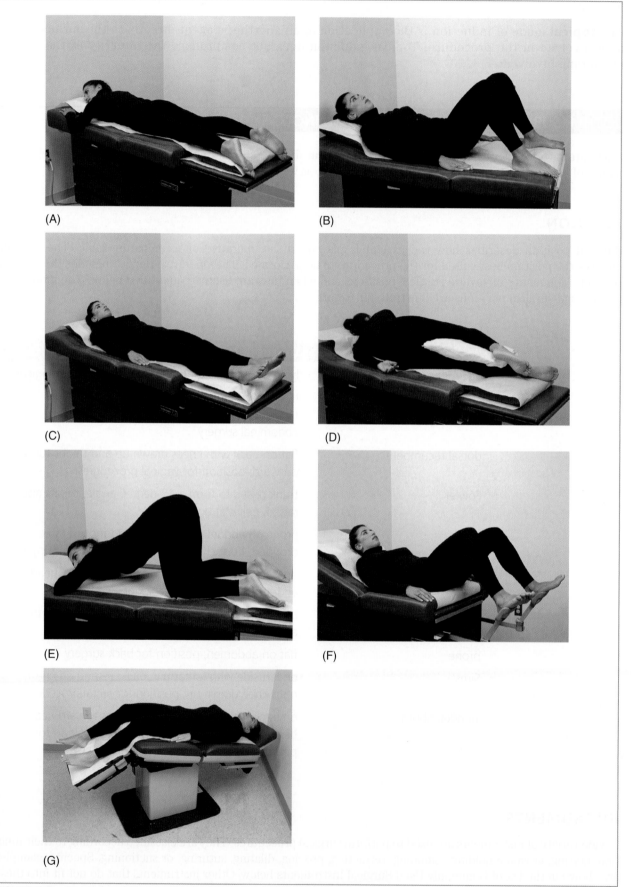

FIGURE 7-2 Surgical and Examination Positions: (A) prone; (B) dorsal recumbent; (C) supine; (D) Sims'; (E) knee-chest; (F) lithotomy; (G) Trendelenburg

COMMONLY USED SURGICAL INSTRUMENTS

Name	Pronunciation	Description
aspirator	ăs'pĭ-rā'tōr	instrument that suctions fluid or gas
cannula	kăn'ū-lă	tube fitted with a trocar for insertion into a duct or cavity; the trocar is removed and the fluids are drained
catheter	kăth'ĕ-tĕr	tubular instrument inserted into a vessel or body cavity structure
clamp		instrument for gripping, joining, supporting, or compressing an organ or vessel
curette, curet	kū-rĕt'	spoon-shaped instrument for scraping and removing tissue
dilator	dī-lā'tōr	instrument used to enlarge an opening by stretching
drains		tubes used for removal of air and/or fluids from a surgical site; may be active or passive (e.g., Penrose, T-tubes, Jackson Pratt)
forceps	fōr'cĕps	instrument for holding, seizing, or extracting tissue or organs
hemostat	hē'mō-stăt	instrument used to stop the flow of blood
insufflator	ĭn'sŭ-flā"tor	infuses CO_2 gas into the abdominal cavity for laproscopic procedures
irrigation/aspiration units (I/A)	ăs-pĭ-rā'shŭn	device powered by nitrogen gas utilized to remove foreign material or tissue from a traumatic or infected wound
retractor	rē-trăk'tōr	instrument for pulling back the edges of a wound or incision
scalpel	skăl'pĕl	small, straight knife
syringes		plastic or glass devices fitted with a needle; used to irrigate wounds, aspirate fluids, or inject medications; vary in capacity from 3–60 cc (most common is 10 cc)
tenaculum	tĕ-năk'ū-lŭm	hooklike instrument for seizing and holding
trocar	trō'căr	sharply pointed instrument with cutting edges inserted in a cannula; used to penetrate a body cavity to permit drainage of the fluid

Cutting instruments are used for incision, sharp dissection, or excision and include knives, scalpels, scissors, and bone-cutting instruments. Scalpel handles come in several sizes (#3, #4, #7, and #9) and are usually not disposable (Figure 7-3A). The blades are disposable and fit a specific handle (Figure 7-3B). The #10 blade is the most frequently used. Scissors are designed for specific cutting purposes: tissue, suture, wire, or bandage/dressings (Figure 7-4).

Grasping and holding instruments are designed to stabilize fractured bone or to facilitate dissection or suturing. They vary in type and length, and the gripping surfaces may have teeth, serrations, or be smooth. Common examples include Adson, Ferris-Smith, DeBakey, Brown, Russian, Geral, Cushing bayonet forceps, Allis, Babcock, and Kocher.

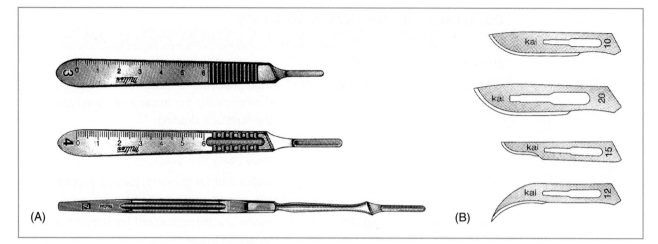

FIGURE 7-3 (A) Scalpel Handles: #3, #4, and #7; (B) Scalpel Blades: #10, #20, #15, and #12 (Courtesy of Miltex Surgical Instruments)

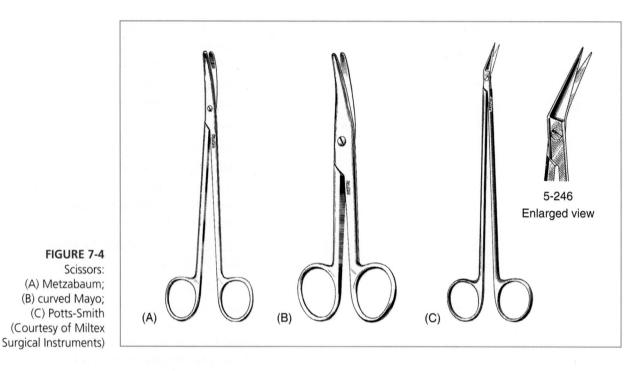

FIGURE 7-4
Scissors:
(A) Metzabaum;
(B) curved Mayo;
(C) Potts-Smith
(Courtesy of Miltex
Surgical Instruments)

Clamping instruments are designed to constrict tissue. Figure 7-5 shows finger rings and ratchets engineered to lock the instrument in place.

Retracting instruments are used to allow the surgeon to see the operative site (Figure 7-6). Sizes and shapes vary according to the surgical site. For example, wide curved retractors are used to retract abdominal walls.

Suturing instruments called needle holders are used to hold a curved suturing needle (Figure 7-7). Most holders are scissorlike clamps (A) with a ratchet or other locking device to lock the needle within the blades. The blades (B) are usually straight, but may be curved to meet special needs. For the subtle maneuvers needed for microsurgical, ophthalmic, and some vascular procedures, the holder is designed with a spring-action ratchet to protect the delicate suture needles.

Suctioning instruments remove blood and body fluids from the operative site. The suction instruments in Figure 7-8 are representative of the many standard and specialized devices available.

Other specialized equipment includes endoscopes, power tools, and lasers. Flexible endoscopes, for example, may be used before, during, or after a surgical procedure for diagnosis, biopsy, visualization, and/or repair of a structure within a body cavity. Power tools may be driven by compressed air or nitrogen, electricity, or battery and are used to cut, drill, or reshape bones. They may also be used to cut skin (grafting) or grind skin (dermabrasion).

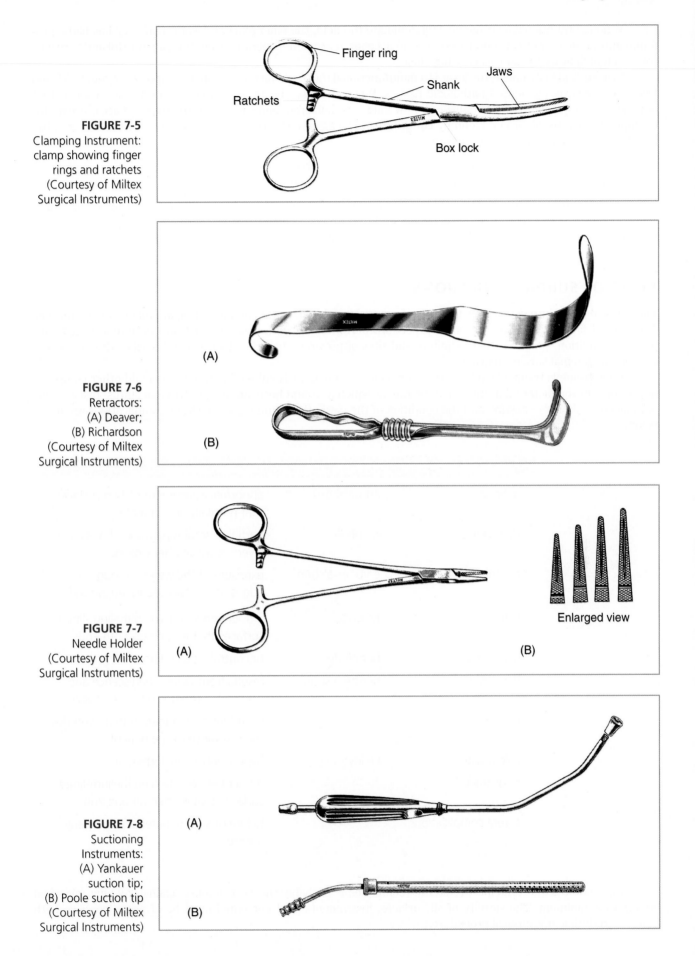

FIGURE 7-5
Clamping Instrument: clamp showing finger rings and ratchets (Courtesy of Miltex Surgical Instruments)

Finger ring
Shank
Jaws
Ratchets
Box lock

FIGURE 7-6
Retractors:
(A) Deaver;
(B) Richardson
(Courtesy of Miltex Surgical Instruments)

(A)

(B)

FIGURE 7-7
Needle Holder
(Courtesy of Miltex Surgical Instruments)

(A)

(B)

Enlarged view

FIGURE 7-8
Suctioning Instruments:
(A) Yankauer suction tip;
(B) Poole suction tip
(Courtesy of Miltex Surgical Instruments)

(A)

(B)

Although traditional instruments still dominate the field, the emergence of laser technology has had a profound impact on a variety of operative procedures. **Laser** instruments operate by emitting a powerful and very narrow beam of light that produces very high heat.

As a surgical instrument, the laser is a multifunctional tool that can cut, coagulate, vaporize tissue, weld, and selectively destroy pigmented pathologic tissues. When the laser beam is focused on the tissue, what it does depends on how much power is delivered, how long it is delivered, and the size of the exposed area. It can, for example, harden tissue or clot blood by **coagulation** (kō-ăg'ū-lā'-shŭn) or perform surgical cuts with very little bleeding. Some types of laser devices are

| Ho:YAG | CO_2 | argon |
| Nd:YAG | KTP | excimer |

Laser technology does, however, present unique safety considerations because laser light can be harmful to skin and eyes. For this reason, both the patient and the surgical team must keep these areas adequately covered. Fire also is a real hazard, and appropriate extinguishing materials must be readily available.

TYPES OF SURGICAL INCISIONS

The surgical procedure determines the type of surgical incision. Location and direction are major considerations. A variety of factors affect the decision: procedure performed, access desired, surgeon's preferences, patient's physical condition, speed of entry required, and sites of previous surgeries. Figure 7-9 describes the location of common abdominal surgical incisions.

When tissue is traumatized by surgery or accident, a patient is vulnerable to infection and other complications. Some of the factors that influence the rate at which a wound heals are age, nutritional status, disease, use of tobacco, radiation exposure, and the condition of the patient's immune system. Other complications are listed below.

Complication	Pronunciation	Description
adhesion	ăd-hē'zhŭn	abnormal attachment of two surfaces that normally are separate
dehiscence	dē-hĭs'ĕns	partial or total separation of a layer or layers of tissue after closure
evisceration	ē-vĭs"ĕr-ā'shŭn	exposure of the viscera through the edges of a totally separated wound
fistula	fĭs'tū-lă	a tract between two epithelium-lined surfaces that is open on both ends
hemorrhage	hĕm'ĕ-rĭj	uncontrolled bleeding
herniation	hĕr-nē-ā'shŭn	results from wound dehiscence and occurs 2–3 months postoperatively
infection		microbial contamination that overrides the resistance of the patient
keloid scar	kē'lŏyd	hypertrophic scar formation
sinus tract		a tract between two epithelium-lined surfaces that is open on one end
suture complications		failure of suture material to properly absorb

Application of the principles of sterile techniques is probably the best defense against keeping microbial counts to a minimum. The sterility of all surfaces, instruments, and personnel must be of prime concern both before and during any surgical procedure.

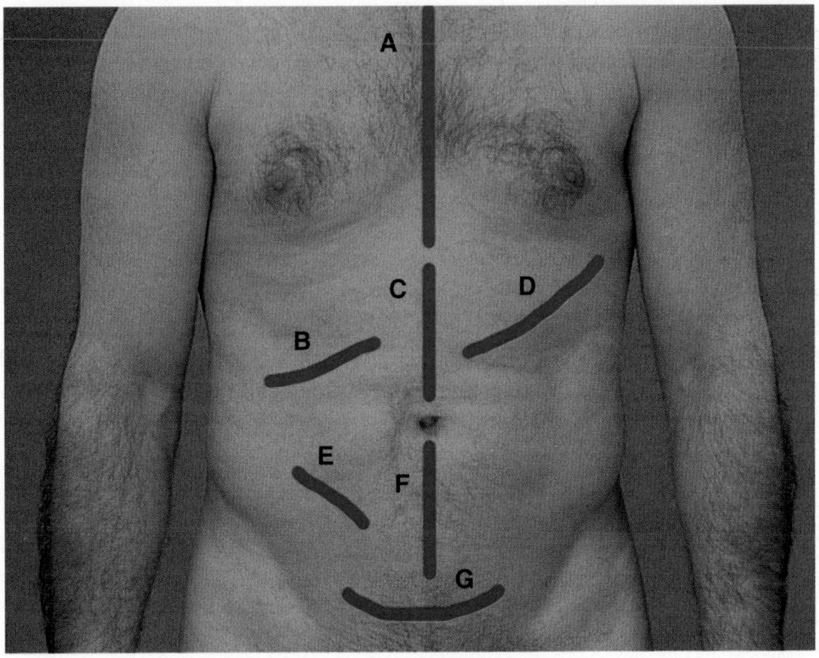

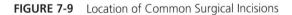

INCISION	LOCATION	ORGAN
A. Sternal Split	Begins at the top of the sternum and extends downward to the sternal notch.	Heart
B. Oblique Subcostal	Begins in the epigastric area and extends laterally and obliquely below the lower costal margin.	Right side: Gallbladder, Biliary Left side: Spleen
C. Upper Vertical Midline	Begins below the sternal notch and distally around the umbilicus.	Stomach, Duodenum, Pancreas
D. Thoracoabdominal	Begins midway between the xiphoid process and the umbilicus and extends across the seventh or eighth intercostal space to the midscapular line.	Thorax, Heart
E. McBurney	Begins below the umbilicus, goes through McBurney's point, and extends toward the right flank.	Appendix
F. Lower Vertical Midline	Begins below the umbilicus, downward toward the symphysis pubis.	Bladder, Uterus
G. Pfannenstiel	Begins 1.5 inches above the symphysis pubis with a curved transverse cut across the lower abdomen.	Uterus, Fallopian tubes, Ovaries

FIGURE 7-9   Location of Common Surgical Incisions

SUTURE MATERIALS

Suture materials are threads, wires, or other materials used to stitch parts of the body together. Some suture materials are absorbable and others are not. Absorbable material will dissolve in the body fluids and then disappear. The rate of absorption depends on the type of material used. Absorbable sutures do not have to be removed by the surgeon or physician. Nonabsorbable suture material remains intact until it is removed. Suture materials are described by size and composition, as follows.

Size

Suture material size has been standardized by governmental regulations. The thickest or largest available size is #5, about the size of commercial string. Sizes progress downward from #5 to #0 and then from #2-0 to #11-0, the smallest. This "n-0" format was chosen as a more convenient way to express the number of zeros in the finer, more delicate suture sizes. For example, suture size 0000 is written as 4-0. Suture material is available in lengths from 13 cm to 150 cm.

Composition

Natural and synthetic materials are used for sutures. Natural materials include plain catgut, surgical cotton and silk, and chromic catgut. Synthetic materials include nylon and polyester. There are many types of natural and synthetic suture materials. The surgeon chooses the type of material best suited to the tissue being sutured.

In many cases surgical staples are used to close incisions. Staples can be made of surgical steel, plastic, or a Teflonlike material. Below are some of the more commonly used suture materials.

catgut	Dexon	Nurolon	surgical cotton
chromatic catgut	Ethilon	nylon	surgical silk
Dacron	Mersilene	PDS II	Tantalum
Dermalene	Monocryl	Prolene	Vicryl
Dermalon	Novafil	stainless steel	

SUTURE TECHNIQUE

Suture technique refers to the method used to unite parts. There are two basic suturing methods: continuous and interrupted. A continuous suture runs from one end of the incision to the other without being snipped or tied between. The interrupted suture is tied and cut with each completed stitch so that each stitch is independent of any other stitch. Figure 7-10 illustrates the continuous and interrupted suture methods.

There are many types of suture techniques. Most are modifications of the continuous or interrupted methods. Suture techniques are often named for the general appearance of the suture or for the person who developed the technique. Below are some of the more interesting names of suture techniques. It is easy to imagine what these sutures look like.

baseball	chain	fish hook	pursestring
blanket	circular	mattress	sliding
button	crown	noose	zipper

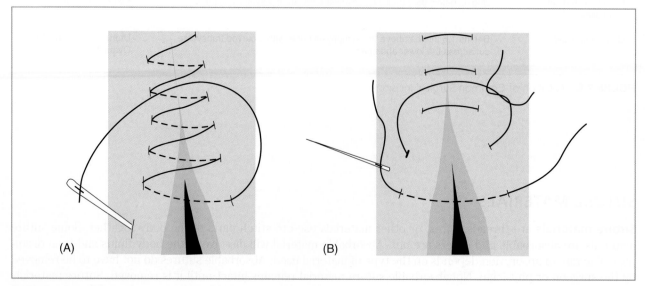

FIGURE 7-10   (A) Continuous Sutures; (B) Interrupted Sutures

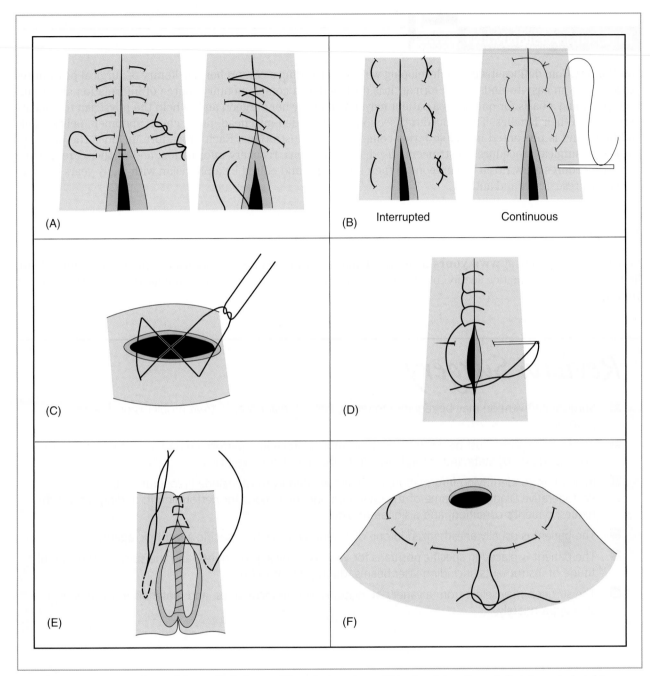

FIGURE 7-11 Commonly Used Suture Techniques: (A) vertical mattress; (B) horizontal mattress (left: interrupted; right: continuous); (C) figure-of-eight; (D) lock-stitch; (E) Connell; (F) pursestring

Some of the more commonly used suture techniques are illustrated in Figure 7-11.

REFERENCES

This chapter presents the basic information needed to use and understand surgical terminology. For more detailed assistance, the medical secretary and surgical transcriptionist can turn to one of the many surgical word reference books available or the Internet. These sources contain listings of surgical equipment and specific information about surgical specialties.

INTERNET ASSIGNMENT

YourSurgery.Com defines itself as a developing web site providing a comprehensive library of surgical procedures presented in an easy-to-understand format. It is designed as a complementary source of information about surgery, providing a basis for questions a patient may ask of his or her surgeon and to help the physician to educate patients and their families. The Procedures section is subdivided into head, neck, chest, abdomen, pelvis, back, and limbs and is presented in simple terms complete with illustrations. Each procedure includes the anatomy, pathology, surgical procedures, instruments used, complications, recovery information, and further care instructions. Procedures are written by surgeons in their specialties and edited by a physician with many years of experience as a researcher and author.

ACTIVITY

Visit YourSurgery.Com at **www.yoursurgery.com** and select Procedures. Click on a treatment procedure identified in the Working Practice section of Chapter 6. Read the entire procedure and summarize one of the parts for your instructor.

Review: Surgery

- Surgical intervention may be required to repair, correct, diagnose, or treat problems or disease processes.

- Operative Reports must be written for every surgical procedure performed and must contain information mandated by state and federal laws and other regulatory agencies.

- In addition to identifying information, an Operative Report must include Preoperative and Postoperative Diagnoses, name of the operation and indications for performing it, findings and techniques, patient's condition, and a signature block.

- The patient is usually anesthetized in one of several ways with a specific anesthetic agent.

- The patient is placed in specific positions for various surgical procedures, and the surgeon uses a multitude of instruments, including laser beams, during the procedure.

- The surgeon may select from a variety of incisions, suture techniques, and materials to close an incision appropriately.

Review of Terminology Presented

Word	Definition
anesthesia	loss of feeling or sensation; may be general, regional, local, or topical
anesthesiologist	physician who specializes in anesthesiology
anesthesiology	branch of medicine that studies anesthesia and anesthetic agents
anesthetic agent	drug used to induce anesthesia

continues

Word	Definition
anesthetist	nurse trained in administering anesthetic agents
block anesthesia	anesthetic agent injected near or along a nerve path to stop nerve impulses to the area supplied by that nerve
bronchus	one of the two larger air passages to the lungs below the trachea
coagulation	clotting of blood or hardening of tissue
endobronchial induction	introduction of gaseous mixture into a large bronchus to produce anesthesia
endotracheal induction	introduction of gaseous mixture into the trachea by a tube to produce anesthesia
epidural block	injection of anesthetic into the epidural space of the spinal column
field block	anesthesia produced by injecting a local anesthetic along the course of a nerve or nerves to prevent pain sensation in the area around the operative site
Findings and Technique	part of the Operative Report that includes type of anesthesia, surgical position, incision, description, closure, patient condition, and signature block
general anesthesia	anesthesia that produces loss of consciousness with an absence of pain sensation over the entire body
incision	surgical cut
Indications	part of the operative report that describes why the procedure was necessary
infiltration	injection of anesthetic into tissue
inhalation	breathing in of a gaseous anesthetic agent
insufflation	introduction of an anesthetic agent through a slender tube into the respiratory tract
intercostal block	anesthesia produced by injecting the anesthetic agent into the nerves along or near the ribs
intravenous	introduction of anesthetic agent into a vein
laser	instrument used to cut, coagulate, or vaporize tissue by way of an intense, narrow light beam that produces heat
local anesthesia	anesthetic agent confined to one part of the body
modes of induction	ways in which anesthetic agents are introduced into the body
nerve block	regional anesthesia that follows a nerve or group of nerves
Operation	part of the Operative Report that describes the procedure(s) performed
Operative Report	written record of a surgical procedure that contains mandated information
perineum	area between the anus and genitalia
Postoperative Diagnosis	part of the Operative Report that states the diagnosis after surgery is completed and gives a short descriptive explanation of what was actually found
Preoperative Diagnosis	part of the Operative Report that describes the diagnosis before surgery is peformed
prognosis	probable outcome
regional anesthesia	anesthetic agent that interrupts nerve conduction from a specific region of the body
saddle block	local anesthesia produced by injecting anesthetic into the area of the spine that affects the buttocks, perineum, and inner aspects of the thighs
spinal block	regional anesthesia produced by injecting anesthetic into the subarachnoid space around the spinal cord

continues

Word	Definition
subarachnoid space	space between the arachnoid and pia layers of the brain and spinal cord
suture materials	threads, wires, or other materials used to stitch parts of the body together
suture technique	method used to unite parts; may be interrupted or continuous
topical anesthesia	anesthetic agent applied to the surface of the area involved
trachea	windpipe

Terminology Review Exercises

Name: _____ Date: _____

SHORT ANSWER*

Supply a short answer to the following:

1. Name and define the major components of an Operative Report.

   _____

   _____

   _____

   _____

   _____

   _____

2. Name three modes of induction for general anesthesia.

   _____

3. Name three modes of induction for regional anesthesia.

   _____

4. Name two modes of induction for local anesthesia.

   _____

COMPLETION*

Complete the following statements.

1. The _____ section of the Operative Report can be a separate paragraph or included in the main body of the report.

2. _____ _____ describes how the patient was placed on the operating table.

3. A surgical cut used to access various parts of the body is called an _____.

4. The _____ and _____ section of the Operative Report includes a detailed and technical narrative of the entire operation.

5. _____ _____ are threads, wires, or other materials used to stitch parts of the body together.

6. The methods used to unite body parts are called _____.

7. A _____ suture runs from one end of the incision to the other.

8. An _____ suture is tied and cut with each completed stitch.

9. As an instrument, the _____ is used to cut, coagulate, or vaporize tissue.

10. The _____ _____ is an accounting for all surgical tools such as sponges, needles, and instruments.

_____

*Answers are in Appendix A.

IDENTIFICATION—MATERIALS AND TECHNIQUES
Identify the following terms as suture material (M) or suture technique (T).

1. mattress   _____
2. Mersilene   _____
3. pursestring   _____
4. Vicryl   _____
5. dacron   _____
6. catgut   _____
7. monocryl   _____
8. sliding   _____
9. Connell   _____
10. lock-stitch   _____

IDENTIFICATION
Identify the following surgical positions.

1. flat on back with legs extended

   _____

2. flat on abdomen; position for back surgery

   _____

3. lying on back with table tilted toward the head, bent at knees

   _____

4. lying on right or left side

   _____

5. lying on back with legs in stirrups

   _____

SPELLING
Rewrite the misspelled words.

1. anestethist   _____
2. epidural   _____
3. currete   _____
4. dialator   _____
5. hemostat   _____
6. scalple   _____
7. insuflation   _____
8. coagulation   _____
9. intravenus   _____
10. perineum   _____

Word Element Review

Root	Meaning	Example	Definition
esthesi/o	feeling, sensation	**esthesiogenic** (es-thē"zē-ō-jĕn'ik)	producing sensation

Prefix	Meaning	Example	Definition
ant-, anti-	against	**antiemetic** (ăn"tǐ-ē-mēt'ǐk)	medication that prevents or alleviates vomiting
hyper-	above, more than	**hyperemia** (hī"per-ē'mē-ah)	excess blood in a part
pro-	before, in front of, favoring	**proptosis** (prŏp-tō'sǐs)	forward displacement or bulging

Suffix	Meaning	Example	Definition
-cele	hernia	**cystocele** (sǐs'tō-cēl)	protrusion of the bladder through the vaginal wall
-centesis	puncture and aspiration of	**thoracentesis** (thŏr"rah-sĕn-tē'sǐs)	surgical puncture of chest wall for aspiration of fluids
-desis	binding, fixation	**arthrodesis** (ăr"thrō-dē'sǐs)	surgical fusion of a joint
-ectomy	surgical removal, excision	**gastrectomy** (găs-trĕk'tō-mē)	surgical removal of the stomach or a portion of it
-lysis	breakdown, destruction, loosening, setting free	**hemolysis** (hē-mŏl'ǐ-sǐs)	destruction of red blood cells with the setting free of hemoglobin
-oid	like, resembling	**dermoid** (der'moid)	skinlike
-oma	tumor, neoplasm	**carcinoma** (kar"sǐ-nō'mah)	malignant new growth or tumor
-ostomy	creation of a new opening	**colostomy** (kŏ-lŏs'tō-mē)	surgical creation of a new opening between the colon and the body surface
-otomy	incision into	**gastrotomy** (găs-trŏt'tō-mē)	incision into the stomach
-pexy	surgical fixation	**hysteropexy** (hǐs'ter-ō-pĕk"sē)	surgical fixation of a displaced uterus
-plasty	surgical correction or repair	**arthroplasty** (ăr'thrō-plăs"tē)	surgical repair of a joint
-rrhaphy	suture of	**herniorrhaphy** (her"nē-ōr'ah-fē)	surgical repair of a hernia, with suturing
-rrhexis	break, burst forth, rupture	**angiorrhexis** (ăn"jē-ō-rĕk'sǐs)	rupture of a blood vessel
-tripsy	crushing, friction	**lithotripsy** (lǐth'ō-trǐp"sē)	crushing of a stone within the bladder or urethra

Word Element Review Exercises

Name: _____ Date: _____

MATCHING*

Match the terms to their meanings.

1. _____ surgical fixation of a displaced uterus
2. _____ creation of a new opening between the colon and the body surface
3. _____ destruction of red blood cells with the setting free of hemoglobin
4. _____ skinlike
5. _____ forward placement or bulging
6. _____ suture of a hernia
7. _____ excision of the stomach or a portion of it
8. _____ rupture of a blood vessel
9. _____ surgical puncture of the chest wall for aspiration of fluids
10. _____ malignant new growth or tumor
11. _____ excess blood in a part
12. _____ crushing of a stone in the bladder or urethra
13. _____ protrusion of the bladder through the vaginal wall
14. _____ incision into the stomach
15. _____ surgical repair of a joint
16. _____ surgical fusion of a joint
17. _____ medication that prevents or eliminates vomiting
18. _____ producing a feeling or sensation

a. angiorrhexis
b. antiemetic
c. arthrodesis
d. arthroplasty
e. carcinoma
f. colostomy
g. cystocele
h. dermoid
i. esthesiogenic
j. gastrectomy
k. gastrotomy
l. hemolysis
m. herniorrhaphy
n. hyperemia
o. hysteropexy
p. lithotripsy
q. proptosis
r. thoracentesis

WORD ELEMENTS AND DEFINITIONS*

In the underlined words below, circle the word element presented in this chapter. Then provide the definition of the word.

1. The patient is scheduled for a <u>gastrotomy</u> tomorrow.

   _____

2. The <u>arthroplasty</u> of her knee allowed her to walk without crutches.

   _____

3. A <u>proptosis</u> of the eye can be corrected by surgery.

   _____

4. We hope the problem will be solved after the patient's scheduled <u>arthrodesis</u>.

   _____

5. <u>Hyperemia</u> was caused by additional swelling around the elastic bandage wrap.

   _____

---

*Answers are in Appendix A.

6. An <u>antiemetic</u> was given after the chemotherapy session.

_____

7. The surgeon found evidence of a <u>carcinoma</u> in the upper abdomen.

_____

SPELLING

Rewrite the misspelled words.

1. herniorhaphy   _____

2. angiorrexis   _____

3. lithotripsy   _____

4. cystosele   _____

5. colostomy   _____

6. dermoyd   _____

WORD ELEMENT MEANINGS

Give the meaning of each word element. Then use your dictionary to find a new word that contains each of the word elements. Specify whether the new word is a noun or an adjective by placing N or A in the last column.

Word Element	Meaning	Word	N or A
1. anti-, ant-			
2. -cele			
3. -centesis			
4. -desis			
5. -ectomy			
6. esthesi/o			
7. hyper-			
8. -lysis			
9. -oid			
10. -oma			
11. -ostomy			
12. -otomy			
13. -pexy			
14. -plasty			
15. pro-			
16. -rrhaphy			
17. -rrhexis			
18. -tripsy			

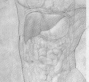

Dictionary Exercises

Name: _____ Date: _____

DICTIONARY EXERCISE 1

Use your dictionary to find the pronunciation and definition of the following words.

	Word	Pronunciation	Definition
1.	ampulla	_____	_____
2.	anastomosis	_____	_____
3.	aponeurosis	_____	_____
4.	bifurcation	_____	_____
5.	cautery	_____	_____
6.	cicatrix	_____	_____
7.	cruciate	_____	_____
8.	electrocoagulation	_____	_____
9.	enucleation	_____	_____
10.	exudate	_____	_____
11.	fulguration	_____	_____
12.	imbricated	_____	_____
13.	intubation	_____	_____
14.	microinstrumentation	_____	_____
15.	peritoneum	_____	_____

DICTIONARY EXERCISE 2

Pronunciation of the words below is provided. Using your dictionary, find the correct spelling and definition of each word.

	Word	Pronunciation	Definition
1.	_____	ā'pĕks	_____
2.	_____	ăs'pĭ-rāt	_____
3.	_____	kah-rī'nah	_____
4.	_____	kŏl'oyd	_____
5.	_____	ĕn-kăp"sū-lā'shŭn	_____
6.	_____	fĭm'brē-āt-ĕd	_____
7.	_____	ĭn-sī'tū	_____
8.	_____	ĭn'dū-rāt"ĕd	_____
9.	_____	lī-gā'shŭn	_____
10.	_____	loo'mĕn	_____
11.	_____	lī'sĭs	_____
12.	_____	rē-flĕk'shŭn	_____
13.	_____	sā'lēn	_____
14.	_____	sē-rō'sah	_____
15.	_____	sē'rŭs	_____

DICTIONARY EXERCISE 3*

Look up the meaning of each italicized word. Write the pronunciation in the space provided. Then rewrite the sentence in your own words.

1. The bleeder was *clamped* and *ligated* (_____).

   _____

2. Several skin conditions can be treated with *cryotherapy* (_____).

   _____

3. The surgeon was able to remove the growth *en bloc* (_____).

   _____

4. A *freely movable mass* was identified during exploratory surgery.

   _____

5. During the colonoscopy, the lining of the colon was very *friable* (_____).

   _____

6. *Hemostasis* (_____) was secured.

   _____

7. Adhesions were removed by *blunt* and *sharp dissection* (_____).

   _____

8. The *Scultetus bandage* (_____) was best suited for the wound.

   _____

9. *Ligatures* (_____) are used by surgeons and orthodontists.

   _____

10. Dilation and *curettage* (_____) are used to remove tumors.

    _____

_____

*Answers are in Appendix A.

Listening Exercise

INSTRUCTIONS

1. Review the spelling, pronunciation, and meaning of the words provided in the preview.
2. Listen to the audio CD and fill in the blank as the word is dictated.
3. At the end of the exercise, check your spelling against the preview words. They appear in the preview in the order in which they are encountered in the exercise.
4. Review and practice the words you missed.
5. Look up words that are not familiar.

PREVIEW OF WORDS FOR LISTENING EXERCISE 7-1

Word	Pronunciation	Meaning
hyperalimentation	hī"pĕr-ăl"ĭ-mĕn-tā'shŭn	intravenous infusion of fluids to augment or substitute for nutritional requirements of patients with severe absorption problems in the GI tract
Xylocaine	zī'lō-kāne	anesthetic agent to sterilize surgical site
Trendelenburg	trĕn-dĕl'ĕn-bŭrg	surgical position in which patient's head is low and the body and legs are on an elevated and inclined plane
fluoroscopic	floŏ"or-ō-skŏp'ĭc	pertaining to the use of an x-ray device that allows the surgeon to visualize on a screen the internal area in which the procedure is being done
clavicle	klăv'ĭ-k'l	collarbone
lumen	lū'mĕn	space within a tube, artery, vein, or intestine. In this case, the catheter has a single entrance.

OPERATIVE NOTE

DATE OF PROCEDURE: 8/21/20—

PROCEDURE:

1. Placement of Hickman catheter for _____ and hydration.

SURGEON: Dr. Sean O'Shancy

ANESTHESIA: Versed 3.5 mg, Demerol 50 mg IV, 1% _____ with epinephrine.

INDICATIONS: This is a 65-year-old female with short bowel syndrome who needed intravenous access for IV fluids and hyperalimentation. She had a port removed recently because of persistent infection.

FINDINGS: Normal anatomy, no difficulty in entering the left internal jugular vein.

PROCEDURE: After usual prep and drape, the left internal jugular area was infiltrated with Xylocaine with the patient in _____ position. The needle was introduced into the internal jugular vein without difficulty and a J-wire threaded under _____ guidance. A small incision was made by the J-wire entrance site and subsequently a counter incision was made near the left breast medially about 15 cm below the _____. A tunnel was developed and a single-_____ Hickman by Bard with Vitacath was advanced through the tunnel. Venous dilator and introducer were placed around the J-wire through the superior vena cava and the catheter, which was cut to an appropriate length, was then threaded under fluoroscopic guidance. After position of the catheter, the neck site was closed with 3-0 nylon vertical mattress suture. The catheter was secured with 3-0 nylon tied in a Chinese fingertrap fashion. Betadine ointment was applied to the exit site and dressing was applied. A chest x-ray was ordered.

Signature _____

Sean O'Shancy, MD

CHAPTER 8

The Cardiovascular System

> *Everywhere he feels his heart because its vessels run to all limbs.*
>
> —Anonymous

OBJECTIVES

When you have completed this study of the cardiovascular system, you should be able to

1. Spell and define major system components and explain how they operate.
2. Identify the meaning of related word elements.
3. Spell and define diagnostic procedures, diagnoses, treatment procedures, and abbreviations.
4. Spell the names of commonly used medications.
5. Be familiar with terminology used in reports.

INTRODUCTION

Blood travels through a closed circular system referred to as the cardiovascular system, which is composed of the heart and blood vessels or vascular network. Blood continuously travels through the heart, into the arteries and their smaller branches, then to the capillaries, into the branches of the vein structure, and back to the heart. The heart serves as the pump that keeps the blood moving. A physician who specializes in the study of the heart is a cardiologist.

HEART

The heart is one of the strongest organs in the human body. It does an incredible amount of work during a person's life span. With an average 70 to 80 beats per minute, the heart will beat more than $2\frac{1}{2}$ *billion* times in seventy years. An adult heart pumps about 4,000 gallons of blood a day. Most people do not even recognize this as a strenuous activity.

COMPOSITION

aort/o	aorta	pericardi/o	pericardium
atri/o	atrium	steth/o	chest
brady-	slow	tachy-	fast, rapid
cardi/o	heart	valv/o, valvul/o	valve
coron/o	heart	ventricul/o	ventricle
-megaly	enlargement		

The heart is a muscular organ slightly bigger than a fist. It is located between the lungs, somewhat to the left of the midline of the body.

As shown in Figure 8-1, there are actually three layers in the heart wall. The first is the **endocardium** (ĕn"dō-kăr'dē-ŭm) (1), which is the membrane that lines the interior of the heart. It is also the material that forms the valves of the heart. The second—and thickest layer—is the **myocardium** (mī"ō-kăr'dē-ŭm) (2), which is the muscle of the heart. The third—and outermost layer—is the **epicardium** (ĕp"ĭ-kăr'dē-ŭm) (4). The heart itself is surrounded by the **pericardial** (pĕr"ĭ-kăr'dē-ăl) **sac** (3), whose lining is called the **pericardium** (pĕr"ĭ-kăr'dē-ŭm). In the space between the pericardium and the epicardium there is a small amount of lubricating fluid.

Physicians sometimes refer to the left and right heart because the heart is responsible for two specific types of circulation. The left heart is involved in systemic circulation, which is the movement of blood from the heart to all parts of the body and back to the heart. The right heart is involved in pulmonary circulation, which is the movement of blood from the heart to the lungs and back to the heart.

Imagine the left and right sides of the heart as back-to-back pumps that beat or function as one. The two sides are completely separated by a partition called the **septum** (sĕp'tŭm). Note in Figure 8-2 that the upper part of the partition is called the **interatrial** (ĭn"ter-ā'trē-ăl) **septum** (8), and the lower portion is called the **interventricular** (ĭn"ter-vĕn-trĭk'ū-lăr) **septum** (9). The septum prevents the blood in the two sides of the heart from mixing. In fact, to get from one side of the heart to the other, blood must go through the entire body.

Each side of the heart has two chambers or sections. One is a receiving chamber and the other is a pumping chamber. The **left atrium** (ā'trē-ŭm) (4), one of the upper chambers of the heart, receives blood high in oxygen

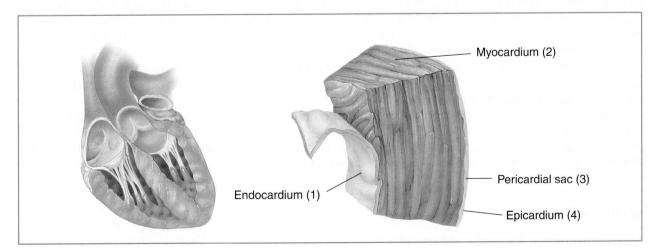

FIGURE 8-1 Layers of the Heart Wall

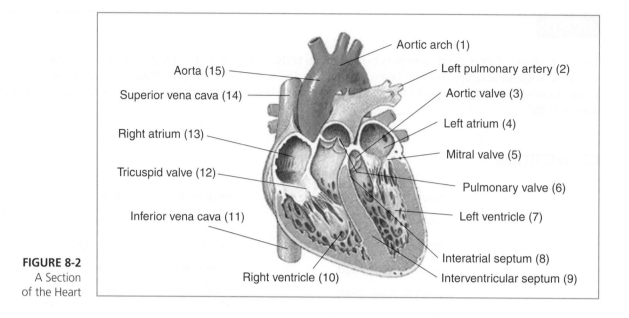

FIGURE 8-2
A Section
of the Heart

content as it returns from the lungs by way of the pulmonary veins. The pulmonary vein is the only vein that carries oxygen-rich blood. The blood then moves to the lower chamber or **left ventricle** (věn'trĭ-k'l) (7)—which has the thickest walls of all the chambers—where newly oxygenated blood is pumped to all parts of the body.

Blood leaves the left ventricle and goes through the arteries via the **aorta** (ā-or'tah) (15), called the great artery. The aorta curves in a great **aortic arch** (1) up from the heart, down the spine, and into the abdomen. From there several smaller arterial systems carry the blood to the head, digestive organs, arms, legs, and other body parts, where it discharges its load of nutrients and oxygen.

The blood then collects carbon dioxide and castoffs from cells and flows into the venules. From there it makes its way back to the heart through the two largest veins of the body called **venae cavae** (vē'nē kā'vē). The **superior vena cava** (vē'nah kā'vah) (14) drains blood from the upper part of the body, and the **inferior vena cava** (11) carries blood from the lower part of the body. Both drain this "used" blood into the upper chamber of the heart or **right atrium** (13).

The blood next moves into the lower chamber or **right ventricle** (10), which contracts to send the deoxygenated blood to the **pulmonary** (pul'mō-něr"ē) **artery** (2). The pulmonary artery takes the blood back to the lungs, where it absorbs fresh oxygen. This whole process, which takes about one minute, then starts all over.

Each pumping chamber, or ventricle, has two valves, one at the entrance and one at the exit. The purpose of the valves is to seal the chambers tightly so that contracting muscles have something to work against. The valves also prevent a backflow of blood.

The **tricuspid** (trī-kŭs'pĭd) **valve** (12) at the entrance to the right ventricle prevents blood from going back into the right atrium. When the right ventricle has finished emptying itself, the **pulmonary valve** (6) closes to prevent blood pumped out to the lungs from returning to the right ventricle. On the other side of the heart, muscles of the powerful left ventricle begin their contraction, and the **mitral** (mī'trăl) **valve** (5), made of two heavy flaps, closes the chamber's entrance to keep blood from returning to the left atrium. At the end of the contraction, the **aortic valve** (3) closes to prevent the backflow of the enriched aortic blood.

Abnormal heart sounds are called murmurs. Often **murmurs** are due to faulty valve action such as failure to close tightly so that blood will not seep back into a chamber. Another condition giving rise to an abnormal sound is the narrowing, or **stenosis** (stě-nō'sĭs), of a valve orifice.

Many conditions can cause abnormal heart sounds. These sounds, which can be heard with a stethoscope, might be caused by congenital defects, disease, or physiological variation. An abnormal sound caused by a structural change in the heart or the vessels connected with the heart is called an organic murmur. A functional murmur is one that does not necessarily involve an abnormality in the heart structure.

WORK OF THE HEART

Although the right and left sides of the heart are completely separate, they work together. The blood is squeezed through the chambers by a contraction of heart muscle, first in the thin-walled upper chambers (the atria) and then in the thick muscle of the lower chambers (the ventricles). The right and left atria contract together; then the right and left ventricles contract together.

The active phase of contraction, or pumping, is called **systole** (sĭs'tō-lē), and is followed immediately by a short resting period known as **diastole** (dī-ăs'tō-lē). The contraction of the walls of the atria is completed as the contraction of the ventricles begins. Thus, the resting phase (diastole) begins in the atria at the same time the contraction (systole) begins in the ventricles.

Although the heart muscle is capable of contracting in rhythm independent of outside control, impulses from the nervous system are required to cause a beat rapid enough to maintain circulation effectively. The normal heartbeat range for an adult is usually 60 to 100 beats per minute and is referred to as the **pulse rate**.

CONDUCTION SYSTEM OF THE HEART

Specialized masses of tissue in the heart wall form the conduction system of the heart to regulate the order of events. Two of these specialized masses are called nodes, and the third is a branching structure called the **atrioventricular bundle**.

Figure 8-3 shows the **sinoatrial** (sĭ"nō-ā'trē-al) **node** (SA) (1) in the upper wall of the right atrium. Its function is to act as a pacemaker. The second node is called the **atrioventricular** (ā"trē-ō-vĕn-trĭk'ū-lar) **node** (AV) (2) and is located at the septum at the junction between the interatrial portion and the interventricular portion. The atrioventricular bundle, or the **bundle of His** (hĭss) (4), is located in the interventricular septum, with branches extending to all parts of the ventricle walls.

The order in which the impulses travel through the heart is as follows.

1. The beginning of the heartbeat is in the sinoatrial node (1), the pacemaker.
2. The excitation wave travels throughout the muscles of the atria (3 and 7), causing them to contract.
3. The atrioventricular node (2) is stimulated next and transmits a wave to the bundle of His (4) with a rapid spread to all parts of the ventricle walls (5 and 6).
4. The entire ventricular musculature then contracts—practically all at once.

All of these events happen without conscious thought or action. It is easy to see why the function of the heart is so critical to the effective operation of the cardiovascular system.

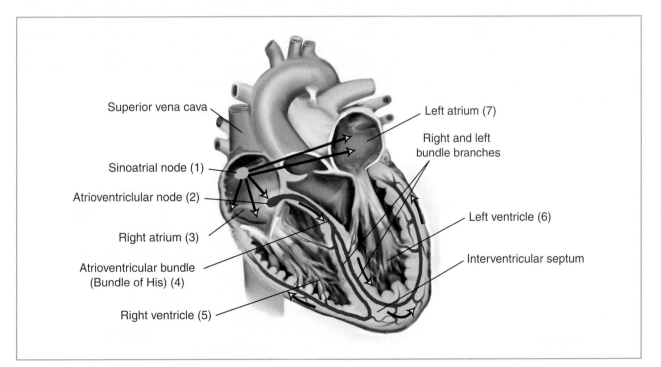

FIGURE 8-3 Conduction System of the Heart

VASCULAR SYSTEM

When the blood leaves the heart, it enters the vascular system. This system is composed of a variety of vessels that transport the blood to all parts of the body, provide for the exchange of certain substances between the blood and body fluids, and eventually return the blood to the heart. Physicians who specialize in surgical procedures performed on veins and arteries are called cardiovascular surgeons.

TYPES OF BLOOD VESSELS

angi/o	blood vessel	phleb/o	vein
arter/o, arteri/o	artery	thromb/o	clot, lump
ather/o	yellowish plaque, fatty substance	vascul/o, vas/o	vessel
furc/o	division, fork	ven/o	vein

On the basis of function, blood vessels may be divided into three groups: arteries, capillaries, and veins, as illustrated in Figure 8-4. **Arteries** (2) (with the exception of the pulmonary artery) carry oxygen-rich blood from the pumping chambers of the heart to the organs and other parts of the body. The pulmonary artery carries deoxygenated blood from the right ventricle of the heart to the lungs. The arteries have the thickest walls and are composed of three layers. These are the **intima** (ĭn'tĭ-mah) (or endothelium), the smooth innermost surface; a bulky layer of involuntary muscle called the **media**; and an outer tunic of supporting connective tissue called the **adventitia** (ăd"vĕn-tĭsh'ē-ah).

The arterial system starts with the aorta. It is the largest artery, with a diameter of about one inch, and also has the thickest wall. Arteries branch and rebranch throughout the body and become smaller and smaller. The smallest subdivision, the **arterioles** (ar-tē'rē-ōls) (1), have thinner walls with little connective tissue and more muscle.

The microscopic branches of these tiny connecting vessels, **capillaries** (3), have the thinnest walls of any vessels—only one cell layer. Because of this thinness, exchanges between the blood and the body cells are possible. During the outbound pass of arterial blood, oxygen leaves the blood and passes freely through these thin capillary walls to enter body cells.

On the return, capillaries drain waste products from tissues into **venules** (vĕn'ūls) (4), the smallest veins. Venules are formed by the union of capillaries; their walls are only slightly thicker than those of the capillaries. Venules then join to form **veins** (5). With the exception of the pulmonary vein, veins carry deoxygenated blood back to the heart. The pulmonary vein carries oxygen-rich blood from the lungs to the left atrium. Like arteries, veins have three layers. They are much thinner than arteries and collapse easily. Therefore, only slight pressure by a tumor or some other mass may interfere with the return blood flow. Essentially arteries and veins are a long, continuous tube, with the capillaries being the smallest portion.

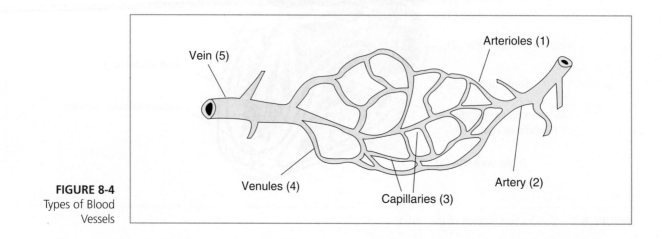

FIGURE 8-4
Types of Blood Vessels

Systemic Arteries

All arteries, carrying oxygen-rich blood, branch from the aorta. In Figure 8-5 is the **aortic arch** (3), which gives rise to the right innominate (ĭ-nŏm'ĭ-nāt) (brachiocephalic) (19), carotid (kah-rŏt'ĭd) (20 and 1), and left subclavian (sŭb-klā'vē-ăn) (18 and 2) arteries. The next section of the descending aorta is the **thoracic** (thō-răs'ĭk) **aorta** (4), located from the arch to the level of the diaphragm. The thoracic aorta consists of nine or ten pairs of intercostal arteries that reach between the ribs, sending branches to the muscles and other structures of the chest wall.

Below the thoracic section and extending downward to the common iliac is the **abdominal aorta** (15) section. This is the longest aortic section and spans the abdominal cavity. Branches of the abdominal aorta may be unpaired or paired. The unpaired vessels have three important parts: the celiac (sē'lē-ăk) (17) trunk, the superior mesenteric (mĕs"ĕn-tĕr'ĭk) (16) artery, and the inferior mesenteric (6) artery. The paired branches are the phrenic (frĕn'ĭk), suprarenal, renal, ovarian or testicular, and lumbar arteries. (These are smaller arteries and are not shown in the drawing.)

The abdominal aorta finally divides into two common iliac (14) arteries. Each extends into the pelvis and subdivides into the internal (13) and external (12) iliac arteries. The internal iliac vessels send branches to the pelvic organs, including the urinary bladder, rectum, and some reproductive organs. The external iliac arteries continue into the thigh, where the name of these tubes is changed to femoral (fĕm'or-ăl) arteries (7 and 11). These vessels branch off in the thigh at the level of the knee and become the popliteal (pŏp-lĭt'ē-ăl) (8) arteries. Below the knee they further subdivide into the tibial (tĭb'ē-ăl) (9 and 10) arteries and extend into the ankle and foot.

Systemic Veins

Although most arteries are located and protected in deep areas, the veins are found both in protected areas and near the surface. Those near the surface are called **superficial veins**, because they lie just beneath the skin and

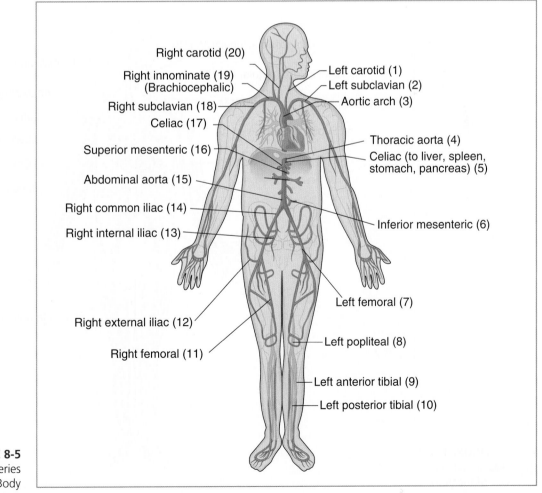

FIGURE 8-5
Major Arteries
of the Body

return blood from the skin and the subcutaneous regions to the deep veins. The **saphenous** (sah-fē'nŭs) **veins**, the longest veins of the body, are in the lower extremities. (These can be used in heart bypass surgery.) The veins on the back of the hand and at the front of the elbow are superficial veins. They are called cephalic (sě-făl'ĭk) (5), basilic (bah-sĭl'ĭk) (4), and median cubital (kū'bĭ-tal) (6) and are illustrated in Figure 8-6.

The deep veins travel alongside an artery and have the same name as the artery, although there are a few exceptions to this pattern. The femoral (7) and iliac (ĭl'ē-ăk) (8) vessels are found in the lower part of the body, and the brachial (brā'kē-ăl) (3), axillary (2), and subclavian (sŭb-klā'vē-ăn) (1) veins are in the upper extremities. Jugular (jŭg'ū-lăr) (12 and 13) veins drain the areas supplied by the carotid arteries. Two brachiocephalic (innominate) veins (11) are formed, one on each side of the neck, by the union of the subclavian and jugular veins.

All veins finally converge into one of two large trunks: the superior vena cava (10) and the inferior vena cava (9). The superior vena cava drains the veins of the head, neck, upper extremities, and chest, and the **azygos** (ăz'ĭ-gŏs) **vein** drains the veins of the chest wall.

The inferior vena cava is much longer than the superior vena cava and drains blood from parts of the body below the diaphragm. The large veins can be divided into two groups, paired and unpaired. The paired veins, such as the lumbar, renal, suprarenal, and hepatic veins, drain paired parts and organs.

The unpaired veins come from parts of the digestive tract and empty into a special vein called the portal tube. The blood coming from the intestines enters the liver through the portal system. Here a good portion of the glucose and protein is extracted and stored for future use. From there the blood flows through the hepatic vein and empties into the inferior vena cava.

PULSE AND BLOOD PRESSURE

Both pulse and blood pressure are good indicators of the efficiency of the cardiovascular system.

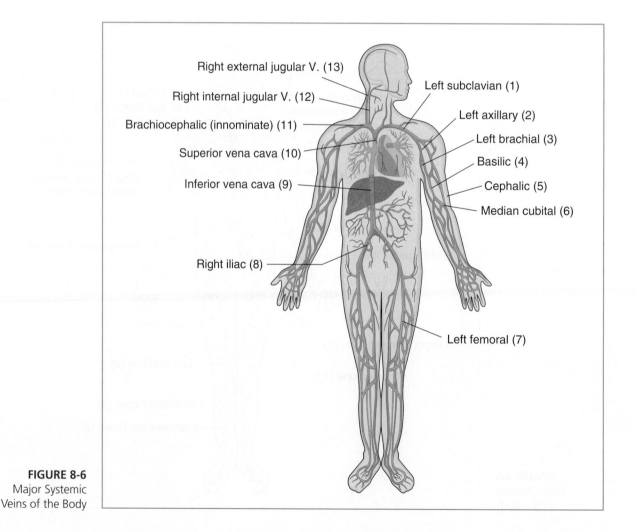

FIGURE 8-6
Major Systemic
Veins of the Body

Pulse

The ventricle pumps blood into arteries at a normal rate ranging from 60 to 100 times per minute. The force of ventricular contraction starts a wave of increased pressure beginning in the heart and traveling through the arteries. This wave is called the pulse. There are several factors that can influence the pulse rate. Here are a few of them.

1. The pulse is somewhat faster in smaller people and usually slightly faster in women than in men.
2. In a newborn infant, the rate may be from 120 to 140 beats per minute.
3. Physical activity influences the pulse rate. The rate can be 100 or higher with strenuous exercise, but may be as slow as 60 beats a minute during sleep.
4. Emotional disturbances can increase the pulse rate.
5. The pulse rate increases with a rise in temperature, such as with infection.

Blood Pressure

Blood pressure is the pressure exerted on the arterial walls by the blood, influenced by the rate of flow and resistance to flow. The instrument used to measure blood pressure is called a **sphygmomanometer** (sfig"mō-mah-nŏm'ĕ-ter) (also called a "cuff"). It takes the following two measurements.

Systolic pressure
The pressure on the arterial walls during the heart muscle contraction. Normal systolic pressure averages around 120 millimeters (mm) of mercury and may vary from 90 to 140 mm of mercury.

Diastolic pressure
The pressure on the arterial walls during relaxation, or the rest period, of the heart muscle. Normal diastolic pressure ranges from 50 to 90 mm of mercury and averages around 80 mm.

Lower-than-normal blood pressure is called **hypotension** (hī"pō-tĕn'shŭn). **Hypertension** (hī"per-tĕn'shŭn) is higher-than-normal blood pressure. The condition of the small arteries may have more effect on the diastolic pressure, thus making it more important than systolic pressure.

INTERNET ASSIGNMENT

healthfinder is a free guide to reliable consumer health and human services information. It was developed by the Office of Disease Prevention and Health Promotion of the U.S. Department of Health and Human Services in collaboration with other Federal agencies. healthfinder can lead you to over 1,800 selected online publications, clearinghouses, data bases, carefully reviewed web sites, and support and self-help groups, as well as government agencies and not-for-profit and professional organizations that produce reliable health information for the public.

The home page provides links to four general topics: health library, just for you, health care, and directory of healthfinder organizations. As an example of topic content, the directory of healthfinder organizations provides a list of related organizations based on a topic you enter. Clicking one of these organizations will bring up a list of organizations concerned about that topic, with links to their home pages. Alternatively, you may click on a letter to browse available topics and then click on a topic of choice and make your specific selection.

ACTIVITY

Access healthfinder at **www.healthfinder.gov**. Click on Health Library to get a list of general categories. You then may either select a category to get a browse list of available topics and choose one, or enter a specific topic in the search field at the top of the page. For this activity, key "how the heart works" into the search window. From the choices presented, select one, cite the source, and summarize the information found for your instructor.

Review: The Cardiovascular System

■ The heart consists of two separate parts that are divided by the septum: The left side receives oxygenated blood and pumps it into the aorta for distribution to the body; the right side receives "used" blood as it returns from the tissues.

■ The period of contraction, when the heart is beating, is referred to as systole; the resting phase of the heart is called diastole.

■ Beating rate is controlled by the sinoatrial node or the pacemaker, the atrioventricular node, and the bundle of His.

■ After blood leaves the heart, a system of arteries, arterioles, capillaries, venules, and veins circulates the blood through the body.

■ The aorta is the largest artery, and the superior and inferior venae cavae are the largest veins.

■ The rate at which blood is pumped is referred to as the pulse rate.

■ Blood pressure readings are a combination of systolic and diastolic pressure readings.

Review of Terminology Presented

Word	Definition
abdominal aorta	longest aortic section; spans the abdominal cavity
adventitia	outermost layer of an artery wall
aorta	great artery; its main trunk arises from the left ventricle
aortic valve	valve that prevents enriched blood from the aorta from returning to the left ventricle
aortic arch	continuation of the ascending aorta that gives rise to the brachiocephalic, carotid, and subclavian arteries
arteries	vessels that carry blood from the heart to the body
arterioles	smallest divisions of arteries
atrioventricular bundle (bundle of His)	specialized bundle of tissue that spreads impulses to all parts of the ventricle walls
atrioventricular node	specialized mass of tissues in the heart wall that carries impulses generated by the sinoatrial node to the bundle of His and ventricle walls
atrium, left and right (*pl.* atria)	upper chambers of the heart
azygos vein	vessel draining the veins of the chest wall into the superior vena cava
capillaries	tiny vessels that connect arterioles and venules to provide for the exchange between oxygenated and deoxygenated blood
diastole	resting phase of the heart
endocardium	membrane that lines the interior of the heart

continues

Word	Definition
epicardium	outermost layer of the heart
hypertension	higher-than-normal blood pressure
hypotension	lower-than-normal blood pressure
intima	innermost structure of an artery wall
media	middle layer of an artery wall
mitral valve	valve that prevents blood from the left ventricle from returning to the left atrium
murmurs	abnormal heart sounds
myocardium	muscle of the heart; middle and thickest layer
pericardial sac	sac surrounding the heart
pericardium	lining of the pericardial sac that surrounds the heart
pulmonary artery	artery that leads deoxygenated blood from the right ventricle to the lungs
pulmonary valve	valve that prevents blood from returning to the right ventricle
pulse rate	number of times per minute that the heart beats
saphenous veins	longest veins of the body located in the lower extremities
septum, interatrial and interventricular	partition that separates the two sides of the heart
sinoatrial node	natural pacemaker of the heart
sphygmomanometer	instrument used to measure blood pressure; a "cuff"
stenosis	narrowing
superficial veins	veins located near the surface
systole	pumping or contracting phase of the heart
thoracic aorta	section of the descending aorta from the aortic arch to the level of the diaphragm
tricuspid valve	valve that prevents blood from the right ventricle from returning to the right atrium
veins	vessels that carry blood from the body to the heart
vena cava, superior and inferior (*pl.* venae cavae)	largest veins of the body
ventricle, left and right	lower chambers of the heart
venules	smallest divisions of veins, formed by the union of capillaries

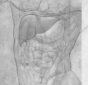

Terminology Review Exercises

Name: _____ Date: _____

SHORT ANSWER*

Supply a short answer to the following.

1. Name the four chambers of the heart and specify the function of each.

    _____

    _____

    _____

    _____

2. Name three types of blood vessels and state their function.

    _____

    _____

    _____

3. Explain the difference between diastolic and systolic blood pressure readings.

    _____

COMPLETION*

Complete the following statements.

1. The two sides of the heart are separated by a partition called the _____.
2. The four valves of the heart are the _____, _____,
    _____, and _____.
3. Abnormal heart sounds are called _____.
4. The active phase of the heart is _____; the resting period is _____.
5. Two types of heart murmurs are _____ and _____.
6. The pulse rate is _____ to _____ beats per minute.
7. The order in which the heart operates is controlled by the _____ system.
8. The sinoatrial node is often referred to as the _____ of the heart.
9. The smallest veins are called _____.
10. The aortic arch sends off three branches; they are the _____, _____,
    and _____.
11. The instrument used to measure blood pressure is called a _____.
12. The two major trunks of veins are the _____ and _____.
13. The largest artery of the body is the _____.
14. The origin of all arteries carrying oxygen-rich blood is the _____.
15. The longest section of the aorta is the _____.

---

*Answers are in Appendix A.

Working Practice

DIAGNOSTIC PROCEDURES

Word	Pronunciation	Definition
General		
cardiac catheterization	kăth"ĕ-tĕr-ĭ-zā'shŭn	intensive study of the heart that uses catheters to perform angiocardiography and/or pressure and flow measurement to determine the severity of suspected cardiac disease
Doppler ultrasound flowmeter		procedure using an apparatus that measures sound waves as echoes bounce off red blood cells
echocardiogram	ĕk"ō-kăr'dē-ō-grăm"	graphic record of reflected ultrasound waves from the heart
electrocardiogram (EKG, ECG)	ē-lĕk"trō-kăr'dē-ō-grăm"	electrical record of heart activity monitored by electrodes placed on the chest wall (Figure 8-7 provides an explanation of a normal tracing.)
Holter monitor		compact recording device that monitors EKG activity over a long period of time by using electrodes attached to a patient's chest; "24-hour EKG"
treadmill exercise tolerance test		evaluation of a patient's heart function as the exercise load on the treadmill is gradually increased
Nuclear Medicine		
angiocardiography	ăn"jē-ō-kăr"dē-ŏg'rah-fē	x-ray of the blood vessels after an injection of radioactive isotope material into the bloodstream
radionuclide angiography (multiple gated acquisition scan [MUGA scan])	rā"dē-ō-nū'klīd ăn"jē-ŏg'rah-fē	x-ray that uses radioactive isotopes injected into the blood vessels to evaluate the condition of the myocardium of the heart
stress thallium test	thăl'ē-ŭm	use of a radioactive tracer given during exercise to detect decreased blood flow to a portion of the heart muscle

continues

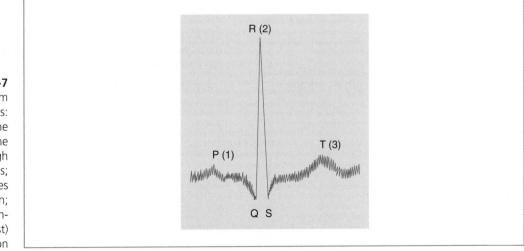

FIGURE 8-7
Electrocardiogram Components:
(1) P wave denotes the electrical impulse from the sinoatrial node through the atrial sinus;
(2) QRS complex denotes ventricle wall contraction;
(3) T wave denotes ventricular recovery (rest) phase after contraction

DIAGNOSTIC PROCEDURES

Word	Pronunciation	Definition
Radiology		
arteriography (angiography)	ăr-tē"rē-ŏg'rah-fē	x-raying of an artery or the artery system after an injection of radiopaque material into the bloodstream
cardiac magnetic resonance imaging (MRI)		test that uses magnetic waves beamed at the heart to produce an image; used to detect detailed information about various heart problems
PA (postero-anterior) and lateral of the chest	pŏs"tĕr-ō-an-tēr'ē-or	routine x-ray views of the lung fields and heart
venography	vē-nŏg'rah-fē	x-ray of the veins after an injection of radiopaque material into the bloodstream
Blood Tests		
arterial blood gases (ABGs)	ăr-tē'rē-ăl	measurement of oxygen, carbon dioxide, and metabolic balance from an arterial blood sample
cardiac enzymes	ĕn'zīms	measurement of the blood for the following: • *AST*—aspartate amniotransferase (ăs-păr'tāt ăm'nē-trănz-fĕr'ās), which is found in its highest concentration in the heart muscle, brain, and liver • *CPK*—creatine phosphokinase (krē'ah-tĭn fŏs"fō-kī'nās), which is released into the blood when the heart or skeletal muscles are injured • *LDH*—lactate dehydrogenase (lăk'tāt dē-hī-drŏj'ĕ-nās), which is an enzyme found primarily in the heart muscles, skeletal muscles, kidneys, liver, and red blood cells • *Troponin I* and *Troponin T*—cardiac-specific enzyme released from dying heart muscle cells
complete blood count (CBC)		measurement of the blood for the following: hemoglobin, hematocrit, red blood count, white blood count, and differential (the types and number of white blood cells present)
electrolytes	ē-lĕk'trō-līts	measurement of the blood for chloride, sodium, and potassium
serum lipids (lipid profile)		measurement of the blood cholesterol, high- and low-density lipoprotein, very low-density lipoprotein, and triglycerides
prothrombin time (PT)	prō-thrŏm'bĭn	tests the coagulation of blood

DIAGNOSES

Word	Pronunciation	Definition
Diseases of the Heart		
angina pectoris	ăn-jī'nah pĕk'tŏr-ĭs	attacks of severe chest pain caused by insufficient blood reaching the heart muscle
arteriosclerotic (coronary) heart disease (ASHD)	ăr-tē"rē-ō-sklĕ-rŏt'ĭk	heart disease produced by coronary artery disease
cardiomyopathy	kăr"dē-ō-mī-ŏp'ah-thē	weakening of the heart muscle
carditis	kăr-dī'tĭs	inflammation of the heart
congenital heart disease	kŏn-jĕn'ĭ-tăl	abnormalities in the heart at birth, such as septal defects, tetralogy of Fallot, and patent ductus arteriosus
congestive heart failure	kŏn-jĕs'tĭv	condition caused by the inability of the heart to pump (beat) adequately, resulting in an accumulation of fluid in tissues (edema or swelling) or in the lungs
hypertensive heart disease	hī"pĕr-tĕn'sĭv	disease characterized by prolonged high blood pressure with varying degrees of heart failure
hypertrophic obstructive cardiomyopathy	hī"pĕr-trŏf'ĭk, kăr"dē-ō-mī-ŏp'ah-thē	abnormal thickening of the heart muscle resulting in a restriction of the flow of blood from the heart
ischemia	ĭs-kē'mē-ah	inadequate flow of blood to a part of the body, caused by constriction or blockage of the blood vessels supplying it (See Figure 8-8)
myocardial infarction (MI)	mi"ō-kăr'dē-ăl ĭn-fărk'shŭn	heart attack; blood clot blocks the flow in one or more coronary arteries
myocarditis	mi"ō-kăr'dī'tĭs	inflammatory disease of the myocardium
pericarditis	per"ĭ-kăr'dī'tĭs	inflammatory disease of the pericardium
septal defect	sĕp'tăl	small holes in the septa between the artria or the ventricles

continues

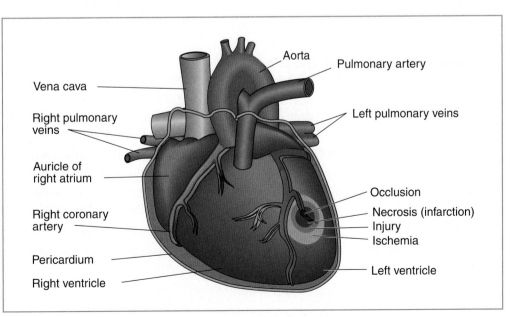

FIGURE 8-8
Areas of Ischemia After
Myocardial Infarction

DIAGNOSES		
Word	Pronunciation	Definition

Diseases of Heart Valves

infective endocarditis	ĭn-fec'tĭv ĕn"dō-kăr-dī'tĭs	inflammatory disease of the endocardium
mitral valve prolapse	mī'trăl, prō'lăps	extra clicking sound caused by failure of heart valves to close properly
murmur		abnormal sound in the heart or vascular system
regurgitation	rē-gŭr"jĭ-tā'shŭn	a backward flowing through a defective heart valve
rheumatic heart disease	roo-mă'tĭk	disease produced by rheumatic fever, particularly involving the valves
stenosis	stĕn-ō'sĭs	impairment of blood flow due to narrowing of a passage or valve
valvular insufficiency, valvular heart disease	văl'vū-lăr	failure of the heart valves (aortic, mitral, tricuspid, or pulmonic) to close completely, causing leakage

Disorders of Heart Rate and Rhythm

arrhythmia (dysrhythmia)	ah-rĭth'mē-ah (dĭs-rĭth'mē-ah)	irregular heartbeat; cause may be for one of several reasons
• *ectopic*	ĕk-tŏp'ĭk	small variation in the heartbeat, often called extrasystoles
• *atrial fibrillation*	ā'trē-ăl fĭ'brĭl-ā'shŭn	uncoordinated muscle contractions in the atria
• *atrial flutter*	ā'trē-ăl	atria contract too often
• *paroxysmal atrial tachycardia*	păr"ŏk-sĭz'măl ā'trē-ăl tăk"ē-kăr'dē-ă	rapid heart beat
• *ventricular tachycardia and fibrillation*	vĕn-trĭk'ū-lăr tăk"ē-kăr'dē-ă fĭ'brĭl-ā'shŭn	muscle fibers of ventricles are uncoordinated
bradycardia	brăd"ē-kăr'dē-ah	slow heart beat
sick sinus syndrome		sinus node initiates beats too slowly, pauses too long between beats, or stops producing beats

Disorders of Arteries, Veins, and Circulation

acrocyanosis	ăk"rō-sī-ă-nō-sĭs	bluish discoloration of the extremities caused by lack of oxygen to these parts
aneurysm	ăn'ū-rĭzm	weakness in the wall of a blood vessel, which causes the vessel to bulge or enlarge abnormally (See Figure 8-8)
atherosclerosis	ăth"ĕr-ō-klĕ-rō'sĭs	hardening of the arteries caused by deposits of cholesterol and calcium in the arterial walls (See Figure 8-9)
coarctation of the aorta	kō"ărk-tā'shŭn	malformation of the muscular wall of the aorta, which constricts to make the vessel narrower
coronary artery disease		narrowing of arteries that supply blood to the heart muscle
deep venous thrombosis (DVT)	thrŏm-bō'sĭs	clotting occurring in femoral and pelvic veins

continues

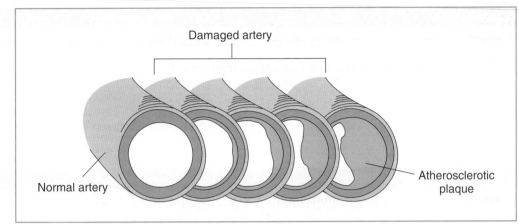

FIGURE 8-9
Artery Damaged
by Atherosclerotic Plaque

Word	Pronunciation	Definition
DIAGNOSES		
Disorders of Arteries, Veins, and Circulation *(continued)*		
embolism	ĕm'bō-lĭzm	free-moving clot or debris from a buildup of atherosclerotic plaque that may plug an artery
gangrene	găng'grēn	death of tissue resulting from deficient or absent blood supply
hypertension	hī"pĕr-tĕn'shŭn	high blood pressure; may be *primary or essential*—idiopathic gradual onset; or *secondary*—due to another problem
hypotension	hi"pĕr-tĕn'shŭn	low blood pressure
infarct	ĭn'fărkt	death of tissue resulting from inadequate blood supply
lymphedema	lĭmf-ĕ-dē'mah	abnormal accumulation of tissue fluid, often caused by venous obstruction
peripheral (hypertensive) vascular disease (PVD)		persistent high blood pressure caused by one of several diseases of the arteries
phlebitis	flĕ-bī'tĭs	inflammation of a superficial vein
Raynaud's phenomenon	rā-nōz' fĕ-nŏm'ĕ-nŏn	short episodes of pallor and numbness in the fingers and toes due to the temporary constriction of arterioles in the skin (See Figure 8-10)

continues

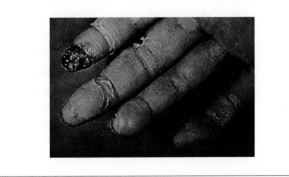

FIGURE 8-10 Arterial
Ulcers as a Result of
Raynaud's Phenomenon
(Courtesy of Marvin
Acerman, M.D.,
Scarsdale, NY)

DIAGNOSES

Word	Pronunciation	Definition
Disorders of Arteries, Veins, and Circulation (*continued*)		
thrombophlebitis	thrŏm″bō-flĕ-bi′tĭs	development of a clot in an inflamed vessel
thrombus	thrŏm′bŭs	fixed blood clot
varicose veins	văr′ĭ-kōs	abnormally swollen veins, usually occurring in the legs

TREATMENT PROCEDURES

Word	Pronunciation	Definition
aneurysmectomy	ăn″ū-rĭz-mĕk′tō-mē	surgical removal of an aneurysm
angioplasty	ăn′jē-ō-plăs″tē	surgical repair of a blood vessel
artery graft		replacement of a portion of an artery by another open structure (e.g., aortofemoral bypass graft, which is a graft between the abdominal aorta and the femoral artery)
atherectomy	ăth-ĕr-ĕk′tō-mē	technique using high-speed drills to remove atheromatous plaque from arteries
cardiomyoplasty	kăr″dē-ō-mī′ō-plăs-tē	surgical implantation of skeletal muscle to either supplement or replace myocardial muscle
cardiopulmonary resuscitation (CPR)	kăr″dē-ō-pŭl′mō-nĕr-ē rē-sŭs″ĭ-tā′shŭn	mouth-to-mouth breathing and chest compression
cardiotomy	kăr″dē-ŏt′ō-mē	surgical incision or opening of the heart for repair
cardioversion (defibrillation)	kar′dē-ō-vĕr″zhŭn (dē-fĭb″rĭ-lā′shŭn)	brief charges of electricity applied to the chest to stop cardiac arrhythmia
commissurotomy	kŏm″ĭ-shūr-ŏt′ō-mē	surgical incision of the connecting bands of a commissure; done to correct valvular stenosis (narrowing)
coronary artery bypass	kor′ŏ-nā-rē	open-heart surgery for the purpose of bypassing an obstructed coronary artery (See Figure 8-11)
correction of atrial septal defect	ā′trē-ăl sĕp′tăl	closure of an abnormal opening in the interatrial septum
correction of ventricular septal defect	vĕn-trĭk′ū-lăr	repair of an abnormal opening in the interventricular septum
defibrillation	dē-fĭb″rĭ-lā′shŭn	delivery of electric shock during emergency situation to return heart to normal rhythm
embolectomy	ĕm″bō-lĕk′tō-mē	removal of an embolus (a plug or clot) from a blood vessel
endarterectomy	ĕnd″ăr-ter-ĕk′tō-mē	removal of the interior portion of an artery and occluding fatty deposits
extracorporeal circulation	ĕks″tră-kŏr′ē-ăl	circulation of blood outside of the body for purposes of removing or exchanging substances
heart transplantation		replacement of the patient's malfunctioning heart with a donor's heart

continues

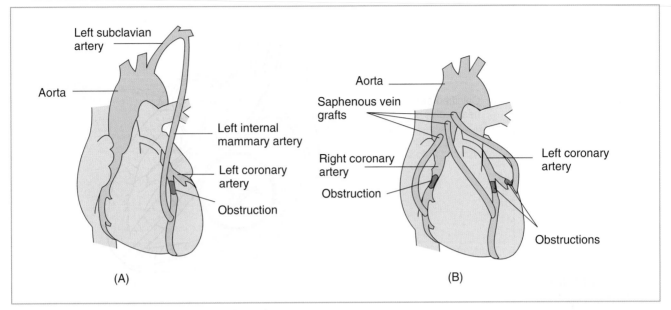

FIGURE 8-11   Coronary Bypass: (A) single; (B) triple

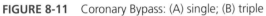

TREATMENT PROCEDURES		
Word	**Pronunciation**	**Definition**
heart valve valvuloplasty	văl'ŭ-lō-plăs"tē	insertion of a guidewire (with a balloon on its tip) through an artery to a diseased valve where the balloon is inflated (Figure 8-12 illustrates this procedure.)
internal cardioverter-defibrillator (ICD)	kăr'dē-ō-věr"těr dē-fĭb"rĭ-lā'tŏr	battery-driven device implanted in the chest to sense abnormal heart rhythm and emit a signal to bring it back to normal
intra-aortic balloon pump (IABP)	ĭn"tră-ā-or'tĭc	mechanical device to help improve coronary blood flow and systemic circulation in weak hearts
left ventricular assist device (LVAD)	věn-trĭk'ū-lăr	external circulatory support device used after bypass surgery to ensure unidirectional blood flow
pacemaker cardiac defibrillator (PCD)	dē-fĭb"rĭ-lă'tŏr	small electronic device consisting of a battery and an electrode implanted in the chest and heart, respectively, that provides an electrical signal to ensure a steady heartbeat and to defibrillate the heart in case of severe arrhythmia
percutaneous transluminal coronary angioplasty (PTCA)	per"kū-tā'nē-ŭs trăns-loo'mĭ-năl kor'ŏ-nā-rē ăn'jē-ō-plăs"tē	opening an obstructed coronary artery with a balloon catheter (See Figure 8-13)
pericardiectomy	pĕr"ĭ-kăr"dē-ĕk'tō-mē	incision and partial removal of the pericardium to relieve the heart of adhesions
pericardiocentesis	pĕr"ĭ-kăr-dē-ō"sĕn-tē'sĭs	procedure to aspirate excess fluid from the pericardial space

continues

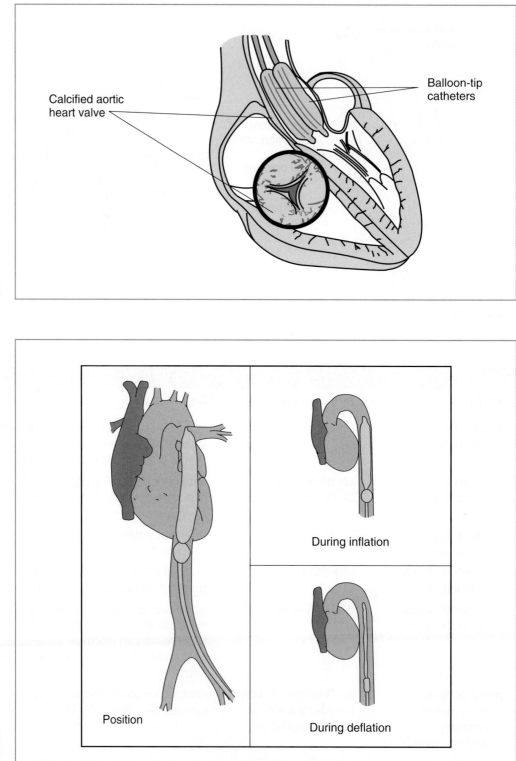

FIGURE 8-12
Heart Valve Valvuloplasty

Calcified aortic heart valve

Balloon-tip catheters

FIGURE 8-13
Intra-aortic Balloon Pump Catheter

Position

During inflation

During deflation

TREATMENT PROCEDURES

Word	Pronunciation	Definition
permanent pacemaker (PPM)		small electronic device consisting of a battery and electrode implanted in the chest and heart, respectively, that provides an electrical signal to ensure a steady heartbeat
phlebectomy	flĕ-bĕk'tō-mē	excision or resection of a vein
phlebotomy	flĕ-bŏt'o-mē	cutting into a vein
sclerotherapy	sklĕr"ō-thĕr'ă-pē	treatment that injects a chemical into a vein to harden, fill, or destroy it
stent	stĕnt	device placed in an artery after angioplasty surgery to keep it from narrowing again (See Figure 8-14)
thrombectomy	thrŏm-bĕk'tō-mē	surgical removal of a clot from a blood vessel
thrombolytic therapy	thrŏm-bō-lĭt'-ĭk	procedure where drugs that dissolve clots are injected into bloodstream
valve replacement		excision of a diseased, incompetent valve, which is replaced with a prosthetic (artificial) valvular structure
vein ligation	lī-gā'shŭn	tying off an involved section of vein with a suture
venipuncture	vĕn'ĭ-pŭnk"tūr	surgical puncture of a vein
vein stripping		removal of a diseased portion of a vein

MEDICATIONS PRESCRIBED

Trade Name	Generic Name
Diuretics	
Aldactazide	spironolactone with HCTz
Aldactone	spironolactone

continues

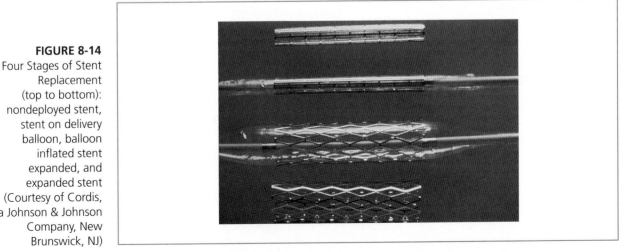

FIGURE 8-14
Four Stages of Stent Replacement (top to bottom): nondeployed stent, stent on delivery balloon, balloon inflated stent expanded, and expanded stent (Courtesy of Cordis, a Johnson & Johnson Company, New Brunswick, NJ)

MEDICATIONS PRESCRIBED

Trade Name	Generic Name
Diuretics (continued)	
Bumex	bumetanide
Diuril	chlorothiazide
Dyazide	triamterene/HCTz
Dyrenium	triamterene
Enduron	methyclothiazide
HydroDIURIL, Esidrix	hydrochlorothiazide (HCTz)
Hygroton	chlorthalidone
Lasix	furosemide
Lozol	indapamide
Midamor	amiloride hydrochloride
Zaroxolyn	metolazone
Alpha-adrenergic Blockers	
Aldomet	methyldopa
Cardura	doxazosin mesylate
Catapres	clonidine hydrochloride
Minipress	prazosin hydrochloride
Regitine	phentolamine mesylate
Hytrin	terazosin hydrochloride
ACE Inhibitors	
Capoten	captopril
Vasotec	enalapril maleate
Zestril	lisinopril
Angiotensin II Receptor Blockers (ARBs)	
Atacand	candesartan cilexetil
Cozaar	losartan
Beta-adrenergic Blockers	
Blocadren	timolol
Inderal	propranolol hydrochloride
Lopressor	metoprolol
Tenormin	atenolol
Toprol XL	metoprolol succinate

continues

MEDICATIONS PRESCRIBED

Trade Name	Generic Name
Calcium Channel Blockers	
Calan, Isoptin	verapamil
Cardene	nicardipine
Cardizem	diltiazem hydrochloride
Norvasc	amlodipine
Procardia	nifedipine
Peripherally Acting Adrenergic Antagonists	
Serpasil	reserpine
Direct Vasodilators	
Apresoline	hydralazine hydrochloride
Hyperstat	diazoxide
Nipride	nitroprusside sodium
Other Cardiac Medications	
Adrenalin	epinephrine
Cordarone, Pacerone	amiodarone hydrochloride
Lanoxin	digoxin
Mexiletine	mexiletine hydrochloride
Nitrostat	nitroglycerine
Norpace	disopyramide phosphate
Pronestyl	procainamide hydrochloride
Quinidex	quinidine
Rythmol	propafenone hydrochloride
Tambocor	flecainide acetate
Thrombolytic Agents	
Abbokinase	urokinase
Activase	alteplase
Retavase	reteplase
Streptase	streptokinase
Anticoagulants	
—	heparin
Coumadin	warfarin sodium
Fragmin	dalteparin

continues

MEDICATIONS PRESCRIBED

Trade Name	Generic Name
Anticoagulants (*continued*)	
Lovenox	enoxaparin
Antibiotics	
Amoxil	amoxicillin
Cipro	ciprofloxacin
Garamycin	gentamicin sulfate
Kefzol	cefazolin
Vancocin	vancomycin hydrochloride
V-Cillin K	penicillin V potassium
Other Supplements or Removing Agents	
Colestid	colestipol
K-Lor, Slow-K, Kay Ciel, Klor-Con, K-Tab, Ten-K, Micro-K	potassium chloride
Lipitor	atorvastatin
Lopid	gemfibrozil
Mevacor	lovastatin
Questran	cholestyramine
Pravachol	pravastatin sodium
Zocor	simvastatin

ABBREVIATIONS

ABG, ABGs	arterial blood gas(es)
AI	aortic insufficiency
AS	aortic stenosis
ASD	atrial septal defect
ASHD	arteriosclerotic heart disease
AV, A-V	atrioventricular
BP	blood pressure
CABG	coronary artery bypass graft
CAD	coronary artery disease
cath	catheterization
CCU	coronary care unit
CHD	coronary heart disease
CHF	congestive heart failure

continues

ABBREVIATIONS

CPR	cardiopulmonary resuscitation
CVD	cardiovascular disease
DSA	digital subtraction angiography
DVT	deep venous thrombosis
ECC	extracorporeal circulation
ECG, EKG	electrocardiogram
ECHO	echocardiography
ETT	exercise tolerance test
HDL	high-density lipoprotein
IABP	intra-aortic balloon pump
ICD	internal cardioverter-defibrillator
LDL	low-density lipoprotein
LVAD	left ventricular assist device
MI	mitral insufficiency, myocardial infarction
MR	mitral regurgitation
MS	mitral stenosis
MUGA	multiple-gated acquisition scan
MVP	mitral valve prolapse
PAC	premature atrial contraction
PAT	paroxysmal atrial tachycardia
PCD	pacemaker cardiac defibrillator
PPM	permanent pacemaker
PTCA	percutaneous transluminal coronary angioplasty
PVC	premature ventricular contraction
PVD	peripheral vascular disease
SA, S-A	sinoatrial
VSD	ventricular septal defect

LIST OF THE MORE COMMON ARTERIES AND VEINS

Arteries

alveolar	brachial	cervical	coronary
anastomotic	bronchial	circumflex	digital
aorta	buccal	• femoral	• plantar
auditory	carotid	• iliac	• radial
auricular	celiac	• scapular	dorsalis pedis
axillary	cerebellar	collateral	epigastric
basilar	cerebral	conjunctival	episcleral

continues

LIST OF THE MORE COMMON ARTERIES AND VEINS

Arteries (continued)

esophageal	mesenteric	sacral	tarsal
ethmoidal	occipital	saphenous	temporal
femoral	ophthalmic	scapular	testicular
gastric	ovarian	sciatic	thoracic
gastroduodenal	perforating	scrotal	thyroid
hepatic	perineal	septal	tibial
hypogastric	peroneal	sigmoid	transverse
iliac	pharyngeal	spermatic	tympanic
intercostal	phrenic	splenic	ulnar
intestinal	plantar	sternocleidomastoid	uterine
lumbar	popliteal	subclavian	vaginal
malleolar	pulmonary	subcostal	vertebral
mammary	radial	sublingual	vesical
mediastinal	renal	suprarenal	volar arch

Veins

auricular	esophageal	pancreatic	sigmoid sinus
axillary	femoral	parumbilical	subclavian
azygos	gastric	peroneal	superficial
brachial	gluteal	pharyngeal	temporal
bronchial	hemorrhoidal	phrenic	thoracic
cardiac	hepatic	popliteal	thyroid
cephalic	iliac	pulmonary	tibial
cerebral	intercostal	pyloric	ulnar
cervical	intervertebral	radial	umbilical
coronary sinus	jugular	rectal	vena cava
digital	lumbar	sacral	vertebral
epigastric	mesenteric	saphenous	

Working Practice Review Exercises

Name: _____ Date: _____

MATCHING*
Match the terms to their meanings.

1. _____ recording device attached to the chest to monitor heart activity for a long period of time
2. _____ bypass of an obstructed coronary artery
3. _____ x-ray visualization of the heart and blood vessels after contrast material is injected into the bloodstream
4. _____ surgical incision of connecting bands of commissure
5. _____ measurement of oxygen, carbon dioxide, and metabolic balance from an arterial blood sample
6. _____ while an exercise load on a treadmill is gradually increased, heart function is evaluated
7. _____ removal of a diseased portion of a vein
8. _____ surgical removal of a clot from a blood vessel
9. _____ removal of the interior portion of an artery
10. _____ excision or restriction of a vein
11. _____ replacement of a portion of an artery by another open structure
12. _____ tests the coagulation of blood

a. angiocardiography
b. arterial blood gases
c. artery graft
d. commissurotomy
e. coronary artery bypass
f. endarterectomy
g. Holter monitor
h. phlebectomy
i. prothrombin time
j. thrombectomy
k. treadmill exercise tolerance test
l. vein stripping

SPELLING*
Rewrite the misspelled words.

1. electrolights _____
2. enzemes _____
3. sodium _____
4. trigylcefides _____
5. potassium _____
6. hematocrit _____
7. cholesterol _____
8. prothronbin _____
9. extracorpeal _____
10. stint _____
11. translumenal _____

IDENTIFICATION
Identify the following diagnoses.

1. irregularity of the heartbeat _____
2. disease characterized by prolonged high blood pressure _____

_____

*Answers are in Appendix A.

3. heart disease produced by
    coronary artery disease

4. inflammatory disease of the
    endocardium

5. abnormality in the heart at
    birth

6. condition caused by a
    weakened heart resulting
    in an accumulation of fluid
    in tissues

7. low blood pressure

8. fixed blood clot

9. clotting and associated
    inflammation in the vein

10. fast heart rate

ABBREVIATIONS

Give the abbreviation for each of the following.

1. arteriosclerotic heart disease

2. atrioventricular

3. mitral insufficiency; myocardial infarction

4. premature ventricular contraction

5. sinoatrial

6. digital subtraction angiography

7. exercise tolerance test

8. internal cardioverter-defibrillator

9. permanent pacemaker

10. congestive heart failure

COMPLETION

Complete the following statements.

1. An _____ results when inadequate blood supply causes death of tissue.

2. When a blood vessel bulges or enlarges abnormally, an _____ results.

3. Disease of an artery, causing high blood pressure, often results in _____.

4. A malformation in the muscular wall of the aorta that makes it narrow is referred to as
    _____.

5. Abnormally swollen veins are _____ veins.

6. The removal of a diseased portion of a vein is _____.

7. Failure of a heart valve to close completely is called _____.

Word Element Review

Root	Meaning	Example	Definition
angi/o	blood vessel	**angiitis** (ăn″jē-ī′tĭs)	inflammation of a blood vessel
		angioma (ăn″jē-ō′mah)	tumor made of blood or lymph vessels
aort/o	aorta	**aortorrhaphy** (ā″ŏr-tor′ah-fē)	suture of the aorta
arter/o, arteri/o	artery	**arterioplasty** (ăr-tē″rē-ō-plăs′tē)	surgical repair of an artery
		arteriorrhaphy (ăr-tē″rē-or′ah-fē)	suture of an artery
ather/o	yellowish plaque, fatty substance	**atheroma** (ăth″er-ō′mah)	mass of plaque of degenerated, thickened arterial intima (inner lining of an artery), occurring in atherosclerosis
atri/o	atrium	**atrial** (ā′trē-ăl)	pertaining to an atrium
		atriomegaly (ā″trē-ō-mĕg′ah-lē)	abnormal enlargement of an atrium of the heart
cardi/o	heart	**cardiomyopathy** (kăr″dē-ō-mī-ŏp′ah-thē)	diagnostic term designating myocardial disease
		myocardial infarction (mī″ō-kăr′dē-ăl ĭn-fărk′shŭn)	a "heart attack"
coron/o	heart	**coronary** (kor′ŏ-nā-rē)	applying to arteries of the heart and the pathology of them
furc/o	division, fork	**bifurcation** (bī′fur-kā′shŭn)	division into two parts
		furcal (fur′kăl)	shaped like a fork
pericardi/o	pericardium	**pericardiectomy** (pĕr″ĭ-kăr″dē-ek′tō-mē)	removal of a portion of the pericardium
phleb/o	vein	**phlebitis** (flĕ-bī′tĭs)	inflammation of a vessel
		phlebostenosis (flĕb″ō-stĕ-nō-′sĭs)	narrowing of a vein
steth/o	chest	**stethoscope** (stĕth′ō-skōp)	instrument for listening to body sounds
thromb/o	clot, lump	**thrombosis** (thrŏm-bō′sĭs)	formation of a blood clot in a vessel or an organ
		thrombus (thrŏm′bŭs)	clot in a blood vessel formed by coagulation of the blood (note the similarity in sound, spelling, and meaning of these two words)

continues

Root	Meaning	Example	Definition
valv/o, valvul/o	valve	**valvular** (văl'vū-lăr)	pertaining to a valve
vascul/o, vas/o	vessel	**vascular** (văs'kū-lăr)	pertaining to a blood vessel
		vasodilator (văs"ō-dī-lāt'or)	agent that dilates the blood vessels
ven/o	vein	**venous** (vē'nŭs)	pertaining to a vein
ventricul/o	ventricle	**ventriculotomy** (věn-trĭk"ū-lŏt'ō-mē)	incision into the ventricle of the heart

Prefix	Meaning	Example	Definition
brady-	slow	**bradycardia** (brăd"e-kăr'dē-ah)	slow heartbeat
tachy-	fast, rapid	**tachycardia** (tăk"ē-kăr'dē-ah)	fast heart rate

Suffix	Meaning	Example	Definition
-megaly	enlargement	**cardiomegaly** (kăr"dē-ō-měg'ah-lē)	condition characterized by an enlarged heart

Word Element Review Exercises

Name: _____ Date: _____

COMPLETION*

Complete the following statements.

1. _____ is a rapid heartbeat.

2. _____ applies to arteries of the heart and the pathology of them.

3. A _____ is commonly known as a "heart attack."

4. A _____ is an instrument for listening to the heart and other body sounds.

5. Suture of the aorta is _____; suture of an artery is _____.

6. _____ refers to a valve.

7. The clot in a blood vessel is a _____, but the formation of a clot is a
   _____.

8. A diagnostic term designating myocardial diseases is _____.

9. _____ is the abnormal enlargement of an atrium of the heart.

10. Removal of a portion of the pericardium is _____.

11. _____ is shaped like a fork.

SPELLINGS AND DEFINITIONS*

Mark any spelling errors in these words. Then define each and specify whether it is a noun or an adjective by placing an N or A in the last column.

		Definition	**N or A**
1.	cardiomegaly	_____	_____
2.	bradicardia	_____	_____
3.	tachicardia	_____	_____
4.	ventriclotomy	_____	_____
5.	venus	_____	_____

DEFINITIONS*

Provide the medical term for the following definitions.

1. surgical repair of an artery   _____
2. division into two parts   _____
3. inflammation of a vessel   _____
4. narrowing of a vein   _____
5. pertaining to a blood vessel   _____
6. agent that dilates the blood vessels _____

*Answers are in Appendix A.

WORD ELEMENT AND MEANING

In the following terms, circle the word element presented in this chapter. Then provide the definition of the term.

1. cardiomyopathy _____
2. atrial _____
3. coronary _____
4. vasodilator _____
5. angioma _____
6. atheroma _____

WORD ELEMENT MEANINGS

Give the meaning of each word element. Then use your dictionary to find a new word that contains each of the word elements. Specify whether the new word is a noun or an adjective by placing N or A in the last column.

Word Element	Meaning	Word	N or A
1. angi/o			
2. aort/o			
3. arter/o			
4. arteri/o			
5. ather/o			
6. atri/o			
7. brady-			
8. cardi/o			
9. coron/o			
10. furc/o			
11. -megaly			
12. pericardi/o			
13. phleb/o			
14. steth/o			
15. tachy-			
16. thromb/o			
17. valv/o			
18. valvul/o			
19. vas/o			
20. vascul/o			
21. ven/o			
22. ventricul/o			

Dictionary Exercises

Name: _____ Date: _____

DICTIONARY EXERCISE 1*

Use your dictionary to find the pronunciation and definition of the following words.

	Word	Pronunciation	Definition
1.	precordium		
2.	atrophy		
3.	auricle		
4.	bigeminal		
5.	bundle branch block		
6.	Purkinje fibers		
7.	cardiac massage		
8.	cardiomotility		
9.	cor pulmonale		
10.	dilatation		
11.	cusp		
12.	lumen		
13.	occlusion		
14.	pneumopericardium		
15.	sinus arrest		
16.	ventricular septal defect		
17.	atresia		
18.	ductus arteriosus		
19.	patent ductus arteriosus		
20.	transposition		
21.	hemodynamics		
22.	bruit		
23.	coarctation		
24.	pallor		

_____

*Answers are in Appendix A.

DICTIONARY EXERCISE 2

Pronunciation of the words below is provided. Using your dictionary, find the correct spelling and definition of the words.

	Word	**Pronunciation**	**Definition**
1.	_____	ăth"ĕr-ō-sklē-rŏt'ĭk	_____
2.	_____	păr"ŏk-sĭz'măl ā'trē-ăl	_____
	_____	tăk"ē-kăr'dē-ah	_____
3.	_____	kăr'dē-ak tăm"pŏn-ād'	_____
4.	_____	kăr'dē-ō-vĕr"zhŭn	_____
5.	_____	kŏm'ĭ-shūr	_____
6.	_____	dē-fĭb"rĭ-lā'tŏr	_____
7.	_____	dĭsp'nē-ah	_____
8.	_____	prē-kŏr'dē-ah	_____
9.	_____	pŭl-mŏn'ĭk stĕ-nō'sĭs	_____
10.	_____	păl-pĭ-tā'shŭn	_____
11.	_____	rē-sŭs"ĭ-tā'shŭn	_____
12.	_____	sī'nŭs ah-rĭth'mē-ah	_____
13.	_____	tĕ-trăl'ō-jē of făl-ō'	_____
14.	_____	sĭn'kō-pē	_____
15.	_____	ah-năs"tō-mō'sĭs	_____
16.	_____	klaw"dĭ-kā'shŭn	_____
17.	_____	eks-trăv"ah-sā'shŭn	_____
18.	_____	plăk	_____
19.	_____	văs"ō-kŏn-strĭk'shŭn	_____
20.	_____	pĕr-fū'zhŭn	_____
21.	_____	ăn"ah-săr'kah	_____

DICTIONARY EXERCISE 3

Rewrite the following sentences in your own words. Provide the pronunciation of the italicized words where indicated.

1. The patient arrived in *cardiac arrest* and *resuscitation* (_____) measures were performed.

_____

2. Diagnosis suggested *aortic regurgitation* (_____).

_____

3. The doctor heard a *gallop rhythm.*

_____

4. The patient experienced *paroxysmal ventricular tachycardia* (_____).

_____

5. Her doctor suspected *subacute bacterial endocarditis* (_____).

_____

6. *Sinus rhythm* was normal.

   _____

7. Problems may be attributed to a *heart block.*

   _____

8. The physician heard *atrial fibrillation* (_____).

   _____

9. Unfortunately the baby was born with an *atrial septal defect* (_____).

   _____

10. *Central venous pressure* was elevated.

   _____

11. *Coronary artery perfusion* will be performed on Monday.

   _____

12. The patient's problem arose from an *embolus* (_____).

   _____

13. Upon physical examination, the patient was noted to have *pitting edema* in her ankle.

   _____

14. The physician prescribed *digitalis* (_____).

   _____

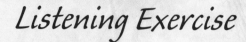

Listening Exercise

Name	Date

INSTRUCTIONS

1. Review the spelling, pronunciation, and meaning of the words provided in the preview.

2. Listen to the audio CD and fill in the blank as the word is dictated.

3. At the end of the exercise, check your spelling against the preview words. They appear in the preview in the order in which they are encountered in the exercise.

4. Review and practice the words you missed.

5. Look up words that are not familiar.

PREVIEW OF WORDS FOR LISTENING EXERCISE 8-1

Word	Pronunciation	Meaning
thrombolytic therapy	thrŏm″bō-lĭt′ĭk	treatment designed to break up a thrombus
ventriculogram	vĕn-trĭk′ū-lō-grăm	radiogram of the ventricles of the heart
percutaneous	pĕr″kū-tā′nē-ŭs	accomplished through the skin
gradient	grā′dē-ĕnt	an increase or decrease of varying degrees
hypokinesia	hī″pō-kī-nē′zē-ă	decreased motor activity
circumflex	sĕr′kŭm-flĕks	curved like a bow; spiraling around
arteriosclerotic heart disease	ăr-tē″rē-ō-sklĕ-rŏt′ĭk	heart disease produced by coronary artery disease

Cardiac Catheterization and Angiography Report

PATIENT PROFILE: The patient is a 51-year-old woman with an acute anterior wall myocardial infarction treated with

_____   _____ .

PROCEDURE: Left heart catheterization with left _____ and coronary arteriography with

_____ transluminal coronary angioplasty of the proximal left anterior descending and placement of an intracoronary stent and intracoronary nitroglycerin administration was performed without complication.

FINDINGS: Left ventricular pressure prior to left ventriculogram was 119/-1, 11 mm/Hg and following left ventriculogram was 121/0, 9 mm/Hg. Aortic pressure following left ventriculogram was 121/63 mm/Hg with a mean of 87 mm/Hg. There was no systolic _____ . The left ventriculogram demonstrated mild _____ of the anterior wall of the left ventricle with an overall normal ejection fraction of 61%. There was no mitral insufficiency. The coronary arteriogram demonstrated no significant disease of the left main and left _____ coronary arteries. There was an 80% proximal stenosis of the left anterior descending coronary artery before the septal perforator branch and a 50% proximal stenosis of a small intermediate coronary artery. There was no significant disease of the right coronary artery. The left anterior descending coronary artery was dominant.

The 80% proximal stenosis of the left anterior descending coronary artery was reduced to a residual 0% stenosis following placement of a 3.0 mm J&J stent that was deployed at 6 atmospheres and extended at 14 atmospheres with a 3.0 mm non-compliant Ranger balloon catheter.

IMPRESSION:

1. _____ _____ _____ , acute anterior wall myocardial infarction treated with thrombolytic therapy, mild hypokinesia of the anterior wall of the left ventricle with a normal ejection fraction, normal left ventricular filling pressure with a significant proximal stenosis of the left anterior descending coronary artery.

2. Successful angioplasty of the proximal left anterior descending coronary artery using an intracoronary stent.

_____ _____

Chan Zhou, MD

CHAPTER

9

The Blood and Lymph Systems

Blood is a very special juice.

—GOETHE

INTRODUCTION

Blood is essential to our existence. It travels literally miles in our veins and arteries, performing many functions grouped primarily into transportation and protection. Blood transports oxygen, carbon dioxide, nutrients, glucose, amino acids, fats, waste products, hormones, electrolytes, and heat from one part of the body to another. When disease or infection invades the body, chemical substances called antibodies move within the blood and take defensive action where needed.

Because blood flows through, around, and among body tissues, organs, and other blood vessels, certain diseases can be diagnosed with the aid of specific blood tests. The study of blood, **hematology** (hē"mah-tŏl'ō-jē), requires knowledge about the bone marrow, spleen, lymph nodes, and all the components of blood. Physicians who specialize in the study and treatment of the blood system are called **hematologists** (hē"mah-tŏl'ō-jĭsts).

COMPOSITION OF BLOOD

bas/o	base	hemat/o, hem/o	blood
blast/o	primitive cell	leuk/o	white
cyt/o	cell	mega-	large
-emia	blood condition	neutr/o	neutral
erythr/o	red	sangui/o	blood

The average adult has about six quarts of blood. Blood is composed of two prime elements, a liquid called plasma and a solid called formed elements, or cells.

PLASMA

Plasma is the fluid component of blood. About fifty-five percent of blood is plasma, and the plasma itself is composed of about ninety percent water. The remaining part of the plasma contains approximately 100 different substances dissolved or suspended in this watery medium. The largest component, about seven percent, is a group of proteins made up of **serum albumin** (ăl-bū'mĭn), **serum globulin** (glŏb'ū-lĭn), **fibrinogen** (fī-brĭn'ō-jĕn), and coagulation proteins such as **prothrombin** (prō-thrŏm'bĭn). There are three types of globulin: alpha, beta, and gamma. They are identified by a process called **electrophoresis** (ē-lĕk"trō-fō-rē'sĭs). The gamma globulin fraction is especially important because it contains antibodies.

Sodium, calcium, potassium, magnesium, phosphorus, and other minerals comprise about one percent of the plasma; they are the **inorganic constituents**. Major **organic constituents** are amino acids, glucose, neutral fats (phospholipids [fŏs"-fō-lĭp'ĭds] and cholesterol [kō-lĕs'ter-ŏl]), and waste products (urea, uric acid, creatinine [krē-ăt'ĭ-nĭn], ammonia, and lactic acids). Plasma carries the nutrients to body cells for nourishment purposes and returns with waste products such as carbon dioxide, which it takes to the kidneys, bowels, intestines, lungs, or skin for excretion. Internal secretions, or hormones, antibodies, and enzymes, make up the remainder of the plasma.

CELLS

The basic unit of the body, the **cell**, varies in size and purpose. (For a review of cells, see Chapter 2.) Three types of blood cells flow freely suspended in the plasma shown in Figure 9-1: erythrocytes, leukocytes, and platelets (thrombocytes). They are formed in the red bone marrow found in the ends of long bones and in the pelvic and other flat bones.

Erythrocytes

Erythrocytes (ĕ-rĭth'rō-sīts) (1) are tiny disk-shaped red blood cells with a central area that is thinner than the edges. On average there are 4.5 million to 6 million erythrocytes per cubic millimeter of blood. Erythrocytes live for about 120 days in the bloodstream; then some of the elements are recycled as new ones are produced.

The main purpose of red blood cells is to carry oxygen from the lungs to the tissues. **Hemoglobin** (hē'mō-glō"bĭn), the primary ingredient of these cells, absorbs oxygen. Hemoglobin also carries about ten percent of the body's carbon dioxide back to the lungs. The normal hemoglobin measurement in the blood of males is from 14 to 18 grams per 100 milliliters; in the blood of females, it is from 12 to 16 grams per 100 milliliters. Iron is an essential constituent of hemoglobin. If iron is lacking, the size, color, and number of red blood cells are affected.

A **hematocrit** (hē-măt'ō-krĭt) is a measurement of red blood cells. It is done by comparing the volume of red blood cells with the total volume of blood. The normal range for men is forty to fifty-four percent; for women, it is thirty-seven to forty-seven percent.

Leukocytes

Leukocytes (lū'kō-sīts) (3) are white blood cells, pale in color with an irregular, ball-like shape, that contain nuclei of varying shapes and sizes. The normal number of leukocytes per cubic centimeter of blood ranges from 5,000 to 10,000.

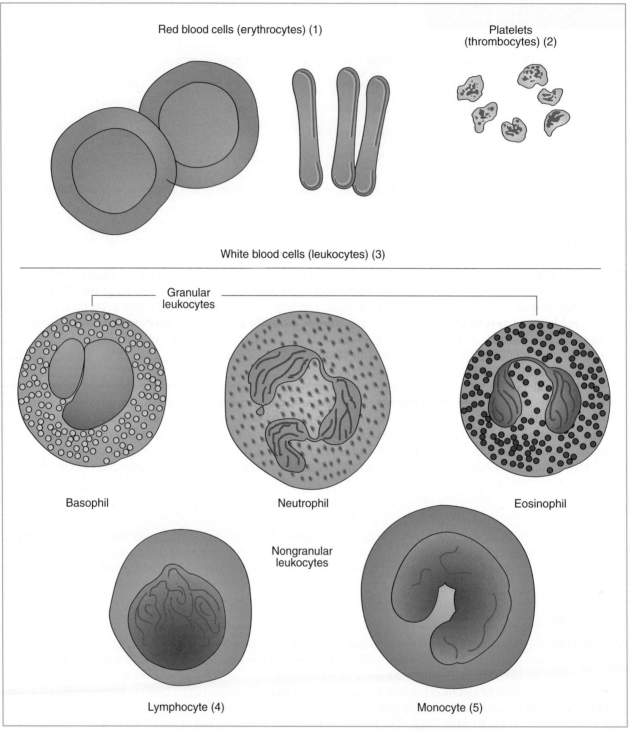

FIGURE 9-1 The Classification of Blood Cells

There are two major types of leukocytes. The most numerous type is **granulocyte** (grăn'ū-lō-sīt"), or **polymorphonuclear** (pŏl"ē-mor"fō-noo'klē-ar) **leukocyte**. These grainy cells are classified as neutrophils (nū'trō-fĭls), eosinophils (ē"ō-sĭn'ō-fĭls), or basophils (bā'sō-fĭls), based on their various staining qualities with specific dyes. Granulocytes are produced in the red bone marrow. When infection invades the body, production of granulocytes in the blood increases. As shown in Figure 9-2, these cells then pass through blood vessel walls and collect in the area of infection. Cells that gather here form pus or a purulent discharge.

The other type of leukocyte is the **mononuclear** (mŏn"ō-noo'klē-ar) **cell**, which includes monocytes (5) and lymphocytes (lĭm'fō-sīts) (4), as shown in Figure 9-1. Monocytes respond to many different types of infection and

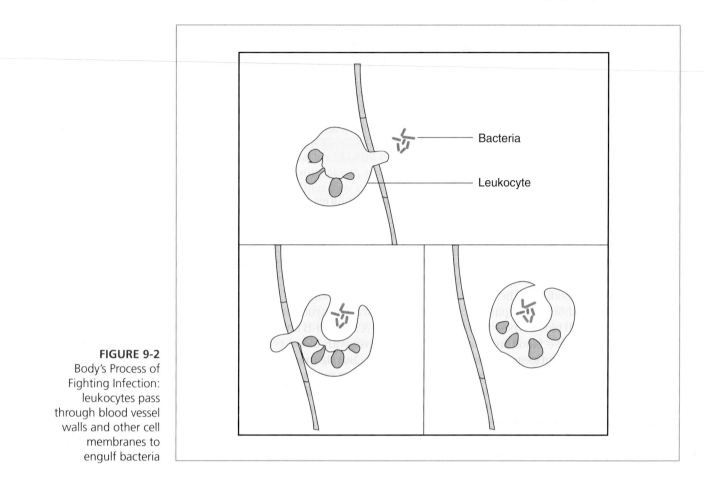

Bacteria

Leukocyte

FIGURE 9-2
Body's Process of Fighting Infection: leukocytes pass through blood vessel walls and other cell membranes to engulf bacteria

defend the body by engulfing foreign substances. Lymphocytes contain B cells and T cells and react to specific infecting agents. T cells are the attack cells. B cells produce antibodies as their contribution to the body's defense.

Platelets

Platelets, or **thrombocytes** (thrŏm'bō-sīts) (2) (see Figure 9-1), are essential for coagulation. If it were not for them, we would bleed to death from even the slightest cut. When a blood vessel is damaged, the platelets gather at that point and form a plug that closes the hole in the vessel. At the same time, platelets release a chemical that helps activate the formation of a protein called **fibrin** (fī'brĭn). Fibrin has the appearance of fine threads tangled together. As red cells are caught in the tangle of fibrin threads, they form the clot and give it its characteristic red color.

Platelets, or thrombocytes, are produced in the bone marrow from a white blood cell called a **megakaryocyte** (mĕg"ah-kăr'ē-ō-sīt). This cell is many times larger than other white blood cells and forms small particles in the cytoplasm around its nucleus as it develops. Once particles break out of the cell and enter the bloodstream, they are called platelets.

BLOOD TYPING AND TRANSFUSIONS

agglutin/o   clumping, sticking together

There are many protein substances, or **antigens** (ăn'tĭ-jĕns), on the surface of the red blood cell that cause the blood of one person to be different from that of another. Antigens are substances that induce the formation of antibodies, which interact specifically with the antigens. The major antigens are referred to as A, B, and Rh. The presence or absence of the A and B antigens determines a person's blood type or group. Here is a summary of the characteristics of the four blood types.

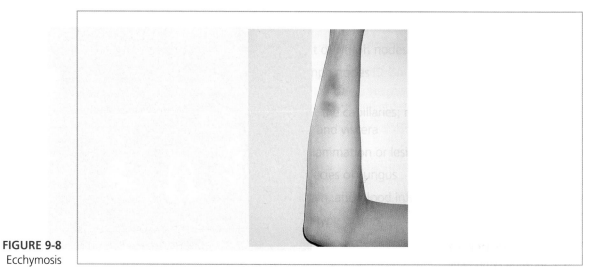

FIGURE 9-8
Ecchymosis

TREATMENT PROCEDURES

Word	Pronunciation	Definition
apheresis	ă-fĕr'ē-sĭs	removal of blood from a patient or donor; separating and retaining certain components (such as plasma, platelets, or abnormal elements), some of which are retained; and then reinfusing elements into the donor
blood transfusion		after testing to ensure a close match of red cells or platelet type, whole blood or cells from an individual are infused into the recipient; may be *homologous* (from another) or *autologous* (from self)
bone marrow transplant		bone marrow cells from a donor whose tissue and blood cells closely match those of the patient are infused into the recipient
erythrocytopheresis	ĕ-rĭth"rō-fĕr-ē'sĭs	procedure that removes abnormal red blood cells and replaces them with healthy red blood cells
immunotherapy	ĭm"ū-nō-thĕr'ă-pē	treatment to suppress or enhance immunological functioning to identified allergens
phlebotomy	flĕ-bŏt-ō-mē	removal of blood from a vein
splenectomy	splē-nĕk'tō-mē	surgical removal of an enlarged spleen

MEDICATIONS PRESCRIBED

Trade Name	Generic Name
Chemotherapeutic Agents	
Adriamycin	doxorubicin HCl
Anzemet	dolasetron
Arimidex	anastrozole

continues

MEDICATIONS PRESCRIBED

Trade Name	Generic Name
Chemotherapeutic Agents *(continued)*	
BCNU, BiCNU	carmustine
Blenoxane	bleomycin sulfate
Camptosar	irinoteca
Casodex	bicalutamide
CeeNu, CCNU	lomustine
Cerubidine	daunorubicin
Cytoxan	cyclophosphamide
Decadron	dexamethasone
Deltasone, Orasone, Cordrol	prednisone
DTIC-Dome	dacarbazine
Elspar	asparaginase
Emcyt	estramustine
Epogen	epoetin alfa (synthetic)
Eulexin	flutamide
Fareston	toremifine
Femara	letrozole
Fludara	fludarabine
Gemzar	gemcitabine
Herceptin	trastuzumab
Hycamtin	topotecan
Hydrea	hydroxyurea
IFEX	ifosfamide
IGIV	immune globulin IV
Intron A, Roferon-A	interferon alfa
Kytril	granisetron
Leucovorin calcium	folinic acid
Leukeran	chlorambucil
Leukine	sargramostim
Lupron	leuprolide acetate
Lysodren	mitotane
Matulane	procarbazine
Medrol	methylprednisolone
Megace	megestrol
MESNEX	mesna
Mithracin	plicamycin

continues

MEDICATIONS PRESCRIBED

Trade Name	Generic Name
Chemotherapeutic Agents *(continued)*	
Mustargen	mechlorethamine
Mutamycin	mitomycin
Myleran	busulfan
Navelbine	vinorelbine
Neupogen	filgrastim (G-CSF)
Nolvadex	tamoxifen
Novantrone	mitoxantrone
—	oxaliplatin
Paraplatin	carboplatin
Platinol	cisplatin
Procrit	epoetin alfa
Rituxan	rituximab
Sandostatin	octreotide acetate
Solu-Cortef	hydrocortisone
Taxol	paclitaxel
Taxotere	docetaxel
Temodal	temozolomide
Thalomid	thalidomide
Velban	vinblastine sulfate
VePesid	etoposide
Xeloda	capecitabine
Zofran	ondansetron HCl
Zoladex	goserelin
5-FU	fluorouracil
AIDS Medications	
Crixivan	indinavir sulfate
Epivir	laminudine
Fortovase, Invase	saquinavir mesylate
Hivid	zalcitabine
Norvir	ruonavir
Rescriptor	delavirdine
Retrovir	zidovudine
Sustiva	efavirenz
Videx	didanosine
Viracept	nelfinavir mesylate

continues

MEDICATIONS PRESCRIBED

Trade Name	Generic Name
AIDS Medications (*continued*)	
Viramune	nevirapine
Zerit	stavudine
Ziagen	abacavir
Other Medications/Preparations	
Alupent	metaproterenol sulfate
Amicar, Immunex	aminocaproic acid
Aminophylline	aminophylline
Benadryl	diphenhydramine
Coumadin	warfarin sodium
Cyklokapron	tranexamic acid
DDAVP	desmopressin acetate
Fergon, Ferralet, Simron	ferrous gluconate
Feosol, Ferosul, Slow Fe	ferrous sulfate
Intropin	dopamine
Levophed	norepinephrine bitartrate
Mestinon	pyridostigmine bromide
Persantine	dipyridamole
Prostigmin	neostigine bromide
Proventil	albuterol
Streptase	streptokinase
Trental	pentoxifylline
Vitamin B$_{12}$	cyanocobalamin
Zyloprim	allopurinol

ABBREVIATIONS

AIDS	acquired immune deficiency; acquired immunodeficiency syndrome
ALL	acute lymphocytic leukemia
AML	acute myelogenous leukemia
ARC	AIDS-related complex
baso	basophil(s)
CBC	complete blood count
CGL	chronic granulocytic leukemia
CLL	chronic lymphocytic leukemia
CML	chronic myelogenous leukemia

continues

ABBREVIATIONS

DIC	disseminated intravascular coagulation
diff	differential blood count
eos, eosins	eosinophil(s)
ESR, Sed rate	erythrocyte sedimentation rate
Hb, Hgb	hemoglobin
Hct	hematocrit
HIV	human immunodeficiency virus
IgA, IgD, IgE, IgG, IgM	immunoglobulins
lymph	lymphocyte
MCH	mean corpuscular hemoglobin (amount of hemoglobin per cell)
MCHC	mean corpuscular hemoglobin concentration (average concentration of hemo-globin per red cell)
MCV	mean corpuscular volume (average volume of a red blood cell)
mono	monocyte
PMN, PMNL	polymorphonuclear neutrophil leukocytes
PT	prothrombin time
PTT	partial thromboplastin time
RBC	red blood cell, red blood count
WBC	white blood cell, white blood count

Working Practice Review Exercises

Name: _____ Date: _____

DEFINITIONS*

Define the following diagnoses.

1. leukocytosis

   _____

2. lymphoma

   _____

3. multiple myeloma

   _____

4. lymphadenopathy

   _____

5. purpura

   _____

MATCHING

Match the terms to their meanings.

1. _____ x-rays follow dye injected into the foot as lymph moves into the chest
2. _____ test to detect presence of HIV virus
3. _____ rate at which red cells settle to the bottom of a test tube when mixed with an anticoagulant
4. _____ decrease in red corpuscles or the iron in them
5. _____ impaired coagulation of blood
6. _____ pinpoint hemorrhages under the skin
7. _____ determine the length of life of red blood cells
8. _____ inserting a large needle to aspirate marrow or using a large cutting needle to remove a small core of bone
9. _____ disorder resulting from overreaction of the immune system to an antigen or allergen
10. _____ test for eleven of thirteen blood clotting factors
11. _____ abnormal increase in the number of granulocytes in blood
12. _____ decrease in red blood cells
13. _____ advanced stage of HIV
14. _____ low blood volume
15. _____ occurs when bone marrow produces too many red cells

a. AIDS
b. allergies
c. anemia
d. bone marrow aspiration and biopsy
e. chromium^{51} RBC survival
f. erythrocyte sedimentation rate
g. erythrocytopenia
h. granulocytosis
i. hemophilia
j. hypovalemia
k. lymphangiogram
l. partial thromboplastin
m. petechiae
n. polycythemia vera
o. Western blot

_____

*Answers are in Appendix A.

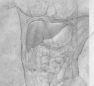

Word Element Review

Root	Meaning	Example	Definition
agglutin/o	clumping, sticking	**agglutination** (ah-gloo″tĭ-nā′shŭn)	clumping together of particular elements in the blood
bas/o	base	**basophil** (bā′sō-fĭl)	granular leukocyte
blast/o	primitive cell	**blastoma** (blăs-tō′mah)	new, abnormal growth of tissue composed of immature cells derived from the blastema of an organ or a tissue
coagul/o	clotting	**coagulant** (kō-ag′ū-lănt)	agent accelerating the formation of a clot
cyt/o	cell	**cytogenic** (sī-tō-jĕn′ĭk)	forming cells
eosin/o	red	**eosinopenia** (ē″ō-sĭn″ō-pē′nē-ah)	abnormal deficiency of eosinophils in the blood
erythr/o	red	**erythematous** (ĕr-ĭ-thĕm′ah-tŭs)	characterized by redness of the skin
granul/o	granules	**granuloblast** (grăn′ū-lō-blăst″)	immature granulocyte
hemat/o, hem/o	blood	**hematoma** (hĕm″ah-tō′mah)	localized collection of blood in an organ, a space, or a tissue; a bruise
immun/o	immune, protection	**immunosuppression** (ĭm″ū-nō-sŭ-prĕsh′ŭn)	artificial prevention of the immune response
kary/o	nucleus	**karyomegaly** (kăr″ē-ō-mĕg′ah-lē)	abnormal enlargement of a cell nucleus
leuk/o	white	**leukocytogenesis** (loo″kō-sī″tō-jĕn′ĕ-sĭs)	formation of white cells (leukocytes)
lymph/o	lymph	**lymphogranulomatosis** (lĭm″fō-grăn″ū-lō″mah-tō′sĭs)	Hodgkin's disease
mon/o	single	**monocyte** (mŏn′ō-sīt)	mononuclear, phagocytic leukocyte
myel/o	bone marrow	**myeloma** (mī″ĕ-lō′mah)	tumor composed of cells of the type normally found in the bone marrow
neutr/o	neutral	**neutrophil** (nū′trō-fĭl)	leukocyte that stains easily with neutral dyes
phag/o	eat, swallow	**phagocyte** (făg′ō-sīt)	any cell that eats another
sangui/o	blood	**sanguineous** (săng-gwĭn′ē-ŭs)	bloody; having an abundance of blood
splen/o	spleen	**splenic** (splĕn′ĭk)	pertaining to the spleen
thym/o	thymus	**thymectomy** (thī-mĕk′tō-mē)	surgical removal of the thymus

continues

Prefix	Meaning	Example	Definition
mega-	large	**megakaryocyte** (mĕg"ă-kăr'ē-ō-sīt")	large bone marrow cell with large nuclei

Suffix	Meaning	Example	Definition
-blast	immature	**myeloblast** (mī'ĕ-lō-blăst")	immature cell of bone marrow
-cytosis	abnormal condition of cells	**leukocytosis** (loo"kō-sī-tō'sĭs)	temporary abnormal increase in the number of circulating white cells
-emia	blood condition	**anemia** (ah-nē'mē-ah)	reduction in the number of erythrocytes, quantity of hemoglobin, or volume of packed red cells
-lytic	pertaining to destruction	**thrombolytic** (thrŏm"bō-lĭt'ĭck)	pertaining to destruction of a blood clot
-penia	deficiency	**neutropenia** (nu"trō-pē'nē-ah)	diminished number of neutrophils in the blood
-philia	attraction for	**eosinophilia** (ē"ō-sīn"ō-fĭl'ē-ah)	formation of an abnormally large number of eosinophils in the blood
-phoresis	carrying	**electrophoresis** (ē-lek"trō-fō-rē'sĭs)	technique involving movement of charged particles suspended in a liquid under the influence of an applied electric field
-poiesis	formation	**erythropoiesis** (ē-rĭth"rō-poi-ē-sĭs)	formation of erythrocytes (red cells)
-stasis	stop, control	**hemostasis** (hē"mō-stā'sĭs)	arrest of bleeding

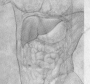

Word Element Review Exercises

Name: _____ Date: _____

COMPLETION*

Complete the following statements.

1. Two of the word elements stand for blood; they are _____ and _____.

2. Two of the elements refer to cells; they are _____ and _____.

3. Two elements designate color. Red is indicated by _____ and _____, and white is indicated by _____.

4. Four elements refer to parts of the lymph system; they are _____, _____, _____, and _____.

5. "Sticking together" is designated by the word element _____.

6. A word element that may serve as a root and a suffix is _____.

MATCHING*

Match the terms to their meanings.

1. _____ agent accelerating the formation of a clot
2. _____ a bruise
3. _____ abnormal enlargement of a cell nucleus
4. _____ pertaining to the spleen
5. _____ tumor composed of cells of the type normally found in bone marrow
6. _____ pertaining to destruction of a blood clot
7. _____ formation of red cells or erythrocytes
8. _____ formation of white cells
9. _____ arrest of bleeding
10. _____ an immature granulocyte

a. coagulant
b. erythropoiesis
c. granuloblast
d. hematoma
e. hemostasis
f. karyomegaly
g. leukocytogenesis
h. myeloma
i. phagocyte
j. splenic
k. thrombolytic

SPELLING

Rewrite the misspelled words.

1. neutraphil _____
2. annemia _____
3. megacaryocyte _____
4. sanguneous _____
5. electroforesis _____
6. myeloblast _____
7. leukocytosis _____
8. eosinophillia _____
9. monocyte _____
10. phagacyte _____

*Answers are in Appendix A.

11. neutropennia   _____

12. agglutinatation   _____

WORD ELEMENT MEANINGS

Give the meaning of each word element. Then use your dictionary to find a new word that contains each of the word elements. Specify whether the new word is a noun or an adjective by placing N or A in the last column.

Word Element	Meaning	Word	N or A
1. agglutin/o			
2. bas/o			
3. blast/o			
4. -blast			
5. coagul/o			
6. cyt/o			
7. -cytosis			
8. -emia			
9. eosin/o			
10. erythr/o			
11. granul/o			
12. hemat/o			
13. hem/o			
14. immun/o			
15. kary/o			
16. leuk/o			
17. lymph/o			
18. -lytic			
19. mega–			
20. mon/o			
21. myel/o			
22. neutr/o			
23. -penia			
24. phag/o			
25. -philia			
26. -phoresis			
27. -poiesis			
28. sangui/o			
29. splen/o			
30. -stasis			
31. thym/o			

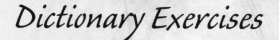

Dictionary Exercises

Name: _____ Date: _____

DICTIONARY EXERCISE 1*

Use your dictionary to find the pronunciation and definition of the following words.

	Word	**Pronunciation**	**Definition**
1.	agranulocytosis	_____	_____
2.	antibody	_____	_____
3.	elliptocytosis	_____	_____
4.	erythropoiesis	_____	_____
5.	granulopoiesis	_____	_____
6.	erythroblast	_____	_____
7.	viscosity	_____	_____
8.	macrocytic anemia	_____	_____
9.	metamyelocyte	_____	_____
10.	Pel-Ebstein fever	_____	_____
11.	poikilocytosis	_____	_____
12.	hemolysis	_____	_____
13.	thrombocytopenic purpura	_____	_____

DICTIONARY EXERCISE 2

Select the correct meaning and provide the pronunciation where indicated.

1. elliptocyte (_____)
   a. elliptical red blood cell
   b. cause of lupus erythematosus, a cutaneous or connective tissue disease

2. erythroblast (_____)
   a. condition in which the capillary vascular channels are more fragile than normal
   b. immature red blood cell still having a nucleus

3. hematopoiesis (_____)
   a. production and development of blood cells
   b. presence of red blood cells of a variety of shapes

4. hypochromic (_____) anemia
   a. anemia in which red cells tend to be larger than normal
   b. anemia characterized by a hemoglobin deficiency in the red blood cells

5. phagocytosis (_____)
   a. process of a cell engulfing and destroying bacteria
   b. any phagocyte cell involved in the defense against infection

6. polychromatophilia (_____)
   a. disorder resulting from excess porphyrins in the blood
   b. quality of staining in which erythrocytes show various shades of blue or pink tinges

7. leukopoiesis (_____)
   a. production of leukocytes
   b. passage of leukocytes through blood vessel walls

*Answers are in Appendix A.

8. fibrinogen (_____)
   a. coagulation factor
   b. resembling fibrin

9. reticulocyte (_____)
   a. cells that mature in the thymus
   b. an immature erythrocyte

DICTIONARY EXERCISE 3

Pronunciation of the words below is provided. Using your dictionary, find the correct spelling and definition of the words.

	Word	**Pronunciation**	**Definition**
1.	_____	grăn"ū-lō-sī"tō-pē'nē-ah	_____
2.	_____	hĕt'ĕr-ō-fĭl" antibody	_____
3.	_____	lĭp"ō-prō'tē-ĭn	_____
4.	_____	lĭm'foid tissue	_____
5.	_____	mī'ĕ-loid tissue	_____
6.	_____	pŏr-fē'rē-ah	_____
7.	_____	hī"pĕr-lĭp-ē'mē-ah	_____
8.	_____	hē"mō-glō"bĭ-nū'rē-ah	_____
9.	_____	ē"ō-sĭn"ō-fĭl'ē-ah	_____
10.	_____	ăn-ī"sō-sī-tō'sĭs	_____

IMPRESSIONS:

1. Thrombocytopenia. The patient did not have any physical findings nor does she have any history that would suggest a cause for her thrombocytopenia. The atenolol and Dyazide have been associated with thrombocytopenia and they have been discontinued. She has not had any recent viral infections nor has she experienced any rheumatologic complaints that might suggest underlying diagnosis of lupus. She has had no lymphadenopathy or systemic symptoms that might suggest an underlying _____ _____. Based on these findings, I would think that the most likely diagnosis would be chronic ITP.

RECOMMENDATIONS:

1. Arrangements will be made for the other studies necessary.

Mark J. Black, MD
Comprehensive consult findings sent to: Vito Mansetti, MD

Oncology

The best of healers is good cheer.

—PINDAR

OBJECTIVES

When you have completed this chapter on oncology, you should be able to

1. Explain the development of cancer cells.
2. Identify and define three types of cancer.
3. Define tumor staging and grading.
4. Identify and define methods of cancer treatment.
5. Spell common anticancer drug combinations.
6. Be familiar with terminology used in medical reports.

INTRODUCTION

Oncology (ŏng-kŏl'ō-jē) is the sum of knowledge regarding tumors. **Tumors**, which may be benign or malignant, are abnormal masses of tissue that result from excessive cell division. Benign tumors are seldom a threat to life because they do not spread to other parts of the body. A malignant tumor, on the other hand, is referred to as *cancer*, and its growth is uncontrollable and marked by the spread of abnormal cells. When cancer cells break away from the primary site and start secondary growths in other parts of the body, the process is referred to as **metastasis** (mĕ-tăs'tah-sĭs). Physicians who specialize in the treatment of malignant tumors are called **oncologists** (ŏng-kŏl'ō-jĭsts).

Oncogenes (ŏng'kō-jēnz) arise when proto-oncogenes mutate. While oncogenes physically resemble the proto-oncogenes, they differ in that they instruct cells to make proteins that stimulate excessive cell growth and cause cells to divide abnormally. Essentially they code for an altered version of the growth-control proteins leading to hyperactivity within a cell. Sometimes more than one oncogene is present in a cell.

Tumor suppressor genes (sometimes called antioncogenes) are normal genes whose function is to instruct cells to produce proteins that inhibit cell growth and division. If they are not present, the loss of the proteins they produce allows a cell to grow and divide uncontrollably and results in cancer. For example, the p53 protein coded by one of the suppressor genes can trigger cell suicide, thus preventing a genetically damaged cell from growing out of control.

DNA repair genes code proteins that will correct DNA cell duplication errors prior to cell division. If a mutation occurs in a DNA repair gene, the gene may fail to repair the DNA, thus allowing the mutations in the tumor suppressor genes and proto-oncogenes to accumulate.

An accumulation of mutations involving all three of these factors often leads to cancer. Figure 10-3 illustrates the difference between the growth of normal cells and cancerous cells.

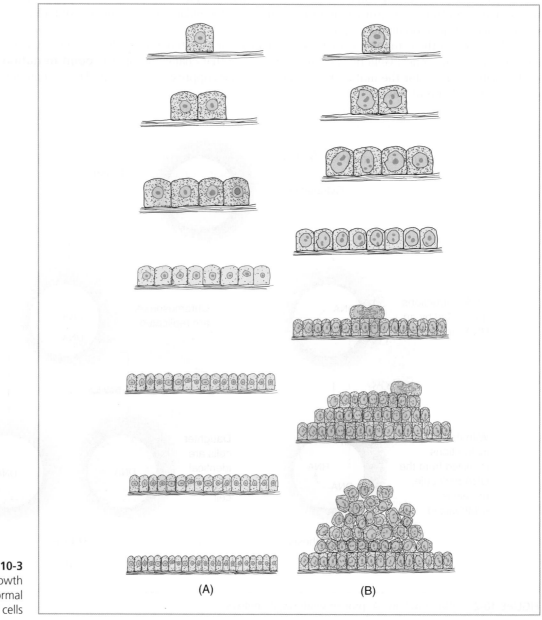

FIGURE 10-3
Cellular Growth Patterns: (A) normal cells; (B) cancer cells

(A)　　　　(B)

MUTATIONS, HEREDITY, AND CARCINOGENS

Many disorders or diseases appear to stem from mutated genes received from the mother and/or father. These mutations are called **germline mutations** because the change exists in the reproductive cells of the parent. Estimates indicate about five percent of all cancers in the United States may be explained by inherited genetic mutations.

Another type of mutation is called an **acquired**, or **somatic**, **mutation**. This disruption of the normal genetic programming of a cell—with its potential of producing a malignancy—may occur any time in a person's life. This kind of mutation is passed only to direct descendants of an altered cell.

A mutation may crop up during cell division or be the by-product of environmental stresses. The most common **carcinogen** (kăr"sĭn'ō-jĕn) results from the use of tobacco products. It causes as many as one of three deaths in any given year. In some cases, infectious, cancer-inducing viruses inject their own oncogenes into normal cells, which then seem to become unregulated by the normal cell process. Examples are cervical cancer, liver cancer, certain lymphomas, leukemia, and sarcomas. In other cases, bacterium such as *H. pylori* may be related to stomach cancer.

Prolonged or repeated exposure to certain types of radiation can cause cancer. Exposure to low-level sources such as sunlight—which delivers ultraviolet rays—most often results in skin cancer. Exposure to high-level radiation, such as those from x-rays or radioisotopes, is more likely to cause not-so-evident internal damage. (Note that dental x-rays and diagnostic body x-rays are considered low-level radiation and therefore not generally harmful when used with appropriate safety procedures.)

Chemicals also can be dangerous carcinogens. Examples include alkylating agents, arsenic, asbestos, benzene, hydrocarbons, and vinyl chloride. Many of these chemicals are "hidden" in common, everyday products. Others, like cigarette smoke, exhaust fumes from vehicles, insecticides, and asbestos insulation, are found in the environment.

GENETIC TESTING, MAPPING, AND SPLICING

Genetic testing can identify individuals or families with a possible predisposition to a disease or to confirm a suspected mutation. Testing is done by examining a person's DNA, which may be taken from cells in blood, tissue, or other body fluids. Several types of tests (with examples) are currently used: newborn screening (phenylketonuria), carrier testing (Tay-Sachs disease), prenatal diagnosis (Down syndrome), cancer/precancerous cells for early detection (familial adenomatous polyposis), diagnosis (leukemia), and prognosis (p53 tumor-suppressor gene).

Predictive gene testing is a newer development and focuses on identifying people who are at risk of getting a disease before any symptoms appear. To make this possible, a massive international collaboration called the Human Genome Project was undertaken in 1990. Its aim has been to map each of the 50,000 to 100,000 genes and the spaces between them, as well as the sequence of the estimated 3 billion chemical bases. Completion of the project with publishing of the DNA sequence of the human genome is scheduled for June 2003. Biomedical research and medical practice will be dramatically affected by the project findings.

Since 1974, **gene-splicing technology** has allowed DNA from a different organism to be spliced or recombined to form a new organism. By 1983, a laboratory method for reproducing DNA quickly led to the identification of the first genetic marker for cystic fibrosis. And in 1986, tumor suppressor genes were discovered. Using these three key discoveries, coupled with genetic engineering, scientists can isolate and manipulate the action of individual cancer-causing genes to create models of human disease and pinpoint genes that are solely responsible for specific types of cancer.

Ongoing research is adding rapidly to our knowledge about the biology of cancer cells and the effect of various carcinogens in developing cancer.

TYPES OF CANCER

-blast	immature	-plasia	formation, growth
-oma	mass, tumor	-plasm	formation, growth

Currently recognized varieties of cancer can be grouped into three basic categories according to the type of tissue from which the tumor cells have arisen: carcinomas, sarcomas, and mixed-tissue tumors.

STAGING AND GRADING TUMORS

cyst/o	sac of fluid	papill/o	papillary
fibr/o	fibers	polyp/o	polyp
fung/o	fungus, mushroom	scirrh/o	hard
medull/o	soft, inner part		

Once a pathologist has diagnosed the type of cancer, the malignant tumor is categorized using a classification such as the American Joint Committee on Cancer (AJCC) or Union Internationale Contre le Cancer (UICC) classification. These classifications are based on the belief that cancers of similar **histology** (hĭs-tŏl'ō-jē) (the science of diseased tissue) or site of origin share similar patterns of growth and extension. Determination of stage and grade will have an impact on treatment.

Stage

A **stage** is based on the extent of invasion or spread of an untreated primary cancer and is an important indicator of prognosis. The **TNM staging system** is commonly used. *T* (0–4) refers to the size of the primary tumor. It also indicates the degree to which it has invaded the local area. *N* (0–3) refers to the regional lymph nodes that have been involved by the tumor. *M* (0–3) refers to the presence or absence of distant metastasis of the tumor cells. This usually occurs when the cancer has existed undetected for an extended period of time and has spread to other parts of the body. Staging can be determined by clinical examination, but it might be classified differently after a surgical procedure and histologic examination. Staging of recurrent cancers may have different significance when considering therapy or determining prognosis.

Grade

Grade is an assessment of the extent to which a tumor resembles the normal tissue in a site and reflects an indication of prognosis. In general, the following classifications can be made.

GX	grade cannot be assessed
G1	well differentiated (least malignant)
G2	moderately differentiated
G3	poorly differentiated
G4	undifferentiated (malignant)

As indicated, the higher the grade the more serious the condition has become and the more difficult it is to treat. It should be noted that grading is not necessarily applied the same way to all types of cancer. One type—melanomas of the conjunctiva or adenocarcinomas—use only three grades. Also be aware that grading is not applied at all to some cancers, examples being carcinomas of the thyroid and some other locations.

Additional Descriptors

Cases needing separate analysis use the symbols m, y, r, and a. The m symbol in parentheses indicates the presence of multiple primary tumors in a single site. The y symbol is used during or following initial multiple methods of therapy. The r symbol is used when a patient has been staged *after* a disease-free interval. The a symbol indicates the classification was first determined during autopsy.

The following table lists the classification possibilities the TNM staging system offers.

TNM STAGING SYSTEM	
Tumor	Meaning
T_0	no evidence of primary tumor
T_{IS}	carcinoma in situ
T_1, T_2, T_3, T_4	progressive increase in tumor size and involvement
T_x	tumor cannot be assessed
Node	Meaning
N_0	regional lymph nodes not demonstrably abnormal
N_1, N_2, N_3, N_4	increasing numbers or increasing distant location of spread to regional lymph nodes
N_x	regional lymph nodes cannot be assessed clinically
Metastasis	Meaning
M_0	no evidence of distance metastasis
M_1, M_2, M_3	ascending degrees of distant metastasis

Other staging systems for tumors have the same general meaning. The most complete reference about tumor definitions is the *Atlas of Tumor Pathology*, published in many volumes by the Armed Forces Institute of Pathology, Washington, D.C.

METHODS OF TREATMENT

chem/o	chemical, drug	radi/o	rays, x-rays
immun/o	immune, immunity	-therapy	treatment

Early diagnosis is a key factor in successfully treating cancer. The American Cancer Society has developed seven cancer "early warning" signs. If any of these symptoms are a problem, one should seek a physician's advice.

1. Change in bowel or bladder habits
2. Sore that does not heal
3. Unusual bleeding or discharge
4. Thickening or lump in a breast or elsewhere in your body
5. Indigestion or swallowing difficulty
6. Obvious change in a wart or mole
7. Nagging cough or hoarseness

During examination, the physician can perform several tests to locate a malignancy. Common procedures are computed tomography (CT) scans, angiograms (to see if there are blockages or abnormal placement of blood vessels that may indicate a tumor is present), radioactive isotopes, ultrasound, special tests with tumor markers, laboratory tests, biopsies, or other diagnostic tests. These procedures are presented with each of the systems in this text.

Once a diagnosis has been made, there are several treatment options that may be used alone or in various combinations. Treatment is considered on an individual basis depending on the diagnosis and stage of the disease; the person's age, gender, and general health; and, in women, menopausal status.

Options are considered and a plan, or **protocol**, is developed for the treatment. Treatment options are surgery, radiation therapy, chemotherapy, hormone therapy, and immunotherapy/biological therapies.

Surgery

Surgery is done in more than ninety percent of all cases to diagnose and stage a cancer to determine whether it has metastasized. Additional surgery is done in about sixty percent of all cases to remove cancerous growths or make the growth smaller (debulk the tumor) to improve the effectiveness of chemotherapy or radiation therapy.

Some of the more common procedures are outlined in the following table.

Procedure	Description
incisional biopsies	removal of a piece of a tumor for examination and diagnosis
excisional biopsies	removal of a tumor and a portion of normal tissue for comparison
en bloc resection	removal of a tumor and a large area of surrounding tissue containing lymph nodes
exenteration	removing an organ of origin and surrounding tissue by a wide resection
fulguration	destruction of tissue with electric sparks
electrocauterization	destruction of tissue by burning
cryosurgery	destruction of tissue by freezing

If a tumor cannot be removed or the patient cannot tolerate surgery, other treatments may be tried.

Radiation Therapy

Radiation therapy is a treatment that uses high energy carried by waves or streams of particles to treat cancer. Types of radiation include x-ray (either high-energy proton or low-energy electron), alpha and beta particles, and gamma rays. Radioactive substances include cobalt, iridium, iodine, and cesium. Sometimes it is called radiotherapy, x-ray therapy, or irradiation. Such therapy affects only those cells within the radiation field and will not kill cancerous cells that have spread to other parts of the body.

Radiation therapy may be used during surgery at the completion of resection but before closure (intraoperative radiation), after surgery to shrink a tumor, after surgery to stop the growth of remaining cancer cells (postoperative radiation), or alone or in combination with anticancer drugs to destroy a malignant tumor. Typically, **external radiation** is delivered by a machine called a linear accelerator that directs the high-energy rays at the cancer.

Simulation, performed by a radiation oncologist, is a process involving special x-ray pictures that are used to plan radiation treatment so the areas or fields to be treated are precisely located and marked for treatment and other tissues are protected by lead blocks. During simulation, the **treatment port** (the place on the body at which the radiation beam is aimed) is determined.

Radiation treatment is a team effort involving the radiation oncologist; a **radiation physicist** (fĭz′ĭ-sĭst), who makes sure the radiation machine delivers the right amount of radiation at the treatment site; and a **dosimetrist** (dō″sĭ-mĕt′rĭst), who plans and calculates the proper radiation dose for treatment. Dividing radiation into small, repeated doses—a process called **fractionation**—allows larger total doses to be given with less damage to normal tissue. These treatments are often administered five days a week on an outpatient basis by a **radiology technologist**.

Internal radiation, sometimes called **brachytherapy** (brăk″ē-thĕr′ah-pē), may be delivered through the use of a radiation implant in the body. Doing so enables the doctor to give a higher dose of radiation than is possible with external radiation therapy and to save most of the healthy tissue around it. When the radioactive source is placed directly into tissue rather than a body cavity, the term **interstitial** (ĭn-tĕr-stĭsh′ăl) **implant** is used.

Another form of internal radiation is **intraoperative radiation therapy**, which consists of a high dose of electronic beam therapy given directly to the tumor or tumor bed. This is done via a Lucite cone attached to the head of the treatment machine located in the operation room.

Unfortunately, radiation cannot distinguish between cancerous and noncancerous cells, so both are affected. Side effects are determined by location and amount of radiation used. Drugs called **radiosensitizers** are currently being studied to boost the effect of radiation therapy by increasing the sensitivity of the tumor to x-rays.

Chemotherapy

Chemotherapy (kē"mō-thĕr'ă-pē) involves using anticancer drugs alone or in various combinations to treat cancer. These drugs may be administered by mouth, by injection, or intravenously. Some of the drugs may be given in cycles of treatment and rest. These drugs find their way into the bloodstream, which carries them through the entire body. Therefore, chemotherapy is called a **systemic treatment**. It, too, can affect normal tissue, especially in the bone marrow, gastrointestinal tract, reproductive system, and hair follicles.

When chemotherapy is used after potentially curative radiation or surgery in an attempt to kill remaining cancer cells, it is called **adjuvant** (ăd'jū-vănt) **chemotherapy**. Hair loss and other side effects may occur with some anticancer drugs, but these side effects are generally temporary.

Categories of chemotherapeutic agents are alkylates, antibiotics, antimetabolites, antimitotics, and hormonal. **Alkylating** (ăl'kĭ-lāt-ĭng) **agents** are combinations of synthetic compounds that interfere with the process of DNA synthesis by attacking the DNA molecules. **Antibiotics** bind to the DNA in a cell and promote DNA strand breaks and prevent normal replication. **Antimetabolites** (ăn"tĭ-mĕ-tăb'ō-lītz) inhibit the synthesis of substances that are necessary components of DNA or they may block the replication of DNA. **Antimitotics** (ăn"tĭ-mī-tŏt'ĭks) are natural products and marine extracts that block the function of the cell's structural protein, which is essential for mitosis.

Hormone therapy uses hormones, a class of chemicals made by the endocrine glands in the body (e.g., corticosteroids and prednisone). Because hormones attach to receptor proteins in target tissue, they are key factors in inhibiting certain kinds of cancer such as breast cancer and leukemia. Other hormones block hormonal action and cause regression, as in prostate cancer. They can cause a number of side effects. Fluid retention, weight gain, nausea and vomiting, and changes in appetite are the more common symptoms. In women, they may interrupt the menstrual cycle and cause vaginal dryness. In men, they may cause impotence, loss of sexual desire, and/or fertility. These changes may be temporary, long lasting, or permanent.

Common Drugs Used in Cancer Treatment

Over the years **clinical trials**, an inherently slow process, have made important contributions in the treatment of cancer. With the introduction of a new drug, laboratory tests and animal studies are conducted. When the drug shows promise, a clinical trial is conducted with cancer patients to evaluate the safety and effectiveness of the treatment. Although progress in the treatment of cancer has improved in recent years, early diagnosis still remains the key to successful treatment. Survival rates are far better when intervention occurs early in the disease process.

The following table identifies medications used in cancer therapy. In addition to chemotherapy drugs, hormones, cell protectants, antidotes, and antiemetics are included. Note that some medications are used in the treatment of conditions or disease processes not related to cancer.

MEDICATIONS USED IN CANCER THERAPY*	
Trade Name	Generic Name
—	oxaliplatin
5-FU	fluorouracil
Adriamycin	doxorubicin hydrochloride
Adrucil	fluorouracil
Alkeran	melphalan
Anzemet	dolasetron
Arimidex	anastrozole
BCNU, BiCNU	carmustine
Blenoxane	bleomycin sulfate
Camptosar	irinoteca
Casodex	bicalutamide
CeeNu, CCNU	lomustine
Cerubidine	daunorubicin

continues

MEDICATIONS USED IN CANCER THERAPY*

Trade Name	Generic Name
Cosmegen	dactinomycin
Cytosar-U	cytarabine
Cytoxan	cyclophosphamide
Decadron	dexamethasone
Deltasone, Orasone, Cordrol	prednisone
Depo-Provera	medroxyprogesterone acetate
DES	diethylstilbestrol
DTIC-Dome	dacarbazine
Elspar	asparaginase
Emcyt	estramustine
Epogen	epoetin alfa (synthetic)
Eulexin	flutamide
Fareston	toremifine
Femara	letrozole
Fludara	fludarabine
Gemzar	gemcitabine
Herceptin	trastuzumab
Histerone, Testoderm	testosterone
Hycamtin	topotecan
Hydrea	hydroxyurea
IFEX	ifosfamide
IGIV	immune globulin IV
Intron A, Roferon-A	interferon alfa
Kytril	granisetron
Leucovorin Calcium	folinic acid
Leukeran	chlorambucil
Leukine	sargramostim (GM-CSF)
Lupron	leuprolide acetate
Lysodren	milotane
Matulane	procarbazine
Medrol	methylprednisolone
Megace	megestrol acetate
MESNEX	mesna
Methotrexact, Trexall	methotrexate
Mexate	methotrexate
Mithracin	plicamycin
Mustargen	mechlorethamine

continues

MEDICATIONS USED IN CANCER THERAPY*

Trade Name	Generic Name
Mutamycin	mitomycin
Myleran	busulfan
Navelbine	vinorelbine
Neupogen	filgrastim (G-CSF)
Nolvadex	tamoxifen
Novantrone	mitoxantrone
Oncovin, Vincasar	vincristine sulfate
Paraplatin	carboplatin
Platinol	cisplatin
Purinethol, 6-MP	6-mercaptopurine
Rituxan	rituximab
Sandostatin	octreotide acetate
Solu-Cortef	hydrocortisone
Taxol	paclitaxel
Taxotere	docetaxel
Temodal	temozolomide
Thalomid	thalidomide
Thiotepa	thiotepa
Velban	vinblastine sulfate
VePesid	etoposide
Xeloda	capecitabine
Zofran	ondansetron hydrochloride
Zoladex	goserelin

*For a complete current list of approved cancer drugs, see **www.fda.gov/cder/
cancer/index**, the Food and Drug Administration web site.

The names of many of these drugs, because they are frequently used in combination, have been abbreviated to provide a quick way to refer to these long words. Some of the more common combinations are listed in the following table.

ABBREVIATIONS FOR FREQUENTLY USED COMBINATIONS

Abbreviation	Drug Combination
CAE	cyclophosphamide, doxorubicin, etoposide
CAMP	cyclophosphamide, doxorubicin, methotrexate, procarbazine
CMF±P	cyclophosphamide, methotrexate, fluorouracil, prednisone
CVP	cyclophosphamide, vincristine, prednisone
FAC	fluorouracil, doxorubicin, cyclophosphamide
MOPP	mechlorethamine, vincristine, procarbazine, prednisone

Immunotherapy/Biological Therapies

Another method (modality) of treating cancer is **immunotherapy** (ĭm"ū-nō-thĕr'ă-pē) or biological therapies, which use the body's own defense system. The **immune system** is considered a complex group of cells and organs that defend the body from foreign substances that might cause infection or disease. Activity of the immune system against these foreign substances is referred to as **immune response**.

According to the National Cancer Institute, **biological response modifiers** are the latest addition to the traditional cancer treatment methods. These are agents that boost, direct, or restore the normal defenses of the body and inhibit the growth of tumor cells. Among other things, they enhance a cancer patient's immune system in its fight against the growth of cancer cells, make the cancer cells more sensitive to destruction by the patient's own immune system, and block the process that changes a normal cell into a precancerous or cancerous cell.

This particular arsenal of cancer-fighting weapons includes four types of biological response modifiers. **Interferon** (ĭn-tĕr-fĕr'ŏn) stimulates the body's immune system to fight cancer cells. **Interleukin** (ĭn'tĕr-loo"kĭn) is a protein that regulates cell growth and stimulates the immune system to destroy tumors. **Monoclonal** (mŏn"ō-klōn'ăl) **antibodies** are substances that can locate cancer cells and bind to them. They carry radioactive agents or poisons to the cells and destroy them. **Colony-stimulating factors** (CSFs) stimulate blood-forming cells to combat the myelosuppressive side effects.

Other therapies used are **bone marrow transplantation** (BMT) or **peripheral stem cell transplantation** (PSCT). Both procedures replace bone marrow destroyed by treatment using radiation or high-dose chemotherapy with healthy stem cells. An **autologous** (aw-tŏl'ō-gŭs) **transplant** uses the patient's own marrow that was saved before treatments. There are four other sources of bone marrow and stem cells. A **syngenic** (sĭn-jĕn'ĭk) **transplant** is where an identical twin donates the marrow or cells. An **allogenic** (ăl"ō-jĕn'ĭk) **transplant** is where a sibling is usually the donor. A **matched unrelated donor transplant** is like an allogenic transplant except the donor and recipient are not related. Finally, **cord stem cells**, which are derived from umbilical cords, are also being used.

Research on biological response modifiers is promising. Their major value is that doses that kill cancer cells are well below dose levels that create severe side effects.

Regardless of the treatment, problems are caused when healthy cells in the body are affected. Side effects develop. Common side effects are fatigue, nausea, vomiting, decreased blood cell counts, and mouth sores. Recently developed pharmaceutical products have helped to control some of the symptoms. After treatment, cells usually recover.

As a result of treatment, cancer symptoms may disappear temporarily or permanently. The cancer is then said to be in **remission**. Sometimes the treatment used will simply relieve symptoms without being able to successfully achieve remission. When this is the case, the treatment is referred to as a **palliative** (păl'ē-ă"tĭv) **therapy**.

INTERNET ASSIGNMENT

The American Cancer Society (ACS) is the nationwide, community-based voluntary health organization dedicated to eliminating cancer as a major health problem. It also has an international mission, which concentrates on developing cancer societies and on collaboration with cancer-related organizations throughout the world in carrying out the strategic directions of the American Cancer Society.

The ACS consists of a National Society, with chartered divisions throughout the country and over 3,400 local units utilizing over 2 million volunteers nationwide. The organization fights to conquer cancer through research, prevention, patient services, public policy, and advocacy programs. For example, the Society's advocacy initiative strives to influence public policies at all levels on issues such as

- the use, sale, distribution, marketing, and advertising of tobacco products, particularly to youth
- improved access for all Americans, particularly poor and underserved Americans, to a range of health care services for the prevention, early detection, diagnosis, and treatment of cancer and care of cancer patients
- increased federal funding and incentives for private sponsorship of cancer research to prevent and cure cancer, and
- advocacy for the rights of cancer survivors.

A visit to the ACS homepage at **www.cancer.org** finds information groups for Patients, Family, Friends; Survivors; ACS Supporters; Health Information Seekers; and Professionals, in addition to current news items concerning cancer.

ACTIVITY

Access the American Cancer Society site at **www.cancer.org**. Click Learn About Cancer, All About Cancer, and then Detailed Guide. Now find the answers to the following questions:

1. Who gets cancer?
2. How is cancer treated?
3. What are some of the questions you should ask your physician about cancer?
4. What did you learn about clinical trials?

Submit your answers in a report to your instructor.

Review: Oncology

■ DNA is composed of a sequence of four chemical subunits that instruct a cell to make a specific protein for a specific purpose.

■ Chromosomes are composed of paired strands of DNA spiraled around one another in the shape of a double helix.

■ Genes are the chemical subunits that identify a specific protein and are the basic unit of the heredity code.

■ Changes in proto-oncogenes of cells cause the cells to grow abnormally and cause cancer.

■ Three types of cancers are carcinomas (the largest group), sarcomas, and mixed-tissue tumors.

■ Tumor staging and grading refer to the extent of invasion of the cancer and degree to which a tumor resembles normal tissue.

■ Cancer may be treated with surgery, radiation therapy, chemotherapy (including hormone therapy), and biological therapies (immunotherapy).

■ Clinical trials provide opportunities to test experimental drugs on cancer patients to determine new safe and effective methods of treatment.

Review of Terminology Presented

Word	Definition
acquired mutations (somatic)	changes in DNA that develop throughout a person's life
adenocarcinoma	type of carcinoma
adjuvant chemotherapy	treatment used after radiation to kill remaining cancer cells
alkylating agents	combinations of synthetic compounds that attack DNA molecules
allogenic transplant	replacement using bone marrow or stem cells donated by a sibling or close relative
antibiotics	agents that bind to DNA, promote strand breaks, and prevent normal replication of microorganisms

continues

Word	Definition
antimetabolites	agent that inhibits synthesis of substances that are necessary components of DNA or block replication of DNA
antimitotics	natural products that block the function of the cell's structural proteins, which are essential for mitosis
autologous transplant	replacement using the patient's own bone marrow gathered before treatment
biological response modifiers	agents that boost, direct, or restore the normal defenses of the body to fight cancer
bone marrow transplantation (BMT) or peripheral stem cell transplantation (PSCT)	replacement of bone marrow destroyed by treatment using radiation or high-dose chemotherapy with healthy stem cells
carcinogens	factors that cause changes that lead to cancer
carcinoma	malignant new growth of epithelial cells
chemotherapy	treatment with anticancer drugs used alone or in combinations; may use alkylating agents, antibiotics, antimetabolics, antimitotics, or hormones
chromosomes	linear strands composed of DNA and proteins that carry genetic information
clinical trials	determining the clinical efficacy and pharmacological effects of a drug when administered to human subjects under carefully designed and executed conditions
colony-stimulating factor (CSF)	substance that stimulates blood-forming cells to combat myelosuppressive side effects
cord stem cell transplant	placement of stem cells derived from an umbilical cord
DNA (deoxyribonucleic acid)	the chemical code that determines the sequence of amino acids in a protein
DNA repair genes	genes that code proteins that will correct DNA cell duplication errors prior to cell division
dosimetrist	health professional who calculates and plans the proper radiation dosage for treatment
external radiation	radiation treatment delivered by a linear accelerator
fractionation	division of radiation into safe, small doses thereby resulting in larger total doses with less damage to normal tissue
gene	basic unit of heredity found in DNA; carries coded instructions for producing a specific protein; each gene occupies a specific location on a chromosome
gene-splicing technology	splicing or recombining of DNA from different organisms to form a new organism
genetic testing	testing done by examining DNA taken from cells in blood, tissue, or body fluids
germline mutations	mutations in reproductive cells
grade	degree to which a tumor resembles normal tissue
histology	science of diseased tissue
human genome	total collection of an individual's genes
immune response	activity of the immune system against foreign substances
immune system	complex groups of cells and organs that defend the body from foreign substances that might cause infection or disease

continues

Word	Definition
immunotherapy (biological therapies)	treatment that uses the body's own defense systems to fight cancer
interferon	substance that stimulates the body's immune system to fight cancer cells
interleukin	protein substance that regulates cell growth
internal radiation (brachytherapy)	treatment with internally placed source of radiation
interstitial implant	radioactive source placed directly into tissue rather than into a body cavity
intraoperative radiation therapy	treatment with a high dose of electron beams delivered directly to the tumor or tumor bed
matched unrelated donor transplant	replacement using bone marrow or stem cells donated by someone other than a close relative
metastasis	process whereby cancer cells break away from the primary site and begin secondary growths in other parts of the body
mitosis	process of cellular reproduction that occurs in the nucleus when it forms two identical daughter cells
mixed-tissue tumors	cancers arising from tissue that is capable of differentiating into epithelial and connective tissue
monoclonal antibodies	substances that locate cancer cells, bind to them, and carry radioactive agents or poisons to these cells
nucleus	core of a cell
oncogenes	special kind of genes that may cause cells to divide abnormally
oncologist	physician specializing in the treatment of malignant tumors
oncology	sum knowledge regarding tumors
palliative therapy	treatment to relieve cancer symptoms even though remission seems unlikely
point mutation	point where one of the components of a gene is changed
predictive testing	testing to identify individuals who are at risk of getting a disease *before* any symptoms appear
proto-oncogenes	normal form of an oncogene
protocol	plan for treatment
radiation physicist	technician who makes certain the machine delivers the right amount of radiation to a treatment site
radiation therapy	treatment that uses high energy radiation to treat cancer
radiology technologist	technician who administers radiation treatment to a patient
radiosensitizers	drugs being studied that will boost the effect of radiation therapy
remission	temporary or permanent absence of cancer symptoms
sarcoma	malignancy of supporting tissues
simulation	process involving special x-ray pictures that are used to plan radiation treatment so the target area is precisely located
squamous cell	type of carcinoma
stage	extent of invasion of an untreated primary cancer

continues

Word	Definition
syngenic transplant	replacement using bone marrow or stem cells donated by an identical twin
systemic treatment	treatment of cancer by chemotherapy through the bloodstream
TNM staging system	system used to refer to the size and degree of invasion of a tumor in the local area, nodes, or distant sites
treatment port	place on the body at which radiation is aimed
tumor	abnormal mass of tissue resulting from excessive cell division
tumor suppressor genes	genes whose function is to instruct cells to produce proteins that restrain cell growth and division

Terminology Review Exercises

Name: _____ Date: _____

MATCHING*

Match the terms to their meanings.

1. _____ point where one of the components of a gene is changed
2. _____ factors that cause changes that lead to cancer
3. _____ substance that stimulates the body's immune system to fight cancer cells
4. _____ agents that boost, direct, or restore the normal defenses of the body to fight cancer
5. _____ treatment of cancer by chemotherapy through the bloodstream
6. _____ treatment used after radiation treatment to kill remaining cancer cells
7. _____ body's defense system
8. _____ treatments conducted on cancer patients after careful laboratory testing to determine effectiveness and safety for the general population
9. _____ substance that locates cancer cells and carries radioactive agents or poisons to them
10. _____ the science of diseased tissue
11. _____ ways of referring to size and degree of invasion of a cancer
12. _____ normal form of an oncogene
13. _____ radiation treatment delivered by a linear accelerator
14. _____ temporary or permanent absence of cancer symptoms
15. _____ activity of immune system against foreign substances
16. _____ abnormal masses of tissue resulting from excessive cell division
17. _____ mutations in reproductive cells
18. _____ total collection of an individual's genes
19. _____ double strand spiraled into a helix composed of millions of chemical building blocks
20. _____ instructs cells to produce proteins that restrain cell growth and division

a. adjuvant chemotherapy
b. DNA molecule
c. interferon
d. human genome
e. biological response modifiers
f. carcinogens
g. clinical trials
h. external radiation
i. germline mutations
j. histology
k. immune system
l. immune response
m. monoclonal antibodies
n. point mutation
o. proto-oncogenes
p. remission
q. systemic treatment
r. TNM staging system
s. tumors
t. tumor suppressor gene

COMPLETION*

Complete the following statements.

1. The process whereby cancer cells break away from the primary site and begin secondary growths at distant locations in the body is referred to as _____.

2. _____ is based on the extent of invasion of an untreated primary cancer; the degree to which a tumor resembles the normal tissue in a site is _____.

3. A cancer arising from tissue that is capable of differentiating into epithelial and connective tissue is said to be a _____ tumor.

---

*Answers are in Appendix A.

4. Two types of carcinomas are _____ and _____.

5. Malignancies of epithelial cells are _____; malignancies of supporting tissues are _____.

6. _____ mutations are changes in DNA that develop throughout a person's life; _____ mutations are in reproductive cells.

7. The sum of knowledge regarding tumors is _____.

8. The categories of chemotherapeutic agents are: _____, _____, _____, _____ and _____.

9. Linear strands composed of DNA and proteins that carry genetic information are called _____.

10. Subunits of DNA are called _____.

11. The core of a cell is the _____.

12. _____ is treatment with a source of radiation located within the body.

13. _____ is using the body's own defense systems to fight cancer.

14. A plan for treatment of cancer is called a _____.

15. Treatment to relieve cancer symptoms even though the possibility of remission seems unlikely is called _____.

16. _____ are drugs being studied that will boost the effect of radiation therapy.

17. A _____ is the place on the body at which the radiation beam is aimed.

SHORT ANSWER

Supply a short answer to the following:

1. Compare the three types of genes that are possible sources of proto-oncogene mutations.

   _____

   _____

   _____

2. Explain the difference between intraoperative radiation therapy and an interstitial implant.

   _____

   _____

   _____

3. What is the role of the immune system?

   _____

   _____

   _____

4. Briefly explain fractionation and its benefit to a patient.

   _____

   _____

   _____

Word Element Review

Root	Meaning	Example	Definition
aden/o	gland	**adenopathy** (ad"ĕ-nŏp'ah-thē)	enlargement of glands, especially lymph nodes
blast/o	immature, embryonic	**blastoma** (blăs-tō'mah)	neoplasm composed of immature cells derived from the blastema of an organ or a tissue
carcin/o	cancerous	**carcinogenic** (kăr"sĭ-nō-jĕn'ĭk)	causing cancer
		carcinomatous (kăr"sĭ-nŏm'ah-tŭs)	pertaining to cancer; malignant
chem/o	chemical, drug	**electrochemistry** (ē-lek"trō-kĕm'ĭs-trē)	study of chemical changes resulting from electric action
cyst/o	sac of fluid	**cystalgia** (sĭs-tăl'jē-ah)	pain in the bladder
fibr/o	fibers	**fibrinogen** (fī-brĭn'ō-jĕn)	kind of protein found in the blood
immun/o	immune, immunity	**immunogen** (ĭm'ū-nō-jĕn)	any substance capable of eliciting an immune response
medull/o	soft inner part	**medullization** (mĕd"ū-lī-zā'shŭn)	enlargement of marrow spaces
mut/a	genetic change	**transmutation** (trăns"mū-tā'shŭn)	evolutionary change of one species into another
mutagen/o	causing genetic change	**mutagenesis** (mū"tah-jĕn'ĕ-sĭs)	induction of genetic mutation
onc/o	tumor	**oncogenic** (ŏng"kō-jĕn'ĭk)	giving rise to tumors
papill/o	papillary	**papillated** (păp'ĭ-lāt-ĕd)	containing small, nipple-shaped projections or elevations
plas/o	formation	**plasma** (plăz'mah)	fluid portion of blood from which all solids have been removed
polyp/o	polyp	**polypoid** (pŏl'ē-poid)	resembling a polyp
radi/o	rays, x-rays	**radiotherapy** (rā"dē-ō-thĕr'ah-pē)	treatment of disease with x-rays, radium, and other radiations
sarc/o	flesh	**sarcomas** (săr-kō'măhs)	malignant tumors of supporting tissues
scirrh/o	hard	**scirrhous** (skĭr'ŭs)	hard or indurated

Prefix	Meaning	Example	Definition
meta-	beyond, change	**metastasis** (mĕ-tăs'tah-sĭs)	transfer of disease from one part of the body to another that is not directly connected to it

continues

Suffix	Meaning	Example	Definition
-blast	immature	**medulloblast** (mĕ-dŭl'ō-blăst)	undifferentiated cell of the neural tube, which may develop into a neuroblast or spongioblast
-plasia	formation, growth	**neoplasia** (nē"ō-plā'zē-ah)	formation of a neoplasm (tumor)
-plasm	formation, growth	**neoplasm** (nē'ō-plăzm)	tumor; any new or abnormal growth
-therapy	treatment	**chemotherapy** (kē"mō-thĕr'ah-pē)	use of drugs to kill cancer cells

Word Element Review Exercises

Name: _____ Date: _____

IDENTIFY WORD ROOTS*

Write the word root of each of the following words and give its meaning.

	Word	Root	Meaning
1.	adenopathy	_____	_____
2.	papillated	_____	_____
3.	scirrhous	_____	_____
4.	sarcomas	_____	_____
5.	blastoma	_____	_____
6.	immunogen	_____	_____
7.	medullization	_____	_____
8.	cystalgia	_____	_____
9.	fibrinogen	_____	_____

IDENTIFY DEFINITIONS*

Provide the terms for the following definitions.

1. causing cancer _____
2. treatment of disease with x-rays, radium, and other radiations _____
3. transfer of disease from one part of the body to another that is not directly connected to it _____
4. resembling a polyp _____
5. evolutionary change of one species into another _____
6. induction of genetic mutation _____
7. giving rise to tumors _____
8. fluid portion of blood from which all solids have been removed _____
9. study of chemical changes resulting from electric action _____
10. pertaining to cancer _____
11. formation of a neoplasm _____
12. undifferentiated cells of the neural tube _____
13. tumor; any new or abnormal growth _____
14. use of drugs to kill cancer cells _____

_____

*Answers are in Appendix A.

MATCHING

Match the word elements to their meanings.

1. _____ beyond, change   a. -blast

2. _____ treatment   b. meta-

3. _____ immature   c. -plasia

4. _____ formation, growth   d. -plasm

     e. -therapy

WORD ELEMENT MEANINGS

Give the meaning of each word element. Then use your dictionary to find a new word that contains each of the word elements. Specify whether the new word is a noun or an adjective by placing N or A in the last column.

Word Element	Meaning	Word	N or A
1. aden/o			
2. blast/o			
3. -blast			
4. carcin/o			
5. chem/o			
6. cyst/o			
7. fibr/o			
8. immun/o			
9. medull/o			
10. meta-			
11. mut/a			
12. mutagen/o			
13. onc/o			
14. papill/o			
15. plas/o			
16. -plasia			
17. -plasm			
18. polyp/o			
19. radi/o			
20. sarc/o			
21. scirrh/o			
22. -therapy			

Dictionary Exercises

Special vocabulary evolves with new procedures, and such terms may not appear in the dictionary. Study these words and then answer the exercise questions.

Word	Pronunciation	Definition
allogeneic transplantation	ăl"ō-jĕ-nē'ik	procedure in which bone marrow donor and recipient are not genetically identical
antithymocyte globulin	an"tĭ-thī'mō-sīt	protein preparation used to prevent and treat graft versus host disease
apoptosis	ă-pŏp-tō'sĭs	self-destruction
autologous transplantation	aw-tŏl'ō-gus	procedure in which marrow is removed from a patient and reinfused into that patient at a later time
B cells		white blood cells that develop in bone marrow and are the source of antibodies
marrow harvest		removal of a portion of the bone marrow for later transplantation
colony-stimulating factors		proteins that stimulate the development of cells in bone marrow
engraftment		process in which transplanted bone marrow begins to manufacture new white cells, red blood cells, and platelets in the patient's marrow cavities
germ cell tumor		tumor arising from the reproductive cells
graft-versus-host disease		reaction of donated bone marrow or peripheral stem cells against the patient's own tissue
growth factor		agent that stimulates the growth of cells
human leukocyte antigen (HLA)	loo'kō-sīt	series of antigen tests used to assess the similarity of the tissue of different people
immuno-suppression	ĭm"ū-nō-sū-prĕsh'ŭn	use of drugs or techniques that interfere with the body's immune response, thus making the body less able to fight infection; used in transplants to help protect against rejection of the tissue
morbidity	mŏr-bĭd'ĭ-tē	condition of being diseased
neoadjuvant therapy	nē-ō-ăd'jū-vănt	treatment given before the primary treatment
NK (natural killer) cells		large lymphocytes (lĭm'fō-sīts) that attack tumor cells and infected cells
purging		removal of tumor cells from marrow before autologous transplantation
severe combined immuno-deficiency disease (SCID)	ĭm"ū-nō-dĕ-fĭsh'ĕn-sē	disorder characterized by complete absence or marked deficiency of B and T cells, types of white blood cells
stem cells		cells from which all blood cells develop
syngeneic transplantation	sĭn"jĕ-nē'ĭk	grafting between identical twins
T cells		white blood cells important in body's immune system

Dictionary Exercises continued

DICTIONARY EXERCISE 1*
What relationships can you see between any of the words in the previous list?

Example: B and T cells are both white blood cells.

1. _____
2. _____
3. _____
4. _____
5. _____
6. _____
7. _____
8. _____
9. _____
10. _____
11. _____
12. _____

DICTIONARY EXERCISE 2
Pronunciation of the words below is provided. Using your dictionary, find the correct spelling and definition of these words.

	Word	**Pronunciation**	**Definition**
1.	_____	lĭm-fō'mah	_____
2.	_____	mĕl"ah-nō'mah	_____
3.	_____	pŏl'ĭp	_____
4.	_____	rē-frăk'tō-rē	_____
5.	_____	făg"ō-sī-tō'sĭs	_____
6.	_____	thrŏm"bō-sī"tō-pē'nē-ah	_____
7.	_____	kor"tĭ-kō-stĕr'oyd	_____
8.	_____	ăn'tĭ-jĕn	_____
9.	_____	ah-plăs'tĭk ah-nē'mē-ah	_____
10.	_____	ĭn-fū'zhun	_____
11.	_____	loo"kō-pē'nē-ah	_____
12.	_____	făg'ō-sīt	_____
13.	_____	ă-pŏp-tō'sĭs	_____
14.	_____	mŏr-bĭd'ĭ-tē	_____
15.	_____	ĕn-kăp'sŭ-lā"tĕd	_____
16.	_____	stĕr'oyd	_____

*Answers are in Appendix A.

282 ■ *Chapter 10*

Listening Exercise

INSTRUCTIONS

1. Review the spelling, pronunciation, and meaning of the words provided in the preview.

2. Listen to the audio CD and fill in the blank as the word is dictated.

3. At the end of the exercise, check your spelling against the preview words. They appear in the preview in the order in which they are encountered in the exercise.

4. Review and practice the words you missed.

5. Look up words that are not familiar.

PREVIEW OF WORDS FOR LISTENING EXERCISE 10-1

Word	Pronunciation	Meaning
irradiation	ĭ-rā-dē-ā'shŭn	exposure to radiant energy for therapeutic purposes
adenocarcinoma	ăd"ĕ-nŏ-kăr"sĭn-ō'mă	cancer derived from glandular tissue
symptomatology	sĭmp"tō-mă-tŏl'ō-jē	the combined symptoms of a disease
fibrosis	fī-brō'sĭs	formation of fibrous tissue
organomegaly	or"gă-nō-mĕg'ă-lē	enlargement of organs
telangiectasias	tĕl-ăn"jē-ĕk-tă'zē-ă	vascular lesions formed by dilation of a group of small blood vessels

Letter of Consultation

Dr. Antonio Rameriz:

I had the opportunity to visit with our mutual patient, Katrina Switzgoebel, on 3/3/20—. She is now nine months after completion of her whole abdominal _____, which followed her second-look laparotomy for a grade 2 ovarian _____.

I am glad you referred her to a dietitian who has been working with her to modify her diet and, therefore, has decreased her _____. She has not had any vomiting since January and only intermittent cramping associated with certain foods. She denied the presence of blood in the stool, urine, or vagina. She does have a significant weight loss since we last saw her in December.

Her physical exam was remarkable for a weight of 61.7 kg, which is down from 70.8 kg on 9/6 of the previous year. She did not have any palpable lymphadenopathy. Breast exam was unremarkable. There was no back tenderness to percussion. Her abdomen showed _____ in the low abdominal area beneath the abdominal incision, but no masses or _____. Her pelvic exam was remarkable for an atrophic vagina, which presented dryness and _____ consistent with her estrogen deficient state and postradiation status.

Her laboratory evaluation was unremarkable except for an alkaline phosphatase of 260 (normal range 90–234), creatinine 1.2 (normal range 0.6–0.9). The creatinine level has not changed since her last visit and her alkaline phosphatase is actually down from 316 on 12/19. Her hemoglobin was 10.8. The rest of the hematology and chemistry panels were unremarkable. Chest x-ray was normal, as were her mammograms. CA-125 level was 18.8.

Dr. Victor Montagno from GYN Oncology examined Katrina and agreed with my findings. It is our impression that she does not have evidence of recurrent ovarian cancer. She does present RTOG grade 2 gastrointestinal toxicity related to her postoperative irradiation.

I would advise that Katrina continue seeing her dietitian since diet modification has been the only thing that helped her gastrointestinal symptoms. We would like to see her again at the end of May.

Thank you for letting us participate in the care of your patient. If you have questions regarding her visit here, please do not hesitate to write.

Sincerely yours,

Lloyd Livermore, MD

CHAPTER

11

Radiology and Nuclear Medicine

❝ One look is worth a thousand listens. ❞

—MERRILL C. SOSMAN

INTRODUCTION

Modern radiology is the outgrowth of two turn-of-the-twentieth-century discoveries. The first, in 1895, was the identification by Wilhelm Conrad Röntgen of types of radiation called **roentgen** (rĕnt'gĕn) **rays**. Then in 1903 Henri Becquerel and Marie Curie discovered radioactive properties in uranium. Curie recognized and diagrammed three different rays, called alpha and beta particles and gamma rays, which can be used to diagnose and treat disease. Such use of these radioactive substances is referred to as **nuclear medicine**.

There are several areas of specialization in the field of radiology and nuclear medicine. For example, a physician trained in the practice of diagnostic radiology is known as a **radiologist**. A physician or radiologist who focuses on the use of diagnostic nuclear medicine procedures is a **nuclear physician**. A physician who specializes in the practice of radiotherapy (treatment of disease using radiation) is a **radiotherapist** or radiation oncologist.

THE RADIOLOGY REPORT

The radiology report describes what the radiologist finds as a result of a radiologic examination. Other items included in the report are the name of the procedure performed, the name of the patient and date, and any other identification information the hospital or office may require.

When a contrast medium is used, it is noted in the report. The balance of the report details the findings and interpretations made by the radiologist who has reviewed the results of the study. More than one study may be included in one report.

An allied health professional must be aware of several types of information relating to radiology reports. This chapter discusses the use of radiology and nuclear medicine to diagnose and treat various medical problems, as well as x-ray positioning, contrast media, radionuclides, and interventional radiology. Such information will help students to work with radiology reports in their specific medical environment.

DIAGNOSTIC TECHNIQUES USING RADIOLOGY

cine/o	movement	-opaque	obscure
fluor/o	luminous	radi/o	ray
-gram	a record	roentgen/o	x-ray
-graphy	process of recording	tele-	distant
is/o	same, equal	tom/o	to cut
-lucent	to shine		

A radiologist can use x-rays, sound waves, and magnetism to produce images that will assist in the diagnosis of medical problems.

IMAGES PRODUCED BY X-RAYS

The x-ray machine is one of the most basic and familiar tools in radiological diagnostics. It uses penetrating rays derived from high-energy electromagnetic sources rather than the chemical sources found in nuclear medicine.

Body tissues and other substances vary in the way they accept x-rays. If x-rays pass through a substance, it is **radiolucent** (rā"dē-ō-lū'sĕnt). If a substance absorbs the rays, it is **radiopaque** (rā"dē-ō-pāk'). The intensity of the rays used is determined by both the body part and the purpose (diagnostic or treatment) of the x-rays.

Radiographic examinations may consist of **film surveys** only. A technologist prepares the patient, takes the radiograph, and develops the film. Interpretation is then done by a radiologist. This is the familiar x-ray that is administered in a dentist's office, a laboratory, or a hospital. An example of a film is shown in Figure 11-1.

In a **fluoroscopic** (floo"rō-skŏp'ĭk) **examination** a continuous, moving picture gives the radiologist a means of observing how organs are functioning before and after a contrast medium has been introduced. The patient's position can be changed during the examination for a different or better view of the target area. In addition, a permanent record of a fluoroscopic (or x-ray) examination can be obtained by combining cameras and video recorders in a process called **cineradiography** (sĭn"ĕ-rā"dē-ŏg'rah-fē).

Fluoroscopy is also used to assist in certain therapeutic procedures, such as installing catheters that deliver antibiotic or chemotherapy treatment or positioning tubes through the nasal passages to the stomach.

Because fluoroscopic or x-ray technologists face a risk from the cumulative effect of continued exposure to radiation, they are required to wear protective coverings.

The danger to a patient is very low even over a lifetime because exposure is infrequent. *However, because radiation exposure to a pregnant woman in her first trimester may cause congenital problems for the fetus, x-rays are avoided. During the second and third trimesters, x-rays may be used cautiously for special reasons. A woman should tell her doctor or dentist if she suspects being pregnant.*

With **computerized axial tomography** (ak'sē-al tō-mŏg'rah-fē) **(CAT)**, a layer or section of the body is exposed to thousands of small x-ray beams. The quantity of rays penetrating a given layer of tissue is recorded. A computer uses this data to compute the density of thousands of very small layers of tissues and produces an image of a cross

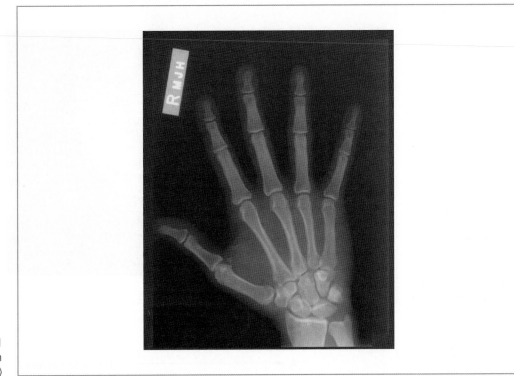

FIGURE 11-1
Example of a Film
Survey (X-ray)

section of the body. This procedure can also be used with a contrast medium. One of the advantages of this option is that it provides a three-dimensional view of a cross section of the body. The procedure is also known as **computed tomography (CT)** or **computer-assisted tomography (CAT)**. See Figure 11-2 for an example of a CAT scan.

Another technique is **tomography**, or **laminography** (lăm″ĭ-nŏg′rah-fē). This procedure permits visualization of a specific layer of the body while blocking out layers in front of and behind it. It is actually an x-ray slice taken at different depths of focus. Calcifications and solid lesions that are missed on conventional x-rays will often be identified on a **tomogram** (tō′mō-grăm), the picture produced by tomography.

Stereoscopy (stē′rē-ŏs′kō-pē) is still another radiographic technique that confers an illusion of depth to an object. The procedure involves two successive radiographs of the part of the body targeted. They are then viewed simultaneously using a stereoscopic viewing device, which gives the appearance of depth to the picture.

X-ray Positioning

X-ray positioning determines the view of an anatomical part being examined. X-rays of certain parts of the body can be taken only from specific body positions. The radiologist has special terms to refer to the direction of the x-ray beam in reference to the patient's position. The four most common terms are:

> **PA [posteroanterior** (pŏs″ter-ō-ăn-tēr′ē-or) **view]**
> patient is positioned with back to the x-ray machine, front close to the film cassette; beam passes from back to front; an example is a chest x-ray (Figure 11-3)
>
> **AP [anteroposterior** (an″tĕr-ō-pŏs-tēr′ē-or) **view]**
> patient is positioned with back to the film plate; beam passes from front to back; an example is a chest x-ray given to a very ill patient in bed (Figure 11-4)
>
> **lateral** (lăt′er-ăl) **view**
> patient is held closely against the film plate; beam passes from one side of the body to the other; an example is an x-ray of the extremities, chest, or abdomen (Figure 11-5)
>
> **oblique** (ŏ-blēk′) **view**
> x-ray beam tube or patient is positioned at an angle that is *not* PA, AP, or lateral (Figure 11-6)

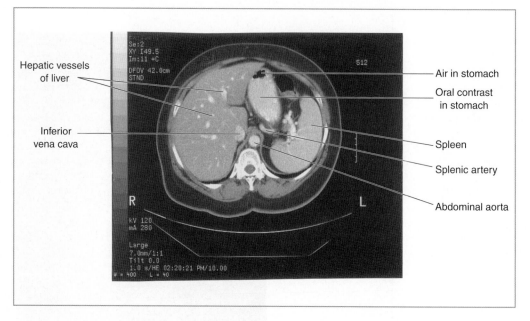

FIGURE 11-2
Computed
Tomography with
Contrast: shows
hepatic vessels, infe-
rior vena cava, aorta,
and splenic artery

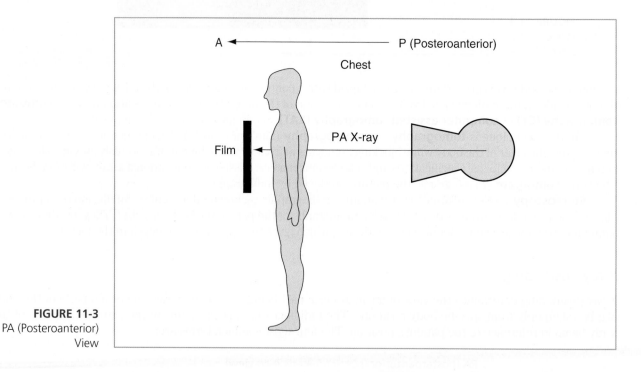

FIGURE 11-3
PA (Posteroanterior)
View

Radiographic Contrast Media

To visualize organs or body parts that are not ordinarily seen, **radiographic contrast media** are used to help the radiologist. They differentiate the organ under study from the surrounding tissue. These media are either injected, ingested, or administered by enema. Contrast media are radiopaque (not permitting passage of x-rays); most are barium- or iodine-based products. Other substances, such as oxygen, carbon dioxide, and air, are nonopaque and are classed as radiolucent (allowing passage of x-rays).

Barium sulfate, a water-soluble salt that does not permit x-rays to pass through it, causes the intestinal tract to stand out. Disorders of the esophagus, duodenum, and small and large intestines are primarily examined by swallowing barium or by barium enema. Most commonly performed tests are the upper GI series, small-bowel follow-through, and barium enema. On occasion a double contrast study is prescribed. This procedure combines both a radiopaque and a radiolucent contrast medium.

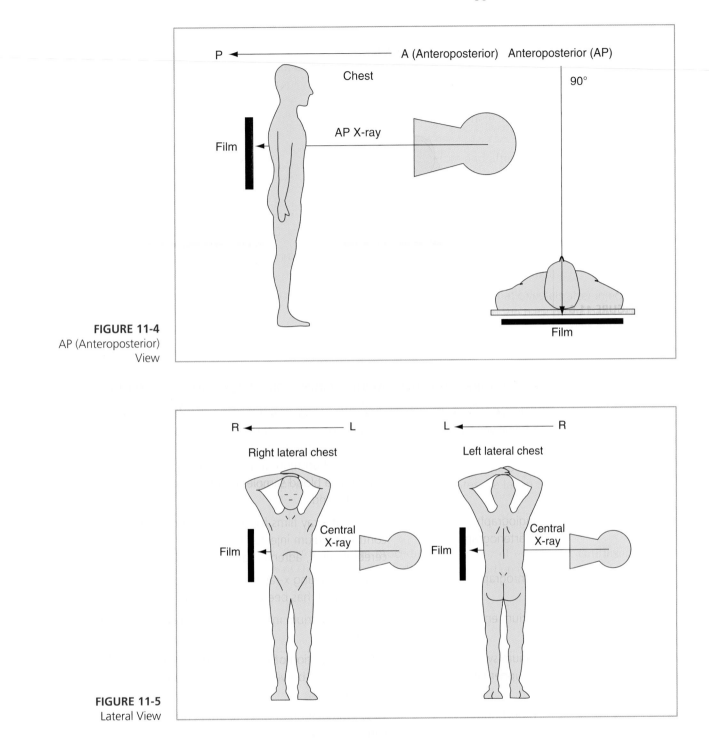

FIGURE 11-4
AP (Anteroposterior)
View

FIGURE 11-5
Lateral View

For a variety of other diagnostic x-ray examinations, **iodinated substances** are combined with other compounds and used as the contrast medium. Three of the most commonly used iodine-based contrast media are diatrizoate (Hypaque, Cardiografin, Renografin), iothalamate (Conray), and Isovue. Diatrizoate and iothalamate both have hyperosmolarity while Isovue has hypo-osmolarity. All are water soluble.

All iodinated contrast media may cause side effects that range from mild to severe. The reason for these adverse reactions is disputed.

Catheters		
Amplatz	Headhunter	Shepherd hook
Bentson	Hickman catheter	Simmons
Chuang	Judkins	Sones
Cobra	Kumpe	straight
Double J stent	Porta catheter	Swan Ganz
Grollman	Rosch	Van Aman

Needles	Introducers	Embolization Materials
Chiba	Greenfield	coils
Micropuncture	Bird	PVA (Ivalon)
Colapinto	S nest	glue
		gelfoam

Guidewires	Stents
solid wire	Wall stent
wrapped wire	Symphony
fixed or movable core	Memotherm
coated or noncoated	Palmaz
J-tip	Z stent
Tomcat	

As in other areas, this field also is affected by the advancement of technology and the resulting changes in procedures and equipment.

IMAGES PRODUCED BY SOUND WAVES

An **ultrasound** scan uses sound waves at ultrasonic levels to obtain images of specific parts of the body. The ultrasonic beam is introduced into the body by an instrument called a transducer placed on the skin. Reflections of the beam can be detected, recorded, and photographed to produce a record, which may be called a **sonogram**, an ultrasound, or an **echogram**. It is useful in detecting the differences between cystic and solid structures in the body.

An ultrasound procedure called **echocardiography** (ĕk"ō-kăr"dē-ŏg'rah-fē) is used to examine the heart to locate aneurysms of the aorta and other abnormalities of the major blood vessels, and to detect and evaluate organs in the abdominal and pelvic cavities and small stuctures like the eye. Obstetricians and gynecologists use it to evaluate fetal size and maturity, fetal and placental position, uterine tumors, and other pelvic masses. An example of a sonogram is shown in Figure 11-8.

IMAGES PRODUCED BY MAGNETISM

Another diagnostic tool is **magnetic resonance imaging** (MRI). Some images created are similar to those produced by computerized axial tomography. However, the images are far more detailed, because one can section the body in multiple planes. In a CAT scan, the computer is linked to images produced by ionizing radiation; in the case of MRI, the computer is linked to images produced by magnetism.

A patient undergoing an MRI scan lies in a cylinder surrounded by a large magnet where the atoms are aligned according to the polarity of the magnet. Radiowaves are sent across the atoms. Each atom absorbs more or less energy from these radiowaves, thus altering the alignment and creating signals that are interpreted by the computer as images. The images are converted to visual displays on a computer screen.

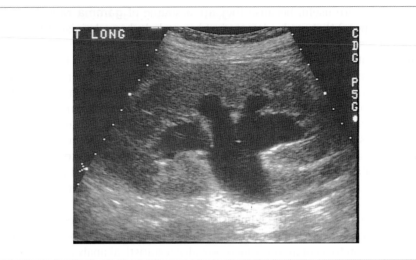

FIGURE 11-8
Ultrasound Showing
Hydronephrosis
in Kidney

The MRI makes it possible to distinguish between normal and abnormal tissue masses within the image. The process has decreased the need for some diagnostic procedures. It has also been especially useful in detecting edema in the brain, in finding tumors in the chest and abdomen, and in visualizing the cardiovascular system. An MRI of the brain can be seen in Figure 11-9.

DIAGNOSTIC TECHNIQUES USING NUCLEAR MEDICINE

vitr/o	glass	viv/o	life

Newer diagnostic tools, based on the radioactive characteristics of various elements, have emerged in the field of nuclear medicine. These diagnostic procedures use radiopharmaceuticals.

A **radiopharmaceutical** (rā"dē-ō-fahr"mah-sū'tǐ-kǎl), or **labeled compound**, is a specific radionuclide (radioisotope) incorporated into a chemical substance. A **radionuclide** (rā"dē-ō-nū'klīd) itself gives off electromagnetic radiation as it disintegrates. The time it takes for this disintegration to occur is called **half-life**, or the time it takes for a substance to lose half its radioactivity. To be effective, the half-life must be long enough to allow for imaging, but short enough to prevent the patient from becoming overexposed to radiation.

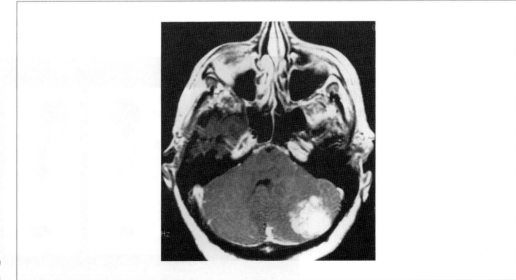

FIGURE 11-9
MRI of the Brain

x-rays against conditions located below the surface of the skin and deep in the body. The linear accelerator and the betatron are two examples of x-ray-based machines.

GAMMA RAYS

Gamma rays are similar to x-rays, but are produced through the disintegration of various radioactive elements. They have short wavelengths, no electric charge, and consist of high-energy photons. Because they can penetrate deep into the body, gamma rays are one of the more valuable agents available to treat cancer in female organs.

RADIOACTIVE ISOTOPES

Radioactive isotopes are unstable variants of several elements, some of which are cobalt, iodine, phosphorus, iron, gold, and strontium. These isotopes give off high-energy particles or rays as they disintegrate. Some are radioactive for just a few hours; others are radioactive for months or even years. One of the most widely used radioactive isotopes is iodine 131. At low levels it is used to test the activity of the thyroid gland; at higher doses, it is used to treat thyroid disease.

Complications are associated with radiotherapy, some of which are reversible. Others may produce long-lasting problems.

INTERVENTIONAL RADIOLOGY

Interventional radiology involves a radiologist introducing and positioning therapeutic devices into the body for diagnostic or corrective purposes. Instruments include catheters, balloons, stents, filters, guide wires, clotting devices, pulse spray devices, and lysing tools. Several new procedures have resulted.

Digital imaging is the most common type of imaging today. Exposure is made using an x-ray tube as is done with taking a film. However, radiation exiting the patient is recorded by a device that intensifies the image and changes it into different intensities of light. This light is directed to a video camera and displayed on a monitor. The images produced also can be stored on disk or tape or be selectively imaged to film. Both vascular and nonvascular procedures may be performed using this method.

Some of the more commonly performed procedures are angioplasty, digital vascular imaging, renal and biliary catheter therapies, organ biopsies, abscess drainages, and vertebroplasty.

Angioplasty, also known as balloon dilatation, is done to open up arteries partially clogged by deposits of fat, cholesterol, and lipids. These arteriosclerotic deposits reduce blood flow and, consequently, the amount of oxygen to a certain organ or group of organs. A catheter with an inflatable balloon tip is positioned so that inflation of the balloon will compress the atherosclerotic material into the wall of the vessel. Blood flow is thus restored in the vessel. This procedure has been successfully performed in coronary arteries and arteries of the legs and kidneys.

Digital vascular imaging uses an arterial or venous injection of iodinated contrast for visualizing arterial vessels. The radiologist positions a venous or arterial catheter and injects the contrast medium. The computer enhances the contrast by subtracting the bones, thereby making the vessels stand out. This latter procedure is referred to as digital subtraction angiography (DSA) and is a form of angiography.

Renal and biliary catheter therapies are possible with interventional radiology. For instance, obstruction of the ureters can be corrected by specialized catheters, or kidney stones can be removed without surgery. Renal and biliary narrowing can also be corrected by the same process used in angioplasty.

Organ biopsies and **abscess drainages** may be accomplished with radiological intervention. First, ultrasound and CT scans locate the abnormality; then a needle aspiration is performed to obtain samples for pathological examination. This procedure eliminates the need for an exploratory surgical procedure. Abscess drainages can be performed in the same way, using larger bore catheters inserted percutaneously.

Vertebroplasty is a treatment procedure to repair a compression fracture in the vertebral body secondary to osteoporosis and sometimes to treat a tumor which does not respond to conventional therapy. An interventional radiologist inserts a needle into the vertebral body and injects a specially formulated cement that will harden and provide support for the weakened bone.

The uses for each body system keep growing. For example, some of the procedures applied to the digestive system include: diagnostic arteriograms, cancer treatment with chemotherapy and/or embolization (vessel occlusion), and transjugular intrahepatic portosystemic shunt (TIPS).

Interventional techniques have been a positive addition to the physician's diagnostic and treatment capability. Some of the benefits include significant reduction of risk, pain, and recovery time; no general anesthesia; and cost effectiveness.

ABBREVIATIONS

These abbreviations are commonly used in reference to radiology or nuclear medicine diagnostic or treatment procedures. See Appendix D for additional abbreviations.

AP	anteroposterior
Ba	barium
BBB	blood-brain barrier
BE	barium enema
CAT	computerized axial tomography, computer-assisted tomography
C-spine	cervical spine film
cGy	centiGray
CT	computer tomography
DSA	digital subtraction angiography
DVI	digital vascular imaging
ERCP	endoscopic retrograde cholangiopancreatography
^{67}Ga	radioactive isotope of gallium*
^{131}I	radioactive isotope of iodine*
IVP	intravenous pyelogram
KUB	kidney, ureter, bladder
MRI	magnetic resonance imaging
NMR	nuclear magnetic resonance
NPO	nothing by mouth
PA	posteroanterior
PET	positron emission tomography
PTC	percutaneous transhepatic cholangiography
rad	radiation absorbed dose
RAI	radioimmunoassay
SBS	small bowel series
SPECT	single-photon emission computed tomography
^{99m}Tc	radioactive isotope of technetium*
^{201}Th	radioactive isotope of thallium*
UGI	upper gastrointestinal (series)
US, U/S	ultrasound

INTERNET ASSIGNMENT

Radiology Info (**www.radiologyinfo.org**) is the public information web site sponsored by the American College of Radiology (ACR) and Radiological Society of North America (RSNA). The site was established to inform and educate the public about radiologic procedures and the role of radiologists in health care. Each section of the site has been created with the guidance of a physician with expertise in the topic presented. All information contained in the web site is further reviewed by an ACR-RSNA committee comprised of physicians with expertise in several radiologic areas. Radiology Info is updated frequently and expanded to include new information as it occurs. The major sections of this web site are Diagnostic Radiology, Interventional Radiology, Radiation Therapy, and Radiation Safety. A glossary of terms and information about professions in radiation and about the RSNA and ACR are also included.

---

*Isotopes of chemical elements may be expressed in either of these formats: ^{201}Th or thallium 201.

ACTIVITY

Access Radiology Info at **www.radiologyinfo.org**. Click on Diagnostic Radiology and a list of body systems and patient groups is displayed. Click on Abdomen and a new screen appears with specific procedures listed. Select CT–Abdomen. Scroll through the questions to What are some common uses of the procedure? Summarize the information you have found.

Go back to the top of the page and select Interventional Radiology from the list at the left. Heart and Vascular Procedures appears. Select Angioplasty & Vascular Stenting. Scroll through the questions until you get to What Are the Limitations of Angioplasty and Vascular Stenting? Summarize the information for this topic.

Next, go back to the top of the page again and select Glossary of Terms from the list at the left. Access to the glossary is through an A–Z index. Select a term from the words introduced in Chapter 11 of the text, click on the appropriate letter, and determine whether the web site provides additional information on the word. Summarize what you have found.

Submit all the information you have gathered to your instructor.

Review: Radiology and Nuclear Medicine

- The discoveries of Röntgen, Curie, and Becquerel at the turn of the twentieth century opened a new field of medicine that uses rays for diagnosis and treatment of a variety of medical conditions.

- Diagnostic techniques include film survey, fluoroscopic examination, computerized axial tomography, ultrasound, tomography, stereoscopy, and magnetic resonance imaging.

- Contrasts, usually barium or iodine, are used to enhance the images obtained in various radiological or nuclear medicine tests.

- Nuclear medicine utilizes radionuclides in two types of diagnostic tests: in vitro and in vivo.

- Treatment of certain medical conditions can be given by therapeutic x-rays, gamma rays, and radioactive isotopes.

- Interventional radiology allows physicians to diagnose and correct certain medical problems without high-risk invasive diagnostic procedures or surgery.

Review of Terminology Presented

Word	Definition
abscess drainages	use of large-bore catheters inserted through the skin to drain infections
angioplasty	use of a catheter and balloon to improve the flow in a blood vessel by compressing the blockage material; balloon dilatation
anteroposterior view (AP)	x-ray position where the beam passes from front to back
barium sulfate	water-soluble salt used as an opaque contrast medium in an x-ray of the digestive tract
cineradiography	use of cameras and video recorders to make a motion picture record of the images appearing on a fluoroscopic screen

continues

Word	Definition
computerized axial tomography (CAT), computed tomography (CT), computer-assisted tomography (CAT)	procedure that uses highly focused x-ray beams and a computer to generate an image of the density of small layers of tissue
digital vascular imaging	use of a computer to enhance images from a contrast medium injected in arterial vessels
echocardiography	method of using ultrasound to examine the heart
echogram	record of an ultrasound scanning procedure
film survey	radiographic film of a body part
fluoroscopic examination	procedure that allows a radiologist to view body organs in motion
gamma rays	powerful photon rays given off by a radioactive substance
half-life	time required for a substance to lose half its radioactivity
in vitro	term referring to testing in a glass unit, such as a test tube, or other artificial environment
in vivo	term referring to testing within a living body
interventional radiology	use of x-rays to introduce and position catheters in the body for diagnostic or corrective purposes
iodinated substances	water-soluble, iodinated contrast media
lateral view	x-ray position where the beam passes from one side of the body to the other
magnetic resonance imaging (MRI)	use of magnetism to create images on a computer screen or tape to distinguish between normal and abnormal tissue changes within the area visualized
nuclear medicine	use of radioactive substances in the diagnosis and treatment of disease
nuclear physician	radiologist who uses diagnostic nuclear medicine procedures
oblique view	x-ray position where the beam passes at an angle that is not PA, AP, or lateral
organ biopsies	needle aspiration of an abnormal area of an organ with the assistance of ultrasound and CT technology
positron emission tomography (PET)	procedure that registers glucose metabolism in a cross section of the brain
posteroanterior view (PA)	x-ray position where the beam passes from back to front
radioactive isotopes	substances that give off high-energy particles or rays as they disintegrate
radiographic contrast media	radiopaque or radiolucent substances used to differentiate organs under study from the surrounding tissue
radiologist	physician who specializes in the practice of diagnostic radiology
radiolucent	permitting the passage of x-rays
radionuclide	radiopharmaceutical substance that gives off high-energy particles as it disintegrates
radiopaque	not permitting the passage of x-rays
radiopharmaceutical (labeled compound)	combination of a radionuclide (radioisotope) with a chemical substance, which is used for diagnostic or therapeutic purposes

continues

MATCHING

Match the terms to their meanings.

1. _____ rate at which a tissue or an organ absorbs a radiopharmaceutical

2. _____ time required for a substance to lose half of its radioactivity

3. _____ an imaging technique using the computer to provide a three-dimensional cross-sectional view of tissues

4. _____ utilizes two successive x-rays of a body part, which are viewed with a device that gives depth to the picture

5. _____ term referring to testing in an artificial environment

6. _____ use of sound to obtain an image of a part of the body

7. _____ use of radioactive materials in the diagnosis and treatment of disease

8. _____ reduces deposits of fat, cholesterol, and lipids in arteries

a. computerized axial tomography

b. in vitro

c. stereoscopy

d. uptake

e. nuclear medicine

f. ultrasound

g. half-life

h. angioplasty

ABBREVIATIONS*

Give the abbreviation for each of the following.

1. barium   _____

2. anteroposterior   _____

3. computerized axial tomography   _____

4. radioactive iodine   _____

5. intravenous pyelogram   _____

6. posteroanterior   _____

7. magnetic resonance imaging   _____

8. digital vascular imaging   _____

9. positron emission tomography   _____

DEFINITIONS

Define the following procedures.

1. radioimmunoassay   _____

2. echocardiography   _____

3. perfusion study   _____

4. radioactive iodine uptake study   _____

5. digital vascular imaging   _____

6. angioplasty   _____

Word Element Review

Root	Meaning	Example	Definition
cine/o	movement	**cineradiography** (sĭn"ĕ-rā"dē-ŏg'rah-fē)	process of making a motion picture record of images produced during a fluoroscopic exam
fluor/o	luminous	**fluorescence** (floo"ō-rĕs'ĕnts)	property of emitting light while exposed to light; usually ultraviolet
is/o	same, equal	**isodose** (ī'sō-dōs')	radiation dose of equal intensity to more than one body area
radi/o	ray	**radiogram** (rā'dē-ō-grăm")	film produced of an x-ray picture
		radioisotopes (rā"dē-ō-ī'sō-tōps)	radioactive forms of elements
roentgen/o	x-ray	**roentgenogram** (rĕnt-gĕn'ō-grăm")	film produced by roentgenography
strict/o	drawing tight, narrowing	**stricture** (strĭk'chur)	abnormal narrowing of a duct or passage
tom/o	cut	**tomography** (tō-mŏg'ră-fē)	any x-ray method that produces images by focusing on a single tissue plane
vitr/o	glass	**vitreous** (vĭt'rē-ŭs)	glassy
viv/o	life	**vividialysis** (vĭv"ĭ-dī-ăl'ĭ-sĭs)	dialysis through a living membrane

Prefix	Meaning	Example	Definition
ab-	away from, not	**abnormality** (ăb"nor-măl'ĭ-tē)	deviation from normal
ante-	before	**anterior** (ăn-tēr'ē-or)	situated in the front
en-	in, within	**encapsulated** (ĕn-kăp'sū-lāt-ĕd)	enclosed in a capsule
post-	after, behind	**posterior** (pŏs-tēr'ē-or)	situated in the back
pre-	before, in front of	**precancerous** (prē-kăn'ser-ăs)	pathological condition that tends to become malignant
sym-, syn-	together, with	**symphysis** (sĭm'fĭ-sĭs)	line of union between two bones
		syndrome (sĭn'drōm)	group of symptoms and signs that collectively characterize a particular disease or abnormal condition
tele-	distant	**teleradiography** (tĕl"ĕ-rā"dē-ŏg'rah-fē)	treatment with the radiation source about two meters from the body

continues

Suffix	Meaning	Example	Definition
-desis	binding, fixation	**syndesis** (sĭn'dĕ-sĭs)	condition of being bound together
-ectasis	expansion, dilation, stretching	**atelectasis** (ăt"ĕ-lĕk'tah-sĭs)	collapse or incomplete expansion of the lung
-gram	record, tracing, picture	**venogram** (vē'nō-grăm)	x-ray of a vein
-graphy	process of recording	**radiography** (rā"dē-ŏg'ră-fē)	making of film records of the internal structure of the body by exposure of x-ray-sensitive film
-lucent	shine	**translucent** (trăns-lū'sĕnt)	allows partial penetration by light rays
-opaque	obscure	**opacity** (ō-păs'ĭ-tē)	condition of being opaque; shadiness
-plasia	developmental	**dysplasia** (dĭs-plā'sē-ah)	abnormal growth development of tissue
		hyperplasia (hī"per-plā'zē-ah)	excessive increase in tissue growth

Word Element Review Exercises

Name: _____ Date: _____

MATCHING*

Match the terms to their meanings.

1. _____ at the back
2. _____ deviation from normal
3. _____ collective symptoms characterizing a disease or abnormal condition
4. _____ equal measure of radiation to more than one body part
5. _____ x-ray of a vein
6. _____ line of union between two bones
7. _____ motion picture record of images
8. _____ collapse of lungs
9. _____ enclosed in a capsule
10. _____ produces images by focusing on a single tissue plane
11. _____ excessive increase in tissue growth
12. _____ situated in front
13. _____ glassy
14. _____ radioactive forms of elements
15. _____ abnormal narrowing of a duct or passage
16. _____ allows partial penetration by light rays
17. _____ shadiness
18. _____ film produced for an x-ray picture
19. _____ dialysis through a living membrane
20. _____ property of emitting light while exposed to light
21. _____ film produced by x-ray
22. _____ bound together
23. _____ abnormal changes in the nature of tissue
24. _____ growth not yet malignant but known to become so if left unattended
25. _____ treatment in which the source of the therapeutic agent is at a distance from the body

a. abnormality
b. anterior
c. atelectasis
d. cineradiography
e. dysplasia
f. encapsulated
g. fluorescence
h. hyperplasia
i. isodose
j. opacity
k. posterior
l. precancerous
m. radiogram
n. radioisotopes
o. roentgenogram
p. stricture
q. symphysis
r. syndesis
s. syndrome
t. teleradiography
u. tomography
v. translucent
w. venogram
x. vitreous
y. vividialysis

_____

*Answers are in Appendix A.

WORD ELEMENT MEANINGS

Give the meaning of each word element. Then use your dictionary to find a new word that contains each of the word elements. Specify whether the new word is a noun or an adjective by placing N or A in the last column.

Word Element	Meaning	Word	N or A
1. ab-			
2. ante-			
3. cine/o			
4. -desis			
5. -ectasis			
6. en-			
7. fluor/o			
8. -gram			
9. -graphy			
10. is/o			
11. -lucent			
12. -opaque			
13. -plasia			
14. post-			
15. pre-			
16. radi/o			
17. roentgen/o			
18. strict/o			
19. sym-, syn-			
20. tele-			
21. tom/o			
22. vitr/o			
23. viv/o			

Dictionary Exercises

Name: _____ Date: _____

DICTIONARY EXERCISE 1*

Use your dictionary to find the pronunciation and definition of the following words.

	Word	Pronunciation	Definition
1.	acoustic impedance		
2.	erg		
3.	proton		
4.	quantum number		
5.	rad		
6.	radon		
7.	rectilinear		
8.	tagging		
9.	atomic weight		
10.	half-life value		
11.	cassette		
12.	tracer studies		
13.	doppler effect		
14.	ionization		
15.	irradiation		

DICTIONARY EXERCISE 2*

Use your dictionary to find the meaning and pronunciation (where indicated) of each term. Then write a sentence that identifies the meaning in your own words.

1. blood-brain barrier (BBB)

_____

2. radioactive contamination

_____

3. Geiger counter (_____)

_____

4. lymphangiography (_____)

_____

5. mammography (_____)

_____

6. planigram (_____)

_____

---

*Answers are in Appendix A.

7. radiation sickness

_____

8. spot film

_____

9. stopcock

_____

10. urography (_____)

_____

11. venogram (_____)

_____

12. lethal

_____

13. transducer

_____

14. multiple-gated acquisitions scan

_____

DICTIONARY EXERCISE 3

Pronunciation of the words below is provided. Using your dictionary, find the correct spelling and definition of each word.

	Word	Pronunciation	Definition
1.	_____	ah-tĕn"ū-ā'shŭn	_____
2.	_____	kal"ĭ-brā'shŭn	_____
3.	_____	ĭ-rā"dē-ā'shŭn	_____
4.	_____	fō'tŏn	_____
5.	_____	sĭn"tĭ-lā'shŭn	_____
6.	_____	dō-sĭm'ē-ter	_____
7.	_____	rĕnt-gĕn'ō-grăm"	_____
8.	_____	kō'bawlt therapy	_____
9.	_____	ăb-sŏrp'shŭn	_____
10.	_____	ăr-tē'rē-ō-grăm"	_____
11.	_____	nu'klē-on	_____
12.	_____	ŏr"thō-vŏl'tĭj mah-chēn'	_____
13.	_____	tāg'ing	_____
14.	_____	mī"ē'lō-sŭ-prĕsh'ŭn	_____
15.	_____	ī'ŏn	_____

DICTIONARY EXERCISE 4

Match the terms to their meanings.

1. _____ a decrease in the number of radioactive atoms in a radioactive substance over time

2. _____ smallest particle of an element capable of entering into a chemical reaction

3. _____ encounter between two subatomic particles that changes the existing momentum and energy conditions

4. _____ a device by which radiant energy can be evaluated

5. _____ specific amount of roentgen rays or other radiation administered

6. _____ determining the amount of ionizing radiation in an area or a substance

7. _____ atom having either a positive or negative charge as a result of having lost or gained an electron

8. _____ changes of direction that subatomic particles or photons undergo as a result of collision or interaction with matter

9. _____ measurement of the ability of the thyroid gland to trap and retain the isotope following the oral ingestion of a tracer dose of radioactive iodine

10. _____ method of introducing a catheter into a vein or an artery

11. _____ a preliminary film taken to check technique, positioning, and patient preparation, as well as to determine what diseases are considered as diagnostic possibilities

12. _____ any protective device used to prevent or reduce the passage of particles of radiation

13. _____ production of an image or picture

14. _____ name for the process of tagging radionuclides and following them through the body

15. _____ number of protons in the nucleus of an atom

a. atom

b. atomic number

c. collision

d. dose

e. imaging

f. ion

g. monitoring

h. radioactive decay

i. radiation detector

j. radioactive iodine uptake determination

k. scattering

l. scout film

m. Seldinger technique

n. shield

o. tracer studies

Listening Exercises

Name		Date

INSTRUCTIONS

1. Review the spelling, pronunciation, and meaning of the words provided in the preview.

2. Listen to the audio CD and fill in the blank as the word is dictated.

3. At the end of the exercise, check your spelling against the preview words. They appear in the preview in the order in which they are encountered in the exercise.

4. Review and practice the words you missed.

5. Look up words that are not familiar.

PREVIEW OF WORDS FOR LISTENING EXERCISES 11-1, 11-2, 11-3

Word	Pronunciation	Meaning
Exercise 11-1, Dx Chest, Two View		
pneumothorax	nū-mō-thō'raks	presence of air in the pleural space outside the lung, but inside the chest
infiltrate	ĭn-fĭl'trāt	an abnormal substance that accumulates gradually in cells or tissues
vasculature	văs'kū-lā-tūr"	the vascular system of the body or any part of it
Exercise 11-2, CT Pelvis, Without		
lobulated	lŏb'ū-lāt-ĕd	made up of lobules or small segments
ileostomy	ĭl"ē-ŏs'tō-mē	surgical creation of an opening into the ileum with a stoma on the abdominal wall
lymphadenopathy	lĭm-făd"ē-nŏp'ă-thē	disease of the lymph nodes
Exercise 11-3, Gallbladder Sonogram		
edema	ě-dē'mă	abnormal accumulation of fluid in the body
common bile duct		union of the hepatic and cystic duct, which leads to the duodenum

Listening Exercises 11-1, 11-2, 11-3

DX Chest, Two View

Clinical Data: PA/LAT CXR

Comparison is made to a study dated 8/3/20—. A central venous catheter is present with the tip in the distal superior vena cava. No _____ is seen. The heart is normal in size. The lungs are free of _____ with normal pulmonary _____. Degenerative changes are seen in the thoracic spine.

IMPRESSION:

1. No change when compared to the study of 8/3/20—.
    No acute process is seen.

CT Pelvis, Without

Clinical Data: CT PELVIS WITHOUT CONTRAST

CT SCAN OF THE PELVIS WITHOUT INTRAVENOUS CONTRAST, 12/21/20—

INDICATIONS:

Rule out pelvic mass/fluid collection

DISCUSSION:

Comparison is with a study dated 12/11/20—. The patient was returned for additional imaging following infusion of contrast material into the bladder and into the rectum. Axial images were obtained prior to infusion of contrast material. Images were obtained following infusion of contrast material into the bladder. Finally, images were obtained following infusion of contrast material into the bladder and into the rectum.

The bladder is well opacified. The bladder is somewhat floppy and _____. The areas previously questioned for the most part do opacify with rectal contrast. There is what appears to be unopacified loops of bowel just below the level of the _____. As they do not fill from below, they are probably jejunum and ileum. No definite fluid collections are identified. No _____ is identified.

IMPRESSION:

1. While some unopacified loops of bowel are seen in the pelvis, specifically left side, no definite fluid collections or masses are identified to suggest an abscess.

2. Gallstones are noted incidentally.

Gallbladder Sonogram

ULTRASOUND OF THE GALLBLADDER:

There are no stones seen in the gallbladder. There is no _____ or thickening of the wall. The _____ is not dilated. Head and body of the pancreas appear normal.

IMPRESSION: 1. A normal study.

CHAPTER 12

The Respiratory System

Some folk seem glad even to draw their breath.

—WILLIAM MORRIS

OBJECTIVES

When you have completed this chapter on the respiratory system, you should be able to

1. Spell and define the major system components and explain how they operate.
2. Identify the meanings of related word elements.
3. Spell and define diagnostic procedures, diagnoses, treatment procedures, and abbreviations.
4. Spell the names of medications commonly used.
5. Be familiar with terminology used in reports.

INTRODUCTION

The respiratory system allows the blood to exchange oxygen and carbon dioxide. This gaseous exchange is known as respiration and is essential for life. Interruption of this cycle for more than a few minutes can cause brain damage or death.

Physicians who specialize in the diagnosis and medical treatment of pulmonary or respiratory diseases are pulmonary disease or chest specialists. Surgeons who specialize in the surgical treatment of chest diseases are called chest or thoracic surgeons.

COMPOSITION OF THE RESPIRATORY SYSTEM

pector/o	chest		-thorax	chest
thorac/o	chest			

The principal organs of the respiratory system discussed in this chapter are the nose, pharynx, larynx, trachea, bronchi, alveoli, and lungs.

NOSE

nas/o	nose		rhin/o	nose

Figure 12-1 illustrates how air enters our nostrils and passes through two **nasal cavities** (2) that are separated by a partition called the **septum**. The septum and walls of the nasal cavity are constructed of cartilage covered with mucous membrane. There are numerous hairs in the nostrils that serve to filter out larger dirt particles as air passes through them. Smaller particles are caught by the mucus secreted by the mucous membranes.

Besides being filtered, inhaled air is conditioned as it moves through the nasal cavities. The airflow is warmed by capillaries in the mucous membrane lining to bring it closer to body temperature, and moisture is added from the membrane secretions.

The nasal cavity itself is separated from the mouth by a partition called the **palate** (păl'ăt) (3). Also within the facial bones are several mucous-membrane-lined, air-filled pockets called **sinuses** (1), which produce the mucus fluids.

PHARYNX

pharyng/o	pharynx, throat

The **pharynx** (far'inks) (13), which is called the throat, is used by both the digestive and respiratory systems. In the respiratory system, the pharynx allows air to pass from the nasal cavity and mouth into the larynx.

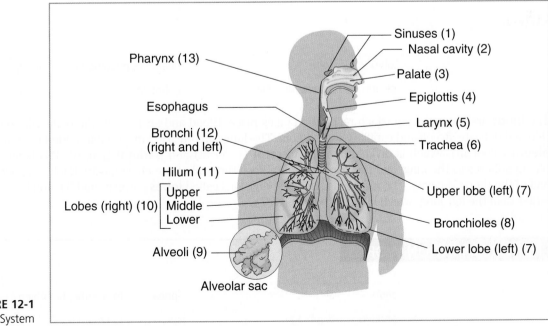

FIGURE 12-1
Respiratory System

LARYNX

epiglott/o	epiglottis	laryng/o	larynx

The **larynx** (lăr'ĭnks) (5), or voice box, is located between the pharynx and the windpipe. The two vocal cords and the opening between them is called the **glottis** (glŏt'ĭs), and the little leaflike structure that closes this opening during swallowing is called the **epiglottis** (ĕp"ĭ-glŏt'ĭs) (4). This way food is kept out of the respiratory tract.

TRACHEA

trache/o	neck

The **trachea** (trā'kē-ah) (6), or windpipe, is a tube that extends from the lower edge of the larynx to the level of the seventh thoracic vertebra. The trachea lies on the anterior (front) surface of the esophagus. The airway passage is kept open by a series of cartilage rings. Its purpose is to conduct air to and from the lungs by way of the bronchi.

BRONCHI AND ALVEOLI

alveol/o	alveolus, air sac	bronchiol/o	bronchiole
bronchi/o, bronch/o	bronchus		

At its lower end the trachea divides into the left and right **bronchi** (brŏng'kī) (12). These bronchi are separated by a tracheal ridge or structure called the **carina** (kah-rī'nah). One bronchus extends to each lung. The notch in the lung that allows the entry of the bronchus and pulmonary vessels is called the **hilum** (hī'lŭm) (11). Within the lung, the bronchus immediately subdivides into branches. These branches are referred to as the **bronchial** (brŏng'kē-ăl) **tree**. Each bronchial tree subdivides again and again into progressively smaller units. The smallest are called **bronchioles** (brŏng'kē-ōls) (8). At the end of the bronchial tree there is a whole cluster of air sacs known as **alveoli** (ăl-vē'ō-lī) (9). An alveolus (singular) is surrounded by networks of capillaries through whose walls an exchange of carbon dioxide and oxygen takes place. There are an estimated 700,000 alveoli.

LUNGS

lob/o	lobe	pneum/o, pneumon/o	lung, air
pleur/o	pleura, rib, side	pulmon/o	lung

The **lungs** are the organs in which respiration takes place. Blood and air meet at the point where the extremely thin and delicate alveoli and capillary walls adjoin. The lungs are encased in a double-folded membrane called the **pleura** (ploor'ah), which is divided into the **visceral** (vĭs'er-ăl) and **parietal** (pah-rī'ĕ-tăl) layers. The visceral pleura adheres to the lung, and the parietal pleura lines the wall of the chest cavity. Each lung occupies its own half of the thoracic cavity. The right lung has three divisions called **lobes**—upper, middle, and lower (10)—and is larger than the left lung, which has only two lobes (7).

HOW RESPIRATION WORKS

aer/o	air	-pnea	to breathe, breathing
phren/o	diaphragm	spir/o	to breathe

The lungs are separated from the abdominal cavity by a muscular partition known as the **diaphragm** (dī'ah-frăm), which is the chief muscle of respiration. There are three cycles in respiration. **Inspiration** is the breathing of air into the lungs, as demonstrated in Figure 12-2A. Figure 12-2B shows **expiration**, or the exhalation of air from the lungs. **Rest** is the interval between expiration and inspiration.

As we breathe, the diaphragm moves down and then up to induce air movement. This is how it works. When the diaphragm contracts and descends, the ribs elevate. The result is a negative thoracic pressure causing air to be drawn into the lungs to equalize the pressure. The diaphragm then relaxes and is drawn upward. This increases the pressure in the thoracic cavity and forces air to be expelled from the lungs. The respiratory center in the brain controls the rhythmic movements produced by respiration.

Respiration involves the exchange of oxygen and carbon dioxide in the lungs. The amount of oxygen retained by the tissues and cells is dependent on several factors, including the needs of the tissues and cells, as well as the age, health, and activity level of the individual.

There are several terms used to indicate lung capacity and airflow volume. **Tidal volume** is the amount of air breathed in and out during quiet or unlabored respiration. **Total lung capacity** is the total volume of air in the lungs at the end of maximum inspiration. **Residual volume** is the amount of air remaining in the lung after a forced expiration. Other terms mentioned frequently in reference to flow volume studies are *expiratory reserve volume* and *inspiratory reserve volume*.

INTERNET ASSIGNMENT

The American Lung Association (ALA), the oldest voluntary health organization in the United States, was founded in 1904 to fight tuberculosis. Today the ALA has widened its scope to include lung disease in all its forms, with special emphasis on asthma, tobacco control, and environmental health. ALA is funded by contributions from the public along with gifts and grants from corporations, foundations, and government agencies. Its web site is located at **www.lungusa.org**.

The homepage of the site shows its comprehensive nature. Click on the Lungs button at the top of the homepage and you are taken to a page that describes how the lungs work and (at the right) lists three sites from which to choose for further information. The Human Respiratory System provides a helpful illustration and explanation of the system. Images of Lungs provides pictures of normal and abnormal lung tissue. Learn About Your Respiratory System takes you through an animated presentation about respiratory functions.

On the left side of the homepage there is a button labeled Diseases A to Z. Clicking here takes you to an index site that lists respiratory diseases. Specific information on a disease is obtained by clicking on the disease name.

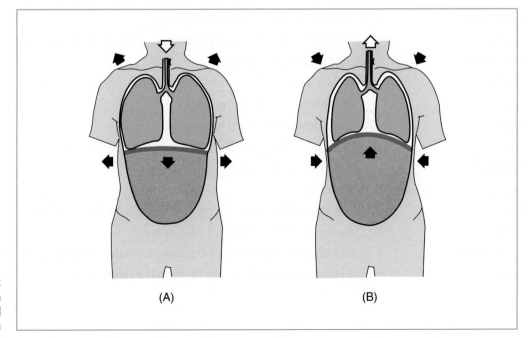

FIGURE 12-2
The Diaphragm in
(A) Inspiration and
(B) Expiration

(A)   (B)

ACTIVITY

Visit the American Lung Association web site at **www.lungusa.org**. Find and read the explanation of how the human respiratory system works. In a short report summarize any new information you found.

Access Images of Lungs and report on the illustrations included.

Access Diseases A to Z and select one of the diagnoses listed in Chapter 12. Click the first letter of that diagnosis and then select the diagnosis from the list. Summarize new information the description provides.

Submit all of your reports to your instructor.

Review: The Respiratory System

■ Respiration provides the oxygen that is essential to life.

■ The components of the respiratory system assist in the exchange of oxygen and carbon dioxide through the walls of capillaries in the lungs.

■ The nose, pharynx, larynx, and trachea carry inhaled (or inspired) air through the bronchi into the lungs.

■ The chief muscle of respiration is the diaphragm, which descends during inspiration and ascends during expiration.

Review of Terminology Presented

Word	Definition
alveoli	clusters of air sacs at the end of the bronchial tree
bronchi	main branches leading from the trachea to the lungs for air movement
bronchial tree	branching of the bronchus after entering the respective lung
bronchioles	smallest divisions of the bronchial tree
carina	ridge at the lower end of the trachea, separating the two bronchi
diaphragm	chief muscle of respiration
epiglottis	leaflike structure that opens and closes over the glottis during swallowing
expiration	exhalation of air from the lungs
glottis	space between the two vocal cords
hilum	notch in the lung where the bronchi and vessels enter
inspiration	breathing of air into the lungs
larynx	voice box
lobes	divisions of the lungs; the right lung has three lobes and the left lung has two
lungs	organs in which respiration takes place
nasal cavities	two cavities—separated by the nasal septum—through which air passes
palate	partition separating the mouth from the nasal cavity

continues

Word	Definition
parietal pleura	membrane that lines the chest cavity
pharynx	airway between the nasal cavity and the mouth and larynx; throat
pleura	double-folded membrane that encases the lungs and lines the chest cavity
residual volume	amount of air remaining in the lung after a forced expiration
rest	interval between expiration and inspiration
septum	partition that separates the nasal cavities
sinuses	pockets in the facial bones
tidal volume	amount of air breathed in and out during quiet or unlabored respiration
total lung capacity	total volume of air in the lungs at the end of maximum inspiration
trachea	tube that extends from the lower edge of the voice box to the level of the seventh thoracic vertebra; windpipe
visceral pleura	membrane that adheres to the lungs

Terminology Review Exercises

Name: _____ Date: _____

SELECTION*

Select the correct word from the list below to complete each of the following statements.

| alveoli | bronchi | bronchioles | carina | diaphragm | epiglottis | expiration | hilum |
| inspiration | lobes | palate | pharynx | pleura | septum | trachea | |

1. The partition between the two nasal cavities is called the _____.
2. The _____ separates the nasal cavity from the mouth.
3. The passageway for food, liquid, and air is the _____.
4. The _____ extends from the lower edge of the voice box and conducts air to and from the lungs.
5. The _____ keeps food out of the respiratory tract.
6. The trachea divides into two _____ and forms the carina.
7. The membrane encasing the lungs is referred to as the _____.
8. The chief muscle of respiration is the _____.
9. The notch where the bronchi and vessels enter the lung is the _____.
10. Air sacs at the end of the bronchial tree are called _____.
11. Exhalation of air out of the lungs is known as _____.
12. Breathing air into the lungs is known as _____.
13. The smallest branches of a bronchial tree are the _____.
14. The bronchi are separated by a structure called the _____.
15. Each lung is divided into two or three _____.

DEFINITIONS

Define each of the following terms.

1. tidal volume

    _____

2. total lung capacity

    _____

3. residual volume

    _____

4. bronchial tree

    _____

---

*Answers are in Appendix A.

DIAGNOSTIC PROCEDURES

Word	Pronunciation	Definition
General		
before and after (B/A) bronchodilator (by and after BCD)	brŏng″kō-dī-lā′tor	breathing test given before and after the use of a bronchodilator that causes dilation of the bronchi to check the effect on airflow
bronchoscopy	brŏng-kŏs′kō-pē	examination that allows direct visualization of the bronchi through a bronchoscope
complete spirometry	spī-rŏm′ĕ-trē	measurement of the breathing capacity of the lungs
fiberoptic bronchoscopy	fī″ber-ŏp′tĭk	procedure using flexible, light-transmitting plastic fibers to visualize the bronchi (See Figure 12-3)
flow volume study		test used to determine obstruction in airflow to the lungs by breathing into a tube until expiration has been completed
laryngoscopy	lăr″ĭng-gŏs′kō-pē	visual examination of the larynx with a scope
lung biopsy	bī′ŏp-sē	biopsy of tissue taken from the lung by bronchoscopy for washing, cytology, and determination of malignancy
pleural biopsy	ploor-ăl	biopsy of tissue from the pleura
pulmonary function test (PFT)	pŭl′mō-nĕr″ē	test used to evaluate how the patient breathes and to determine lung volumes, pulmonary gas exchange, and flow rates
thoracentesis (thoracocentesis)	thō″rah-sĕn-tē′sĭs	procedure in which the chest wall is punctured with a needle to obtain fluid for diagnostic studies
tracheostomy	trā″kē-ŏs′tō-mē	emergency or elective procedure in which an opening through the neck into the trachea is created to permit the insertion of a tube to facilitate the flow of air or drainage of secretions
tuberculin skin tests	too-bĕr′kū-lĭn	application of agents to the surface of the skin (Heaf and tine tests) or by intradermal injection (Mantoux test) to detect the presence of tuberculosis infection

continues

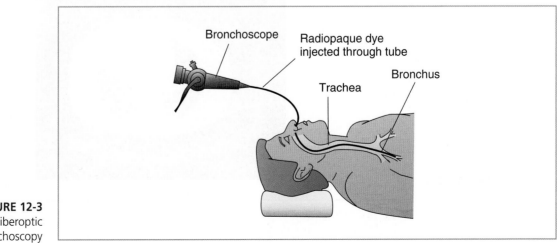

FIGURE 12-3
Fiberoptic
Bronchoscopy

Word	Pronunciation	Definition
Nuclear Medicine		
radioisotope perfusion and ventilation lung scan; ventilation-perfusion scan (V/Q scan)	rā"dē-ō'ī'sō-tōp pĕr-fū'zhŭn	techniques for diagnosing pulmonary embolism and demonstrating perfusion defects in normally ventilated areas of the lung
Radiology		
chest x-ray (PA/lat)		full view of the lungs and heart from the back and side
CT scan of the chest or lungs		computerized reconstruction of x-ray slices of the chest (See Figure 12-4)
MRI scan of the chest or lungs		procedure using magnetic fields to diagnose problems in the chest area (See Figure 12-5)
pulmonary angiography	ăn"jē-ŏg'rah-fē	x-ray technique for studying circulation in the lungs
sinus x-ray	sī'nŭs	face view of the sinus cavity
tomogram (laminogram)	tō'mō-grăm (lăm'ĭ-nō-grăm)	x-ray of a selected layer of the body made by body section roentgenography to examine lung fields
Laboratory Tests		
sputum culture and sensitivity	spū'tŭm	test requiring a patient to cough up sputum from the lungs for laboratory analysis; laboratory incubates the sputum sample to test for the presence and identification of micro-organisms; if organisms are found, a determination is made about which antibodies inhibit the growth of these organisms to aid the physician in prescribing drugs appropriately
sputum cytology	sī-tŏl'ō-jē	test for malignant cells in the sputum

continues

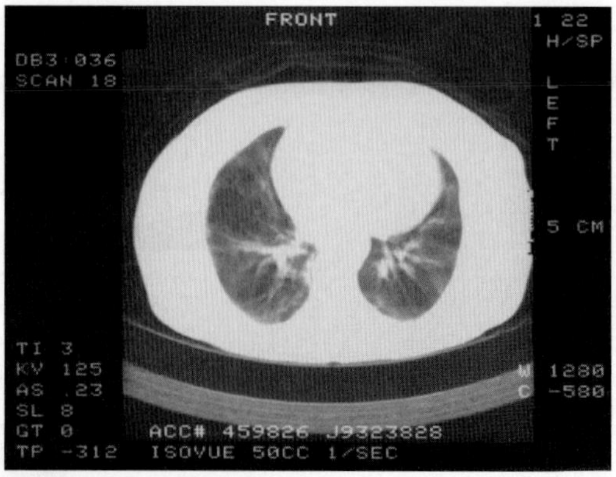

FIGURE 12-4
CT Scan of the Lungs

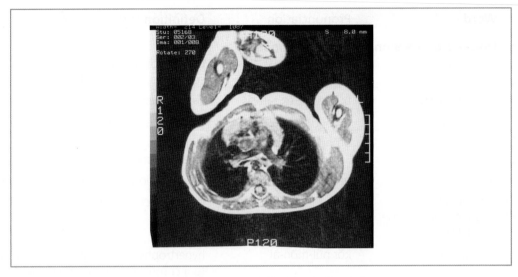

FIGURE 12-5
MRI Scan of the Lungs

Word	Pronunciation	Definition
Blood Tests		
arterial blood gases (ABGs)		measurements of hydrogen, carbon dioxide, pH, and oxygen pressures are obtained from a sample of arterial blood; aids in the determination of acid base balance, oxygen, and carbon dioxide level in arterial blood
Diseases of the Upper Respiratory System		
coryza	kŏ-rī'zah	common head cold; condition causing profuse discharge from nose
croup	kroop	condition seen in children and marked by obstruction, barking cough, hoarseness, and persistent stridor
laryngitis	lăr"ĕn-jī"tĭs	inflammation of the larynx
pertussis	pĕr'tŭs'ĭs	whooping cough
pharyngitis	făr"ĭn-jī'tĭs	inflammation of the throat
rhinitis	rī-nī'tĭs	inflammation of the mucous membrane of the nose; may be acute (common cold) or allergic (hay fever), which is due to an allergy
sinusitis	sī"nŭ-sī'tĭs	inflammation of the sinuses
upper respiratory infection (URI)		broad term referring to several infectious diseases often caused by a group called *Rhinovirus*
Diseases of the Bronchi/Lungs		
adult respiratory distress syndrome (ARDS) (shock lung)		condition that may follow or accompany various serious diseases including pulmonary embolism or sepsis; shock lung
asthma	ăz'mah	condition marked by recurrent attacks of shortness of breath with wheezing due to spasms in the bronchi

continues

Word	Pronunciation	Definition
Diseases of the Bronchi/Lungs *(continued)*		
atelectasis	ăt"ĕ-lĕk'tah-sĭs	collapse of the lung parenchyma due to obstruction from secretions, fluids, or other factors
bronchiectasis	brŏng"kē-ĕk'tah-sĭs	chronic distention of the bronchi or bronchioles
bronchocarcinoma	brŏng"kō-kăr-sĭ-nō'mah	lung cancer arising from the airway or bronchi
bronchiolitis	brŏng"kē-ō'lĭ'ts	respiratory infection that causes bronchioles to become inflamed and secrete an excessive amount of mucus
bronchitis	brŏng"kī'tĭs	inflammation of the bronchi; may be acute or chronic
chronic obstructive pulmonary disease (COPD)		condition characterized by chronic obstruction to airflow in the lungs
cor pulmonale	kŏr pŭl-mŏn-āl'	hypertrophy of the right ventricle of the heart usually due to a chronic condition of airflow obstruction
cystic fibrosis	sĭs'tĭk fī-brō'sĭs	hereditary disease affecting both respiratory and digestive systems
emphysema	ĕm"fĭ-sē'mah	condition marked by presence of increased air in the intra-alveolar tissue of the lungs due to distention of their walls and rupture of the alveoli (See Figure 12-6)
hyline membrane disease (respiratory distress syndrome [RDS])		severe impairment of respiratory function in a newborn
influenza (flu)	ĭn"flū-ĕn'zah	highly contagious viral upper respiratory infection
pneumonia	nū"mō'nē-ah	inflammation of the lungs; may be caused by bacteria, viruses, fungi, or mechanical, physical, or chemical irritants (Figure 12-7 shows comparison of alveoli in normal tissue to various abnormal alveoli.)
pulmonary abscess	pŭl'mō-nĕr"ē ăb'sĕs	collection of pus in the lungs
pulmonary edema	ĕ-dē'mah	swelling of fluid in air sacs and bronchioles
pulmonary embolism	ĕm'bō-lizm	obstruction of the pulmonary artery or one of its branches by a clot or foreign material

continues

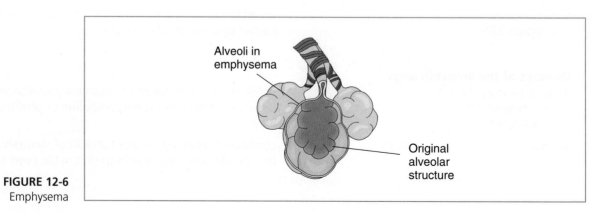

FIGURE 12-6
Emphysema

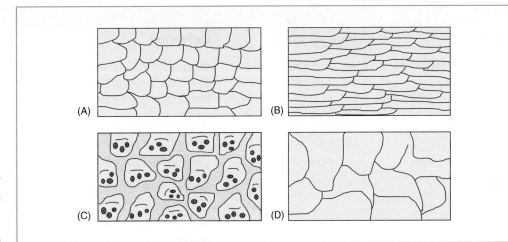

FIGURE 12-7
Alveoli: in (A) normal lung tissue; (B) atelectasis; (C) pneumonia; and (D) emphysema

Word	Pronunciation	Definition
Diseases of the Bronchi/Lungs *(continued)*		
sarcoidosis	săr″koi-dō′sĭs	chronic, progressive, generalized granulomatous reticulosis involving the lungs
tuberculosis	too-bĕr″kū-lō′sĭs	chronic bacterial infection caused by inhaling droplets sprayed into the air by someone infected with Mycobacterium tuberculosis
Diseases of the Pleura and Chest		
empyema	ĕm″pī-ē′mah	condition marked by pus in the pleural space
hemothorax	hē″mō-thō′răks	collection of blood in the chest cavity
pleural effusion (hydrothorax)	ploo′răl ĕ-fū′zhŭn	presence of fluid in the pleural space (See Figure 12-8)
pleurisy	ploor′ĭ sē	inflammation of the pleura
pneumothorax	nū″mō-thō′răks	presence of air in the pleural space outside the lung, but inside the chest due to a ruptured alveolus or bronchus (See Figure 12-9)

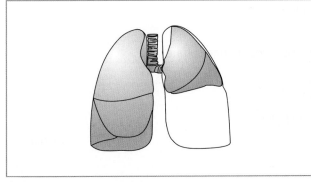

FIGURE 12-8   Pleural Effusion

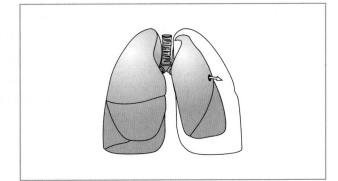
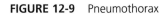

FIGURE 12-9   Pneumothorax

TREATMENT PROCEDURES

Word	Pronunciation	Definition
endotracheal intubation	ĕn"dō-trā'kē-al ĭn"tū-bā'shŭn	procedure that establishes an airway with the insertion of a tube through the nose or mouth, pharynx, and larynx into the trachea
lobectomy	lō-bĕk'tō-mē	resection of a lobe of the lung
pleurectomy	ploor-ĕk'tō-mē	excision of a portion of the pleura
pneumonectomy	nū"mō-nĕk'tō-mē	surgical removal of a lung—total or either right or left lung
thoracostomy	thō"rah-kŏs'tō-mē	surgical insertion of a tube in the chest to drain fluid or air or to aid diagnosis of a disease process
tracheotomy	trā"kē-ŏt'ō-mē	incision into the trachea for the purpose of establishing airflow

MEDICATIONS PRESCRIBED

Trade Name	Generic Name
Antiasthmatic, Antiallergic, Inhalant, or by Mouth	
Intal, Nasalcrom, Gastrocrom	cromolyn Na
Antibiotics	
Amoxil, Augmentin	amoxicillin
Ampicillin, Polycillin	ampicillin
Biaxin	clarithromycin
Ceclor	cefaclor
Ceftin	cefuroxime axetil
Cefzil	cefprozil monohydrate
Cipro	ciprofloxacin
Eryped	erythromycin ethylsuccinate
Keflex	cephalexin
Tequin	gatifloxacin
Antihistamines	
Benadryl	diphenhydramine
Claritin	loratadine
Claritin D	loratadine and pseudophedrine sulfate
Hismanal	astemizole
Phenergan	promethazine
Zyrtec	cetirizine hydrochloride

continues

MEDICATIONS PRESCRIBED

Trade Name	Generic Name
Bronchodilators	
Albuterol, Proventil, Ventolin	albuterol
Alupent, Metaprel	metaproterenol
Aminophylline	aminophylline
Atrovent	ipratropium
Brethine, Brycanyl	terbutaline
Isuprel	isoproterenol
Primatene, Bronkaid, Vaponephrine, Adrenalin	epinephrine
Slo-Phyllin, Slo-bid, Theo-clear, Theo-Dur	theophylline
Combination Products	
Entex	phenylephrine and guaifenesin
Expectorants	
Humabid	guaifenesin
Organidin	iodinated glycerol
Inhalation Steroids	
Azmacort, Nasacort	triamcinolone
Beclovent, Vanceril	beclomethasone
Decadron	dexamethasone
Flovent	fluticasone propionate
Nasalide	flunisolide
Vancenase, Beconase	beclomethasone
Lung Surfactants	
Exosurf	colfosceril palmitate
Survanta	beractant
Nasal Decongestants	
Afrin, Sudafed	pseudoephedrine

ABBREVIATIONS	
Trade Name	Generic Name
ABGs	arterial blood gases
A&P	auscultation and percussion
ARDS	acute respiratory distress syndrome
ARF	acute respiratory failure
Bronch	bronchoscopy
COLD	chronic obstructive lung disease
COPD	chronic obstructive pulmonary disease
CPR	cardiopulmonary resuscitation
DOE	dyspnea on exertion
IPPB	intermittent positive pressure breathing
PFT	pulmonary function test
PND	paroxysmal nocturnal dyspnea
PPD	purified protein derivative
SOB	shortness of breath
TB	tuberculosis
URI	upper respiratory infection
V/Q scan	ventilation-perfusion scan

Working Practice Review Exercises

Name: _____ Date: _____

IDENTIFICATION/PROCEDURES*
Identify the following procedures.

1. x-ray technique for studying circulation
   in the lungs   _____

2. measurement of hydrogen, carbon dioxide,
   pH, and oxygen pressure from arterial blood   _____

3. evaluates how a patient breathes   _____

4. the chest wall is punctured with a needle to
   obtain fluid for diagnostic studies   _____

5. examination of the bronchi with a scope   _____

MEANING
Give the meaning of the underlined words.

1. The patient suffered an <u>asthmatic</u> attack on Friday.

   _____

2. As a result of the automoibile accident, she developed a <u>hemothorax</u>.

   _____

3. We have scheduled her for a <u>thoracostomy</u> tomorrow.

   _____

4. For the past six months the patient has suffered with <u>chronic obstructive pulmonary disease</u>.

   _____

5. (On an x-ray report) Impression: <u>Atelectasis</u>, left lung.

   _____

6. Her lungs were clear to <u>A&P</u>.

   _____

7. It was diagnosed as a <u>URI</u>.

   _____

8. I have ordered a <u>sputum culture and sensitivity</u>.

   _____

9. She will have a <u>V/Q scan</u> later today.

   _____

IDENTIFICATION/ABBREVIATIONS*
Identify the following abbreviations.

1. ARDS   _____

2. COPD   _____

3. IPPB   _____

4. PFT   _____

_____

*Answers are in Appendix A.

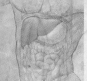

Word Element Review

Root	Meaning	Example	Definition
aer/o	air	**aerial** (ār'ē-ăl)	pertaining to the air
alveol/o	alveolus, air sac	**alveolocapillary** (al-vē"ah-lō-kap'ĭ-lar-ē)	pertaining to pulmonary alveoli and capillaries
bronchi/o, bronch/o	bronchus	**bronchopneumonia** (brŏng"kō-nū-mō'nē-ah)	inflammation of the lungs, beginning at the end of the bronchi
bronchiol/o	bronchiole	**bronchiolitis** (brong"kē-ō-lī'tĭs)	inflammation of the bronchioles due to a viral infection
epiglott/o	epiglottis	**epiglottidectomy** (ĕp"ĭ-glŏt"ĭ-dĕk'tō-mē)	excision of the epiglottis
laryng/o	larynx	**laryngology** (lăr"ĭn-gŏl'ō-jē)	branch of medicine dealing with the throat
		otorhinolaryngology (ō"tō-rī"nō-lăr"ĭn-gŏl'ō-jē)	study of otology, rhinology, and laryngology
lob/o	lobe	**lobar pneumonia** (lō'ber)	inflammation of one or more lobes of the lung
nas/o	nose	**nasopharyngitis** (nā"zō-făr"ĭn-jī'tĭs)	inflammation of the nasopharynx
pector/o	chest	**pectoralis** (pĕk"tō-rā'lĭs)	one of four muscles of the anterior upper portion of the chest
pharyng/o	pharynx, throat	**pharyngocele** (fah-rĭng'gō-sēl)	hernial protrusion of a part of the pharynx
phren/o	diaphragm	**phrenitis** (frĕ-nī'tĭs)	inflammation of the diaphragm
pleur/o	pleura, rib, side	**pleurisy** (ploor'ĭ-sē)	inflammation of the pleura
pneum/o, pneumon/o	lung, air	**pneumonia** (nū-mō'nē-ah)	disease of the lungs
pulmon/o	lung	**pulmonary** (pŭl'mō-nĕr"ē)	pertaining to lungs
rhin/o	nose	**rhinitis** (rī-nī'tĭs)	inflammation of the nose
spir/o	to breathe, breathing	**spirometer** (spī-rŏm'ĕ-ter)	instrument for measuring the volume of air inhaled and exhaled
thorac/o	chest	**thoracic surgeon** (thō-răs'ĭk)	surgeon who specializes in chest surgery
trache/o	windpipe	**tracheostomy** (trā"kē-ŏs'tō-mē)	creation of a new opening into the trachea

continues

Suffix	Meaning	Example	Definition
-pnea	to breathe	**dyspnea** (dǐsp'nē-ah)	labored or difficult breathing
-thorax	chest	**hemothorax** (hē"mō-thō'răks)	collection of blood in the chest

Listening Exercise 7-1

Operative Report

The patient is a 57-year-old white female who was referred by Dr. Steinger for evaluation of increasing shortness of breath as well as progressive _____ of a left _____. The patient was initially admitted and watched closely over the next hour-and-a-half after admission. The patient's respiratory rate increased remarkably and O_2 stats continued to drop. Initial films were obtained from Lakeview Hospital revealing a left lower lobe pneumonia. Repeat films tonight upon arrival here revealed increasing opacification with a left hemothorax. It was suspected there was marked mucous plugging of the left main stem _____. After discussing options with the patient and her daughter, the patient was electively intubated with bronchoscopic evaluation following.

The patient was given Versed for _____ and then Ativan. She underwent bronchoscopic evaluation for both diagnostic as well as therapeutic reasons.

On examination, the patient was in a fair amount of respiratory distress. The patient was given Ativan at 4 mg during the procedure. The P20 bronchoscope was gently inserted through the ET tube. This was held in place by the respiratory therapist and continuous O_2 monitoring as well as blood pressure and EKG monitoring were maintained. The patient was Ambued with 100% oxygen. The bronchoscope was gently inserted through the endotracheal tube. Initially, the endotracheal tube required pulling back approximately 2 cm because it was at the level of the _____. Following this, the right upper, middle, and lower lobe segments were inspected. All segments were _____. The carina was in the midline. The bronchoscope then was reentered into the left main stem bronchus. The entire left main stem bronchus was totally occluded with yellowish mucoid material. This was suctioned. All airways including the lingula, upper lobe, and lower lobe segments were totally occluded with mucus. Again multiple irrigations were instilled and these airways were suctioned. At the end of the procedure, all airways were patent. The bronchoscope was then withdrawn. The patient tolerated the procedure well. No endobronchial lesions were noted during the procedure. The specimens will be sent for Gram's stain and C&S as well as cytology when available.

IMPRESSION:

1. Total occlusion, left main stem bronchus, secondary to pneumonitis.

2. Heavy history of tobacco abuse.

3. Possible poliomyelitis syndrome.

The patient will be followed quite closely.

The Digestive System

*Now good digestion waits on appetite
And health on both!*

—WILLIAM SHAKESPEARE

OBJECTIVES

When you have completed this chapter on the digestive system, you should be able to

1. Spell and define major system components and explain how they operate.
2. Identify the meaning of related word elements.
3. Spell and define diagnostic procedures, diagnoses, treatment procedures, and abbreviations.
4. Spell the names of medications commonly used.
5. Be familiar with terminology used in reports.

INTRODUCTION

The purpose of the digestive or gastrointestinal system is to receive and process food so that it nourishes the body and to eliminate solid waste. Physicians who specialize in the study of the digestive system are known as gastroenterologists.

Terms that apply to this process include digestion, absorption, and elimination. **Digestion** is the process that converts food into nutrients; **absorption** is the process that transfers these nutrients into the bloodstream and body. **Elimination** is the process that concentrates and releases solid waste (feces). The process of digestion and absorption takes 36 hours or more.

The digestive system consists of the mouth or oral cavity, pharynx, esophagus, stomach, small intestine, appendix, and large intestine—all referred to as the **alimentary** (ăl"ĕ-mĕn'tăr-ē) **canal**, illustrated in Figure 13-1. This chapter discusses these organs.

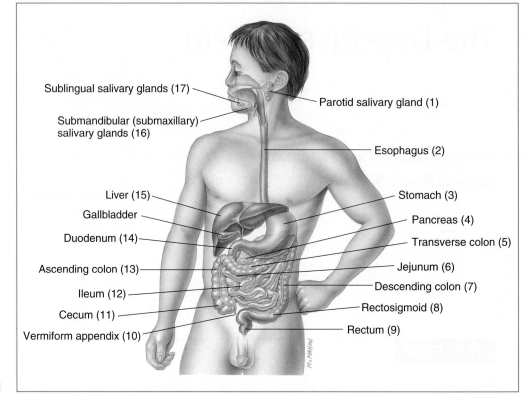

FIGURE 13-1
Alimentary Canal

Sublingual salivary glands (17)

Submandibular (submaxillary) salivary glands (16)

Parotid salivary gland (1)

Esophagus (2)

Liver (15)

Stomach (3)

Gallbladder

Pancreas (4)

Duodenum (14)

Transverse colon (5)

Ascending colon (13)

Jejunum (6)

Ileum (12)

Descending colon (7)

Cecum (11)

Rectosigmoid (8)

Vermiform appendix (10)

Rectum (9)

ORAL CAVITY

cheil/o, chil/o	lip	peritone/o	peritoneum
gingiv/o	gum	phag/o	to eat
gloss/o	tongue	sial/o	salivary
odont/o	tooth	stomat/o, stom/o	mouth

The alimentary canal is a muscular digestive tube that starts in the oral cavity, or mouth, and extends through the entire body. Lodged in the mouth is a muscular organ called the tongue, which aids in chewing and swallowing, as well as in speech and breathing. **Saliva** is produced in the oral cavity and allows food to be swallowed more easily. This fluid is manufactured by three pairs of salivary glands, the first of several accessory organs that aid in the digestive process. The three pairs of major salivary glands are the **parotid** (pah-rŏt'ĭd) (1), **submandibular** (sŭb"măn-dĭb'ū-lăr) or **submaxillary** (sŭb-măk'sĭ-lĕr"ē) (16), and **sublingual** (sŭb-lĭng'gwăl) (17).

Like the rest of the alimentary canal, the oral cavity is lined with a moist mucous membrane.* Beneath this mucous membrane is a layer of connective tissue containing blood vessels and nerves. The parts of the alimentary canal that extend into the abdominal cavity have an additional covering or layer called the **peritoneum** (pĕr"ĭ-tō-nē'ŭm).

PHARYNX

laryng/o	larynx	pharyng/o	pharynx

---

*mucous (adj.)—secreting mucus; mucus (n.)—free slime of the mucous membranes

The **pharynx** (făr'ĭnks), which is situated directly behind the mouth, is the second part of the digestive system. The following seven cavities communicate with the pharynx: the two nasal cavities, the two tympanic cavities (middle ears via the eustachian tubes, commonly called the tympanopharyngeal canals), the mouth or oral cavity, the larynx, and the esophagus. The function of the pharynx in the digestive tract is to carry food to the esophagus.

ESOPHAGUS

esophag/o	esophagus

The **esophagus** (ĕ-sŏf'ah-gŭs) (2) is a passage that extends from the lower part of the pharynx through the diaphragm to the stomach (3). It is lined with stratified squamous epithelial cells. A loosely arranged coat of connective tissue and muscle lie beneath these cells. These layers of involuntary muscles produce a rhythmic, wave-like motion known as **peristalsis** (pĕr"ĭ-stăl'sĭs). This motion—which occurs along the entire length of the alimentary canal—begins in the esophagus where it directs food to the next organ, the stomach.

STOMACH

gastr/o	stomach	pyl/o, pylor/o	pylorus

The stomach is guarded by muscular valves called **sphincters** (sfĭngk'ters), which permit the passage of food in only one direction. The **cardiac valve**, more commonly called the lower esophageal sphincter (LES), encircles the lower end of the esophagus. The valve at the distal (or lower) end of the stomach, where it connects to the small intestine, is called the **pyloric** (pī-lor'ĭk) **sphincter**.

When the stomach is empty, it has folds called **rugae** (roo'gay) in the lining. As food is ingested, these folds open to provide room for food to be mixed with the gastric juices (primarily hydrochloric acid and pepsin) that will begin the digestive process. When the gastric pressure exceeds that of the intestine, the pyloric sphincter relaxes and allows the passage of this slurrylike mixture of partially digested food and digestive secretions (called chyme) into the small intestine. The sphincter then closes to prevent any backup. After this process—which takes 2 to 6 hours—is completed, the rugae return to the folded position.

SMALL INTESTINE

append/o,	appendix	duoden/o	duodenum
appendic/o		enter/o	intestine
bili/o	bile	hepat/o, hepatic/o	liver
celi/o, cel/o	abdomen	ile/o	ileum
cholangi/o	bile or hepatic duct	jejun/o	jejunum
choledoch/o	bile duct	lapar/o	abdominal wall
chol/e, chol/o	bile	pancreat/o	pancreas
cyst/o	bladder, sac	rect/o	rectum

The **small intestine** is the chief organ of digestion and absorption of food products. It is the longest part of the alimentary canal, averaging 20 feet. The lining of the small intestine, or the **mucosa** (mū-kō'sah), is covered with tiny fingerlike projections called **villi** (vĭl'lī).*

---

*villi (n.)—plural; villous (adj.); villus (n.)—singular

The first 10 to 12 inches of the small intestine is called the **duodenum** (dū"ō-dē'nŭm) (14). Secretions from the accessory organs—namely the pancreas (4) and the liver (15)—are received there.

One of the more important secretions is bile, which is produced by the liver and stored in a pouch called the **gallbladder** (7) (Figure 13-2). Bile assists the digestive processing of fats in two ways. Bile causes emulsification, or the break up, of large fat globules into millions of small fat droplets that provide large surface areas for the fat-digesting enzymes to work on. Subsequently, bile combines with the products of fat digestion to form spheres of bile salt molecules called micelles, which bring these end products into closer contact with the absorptive surface of the intestinal wall surface.

Aside from bile production, the **liver** (6)—the second largest glandular organ of the body—performs many other functions, including removal of poisons absorbed from the intestines, final treatment of fats, storage of certain vitamins, and formation of antibodies.

Bile moves through several ducts that are called the **biliary** (bĭl'ē-ā-rē) **tree**. The **hepatic** (hĕ-păt'ĭk) **duct** (2) (**right**, **left**, and **common**) leads from the liver to the duct draining the gallbladder, referred to as the **cystic duct** (1). These two ducts join to form the **common bile duct** (3), which leads to the duodenum. The opening of the common bile duct into the duodenum (5) is the **ampulla of Vater**.

The **pancreas** (4) is a gland situated under the stomach. It produces secretions that aid in the digestion of food and the neutralization of acid produced by the stomach. The main and accessory pancreatic ducts join with the common bile duct before they enter the duodenum through the ampulla of Vater.

Two more divisions of the small intestine (see Figure 13-1) are beyond the duodenum—the **jejunum** (jĕ-joo'nŭm) (6) and the **ileum** (ĭl'ē-ŭm) (12). The ileum joins the large intestine through another muscle valve called the **ileocecal** (ĭl"e-ō-sē'kăl) **valve**.

LARGE INTESTINE

an/o	anal	proct/o	anus, rectum
cec/o	cecum	sigmoid/o	sigmoid colon
col/o, colon/o	colon		

Once digestion and absorption have taken place in the small intestine, the residual liquid is passed to the **large intestine**, also referred to as the **colon**. Water is returned to the body through absorption of most of the fluids, and the residue becomes a solid called **fecal** (fē'kăl) **matter**.

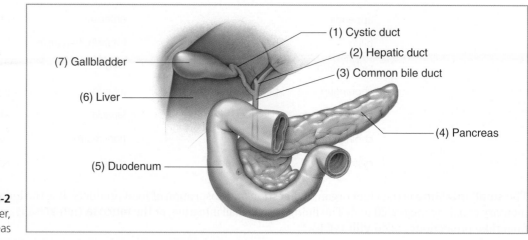

FIGURE 13-2
The Liver, Gallbladder, and Pancreas

(1) Cystic duct
(2) Hepatic duct
(3) Common bile duct
(4) Pancreas
(7) Gallbladder
(6) Liver
(5) Duodenum

The large intestine begins below the ileum and extends to the rectum (see Figure 13-1). It has five divisions in this order—**ascending** (13), **transverse** (5), **descending** (7), **rectosigmoid** (rĕk″tō-sĭg′moid) (8), and **rectum** (9). At the beginning of the large intestine is a pouch called the **cecum** (sē′kŭm) (11). Attached to the cecum is a small, blind tube called the **vermiform** (vĕr′mĭ-form) **appendix** (10). At the lower end the large intestine empties into the rectum. From the rectum the **anal** (ā′năl) **canal** leads out of the body, terminating in an opening called the **anus** (ā′nŭs). The veins in this region are called **hemorrhoidal** (hĕm″ō-roi′dăl) **veins**.

The **mesentery** (mĕs′ĕn-tĕr″ē) is a specialized, double-layered tissue that connects and suspends the intestines in the abdominal cavity. The portion of the mesentery connecting the lower border of the stomach to the transverse colon is called the **greater omentum** (ō-mĕn′tŭm). Sometimes it is referred to as the apron since it is elongated and extends freely into the pelvis. One of its functions is to control the spread of infection inside the abdominal cavity. The **lesser omentum** extends between the stomach and liver.

INTERNET ASSIGNMENT

The American College of Gastroenterology is a professional organization of over 7,000 gastroenterologists in thirty countries. Their mission is to advance the scientific study and medical treatment of disorders of the gastrointestinal tract. The College promotes the highest standards in medical education and is guided by its commitment to meeting the needs of clinical gastroenterology practitioners. One of their goals is to promote patient education on gastrointestinal conditions and digestive health. Their web site is at **www.acg.gi.org** where patient-related links for Patient Information, Site Map, and Site Search can be found at the bottom of the homepage. Other links are directed to clinical practioners.

ACTIVITY

Visit the American College of Gastroenterology site at **www.acg.gi.org**. Click on Patient Information and note the link options available. Select an option that will take you to a digestive system problem or condition and read the information given. Summarize by providing bullets of important information and submit it to your instructor.

Review: The Digestive System

- The digestive system consists of the mouth, pharynx, esophagus, stomach, small intestine, large intestine, and secretory glands (salivary glands, liver, pancreas).

- The mouth prepares food for swallowing; the pharynx and esophagus carry the food to the stomach.

- The stomach breaks up food by a churning action and the addition of hydrochloric acid and gastric juices.

- Bile and pancreatic juices are added to food after it passes through the pyloric sphincter into the duodenum.

- The small intestine absorbs nutrients from processed food.

- Nutrients travel through the lymphatic and vascular channels to the liver for further processing and distribution.

- The large intestine (colon) dehydrates the bowel contents, returns water to the body, and excretes the waste products as fecal material.

Review of Terminology Presented

Review of Terminology Presented

Word	Definition
absorption	process that transfers nutrients into the bloodstream and body
alimentary canal	muscular digestive tube that starts in the oral cavity and extends through the entire body
ampulla of Vater	opening of the common bile duct into the duodenum
anal canal	passage leading to the body opening called the anus
anus	outlet of the anal canal
ascending colon	first section of the large intestine
biliary tree	system of ducts through which bile moves
cardiac valve	lower esophageal sphincter; muscular valve located at the lower end of the esophagus
cecum	pouch at the beginning of the colon or large intestine
colon	part of the digestive system that extends from the cecum to the rectum; large intestine
common bile duct	duct that leads to the duodenum; combination of the hepatic and cystic ducts
cystic duct	duct of the gallbladder
descending colon	third section of the large intestine
digestion	process that converts food into nutrients for the body
duodenum	first 10 to 12 inches of the small intestine
elimination	process that concentrates and releases solid waste (feces)
esophagus	passage from the pharynx through the diaphragm to the stomach
fecal matter	solid waste material left after food intake has been digested and absorbed
gallbladder	storage pouch for bile
greater omentum	portion of the mesentery connecting the lower border of the stomach to the transverse colon; sometimes called the apron
hemorrhoidal veins	veins in the region of the anus
hepatic duct	duct leading from the liver to the cystic duct for the gallbladder; has left, right, and common sections
ileocecal valve	muscular valve that joins the large intestine to the ileum
ileum	third division of the small intestine
jejunum	second division of the small intestine
large intestine	part of the digestive tract that turns residue into fecal matter; colon
lesser omentum	portion of the mesentary that extends between the stomach and liver
liver	second largest glandular organ of the body; produces bile and performs other functions
mesentery	specialized, double-layered tissue that connects and suspends the intestines in the abdominal cavity
mucosa	membrane that lines the alimentary canal
pancreas	gland that secretes juices that aid in the digestion of food and the neutralization of acid produced by the stomach

continues

Word	Definition
parotid glands	glands that produce saliva; located near the ear
peristalsis	rhythmic, wavelike motion produced by involuntary muscles of the alimentary canal to move food through its entire length
peritoneum	additional covering or layer on parts of the alimentary canal that extends into the abdominal cavity
pharynx	throat
pyloric sphincter	valve at the distal end of the stomach where the stomach connects to the small intestine
rectosigmoid colon	fourth section of the large intestine
rectum	lower part of the large intestine
rugae	folds found in the stomach lining
saliva	enzyme-containing secretion produced in the oral cavity to assist in chewing and swallowing
small intestine	chief organ of digestion and absorption
sphincters	ringlike muscular valves that encourage the passage of food in the stomach in only one direction
sublingual glands	glands that produce saliva; located under the tongue
submandibular (submaxillary) glands	glands that produce saliva; located in the lower jaw
transverse colon	second section of the large intestine
vermiform appendix	small, blind tube attached to the cecum
villi	tiny, fingerlike projections in the mucosa that line the small intestine

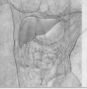

Terminology Review Exercises

Name: _____ Date: _____

DEFINITIONS
Define the following terms.

1. digestion

   _____

2. absorption

   _____

3. peristalsis

   _____

4. rugae

   _____

5. alimentary canal

   _____

6. fecal matter

   _____

7. peritoneum

   _____

8. mesentery

   _____

9. greater omentum

   _____

SHORT ANSWERS
Supply a short answer to the following.

1. Explain the difference between mucus and mucous.

   _____

   _____

   _____

   _____

2. Explain the difference between villi, villus, and villous.

   _____

   _____

   _____

   _____

3. Describe the biliary tree.

_____

_____

_____

4. Explain the difference between the rectum and anus.

_____

_____

_____

COMPLETION*

Complete the following statements.

1. It usually takes food _____ hours to move from the mouth to the anus.
2. The longest part of the alimentary canal is the _____.
3. The chief organ of digestion, absorption, and elimination is the _____.
4. Food is carried to the stomach from the pharynx by the _____.
5. The gallbladder stores _____.
6. The second largest glandular organ of the body is the _____.
7. The portion of the mesentery that extends between the stomach and liver is the _____.
8. Two valves in the stomach ensure that food passes in only one direction; these are the _____ and the _____.
9. The three anatomic divisions of the small intestine are the _____, _____, and _____.
10. Bile is produced in the _____.
11. Saliva is produced in three glands; they are the _____, _____, and _____.
12. The large intestine is also known as the _____.
13. The five anatomic divisions of the colon are the _____, _____, _____, _____, and _____.
14. The fluid produced in the oral cavity that assists digestion is _____.
15. The stomach is guarded by muscular valves called _____.
16. The function of the _____ is to carry food to the esophagus.
17. The lining of the small intestine is the _____.
18. Tiny, fingerlike projections of the small intestine are _____.
19. A muscular valve that joins the large intestine to the ileum is the _____.
20. The _____ is the pouch at the beginning of the colon.

_____

*Answers are in Appendix A.

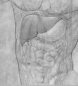

DIAGNOSTIC PROCEDURES

Word	Pronunciation	Definition
General		
colonoscopy	kō″lŏn-ŏs′kō-pē	visual examination of the colon using a flexible colonoscope (See Figure 13-3)
esophageal motility studies	ĕ-sŏf″ah-jē′ăl mō-tĭl′ĭ-tē	diagnostic test that records movement and pressure in the esophagus
esophagogastroduo-denoscopy (EGD) (panendoscopy)	ĕ-sŏf″ah-gō-găs″trō-dū″ŏ-dĕ-nŏs′kō-pē (păn″ĕn-dŏs′kō-pē)	visual examination of the esophagus, stomach, and duodenum with a flexible gastroscope
esophagoscopy	ĕ-sŏf″ah-gŏs′kō-pē	visual examination of the esophagus using an esophagoscope
liver biopsy		removal of a tissue sample from the liver for microscopic examination
paracentesis (abdominocentesis)	păr″ah-sĕn-tē′sĭs (ăb-dŏm″ĭ-nō-sĕn-tē′sĭs)	needle puncture of a cavity to remove fluid from the cavity for laboratory examination
sigmoidoscopy (proctoscopy)	sĭg″moy-dŏs′kō-pē (prŏk-tŏs′kō-pē)	direct examination of the anus, rectum, and part of the sigmoid colon using a sigmoidoscope
Nuclear Medicine		
liver scan		injection of a radioactive substance intravenously, which then circulates through the blood to the liver; a special camera takes a picture of the liver
Radiology		
abdominal magnetic resonance imaging (MRI)		visualization of the contents of the abdomen using magnetic resonance imaging

continues

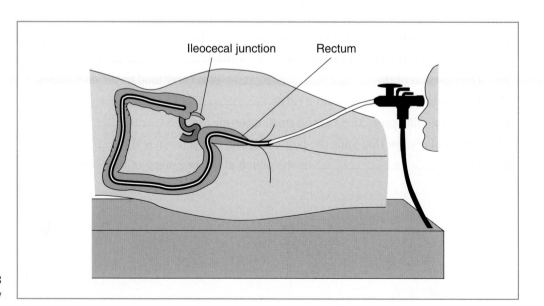

FIGURE 13-3
Colonoscopy

DIAGNOSTIC PROCEDURES

Word	Pronunciation	Definition
Radiology (continued)		
abdominal ultrasonography	ŭl'tră-sŏn-ŏg'ră-fē	record made by imaging abdominal viscera from reflected sound waves
barium enema, air contrast		x-ray procedure that introduces first barium and then air into the colon to give added contrast; provides fine detail
barium enema (BE)		infusion of barium, a radiopaque contrast medium, into the colon to better visualize the lower intestinal tract during x-ray examination (See Figure 13-4)
CT of the abdomen		detailed cross section of tissue structures within the abdomen
endoscopic retrograde cholangiopancre-atography (ERCP)	ĕn-dō-skŏp'ĭk rĕt'rō-grād kō-lăn"jē-ō-păn"krē-ah-tŏg'rah-fē	x-ray of the bile and pancreatic ducts by injecting contrast medium through their opening into the intestinal tract by using an endoscope
fluoroscopy	floo"or-ŏs'kŏ-pē	realtime x-ray examination of organs to study their condition
intravenous cholangiogram	ĭn-tră-vē'nŭs kō-lăn'jē-ō-grăm"	x-ray procedure whereby a special dye is injected intravenously and then excreted into the bile ducts for study of the common bile duct primarily and the gallbladder secondarily
oral cholecystogram	kō"lē-sĭs'tō-grăm	x-ray of the gallbladder, which is made visible by orally administered dye; the dye is absorbed, excreted into the bile, and concentrated by the gallbladder
percutaneous transhepatic cholangiography (PTHC)	pĕr"kū-tā'nē-ŭs trăns-hĕ-pat'ĭk kō-lăn"jē-ŏg'rah-fē	x-ray procedure whereby a contrast medium is injected through the liver into the bile duct to detect an obstruction
small bowel follow-through (SBFT)		x-ray using barium to examine the small intestine at timed intervals

continues

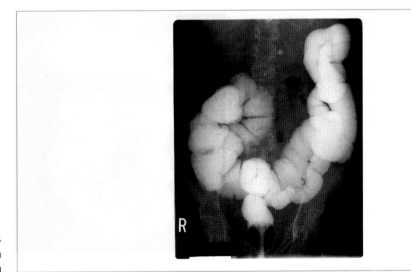

FIGURE 13-4
X-Ray of Colon with Barium Enema

DIAGNOSES

Word	Pronunciation	Definition
Diseases of the Esophagus (*continued*)		
reflux esophagitis	ē-sŏf-ah-gī'tŭs	inflammation of the esophagus caused by backward flow of stomach acid into the esophagus
Diseases of the Stomach		
cancer of the stomach		malignant tumor of the stomach
dyspepsia (indigestion)	dis-pĕp'sē-ah	syndrome with upper abdominal pain, bloating, and nausea
gastritis	găs-trī'ĭs	inflammation of the stomach; may be acute or chronic; may be caused by *Helicobacter*
peptic ulcer		ulceration through the mucous membrane of the esophagus, stomach, or duodenum; called gastric ulcer in the stomach and duodenal ulcer in the duodenum
Zollinger-Ellison syndrome		condition caused by tuberous secretion of gastrin, a hormone that causes gastric hyperacidity with secondary ulcers and/or diarrhea
Diseases of the Small Intestine		
Viral Infections		
rotavirus	rō'tă-vī"rŭs	acute viral infection often found in child care centers and homes for the elderly
Norwalk virus		an acute viral infection, also called winter vomiting disease
cytomegalovirus	sī"tō-mĕg"ă-lō-vī'rŭs	an acute viral infection and common cause of diarrhea in individuals with AIDS; a species-specific herpes virus
Bacterial Infections		
bacterial overgrowth		a condition characterized by diarrhea and malabsorption caused by accumulation of bacteria in the small intestine
Campylobacter infections	kăm"pĭ-lō-băk'tĕr	infections most commonly occurring in children younger than 1 year of age or in young adults; the source seems to be raw foods such as milk and poultry
Salmonella	săl"mō-nĕl'ah	a gram-negative bacteria that may cause intestinal infection; found in meats and dairy products; causes mild to fatal food poisoning
Shigella	shĭ-gĕl'lă	bacteria causing mild to fatal dysentery; found primarily in developing countries and in children ages 1 to 5
Parasitic Infections		
Cryptosporidium	krĭp"tō-spō-rĭd'ē-ŭm	an infection that is the common cause of diarrhea in AIDS patients; may occur in otherwise healthy individuals
Entamoeba histolytica	ĕn"ta-mē'bă hĭs"tō-lĭt'ĭk-ah	a diarrheal infection that is common in the world but not in the United States; common in homosexual men

continues

DIAGNOSES		
Word	**Pronunciation**	**Definition**

Diseases of the Small Intestine (*continued*)

Giardia lamblia	jē-ăr'dē-ah lăm'blē-ah	infection that is one of the most common parasitic causes of diarrhea in the United States; the source is a contaminated water supply

Other GI-related Infections

antibiotic-associated diarrhea		antibiotics may alter the bowel environment resulting in certain bacterial growth and in inflammation
dysentery	dĭs'ĕn-tăr"ē	acute inflammation caused by the invasion of microorganisms into the colon lining; results in diarrhea
food poisoning		a condition caused by eating contaminated foods, which results in the production of toxins such as those produced by *Staphylococcus aureus*, *Bacillus cereus*, and *Clostridium botulinum*
peritonitis	pěr"ĭ-tō-nī'tĭs	an inflammation of the peritoneal lining
celiac sprue	sē'lē-ăk sproo	malabsorption and other difficulties from gluten (a wheat protein) intolerance
Crohn's disease (regional enteritis)	krōnz	chronic inflammatory bowel disease usually affecting the ileum, colon, or both structures; it is one type of *inflammatory bowel disease (IBD).*
duodenal ulcer	dŭ-ō-dē'năl	peptic ulcer in duodenum
gastroenteritis	găs"trō-ĕn-tĕr-ī"tĭs	inflammation of both the stomach and intestines
inguinal hernia	ĭng'gwĭ-năl	a protrusion of a loop of bowel through the groin area; usually requires corrective surgery
malabsorption syndrome		inability of the small intestine to absorb nutrients and minerals

Diseases of the Colon

appendicitis	ă-pēn'dĭ-sī'tĭs	inflammation, swelling, and accumulation of pus in the appendix resulting in abdominal pain, nausea, and/or vomiting; usually requires surgery (See Figure 13-6)
colorectal cancer	kō"lō-rěk'tăl	carcinoma of the colon or rectum
congenital megacolon (Hirschsprung's disease)		a congenital condition marked by enlarged colon (as a result of nerve damage) resulting in the inability of the colon to move feces
diverticulitis	dī"věr-tĭk"ū-lī'tĭs	inflammation of a diverticulum
diverticulosis	dī"věr-tĭk"ū-lō'sĭs	presence of diverticula (See Figure 13-7)
granulomatous colitis	grăn"ū-lŏm'ă-tŭs kō-lī'tĭs	inflammation of the colon characterized by nodules of granular tissue; frequently involves all layers of the intestinal wall; also called Crohn's colitis
ileus	ĭl'ē-ŭs	intestinal obstruction

continues

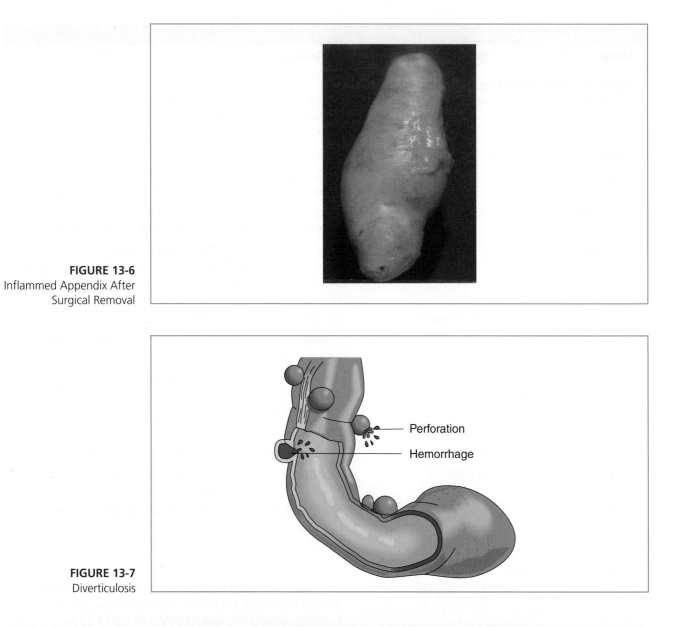

FIGURE 13-6
Inflammed Appendix After
Surgical Removal

FIGURE 13-7
Diverticulosis

DIAGNOSES

Word	Pronunciation	Definition
Diseases of the Colon (*continued*)		
inflammatory bowel disease (IBD)		descriptive term usually referring to ulcerative colitis or Crohn's disease
intestinal obstruction		partial or complete obstruction in small intestine or colon that prevents movement of the products of digestion
intussusception	ĭn"tŭ-sū-sĕp'shŭn	disorder occurring when a portion of the intestine telescopes into another segment of the intestine (See Figure 13-8A)

continues

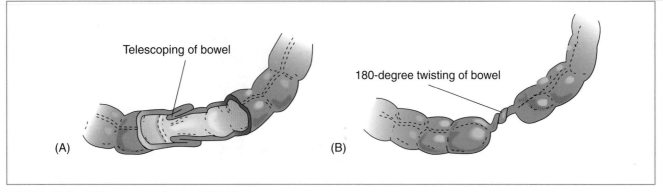

FIGURE 13-8   (A) Intussusception and (B) Volvulus

DIAGNOSES		
Word	Pronunciation	Definition
Diseases of the Colon (continued)		
irritable bowel syndrome (IBS) (spastic colon)		abnormally increased motility of the large and small intestine that may be associated with emotional stress
polyps	pŏl'ĭps	small, tumorlike growths that project from the mucous membrane surface of the alimentary tract (See Figure 13-9)
scleroderma	sklē"rō'dĕr'mah	a condition marked by atrophy of the muscular walls of the intestines and esophagus resulting in impairment of movement of the intestine and the absorption of nutrients
short bowel syndrome		loss of a significant part of the intestines or disease involving a sufficient length of the small intestine with consequent impaired nutrient absorption
ulcerative colitis	ŭl'sĕr-ā-tĭv kō-lī'tĭs	ulceration of the colonic mucosa, cause unknown; it may cause diarrhea, loss of weight, or anemia, and increases the risk of developing colon cancer (See Figure 13-10)
volvulus	vōl'vū-lŭs	twisting or looping of the intestine, often requiring emergency surgery (See Figure 13-8B)
Whipple's disease (intestinal lipodystrophy)	(lĭp"-ō-dĭs'-trō-fē)	a disease characterized by fatty deposits caused by an infectious organism

continues

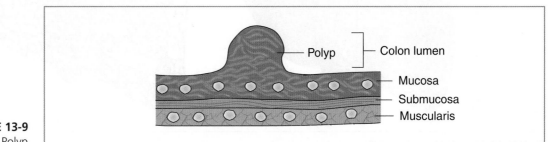

FIGURE 13-9
Colon Polyp

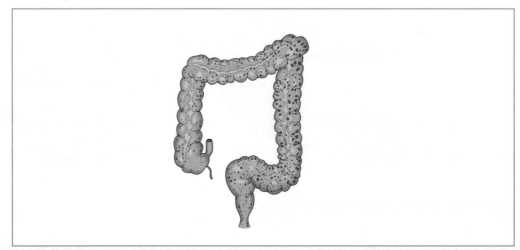

FIGURE 13-10
Ulcerative Colitis

DIAGNOSES

Word	Pronunciation	Definition
Diseases of the Anus and Rectum		
abscess		collection of pus in tissue near the rectum, usually as a result of infected anal glands
fissure	fish'ūr	split in the epithelial surface of the anal canal
fistula	fĭs'tū-lah	abnormal passage between organs
hemorrhoids	hĕm'ō-roydz	varicose dilation of veins in the anal canal or rectum
Diseases of the Liver, Gallbladder, and Pancreas		
Liver		
cirrhosis	sĭ-rō'sĭs	scarring of the liver associated with a destruction of liver cells (See Figure 13-11); complications include varicosities, splenomegaly, GI hemorrhage, ascites, edema, jaundice, and hepatic encephalopathy
hepatitis	hĕp"ă-tī'tĭs	inflammation of the liver; may be Hepatitis A, B, or C

continues

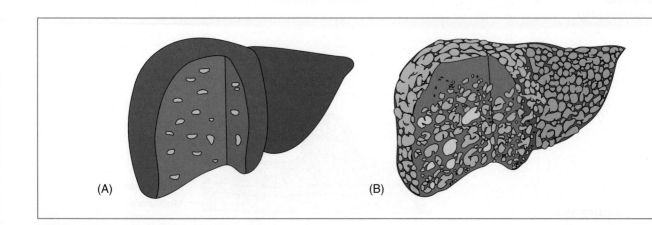

(A)   (B)

FIGURE 13-11   (A) Normal vs (B) Cirrhotic Liver

DIAGNOSES

Word	Pronunciation	Definition
liver cancer		malignant tumor in the liver
Gallbladder		
cholecystitis	kō"lē-sĭs-tī'tĭs	inflammation of gallbladder generally caused by obstruction of bile flow due to a gallstone
cholelithiasis	kō"lē-lĭ-thī-sĭs	presence of gallstones in the gallbladder
Pancreas		
pancreatic cancer	păn'krē-ăs	malignant tumor that occurs in the pancreas
pancreatitis	păn"krē-ă-tī'tĭs	inflammation of the pancreas; may be acute or chronic

TREATMENT PROCEDURES

Word	Pronunciation	Definition
anal fissurectomy	fĭsh-ūr-ĕk'tō-mē	removal of an anal fissure
appendectomy	ăp"ĕn-děk'tō-mē	removal of the appendix
cholecystectomy	kō"lē-sĭs-těk'tō-mē	excision of the gallbladder
colectomy	kō-lěk'tō-mē	excision of the colon
colostomy	kō-lŏs'tō-mē	surgical creation of an opening between the colon and body surface
esophagogastrostomy	ē-sŏf"ă-gō-găs-trŏs'tō-mē	creation of an opening between the esophagus and stomach
esophagostomy	ē-sŏf"ah-gŏt'ō-mē	surgical creation of an opening in the esophagus
excision of Meckel's diverticulum	dī"věr-tik'ū-lūm	surgical removal of a congenital outpouching of the wall of the ileum
herniorrhaphy	hěr-nē-or'ă-fē	surgical repair of a hernia
fistulectomy	fĭs"tū-lěk'tō-mē	surgical removal of a fistula
gastrectomy	găs-trěk'tō-mē	excision of all or part of the stomach
gastrostomy	găs-trŏs'tō-mē	surgical placement of a tube into the stomach
hemorrhoid ligation	hěm'ō-royd lī-gā'shŭn	removal of internal hemorrhoid groupings using a rubber band technique
hemorrhoidectomy	hěm"ō-royd-ěk'tō-mē	excision of a varicose dilation of a vein
extracorporeal shock wave lithotripsy (ESWL)	ěks"tră-kor-por'ē-ăl, lĭth'ō-trĭp"sē	ultrasound crushing of calculi in the gallbladder or kidney
ileo-anal anastomosis	ĭl"ē-ō-ā'năl ă-năs"tō-mō'sĭs	procedure to remove the entire colon and rectum through the abdominal wall, but preserving the sphincter muscles of the anus; a pouch is created in the ileum, which is then attached to the anus; a temporary ileostomy is used to collect fecal material until the juncture is healed

continues

TREATMENT PROCEDURES

Word	Pronunciation	Definition
ileostomy	ĭl"ē-ŏs'tō-mē	a surgical passage through the abdominal wall into the small intestine (ileum) for drainage of fecal material
jejunostomy	jē"jū-nŏs'tō-mē	creation of an opening between the jejunum and the surface of the abdominal wall
laparoscopic cholecystectomy	lăp'ă-rō-skŏp"ĭk kō"lē-sĭs-tĕk'tō-mē	removal of gallbladder by making four punctures for four tiny tubes through which instruments and cameras are placed
liver transplantation		replacement of liver after other treatments have been exhausted
pancreatectomy	păn"krē-at-ĕk'tō-mē	removal of the pancreas
splenectomy	splē-nĕk'tō-mē	removal of the spleen
vagotomy	vă-gŏt'ō-mē	surgical transection of the fibers of the vagus nerve; frequently done to decrease acid secretion of the stomach in patients with ulcers

MEDICATIONS PRESCRIBED

Trade Name	Generic Name
Anthelminthics	
Antepar	piperazine citrate
Antiminth	pyrantel pamoate
Vermox	mebendazole
Antibiotics	
Achromycin, Sumycin	tetracycline
Azulfidine	sulfasalazine
Flagyl	metronidazole
Vancocin	vancomycin HCl
Anticholinergics/Antispasmodics	
Anaspaz, Levsin	l-hyoscyamine sulfate
Bentyl	dicyclomine HCl
Clindex, Clinoxide, Librax	clidinium, chlordiazepoxide
Donnatal	atropine, scopolamine, hyoscyamine, phenobarbital
Pro-Banthine	propantheline bromide
Robinul	glycopyrrolate
Antidiarrheals	
Bacid, Lactinex	lactobacillus

continues

MEDICATIONS PRESCRIBED

Trade Name	Generic Name
Antidiarrheals *(continued)*	
Imodium	loperamide
Lomotil	diphenoxylate with atropine
Pepto-Bismol	bismuth subsalicylate
Digestive Enzymes	
Ultrase, Pancrease	pancrelipase
Creon, Donnazyme	pancreatin
Gallstone Solubilizing Agents	
Actigall	ursodiol
GI Stimulants	
Reglan	metoclopramide
H$_{(2)}$ Antagonists	
Tagamet	cimetidine
Zantac	ranitidine
Axid	nizatidine
Pepcid	famotidine
Other Medications that Lower Acid Secretion and/or Protect Mucosa	
Cytotec	misoprostol
Prilosec	omeprazole
Over-the-Counter Antacids	
Amphojel	
Alternagel	
Gaviscon	
Maalox	
Milk of Magnesia (MOM)	
Mylanta	
Riopan	
Over-the-Counter Laxatives	
Cascara Sagrada	
Chronulac, Duphalac (lactulose)	
Citrucel	

continues

MEDICATIONS PRESCRIBED

Trade Name	Generic Name
Over-the-Counter Laxatives *(continued)*	
Colace (docusate Na)	
Colyte, Golytely	
Dulcolax (bisacodyl)	
Ex-Lax	
Feen-a-mint	
Fleet Prep	
Metamucil	
Milk of Magnesia (MOM)	
Perdiem	
Senokot	
Surfak (docusate Ca)	
X-Prep	
Ulcer Protectant	
Carafate	sucralfate

ABBREVIATIONS

A/G	albumin globulin ration
alb	serum albumin
ALT	alanine aminotransferase
AST	aspartate aminotransferase
BE	barium enema
CEA	carcinoembryonic antigen
EGD	esophagogastroduodenoscopy
ERCP	endoscopic retrograde cholangiopancreatography
GERD	gastroesophageal reflux disease
GGT	gamma-glutamyl transpeptidase
GI	gastrointestinal
IBD	inflammatory bowel disease
IBS	irritable bowel syndrome
IVC	intravenous cholangiogram
LDH	serum lactate dehydrogenase
MRI	magnetic resonance imaging
NG	nasogastric

continues

ABBREVIATIONS

O&P	ova and parasite
ProTime, PT	prothrombin time
PTHC	percutaneous transhepatic cholangiography
SBFT	small bowel follow-through
SPEP	serum protein electrophoresis
TP	serum total proteins
TPN	total parenteral nutrition
UGI	upper gastrointestinal series

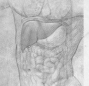

Word Element Review

Root	Meaning	Example	Definition
an/o	anal	**anus** (ā'nŭs)	opening of the anal canal
append/o, appendic/o	appendix	**appendectomy** (ăp"ĕn-dĕk'tō-mē)	surgical removal of the vermiform appendix
bil/i	bile	**biliary** (bĭl'ē-ā-rē)	pertaining to bile
		biliousness (bĭl'yŭs-nĕs)	discomfort characterized by constipation and indigestion
cec/o	cecum	**cecocolostomy** (sē"kō-kō-lŏs'tō-mē)	colostomy consisting of joining the cecum and the colon
celi/o, cel/o	abdomen	**celiac** (sē'lē-ăk)	pertaining to the abdomen
cheil/o, chil/o	lip	**cheilitis** (kī-lī'tĭs)	inflammation of the lip
cholangi/o	bile or hepatic duct	**cholangitis** (kō"lăn-jī'tĭs)	inflammation of a bile duct
choledoch/o	bile duct	**choledochojejunostomy** (kō-lĕd"ō-kō-jĕ-jū-nŏs'tō-mē)	surgical anastomosis of the common bile duct to the jejunum
		choledocholithiasis (kō-lĕd"ō-kō-lĭ-thī'ah-sĭs)	calculi in the common bile duct
chol/e, chol/o	bile	**cholecystitis** (kō"lē-sĭs-tī'tīs)	inflammation of the gallbladder
col/o, colon/o	colon	**colostomy** (kō-lŏs'tō-mē)	surgical creation of an opening to drain the intestines through the abdominal wall
cyst/o	bladder, sac	**cholecystectomy** (kō"lē-sĭs-tĕk'tō-mē)	excision of the gallbladder
duoden/o	duodenum	**duodenitis** (dū"ŏd-ĕ-nī'tĭs)	inflammation of the duodenum
enter/o	intestine	**enteropathy** (ĕn"ter-ŏp'ah-thē)	any disease of the intestines
esophag/o	esophagus	**esophageal** (ĕ-sŏf"ah-jē'ăl)	pertaining to the esophagus
gastr/o	stomach	**gastroenteric** (găs"trō-ĕn-tĕr'ĭk)	pertaining to the stomach and intestines
		gastrointestinal (găs"trō-ĭn-tĕs'tĭ-năl)	pertaining to the digestive system
gingiv/o	gum	**gingiva** (jĭn-jī'vah)	gum of the mouth
gloss/o	tongue	**hypoglossal** (hī"pō-glŏs'ăl)	underneath the tongue

continues

Root	Meaning	Example	Definition
hepat/o, hepatic/o	liver	**hepatology** (hĕp″ah-tŏl′ō-jē)	study of the liver
ile/o	ileum	**ileitis** (ĭl″ē-ī′tĭs)	inflammation of the ileum
		ileocecostomy (ĭl′ē-ō-sē-kŏs′tō-mē)	surgical opening between the ileum and cecum
jejun/o	jejunum	**jejunorrhaphy** (jē″joo-nor′ă-fē)	surgical repair of the jejunum
lapar/o	abdominal wall	**laparotomy** (lăp-ah-rŏt′ō-mē)	incision into the abdomen
laryng/o	larynx	**laryngitis** (lār″ĭn-jī′tĭs)	inflammation of the larynx
		laryngoscope (lah-rĭng′gō-skōp)	instrument for viewing the larynx
odont/o	tooth	**odontic** (ō-dŏn′tĭk)	pertaining to the teeth
pancreat/o	pancreas	**pancreatalgia** (păn″krē-ă-tăl′jē-ă)	pain in the pancreas
peritone/o	peritoneum	**peritoneopathy** (pĕr″ĭ-tō-nē-ŏp′ăth-ē)	any disordered condition of the peritoneum
phag/o	to eat	**dysphagia** (dĭs-fā′jē-ah)	difficulty in swallowing
		phagocyte (făg′ō-sīt)	any cell that "eats" other cells
pharyng/o	pharynx	**pharyngeal** (făh-rĭn′jē-ăl)	pertaining to the pharynx
		pharyngitis (făr″ĭn-jī′tĭs)	inflammation of the pharynx
proct/o	anus and rectum	**proctology** (prŏk-tŏl′ō-jē)	branch of medicine dealing with the anus and rectum
pyl/o, pylor/o	pylorus	**gastropyloric** (găs″trō-pī-lor′ĭk)	pertaining to the stomach and pylorus
		pyloric (pī-lor′ik)	pertaining to the pylorus
rect/o	rectum	**rectoclysis** (rĕk-tŏk′lī-sĭs)	slow introduction of fluid into the rectum
sial/o	salivary	**sialogram** (sī-ăl′ō-grăm)	film produced by sialography
sigmoid/o	sigmoid colon	**sigmoidostomy** (sĭg-moyd-ŏs′tō-mē)	creation of an artificial anus in the sigmoid flexure
stomat/o, stom/o	mouth	**stomatic** (stō-măt′ĭk)	pertaining to the mouth

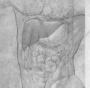

Word Element Review Exercises

Name: _____ Date: _____

WORD ELEMENTS*

Provide the correct word element to complete the following words.

1. branch of medicine dealing with the anus and rectum _____ ology
2. underneath the tongue   hypo _____
3. any cell that "eats" other cells _____ cyte
4. incision into the abdomen _____ otomy
5. the gum of the mouth _____ a
6. pertaining to the esophagus _____ eal
7. any disease of the intestines _____ pathy
8. pertaining to the abdomen _____ iac
9. difficulty in swallowing   dys _____ ia
10. calculi in the common bile duct _____ lithiasis

MATCHING

Match the word elements to their meanings.

1. _____ any disorder of the peritoneum   a. biliary
2. _____ colostomy that joins cecum and colon   b. cecocolostomy
3. _____ excision of gall bladder   c. cheilitis
4. _____ inflammation of the lip   d. cholecystectomy
5. _____ inflammation of the duodenum   e. colostomy
6. _____ inflammation of ileum   f. duodenitis
7. _____ instrument for viewing the larynx   g. hepatology
8. _____ pain in the pancreas   h. ileitis
9. _____ pertaining to teeth   i. laryngoscope
10. _____ pertaining to bile   j. odontic
11. _____ pertaining to the pharynx   k. pancreatalgia
12. _____ pertaining to the mouth   l. peritoneopathy
13. _____ slow introduction of fluid into the rectum   m. pharyngeal
14. _____ study of the liver   n. rectoclysis
15. _____ surgically created opening in the abdominal wall to drain intestines   o. stomatic

*Answers are in Appendix A.

SPELLING*

Rewrite the misspelled words.

1. biliousness _____
2. annus _____
3. laryngitis _____
4. apendectomy _____
5. cholesistitis _____
6. jejunorhaphy _____
7. gastropiloric _____
8. iliosecostomy _____
9. cholangitis _____
10. cholidochojejunostomy _____

WORD ELEMENT

Give the meaning of each word element. Then use your dictionary to find a new word that contains each of the word elements. Specify whether the new word is a noun or an adjective by placing N or A in the last column.

Word Element	Meaning	Word	N or A
1. an/o			
2. append/o			
3. appendic/o			
4. bil/i			
5. cec/o			
6. celi/o			
7. cel/o			
8. cheil/o			
9. chil/o			
10. choledoch/o			
11. chol/e			
12. chol/o			
13. cholangi/o			
14. col/o			
15. colon/o			
16. cyst/o			
17. duoden/o			
18. enter/o			

*Answers are in Appendix A.

7. esophagitis (_____)
   a. inflammation of the stomach
   b. inflammation of the intestine
   c. inflammation of the bile ducts
   d. inflammation of the esophagus

8. paralytic ileus (_____)
   a. loss of peristalsis
   b. resection of the ileum
   c. islets of Langerhans
   d. inflammation of the ileum

9. melena (_____)
   a. referring to the color black, especially with respect to blood in the feces
   b. without teeth
   c. benign tumor of the bile duct
   d. round mass of anything

10. hyperchlorhydria (_____)
    a. failure of any part of the smooth muscle of the gastroenteric tract to relax where one section joins another
    b. absence of hydrochloric acid in the gastric juices
    c. difficulty in swallowing
    d. excessive amount of hydrochloric acid in the gastric juices

11. biliary colic
    a. pain from blocked cystic or common bile duct
    b. malabsorption caused by disease of the absorbing surfaces of the intestine
    c. disease caused by damage to the gallbladder
    d. congenital defect in diverticula of the ileum

12. Salmonella (_____)
    a. excess fat in the feces
    b. various rod-shaped bacteria, many of which may cause food poisoning
    c. condition in which tumors form in the pancreas
    d. intestinal obstruction

13. jaundice (_____)
    a. frequent thirst
    b. an enlarged vein
    c. yellowish coloration of the skin caused by bilirubin in the blood
    d. characteristic foul odor of breath due to disease of the liver

14. steatorrhea (_____)
    a. cramping and straining feeling when passing stool
    b. redness of skin on palm of hand
    c. protrusion of part of an organ through the wall of its natural cavity
    d. excess fat in the feces

DICTIONARY EXERCISE 3

Pronunciation of the words below is provided. Using your dictionary, find the correct spelling and definition of each word.

	Word	Pronunciation	Definition
1.	_____	bē'zōr	_____
2.	_____	bor"bō-rĭg'mŭs	_____
3.	_____	ē-dĕn'tū-lŭs	_____
4.	_____	flăt'ū-lĕns	_____
5.	_____	kīm	_____
6.	_____	ŏb"stĭ-pā'shŭn	_____
7.	_____	fī"tō-bē'zōr	_____
8.	_____	tĕ-nĕz'mŭs	_____
9.	_____	ĕp"ĭ-gǎs'trĭk	_____
10.	_____	hĕp"ah-tō-mĕg'ah-lē	_____
11.	_____	dĕ"gloo-tīsh'ŏn	_____
12.	_____	ĕ-sŏf"ah-jĕk'tō-mē	_____

13. _____ hĕ-păt'ĭk-ĕn-sĕf"ă-
   lŏp'-ă-thē   _____

14. _____ lăp-ah-rŏt'ō-mē   _____

15. _____ lah-vahzh'   _____

DICTIONARY EXERCISE 4*

Rewrite the sentences in your own words. Provide pronunciation marks for each italicized word.

1. The problem was related to *aphagia* (_____).

   _____

2. Failure of the alimentary canal to move the *bolus* (_____) caused a cramping feeling.

   _____

3. They discovered a *cholangioma* (_____).

   _____

4. It was necessary to perform a *choledocholithotomy* (_____).

   _____

5. She was experiencing *polydipsia* (_____), *eructation* (_____), and difficulties with *deglutition* (_____).

   _____

6. Besides dysphagia, the patient had *palmar erythema* (_____).

   _____

7. He was admitted with *icterus* (_____) and *asterixis* (_____).

   _____

8. The physician said she had trouble *defecating* (_____).

   _____

9. One of the symptoms was *fetor hepaticus* (_____).

   _____

10. The symptoms were indicative of *enteritis* (_____).

   _____

11. The digestive problem was directly tied to *emulsification* (_____) of fats.

   _____

12. The patient presented with *gastroduodenitis* (_____).

   _____

13. The patient reported *flatus* (_____) and *constipation* (_____).

   _____

14. The physician noted the pressure of *hyperbilirubinemia* (_____).

   _____

*Answers are in Appendix A.

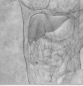

Listening Exercise

Name	Date

INSTRUCTIONS

1. Review the spelling, pronunciation, and meaning of the words provided in the preview.
2. Listen to the audio CD and fill in the blank as the word is dictated.
3. At the end of the exercise, check your spelling against the preview words. They appear in the preview in the order in which they are encountered in the exercise.
4. Review and practice the words you missed.
5. Look up words that are not familiar.

PREVIEW OF WORDS FOR LISTENING EXERCISE 13-1

Word	Pronunciation	Meaning
Hemoccult	hē'mō-kŭlt	trademark for guaiac reagent strip test for occult blood
colonoscopy	kō"lŏn-ŏs'kō-pē	visual examination of the colon using a special instrument
Helicobacter	hēl"ĭ-kō-băk'těr	gram-negative, spiral bacterium that causes gastritis in humans
organomegular	or"gă-nō-měg'ŭ-lăr	visceral organs that have become enlarged
cholelithiasis	ko"lē-lĭ-thī'ă-sĭs	presence or formation of gallstones in the gallbladder
serology	sē-rŏl'ō-jē	the study of antibody reactions in infectious disease

Letter of Consultation

Dr. Rutherford Wiggins

1414 N. Cambria, Suite 245

Duluth, MN

Dear Dr. Wiggins:

Thanks for asking me to see your patient, Signe Nelstrom, because of her family history of early colon cancer. Her mother had that disease at age 24. As you know, we have seen Mrs. Nelstrom over the years for a variety of GI complaints. She had intermittent rectal bleeding, _____ positive stool. She last underwent _____ by Dr. Chan in 1992. The patient also was found to have gastritis due to _____ and was treated in 1994 with triple therapy.

Patient continues to have intermittent epigastric and right upper quadrant pain. It hasn't progressed, but it does bother her regularly. She has no food intolerance, no nausea or vomiting, no change in appetite or weight. Her bowels are still somewhat irregular and she occasionally notices some bright red blood. Her stools have not been tested for occult blood yet this year.

Review of the patient's family history shows no other family members with malignancies.

Physical exam; Weight 175, temperature 97.3, blood pressure is 120/82. Cardiorespiratory exam is negative. Her abdomen is soft. She has mild tenderness to deep palpation in the right upper quadrant. There is no _____ mass, guarding, or rebound. Bowel sounds are normal. Rectal exam is deferred.

IMPRESSIONS: (1) Early colon cancer in first degree relative (mother—age 24) in a patient with chronically irregular bowel habits, abdominal pain, history of Hemoccult positive stool and intermittent bright red rectal bleeding.

(2) Right upper quadrant and epigastric pain. Rule out persisting or recurrent Helicobacter gastritis. Rule out _____.

PLAN: I am going to get _____ for Helicobacter and an ultrasound of the upper abdomen. If the serology is still significantly positive, I'll plan to do an upper GI endoscopy along with her colonoscopy. I agree with your recommendation for colonoscopy because of her family history, as well as her additional symptoms. I'll keep you informed of her progress.

Sincerely yours,

Hector Verandez, MD

chapter 14

Discharge Summaries

> *Patients may not swear, curse, get drunk, behave rudely or indecently on pain of expulsion after the first admonition. There shall be no card playing or dicing and such patients as are able shall assist in nursing others, washing and ironing linen and cleaning the rooms and such other services as the matron may require.*
>
> —Regulation of the Philadelphia General Hospital, 1790

OBJECTIVES

When you have completed this chapter on discharge summaries, you should be able to

1. Define a Discharge Summary.
2. Identify and define the sections of a Discharge Summary.
3. Describe clinical uses of a Discharge Summary.
4. Identify administrative uses of a Discharge Summary.
5. Be familiar with terminology used in reports.

INTRODUCTION

The Discharge Summary, or *Clinical Resumé*, is an important document in the patient's medical record. This document is usually associated with an episode of hospital care. In today's health care environment, many settings require a summarization of the care rendered to the patient. Nursing facilities, outpatient surgical clinics, community mental health centers, outpatient substance abuse centers, home health agencies, and large group practices or specialty centers are called upon to provide a summarization of patient care.

The Discharge Summary is one of the most frequently requested patient reports. It provides a clear description of the treatment the patient received, the patient's response to the treatment, and the condition of the patient at the conclusion of the episode of care. Review organizations, insurance companies, and other health care professionals are just a few of the groups that may need a copy of this document.

The Discharge Summary is usually dictated by the patient's physician. This may also be done by a nurse practitioner or physician assistant, but the report *must* be authenticated by the physician. Although specific headings in the report are determined by the health care agency, the health care industry has identified the types of information that should be included in a quality Discharge Summary. Regulatory and accrediting agencies have provided the impetus for improving the quality of this document.

Keep in mind that the headings used in the report and the organization of the report may vary from agency to agency. This chapter describes and defines the most frequently used and accepted components of a Discharge Summary.

COMPONENTS OF A DISCHARGE SUMMARY

The Discharge Summary includes several sections that provide Patient Identification, indicate the Diagnosis (Admitting and Discharge) and History, and give results of Laboratory Data and other Diagnostic Tests. A summary of the patient's Hospital Course, as well as the Discharge Disposition and Diagnosis, is included. These sections are discussed below. Italicized words used in the examples are defined in the Review of Terminology at the end of this section.

PATIENT IDENTIFICATION

The Patient Identification section must include the patient's name and case number. If the agency does not assign a case number, the date of birth or social security number is often used as secondary Patient Identification. The section usually includes the admission date and the discharge date. Ambulatory surgical centers may even include the time of admission and the time of discharge.

In addition to basic patient data and the admission and discharge dates, the section can include a brief notation about consultations, surgical procedures, and special procedures. Here is an example of a Patient Identification section.

> **EXAMPLE**
>
> PATIENT NAME: Juan Castilla   CASE NUMBER: 55-55-12
> ADMITTED: March 19, 20—   DISCHARGED: March 21, 20—
> CONSULTATIONS: Dermatologist   SPECIAL PROCEDURES: none
> SURGICAL PROCEDURES: none

This first section tells the practitioner that this patient did not have any surgery or special procedures. There would be no need to page through the entire record to find this out. The notation about the consultation would be an indication that there should be a Dermatology Report.

DIAGNOSIS

The Diagnosis section can include the **Admitting Diagnosis** (the reason for the episode of care) and **Discharge Diagnosis** (the diagnosis that is made during the episode of care). When both diagnoses are given, this section is near the beginning of the report. Some agencies put the Admitting Diagnosis at the beginning of the report and the Discharge Diagnosis at the end.

Comparing these diagnoses is of particular interest to regulatory agencies and insurance companies. If there is a substantial difference between the Admitting and Discharge Diagnoses, the documentation in the patient record must clearly support that variation. In all cases, the diagnoses must always be supported by the information in the patient's record.

> **EXAMPLE**
>
> ADMITTING DIAGNOSIS: Acute *erythematous* (er"ĭ-thĕm'ah-tŭs) rash, lower legs.
>   *Ulcerations* (ŭl"sĕ-rā'shŭnz) with *exudate* (ĕks'ū-dāt)
>
> DISCHARGE DIAGNOSIS: *Cellulitis* (sĕl"ū-lī'tĭs) Staph infection

HISTORY

The **History** section may or may not be a separate heading of the Discharge Summary. This section is most commonly used in hospitals and larger ambulatory care agencies. The History is a brief recap of the reason for the episode of care. A brief summary of the patient's current history and physical examination may also be included in the History section. Inclusion of the history and physical summary depends on agency policy and physician training and preference.

> **EXAMPLE**
>
> HISTORY: Mr. Castilla is a 40-year-old man who noticed a rash developing on his legs. He treated the rash with several ointments and creams. He noticed an increase in redness; and when the skin actually began to break down, he sought treatment.

LABORATORY DATA/DIAGNOSTIC TESTS

The **Laboratory Data and Diagnostic Tests** section is the most clinical and technical section of the Discharge Summary. The physician will describe and give the results of all tests performed. Careful attention must be given to the order of this information. Test results are usually presented in chronological order. Similar tests are grouped by date of service, with an explanation of the results. This information is taken from individual laboratory and Diagnostic Reports. The purpose of the summary is to consolidate all of this important information in one convenient location.

> EXAMPLE
>
> LABORATORY DATA: White count on 3/19 was 10,800 and 8,200 on 3/21. On 3/19 hemoglobin was 11 with a hematocrit of 33.3%. The hemoglobin was 12.8 on 3/21, with a hematocrit of 38.7. Culture taken on 3/19 revealed *Staphylococcus aureus* (stăf″ĭ-lō-kŏk'ŭs aw're-ŭs). Urinalysis was negative.

HOSPITAL COURSE

Discharge Summaries are usually associated with hospitalization. The patient's record will have many detailed reports that describe the treatment given and the patient's response. This section, called the **Hospital Course**, highlights the most significant aspects of the treatment process. Expect to find a chronological review of events justifying the hospital stay. This review would reflect on the severity of the illness and note any significant change in the patient's condition while in the hospital and when that change took place. It may also include a summary of important medications taken with the date and duration of their use. In the event that patient care is delivered in an outpatient or ambulatory setting, this section might be called *Treatment Course* or *Summary of Treatment*.

> EXAMPLE
>
> HOSPITAL COURSE: The patient was *febrile* (fēb'rĭl) on admission and started on antibiotic therapy. Culture revealed Staph aureus. An intramuscular injection of 1.2 million units of long-acting benzathine penicillin was given. The patient responded well to this treatment and was started on *cloxacillin* (klŏks″ah-sĭl'ĭn) 250 mg q.i.d. to be continued after discharge. On 3/21 lab work was within normal limits.

DISCHARGE DISPOSITION

The **Discharge Disposition** includes information about the condition of the patient and the plan for follow-up care. This section is mandated by regulatory and accrediting agencies. It may also be called the *Discharge Plan*. Specific information about dose and duration of medications, referrals, plans, and continued treatment is generally found in this section, as well as the name of the primary care or physician specialist who will have overall responsibility for the patient's follow-up care. Any additional appointments are also included. If applicable, identify physical limitations, capacity for self-care, and mental condition. There must also be a notation indicating that the discharge instructions were given to the patient. These instructions may be listed in the Discharge Disposition or documented on a separate form, signed by the patient, and placed in the patient's record.

> EXAMPLE
>
> DISCHARGE DISPOSITION: The patient was discharged on a regular diet. He is to stay off his feet as much as possible. He will continue with the cloxacillin 250 mg q.i.d. for eight days. If he notices any changes in the condition of his legs, Mr. Castilla was advised to contact his attending physician immediately. He has been scheduled for a follow-up visit on March 30, 20—. Mr. Castilla was given discharge instructions, and a copy was placed in his record.

DISCHARGE DIAGNOSIS

Many agencies prefer to list the Discharge Diagnosis as a separate section at the end of the report. Location of the Discharge Diagnosis is dependent on agency policy and physician training and preference. This section is sometimes called *Final Diagnosis*.

EXAMPLE

DISCHARGE DIAGNOSES: 1. Cellulitis
2. Borderline hypertension
3. Psoriasis

The Discharge Summary *must* be authenticated by the physician. If the Discharge Summary is transcribed, the dates of dictation and transcription are required. This information is often checked by survey teams in order to verify compliance with accreditation standards.

Figure 14-1 shows an example of a completed Discharge Summary.

USES OF THE DISCHARGE SUMMARY

The Discharge Summary is a frequently requested report. Health care and administrative agencies can use this report to verify episodes of care, to communicate patient health information, and to monitor compliance with regulatory standards. Specific types of agencies and how they use the Discharge Summary are identified in this section.

HEALTH CARE AGENCIES

Patient care is provided in many different settings. Once a patient has been treated, there is a high probability that the results of that treatment will be sent to other health care professionals. Here are some examples of this process.

Physicians' Offices

Many patients receive services from specialists, regional medical centers, and ambulatory centers. Results of the treatment must be shared with the patient's family physician. The Discharge Summary can play an important role in communicating treatment results and aftercare plans.

Nursing Facilities

As the population ages, there is and will be greater demand for nursing facility care. In the past, nursing facilities were used as the end point of the health care process. Today these establishments may be used as a step between acute care and returning home. When a patient is transferred to a nursing or convalescent center, the Discharge Summary provides valuable information for the continuation of patient care. A thorough Discharge Summary will identify successful treatments, provide data about laboratory tests, and enumerate patient medications and follow-up plans.

Hospitals

Today's highly mobile population has resulted in the need to transfer and share patient information. Individuals may move from one community to another and take their health care concerns with them. Hospitals are able to transmit efficiently information about previous episodes of care with the Discharge Summary.

ADMINISTRATIVE AGENCIES

The Discharge Summary is used in many administrative settings. Various agencies that are involved in monitoring quality of care and cost-containment activities often need patient information. The Discharge Summary is a good way to provide that information. Here are some examples of the administrative uses of the Discharge Summary.

Insurance Companies

Reimbursement for patient care is a complex process. A common practice for health insurance companies is to request verification of patient services. Health care agencies may be able to charge the insurance companies for the cost of reproducing and sending information. If not, the agency must absorb the cost of sending this information;

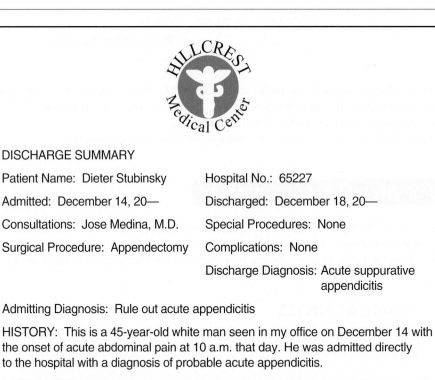

DISCHARGE SUMMARY

Patient Name: Dieter Stubinsky   Hospital No.: 65227

Admitted: December 14, 20—   Discharged: December 18, 20—

Consultations: Jose Medina, M.D.   Special Procedures: None

Surgical Procedure: Appendectomy   Complications: None

Discharge Diagnosis: Acute suppurative appendicitis

Admitting Diagnosis: Rule out acute appendicitis

HISTORY: This is a 45-year-old white man seen in my office on December 14 with the onset of acute abdominal pain at 10 a.m. that day. He was admitted directly to the hospital with a diagnosis of probable acute appendicitis.

LABORATORY DATA: Serum amylase was normal at 64. Cultures of peritoneal fluid at the time of discharge showed no growth. CBC performed as a follow-up on December 16 showed a white count of 12,400 (decreased from 21,000 on December 14). Hemoglobin today is 12 (decreased from 15.5 on the 14th). The remainder of the laboratory data was performed in the office prior to admission.

HOSPITAL COURSE: The patient was admitted and surgical consultation was obtained from Dr. Medina. The patient was taken to surgery the evening of admission where acute appendicitis with a small perforation was found. Pathology confirmed acute appendicitis. The patient convalesced without further difficulties, although he did have a low-grade fever with temperature of 100°F until the morning of December 17. He was discharged on the following medications: Darvocet N-100 one q.6h p.r.n. pain, Keflex 500 mg p.o. q.6h for three days. Diet at the time of discharge is as tolerated. Activities are as tolerated.

DISPOSITION: He will be seen by Dr. Medina in five days. He will be seen in my office in six weeks to be evaluated for possible hypercholesterolemia and possible hypothyroidism.

Ruth L. Samaan, M.D./XX

DD: 12-20-20—
DT: 12-22-20—

FIGURE 14-1
A Discharge
Summary

it may not charge the patient. By providing only the Discharge Summary instead of the entire patient record, the cost of reproduction may be controlled.

Peer Review Organizations

Peer review organizations are concerned with the quality and cost of health care services. These organizations review patient records to determine the adequacy and cost of the care provided. The Discharge Summary is a key document for the review process.

Accrediting, Licensing, and Regulatory Agencies

Accrediting, licensing, and regulatory agencies use patient records as part of the survey process. These agencies look for accurate and timely documentation of patient care. The Discharge Summary is a required report and an important part of overall review activity. Incomplete or missing Discharge Summaries can have a negative impact on the licensing and accreditation process.

The Discharge Summary is an important part of the overall documentation of patient care. A quality report can contribute to continuity of patient care, reimbursement, and various administrative activities.

ABBREVIATIONS

Abbreviations are commonly used in medical reports. While the use of abbreviations is acceptable, health care agencies, accrediting bodies, regulatory agencies, and various allied health professional organizations are actively discouraging their use, especially in the Discharge Summary. Abbreviations that relate to laboratory tests and medications are usually the only abbreviations found in a Discharge Summary. Generally accepted abbreviations for laboratory tests and medications are provided in each system chapter with more specific references in Chapters 3 and 4, respectively.

INTERNET ASSIGNMENT

The authoritative source about report guidelines is The American Health Information Management Association (AHIMA) at **www.ahima.org**. This organization was first identified in Chapter 3 of your text. The AHIMA represents more than 40,000 specially educated health information management professionals who work throughout the health care industry. They are specialists in administering information systems, managing medical records, and coding information for reimbursement and research. More specifically, these professionals are uniquely qualified to

■ ensure health information is complete and available to legitimate users
■ code and classify data for reimbursement
■ analyze information necessary for decision support
■ protect patient privacy and provide information security
■ enhance the quality and uses for data within health care
■ administer health information computer systems
■ comply with standards and regulations regarding health information, prepare health data for accreditation surveys, and
■ analyze clinical data for research and public policy.

In addition to professional issues, the site has information for patients with regard to maintaining their personal medical record.

ACTIVITY

Access the American Health Information Management Association at **www.ahima.org**. Select Your Health Record from the options bar above the main text. Read the information about maintaining your own medical record. Summarize your findings for your instructor.

Review: Discharge Summaries

■ The Discharge Summary is a key document in the patient's record that recaps the treatment provided to the patient.

■ Components of a Discharge Summary include Patient Identification, Admitting and Discharge Diagnoses, History, Laboratory and Diagnostic Test results, Hospital (or Treatment) Course, and Discharge Disposition.

■ Nursing homes, physicians' offices, hospitals, and other health care agencies use the Discharge Summary to communicate clinical and medical information about the patient.

■ The Discharge Summary is used as an administrative tool by insurance companies, professional review organizations, and accrediting and licensing agencies.

■ The Discharge Summary must be accurate, complete, and produced in a timely manner. All information in the Discharge Summary must be supported by documentation elsewhere in the patient's record.

Review of Terminology Presented

Word	Definition
Admitting Diagnosis	reason for the episode of care
cellulitis	inflammation of soft or connective tissue caused by infection
cloxacillin	penicillinase-resistant penicillin
Discharge Diagnosis	diagnosis that is made during the episode of care
Discharge Disposition	information about the condition of the patient and the plan for follow-up care
erythematous	characterized by the redness of skin due to congestion of the capillaries
exudate	fluid filled with cellular debris and protein that has escaped from blood vessels as a result of inflammation
febrile	pertaining to fever; feverish
History	summary of the reason for the episode of care
Hospital Course	summary of the most significant aspects of the treatment process in the hospital
Laboratory Data and Diagnostic Tests	results of all tests performed
Staphylococcus aureus	bacteria that causes infection
ulceration	circumscribed lesion of the skin resulting from necrosis caused by infection or inflammation

Terminology Review Exercises

Name: _____ Date: _____

TERMS
Give the medical term for the following.

1. circumscribed lesion of the skin   _____

2. inflammation of soft or connective tissue   _____

3. pertaining to fever; feverish   _____

4. redness of skin due to capillary congestion   _____

5. fluid filled with cellular debris and protein   _____

MATCHING*
Match the terms to their meanings.

1. _____ diagnosis that is made during the episode of care
2. _____ bacteria that causes infection
3. _____ penicillinase-resistant penicillin
4. _____ reason for the episode of care
5. _____ summary of the reasons for the episode of care
6. _____ summary of the most significant aspects of the treatment process while in the hospital
7. _____ results of all tests performed

a. cloxacillin
b. Discharge Diagnosis
c. Admitting Diagnosis
d. Staphylococcus aureus
e. Hospital Course
f. History
g. Laboratory Data and Diagnostic Tests

IDENTIFICATION
Check the headings that would be found in a discharge summary.

_____ Chief Complaint

_____ History

_____ Patient Identification

_____ Family History

_____ Diagnosis

_____ Plan

_____ Discharge Disposition

_____ Final Diagnosis

_____ Review of Systems

_____ Hospital Course

_____ Laboratory Data

_____ Social History

---

*Answers are in Appendix A.

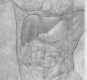

Word Element Review

Prefix	Meaning	Example	Definition
bi-	two	**bifurcation** (bī"fur-kā'shŭn)	separation into two branches
gemin-	two	**geminate** (jĕm'ĭ-nāt)	paired
hypo-	under, below	**hypotension** (hī"pō-tĕn'shŭn)	lowered blood pressure
macro-	large	**macrocyte** (măk'rō-sīt)	abnormally large erythrocyte
mal-	bad	**malformation** (măl"for-mā'shŭn)	deformity
malign-	bad	**malignant** (mah-lĭg'nănt)	tending to become progressively worse
meso-	middle	**mesiad** (mē'zē-ăd)	toward the median or center
micro-	small	**microcephaly** (mī"krō-sĕf'ah-lē)	abnormal smallness of the head
multi-	many	**multicystic** (mŭl"tĭ-sĭs'tĭk)	having many cysts
pan-	all	**panacea** (păn'ah-sē'ah)	remedy for all diseases
poly-	many	**polycythemia** (pŏl"ē-sī-thē'mē-ah)	excessive number of red corpuscles in the blood
semi-	half	**semilunar** (sĕm'ē-lū'năr)	shaped like a crescent or half-moon
tri-	three	**trigeminy** (trī-jĕm'ĭ-ne)	three pulse beats in rapid succession
uni-	one	**unicellular** (ū"nĭ-sel'ū-lar)	made up of a single cell

Suffix	Meaning	Example	Definition
-asthenia	weakness	**myasthenia** (mī"ăs-thē'nē-ah)	weakness of muscles
-coccus	berry-shaped organism	**enterococcus** (ĕn"ter-ō-kŏk'ŭs)	any streptococcus of the human intestine
-penia	decrease, deficiency	**cytopenia** (sī"tō-pē'nē-ah)	deficiency of cellular elements of blood
-(r)rhea	discharge, flow	**rhinorrhea** (rī"nō-rē'ah)	free discharge of thin nasal mucus
-tropin	nourish, develop, stimulate	**somatotropin** (sō"mah-tō-trō'pĭn)	growth hormone

Word Element Review Exercises

Name: _____ Date: _____

CIRCLE AND DEFINE*

Circle and define the word element in the following terms.

1. myasthenia   _____
2. malformation   _____
3. malignant   _____
4. cytopenia   _____
5. panacea   _____
6. hypotension   _____
7. polycythemia   _____
8. macrocyte   _____

MATCHING*

Match the word elements to their meanings.

1. _____ three
2. _____ large
3. _____ bad
4. _____ half
5. _____ under
6. _____ two
7. _____ all
8. _____ weakness
9. _____ decrease, deficiency
10. _____ many

a. bi-, gemin-
b. tri-
c. -penia
d. mal-, malign-
e. macro-
f. poly-, multi-
g. pan-
h. hypo-
i. -asthenia
j. semi-

MEANINGS

In the underlined words below, circle the word element presented in this chapter. Provide the meaning of the word.

1. Myasthenia gravis is an autoimmune disease that affects the legs and arms, as well as other body parts.

   _____

2. Blood tests revealed cytopenia, and the physician prescribed an appropriate treatment.

   _____

3. He required a myelosuppressive therapy to control his polycythemia.

   _____

4. The research team was looking for the ultimate panacea.

   _____

*Answers are in Appendix A.

5. A biopsy performed indicated the tumor was <u>malignant</u>.

_____

6. On examining the infant, the pediatrician noted a <u>malformation</u> of the right ear.

_____

7. Examination of the blood sample determined the presence of a <u>macrocyte</u>.

_____

8. <u>Hypotension</u> is often associated with long life.

_____

WORD ELEMENTS

Give the meaning of each word element. Then use your dictionary to find a new word that contains each of the word elements. Specify whether the new word is a noun or an adjective by placing N or A in the last column.

Word Element	Meaning	Word	N or A
1. -asthenia			
2. bi-			
3. -coccus			
4. gemin-			
5. hypo-			
6. macro-			
7. mal-			
8. malign-			
9. meso-			
10. micro-			
11. multi-			
12. pan-			
13. -penia			
14. poly-			
15. -(r)rhea			
16. semi-			
17. tri-			
18. -tropin			
19. uni-			

Dictionary Exercises

Name: _____ Date: _____

DICTIONARY EXERCISE 1

Use your dictionary to find the pronunciation and definition of the following words.

	Word	Pronunciation	Definition
1.	Candida	_____	_____
2.	Proteus	_____	_____
3.	Pseudomonas aeruginosa	_____	_____
4.	pus	_____	_____
5.	trocar	_____	_____

DICTIONARY EXERCISE 2

Pronunciation of the words below is provided. Using your dictionary, find the correct spelling and definition of each word.

	Word	Pronunciation	Definition
1.	_____	kŭl'tūr	_____
2.	_____	dĭ-zēz'	_____
3.	_____	fŭnk'shŭn-al	_____
4.	_____	or-găn'ĭk	_____

DICTIONARY EXERCISE 3*

Rewrite each sentence in your own words. Provide the pronunciation for the italicized words.

1. Some diseases can be caused by specific *bacteria* (_____).

   _____

2. A *cannula* (_____) can be used by nurses and physicians when they provide care to the patient.

   _____

3. Once the infection had *disseminated* (_____), several medications were needed to bring it under control.

   _____

4. Everyone involved in health care must take every precaution against *sepsis* (_____).

   _____

5. Sometimes the *sequela* (_____) is worse than the disease.

   _____

---

*Answers are in Appendix A.

Listening Exercise

INSTRUCTIONS

1. Review the spelling, pronunciation, and meaning of the words provided in the preview.

2. Listen to the audio CD and fill in the blank as the word is dictated.

3. At the end of the exercise, check your spelling against the preview words. They appear in the preview in the order in which they are encountered in the exercise.

4. Review and practice the words you missed.

5. Look up words that are not familiar.

PREVIEW OF WORDS FOR LISTENING EXERCISE 14-1

Word	Pronunciation	Meaning
aspiration	ăs-pĭ-rā'shŭn	withdrawal of fluid by suction
suspension	sŭs-pĕn'-shŭn	solution where solid particles are *mixed* with the fluid, but *not dissolved* in it
aerosols	ĕr'ō-sŏlz	colloidal solutions suspended in a gas and dispensed in the form of a mist
lethargic	lĕ-thăr'jĭk	abnormally drowsy, sluggish, or indifferent
pulmonary toilet	pŭl'-mō-nĕ-rē	draining of fluids from the lungs

Discharge Summary

Date of Admission: 5/12/20—

Date of Discharge: 5/18/20—

DISCHARGE DIAGNOSIS:

1. Bronchitis.
2. Chronic respiratory insufficiency secondary to recurrent _____ and scarring of the lungs.
3. Cerebral palsy, severe.
4. Severe mental retardation.
5. History of seizure disorder.

RECOMMENDATIONS: The patient will be released on the following medications:

1. Bactrim _____ equivalent of a DS b.i.d. or 20 cc b.i.d.
2. Depakene 250 mg 5 cc at 2 p.m. and 10 cc b.i.d.
3. Organidin 4 cc q. 8 hours.
4. Valium 2 mg. h.s.
5. Beclovent 5 mg. q. 8 hours.
6. Reglan 5 cc q. 6 hours.
7. Theophylline syrup 80 mg in 15 cc, 25 cc q. 12 hours.
8. Albuterol _____ every 4 hours.
9. Nutren 3 cans 1.5 with one can of water.
10. 3 packs of ProMod over 14 hours daily.
11. Beclofen 5 mg t.i.d.
12. Theophylline 25 cc every 12 hours.
13. Natural Tears as needed.

The patient was also receiving 1,500 cc of free water. She is intolerant of Theragran.

Regina is a 15-year-old female who was admitted through the Emergency Room. The patient developed increasing shortness of breath and chest congestion. She had been on Cipro for the last 7–10 days without improvement. The patient has severe mental retardation. Her family was caring for her extremely well, but she continued to deteriorate. When seen in the Emergency Room, the patient was _____. She was in moderate respiratory distress. The patient was admitted for aggressive _____ _____ as well as IV antibiotics. We have attempted on a number of occasions to try to treat her as an outpatient on IV antibiotics, but access has been a major difficulty.

The patient was aggressively started on Fortaz as well as gentamicin. Gentamicin levels were followed closely. The patient continued to gradually improve. The patient over the next 48 to 72 hours improved enough that she was able to smile and her breathing was much improved. The patient is now released to be followed up as an outpatient.

Signature: _____

      Katrina Zemstov, MD

DIAGNOSTIC PROCEDURES

Word	Pronunciation	Definition
Radiology (continued)		
cystography	sĭs-tŏg'rah-fē	contrast media study of the bladder
intravenous pyelography (IVP)	ĭn"trah-vē'nŭs pī"ĕ-lŏg'rah-fē	x-ray study of the kidney, ureter, and bladder using an intravenous contrast medium (See Figure 15-6)
nephrotomography	nĕf"rō-tō-mŏg'răh-fē	body section x-ray for visualization of the kidney
renal artery Doppler		ultrasound study of the renal arteries to aid in the evaluation of renal blood flow
retrograde pyelography	rĕt'rō-grād pī"ĕ-lŏg'rah-fē	contrast media study of the urinary system via catheters introduced into the ureters through a cystoscope
renal ultrasound	ul'trah-sownd	radiologic technique in which the structure of the kidneys is visualized by recording the reflection of ultrasound waves directed into the tissues (See Figure 15-7)
ureterography	ū-rē"ter-ŏg'rah-fē	contrast media study of the ureters
voiding cystourethrography	sĭs"tō-ū-rē-thrŏg'rah-fē	x-ray of the urinary bladder while the patient is voiding
x-ray of kidney, ureter, bladder (KUB)		radiogram done without injection of air or contrast media to demonstrate the size and location of the kidneys

continues

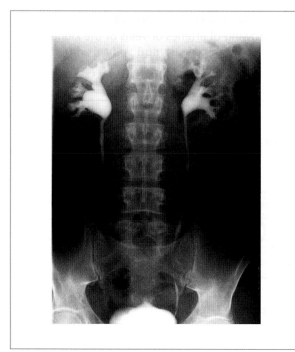

FIGURE 15-6 Intravenous Pyelography

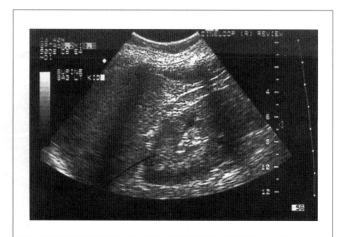

FIGURE 15-7 Renal Ultrasound: preferred imaging modality for suspected pyelonephritis

DIAGNOSTIC PROCEDURES

Word	Pronunciation	Definition
Laboratory Tests		
24-hour specimen		collection of all of an individual's urine into a large container to evaluate kidney function, protein excretion, or the excretion of other substances by the kidney
urinalysis (UA)	ŭ"rĭ-năl'ĭ-sĭs	analysis of the urine to determine its physical, chemical, and microscopic properties; physical properties may include color, appearance, quantity, pH, and specific gravity; chemical properties are protein, sugar, ketone bodies, and bilirubin; a microscopic exam shows red and white blood cells, crystals, casts, and pus
urine culture and sensitivity (C&S)		test to determine the type of bacteria present and which antibiotic is the most effective for treatment
Blood Tests		
acid phosphatase	fŏs'fah-tās"	test that measures an enzyme in the blood when checking for prostate cancer
blood urea nitrogen (BUN)	ū-rē'ah nī'trō-jĕn	test that measures the concentration of urea in the blood
creatinine clearance	krē-ăt'ĭ-nĭn	test that measures the ability of the kidney to remove creatinine from the blood; used as an estimate of glomerular filtration rate
dysmorphic red blood cells	dĭs-mŏr'fĭk	red blood cells seen in the urine that have an irregular shape, indicating an origin in the glomerulus as opposed to the renal collecting system
immunoelectrophoresis	ĭ-mū"nō-ē-lĕk"trō-fō-rē'sĭs	method of distinguishing proteins and antibodies in body fluid on the basis of their electrophoretic mobility and antigenic specificities

DIAGNOSES

Word	Pronunciation	Definition
Urinary Tract Infections/Disorders		
cystitis	sĭs-tī'tĭs	inflammation of the urinary bladder (See Figure 15-8C)
nocturia	nŏk-tū'rē-ah	excessive urination at night
pyelonephritis	pī"ĕ-lō-nĕ-frī'tĭs	inflammation of the renal pelvis, usually due to infection (See Figure 15-8E)
stricture	strĭk'chŭr	narrowing of a urinary structure that interferes with flow of urine to the bladder
uremia	ū-rē'mē-ah	systemic result of the accumulation of toxins normally excreted by the kidneys
ureteritis	ū-rē"tĕr-ī'tĭs	inflammation of the ureter

continues

DIAGNOSES

Word	Pronunciation	Definition
Urinary Tract Infections/Disorders (*continued*)		
urethritis	ū"rē-thrī'tĭs	inflammation of the urethra (See Figure 15-8B)
urinary calculi	kăl'kū-lī	stones occurring anywhere in the urinary tract
urinary tract infection (UTI)		infection of the urinary tract, especially the bladder and urethra; structural and systemic disorders affecting urine flow contribute to the problem (See Figure 15-8A)
vesicoureteral reflux	věs"ĭ-ko-ū-rē'těr-ăl	recurrent urinary tract infections, especially in children, where urine passes through the ureter from the bladder back to the kidney because the valve in the ureter is malfunctioning
Disorders/Disease of the Kidney		
cystinuria	sĭs'tī-nū'rē-ah	persistent excessive urinary excretion of certain amino acids due to impairment of their renal tubular reabsorption
end-stage renal disease (ESRD)		terminal kidney failure requiring dialysis or transplantation
glomerulonephritis	glō-měr"ū-lō-ně-frī'tĭs	inflammation of the glomeruli; may be acute or chronic
hydronephrosis	hī"drō-ně-frō'sĭs	dilation of the pevis of the kidney caused by obstruction of the ureter or lower urinary tract (See Figure 15-9)
interstitial nephritis	ĭn"těr-stĭsh'ăl ně-frī'tĭs	inflammation of the spaces between the glomeruli and tubules in the kidney

continues

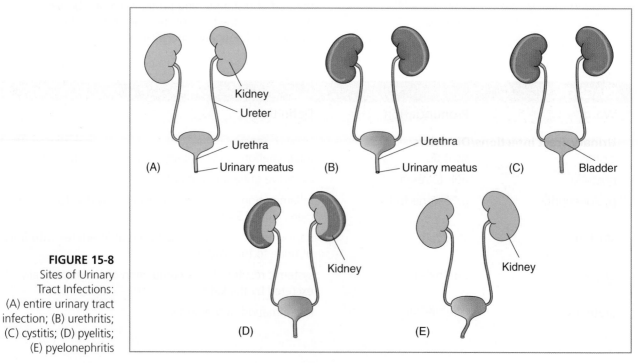

FIGURE 15-8
Sites of Urinary Tract Infections: (A) entire urinary tract infection; (B) urethritis; (C) cystitis; (D) pyelitis; (E) pyelonephritis

DIAGNOSES

Word	Pronunciation	Definition
Disorders/Disease of the Kidney (continued)		
kidney cysts		fluid-filled masses in the kidney
medullary sponge kidney	mĕd'ū-lār-ē	multiple small cysts in the central portion of the renal pyramids
nephrotic syndrome (nephrosis)	nĕ-frŏt'ĭk (nĕf"rō'sĭs)	disorder characterized by protein loss from the kidneys, resulting in edema
nephrolithiasis (renal calculi)	nĕf"rō-lĭth-ī'ah-sĭs (rē'năl kăl'kū-lī)	presence of calculi in the kidney; kidney stones (See Figure 15-10)
nephropathy	nĕ-frŏp'ah-thē	any disease of the kidney
polycystic kidney disease (PKD)	pŏl"ē-sĭs'tĭk	multiple cysts in the kidney (See Figure 15-11)
proteinuria	prō'tē-ĭn-ū'rē-ah	presence of abnormal amounts of protein in the urine
pyelitis	pī"ĕ-lī'tĭs	inflammation of the pelvis of the kidney (See Figure 15-8D)
renal cell carcinoma	kăr"sĭ-nō'mah	malignant growth of the renal parenchyma, composed of tubular cells in varying arrangements
renal failure		decreased function of the kidney
renal tubular acidosis	ăs"ĭ-dō'sĭs	excessive acidity of renal fluids resulting from impairment of the reabsorption of bicarbonate by the renal tubules
Wilms' tumor	vĭlmz	tumor of the kidneys seen in children

continues

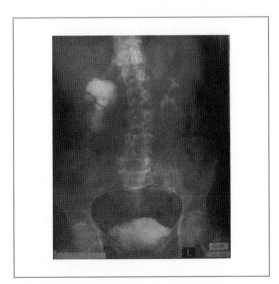

FIGURE 15-9 Pelvis Dilation in Hydronephrosis

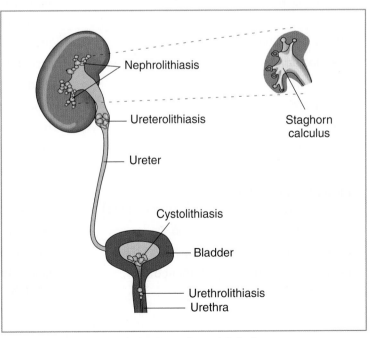

FIGURE 15-10 Types and Locations of Renal Calculi

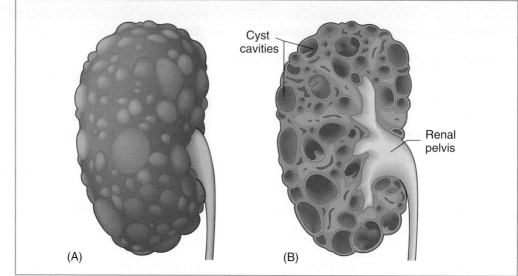

FIGURE 15-11
Polycystic Kidneys:
(A) polycystic;
(B) section through kidney

DIAGNOSES		
Word	**Pronunciation**	**Definition**
Disease/Disorders of the Bladder		
bladder cancer		malignant growth of the bladder
bladder stones		calculi usually formed of crystalline urinary salts that collect in the bladder and other organs
diuresis	dī"ū-rē'sĭs	urine excretion in excess of the usual amount
hematuria	hē"mă-tū'rē-ah	discharge of blood in the urine
neurogenic bladder	nū"rō-jĕn'ĭk	dysfunction due to injury of the nervous system supplying the urinary tract or bladder
urinary incontinence	ĭn-kŏnt'ĭn-ĕns	loss of control of the passage of urine from the bladder
• *nocturnal enuresis*	nŏk-tŭr'năl ĕn"ū-rē'sĭs	incontinence that occurs during sleep
• *overflow*		bladder does not empty properly; leaks when overfull
• *stress*		reaction to laughing, sneezing, coughing, etc.
• *total*		no urine can be retained in the bladder
• *urge*		uncontrollable urge to empty the bladder
Blood Vessel Problems		
acute arterial occlusion	ăr-tē'rē-ăl ō-kloo'zhŭn	sudden, severe blockage of the renal artery
renal artery stenosis	stĕ-nō'sĭs	blockage of the renal artery before it enters the kidney
renal hypertension	hī"pĕr-tĕn'shŭn	high blood pressure resulting from kidney disease
renal vein thrombosis	thrŏm-bō'sĭs	blood clot attached to the wall of the veins draining the kidneys

continues

DIAGNOSES

Word	Pronunciation	Definition
Trauma/Rare Diseases		
interstitial cystitis	ĭn″tĕr-stĭsh'ăl sĭs-tī'tĭs	inflammation of the spaces between the glomeruli and tubules in the kidney
straddle injuries		injury as a result of riding a bike, walking a beam, etc.
toxic injury		injuring results from factors such as drugs, lead-based paints, solvents and fuels, as well as the body's own overproduction of uric acid

TREATMENT PROCEDURES

Word	Pronunciation	Definition
bilateral cutaneous ureterostomy	kū-tā'nē-ŭs ū-rē″tĕr-ŏt'ō-mē	surgical procedures to implant ureters into the abdominal wall
bladder diverticulectomy	dī″ver-tĭk″ū-lĕk'tō-mē	removal of a diverticulum (sac) from the bladder
cystectomy	sĭs-tĕk'tō-mē	partial or complete resection of the urinary bladder
cystostomy	sĭs-tŏs'tō-mē	incision into the urinary bladder, usually for drainage
dialysis	dī-ăl'ĭ-sĭs	artificial means of removing waste products from the blood when kidneys have failed; may be *hemodialysis* (waste removed directly from the blood), *peritoneal* (uses peritoneal cavity in the abdomen to filter the blood), *continuous ambulatory peritoneal dialysis* (CAPD) (abdominal cavity is infused four or five times per day), *continuous cycling peritoneal dialysis* (automatic infusion of dialysis solution in and out of the peritoneal cavity, drains several times during the night), or *intermittent peritoneal dialysis* (IPD) (performed several times a week, usually done at home)
fulguration	fŭl-gū-rā'shŭn	procedure using high-frequency electric sparks to burn lesions off the bladder wall
ileal conduit	ĭl'ē-ăl kŏn'doo-ĭt	surgical procedure to implant ureter into a piece of the ileum, which is attached to the abdominal wall as a stoma
kidney transplantation		replacement of a failed kidney with a kidney from an identical twin (isograft) or another compatible donor (allograft)
litholapaxy	lĭth-ŏl'ă-păks″ē	crushing of a calculus (stone) in the bladder, followed by immediate washing out of fragments through a catheter

continues

TREATMENT PROCEDURES

Word	Pronunciation	Definition
lithotripsy	lĭth'ō-trĭp"sē	procedure to break up or crush stones in the urinary tract; for *extracorporeal shock wave lithotripsy* the body is immersed in water and hundreds of shock waves are administered using the water as the carrier (the body is not harmed); *percutaneous ultrasonic lithotripsy* uses a small ultrasound-producing unit inserted into the kidney through the abdomen; *endoscopic lithotripsy* uses an ultrasound-producing unit passed through the bladder and into the ureter
meatotomy	mē"ah-tŏt'ō-mē	procedure that increases the caliber of urinary meatus
nephrectomy	nĕ-frĕk'tō-mē	removal of a kidney
nephrolithotomy	nĕf"rō-lĭth-ŏt'ō-mē	removal of a calculus from a kidney
nephrostomy	nĕ-frŏs'tō-mē	surgical creation of an opening from the renal pelvis to the outside of the body
percutaneous nephrolithotomy	pĕr"kū-tā'nē-ŭs nĕf"rō-lĭth-ŏt'ō-mē	endoscopic procedure to remove kidney stones
pyelolithotomy	pī"ĕ-lō-lĭ-thŏt'ō-mē	incision into the renal pelvis for removal of calculi
pyeloplasty	pī'ĕ-lō-plăs"tē	repair of the renal pelvis
ureterolithotomy	ū-rē"ter-ō-lĭ-thŏt'ō-mē	incision of the ureter for removal of a calculus
ureterosigmoidostomy	ū-rē"tĕr-ō-sĭg-moyd-ŏs'tō-mē	procedure to implant ureter into the sigmoid colon and creation of a continent stoma with a pouch of bowel; may be Kock, Mainz, or Gilchrist ileocecal reservoir
urethropexy	ū-rē'thrō-pĕk"sē	fixation of the urethra to the posterior aspect of the pubic bone
urethroplasty	ū-rē'thrō-plăs"tē	reconstruction or operative repair of the urethra
urinary catheterization	kăth"ĕ-tĕr-ĭ-zā'shŭn	passing of a flexible tube through the urethra into the urinary bladder

MEDICATIONS PRESCRIBED

Trade Name	Generic Name
Antibiotics, Antimicrobials	
Bactrim, Cotrim, Septra	sulfamethoxazole and trimethoprim
Ceftin	cefuroxime axetil
Cipro	ciprofloxacin
Diflucan	fluconazole
Duricef	cefadroxil
Fortaz	ceftazidime
Furadantin, Macrodantin	nitrofurantoin
Gantrisin	sulfisoxazole

continues

MEDICATIONS PRESCRIBED

Trade Name	Generic Name
Antibiotics, Antimicrobials (continued)	
Garamycin, Genoptic, Gentacidin, Gentak, Pediatric Gentamicin	gentamicin sulfate
Keflex	cephalexin
Monocid	cefonicid
Noroxin	norfloxacin
Omnipen, Principen, Totacillin	ampicillin
Rocephin	ceftriaxone
Tobramycin	aminoglycosides
Vancocin, Vancoled	vanconmycin HCl
Anticholinergics/Anesthetics	
Detrol	tolterodine tarte
Pyridium, Pyridiate, Baridium	phenazopyridine HCl
Urised	methenamine, phenyl salicylate, atropine, hyoscyamine, benzoic acid, and methylene blue
Urispas	flavoxate
Antispasmodics	
Anaspaz, Cystospas, Levbid, Levsin, Levsinex	hyoscyamine sulfate
Ditropan	oxybutynin chloride
Pro-Banthine	propantheline bromide
Renal Failure	
Accupril	quinapril
Aldomet	methyldopa
Apresoline	hydralazine HCl
Bumex	bumetanide
Calderol	calcifedial
Capoten	captopril
Catapres	clonidine HCl
HydroDIURIL	hydrochlorothiazide HCl
Incor	amrinone lactate
Kayexalate	sodium polystyrene sulfonate
Lanoxin	digoxin
Lasix	furosemide
Loniten	minoxidil

continues

MEDICATIONS PRESCRIBED

Trade Name	Generic Name
Procardia	nifedipine
Rocaltrol	calcitrol (synthetic vitamin D)
Vasotec	enalapril maleate

Other Medications

Azo Gantrisin	sulfisoxazole and phenazopyridine
Bicitra, Shohl's solution	sodium citrate, citric acid
Neosporin G.U. irritant	neomycin, polymyxin B
Prostigmin	neostigmine bromide
Renacidin Irrigation	citric acid, magnesium carbonate, gluconodelta-lactone
Urecholine, Duvoid	bethanechol

ABBREVIATIONS

ADH	antidiuretic hormone
ARF	acute renal failure
BUN	blood urea nitrogen
CAPD	continuous ambulatory peritoneal dialysis
cath	catheter, catheterization
CRF	chronic renal failure
C&S	culture and sensitivity
cysto	cystoscopic examination
ESRD	end-stage renal disease
ESWL	extracorporeal shock wave lithotripsy
GFR	glomerular filtration rate
GU	genitourinary
HD	hemodialysis
IPD	intermittent peritoneal dialysis
IVP	intravenous pyelogram
KUB	kidney, ureter, and bladder
PD	peritoneal dialysis
PKD	polycystic kidney disease
SLE	systemic lupus erythematosus
UA	urinalysis
UC	urine culture
UTI	urinary tract infection
VCUG	voiding cystourethrogram

Working Practice Review Exercises

Name: _____ Date: _____

IDENTIFICATION/PROCEDURES*
Identify the following diagnostic procedures.

1. deep structures of the kidney are visualized by recording reflections of sound waves   _____

2. x-ray of the urinary bladder while the patient is voiding   _____

3. body section roentgenography of the kidney   _____

4. x-ray study of the kidney, ureter, and bladder using an intravenous contrast medium   _____

5. contrast medium study of the bladder   _____

6. visual examination of the bladder with a scope   _____

7. removal of a tissue sample from the kidney, usually done with a biopsy needle   _____

8. graphic recording of bladder volumes and changing pressure reactions   _____

IDENTIFICATION/LABORATORY TESTS
Identify the following laboratory tests.

1. analysis of urine   _____

2. measures urea in the blood   _____

3. measures the ability of the kidney to remove creatinine from the blood   _____

4. measures an enzyme in the blood to check for cancer of the prostate   _____

DEFINITIONS
Define and provide the pronunciation for the following surgical procedures.

1. cystostomy   _____

   _____

2. pyelolithotomy   _____

   _____

3. urethroplasty   _____

   _____

4. meatotomy   _____

   _____

5. nephrectomy   _____

   _____

_____

*Answers are in Appendix A.

MATCHING*

Match the meanings to the correct diagnoses.

1. _____ more urine than usual
2. _____ any disease of the kidney
3. _____ stones occurring anywhere in the urinary tract
4. _____ decreased function of the kidneys
5. _____ multiple cysts in the kidney
6. _____ inflammation of the glomeruli
7. _____ inflammation of the urinary bladder
8. _____ protein loss from the kidneys, resulting in edema
9. _____ multiple small cysts in the central portion of the renal pyramids
10. _____ severe blockage of the renal artery
11. _____ terminal kidney failure requiring dialysis or transplantation
12. _____ fluid-filled masses in the kidney

a. polycystic kidney disease
b. cystitis
c. glomerulonephritis
d. nephrotic syndrome
e. urinary calculi
f. diuresis
g. renal failure
h. nephropathy
i. kidney cysts
j. medullary sponge kidney
k. acute arterial occlusion
l. end-stage renal disease

IDENTIFICATION/ABBREVIATIONS

Identify the following abbreviations.

1. IVP _____
2. BUN _____
3. UA _____
4. GU _____
5. GFR _____
6. cath _____
7. ESRD _____

---

*Answers are in Appendix A.

Word Element Review

Root	Meaning	Example	Definition
cali/o, calic/o	calyx (calix)	**calicectasis** (kăl"ĭ-sĕk'tă-sĭs)	dilation of a calyx of the kidney
cyst/o	sac	**cystectomy** (sĭs-tĕk'tō-mē)	excision of a cyst
		endocystitis (ĕn"dō-sĭs-tī'tĭs)	inflammation of the membrane lining of the urinary bladder
glomerul/o	ball, cluster	**glomerulus** (glō-mer'ū-lŭs)	cluster of capillaries within the kidney
		glomeruli (glō-mer'ū-lī)	plural of glomerulus
meat/o	meatus	**meatotomy** (mě"ā-tŏt'ō-mē)	incision of the urinary meatus to enlarge the opening
medull/o	medulla	**medullary** (měd'ū-lār"ē)	pertaining to the medulla; one of the inner parts of the kidney
nephr/o	kidney	**nephrectomy** (ně-frěk'tō-mē)	excision of the kidney
		nephrosis (ně-frō'sĭs)	any condition of the kidney in which there are degenerative changes without the occurrence of inflammation
pyel/o	trough, basin, pelvis	**pyelogram** (pī'ě-lō-grăm")	radiography of the renal pelvis and ureter after the injection of contrast material
		pyelonephritis (pī"ě-lō-ně-frī'tĭs)	inflammation of the kidney and its pelvis due to bacterial infection
ren/o	kidney	**renal insufficiency** (rē'năl ĭn"sŭ-fĭsh'ĕn-sē)	reduced capacity of the kidney to perform its function
ur/o	urinary tract, urine	**urogenital** (ū"rō-jĕn'ĭ-tăl)	pertaining to the urinary and reproductive organs
ureter/o	ureter	**ureteral** (ū-rē'ter-ăl)	pertaining to the ureter
		ureterectasis (ū-rē"ter-ĕk'tah-sĭs)	dilation of the ureter
urethr/o	urethra	**urethritis** (ū"rě-thrī'tĭs)	inflammation of the urethra
		urology (ū-rŏl'ō-jē)	study of the urinary tract of both sexes and the genital tract of the male
urin/o	urine	**urinoma** (ū"rĭ-nō'mă)	cyst containing urine
vesic/o	bladder	**vesicouterine** (věs"ĭ-kō-ū'ter-ĭn)	pertaining to the urinary bladder and uterus

continues

Suffix	Meaning	Example	Definition
-uresis	urination	**enuresis** (ĕn″ū-rē'sĭs)	involuntary discharge of urine
-uria	urination	**dysuria** (dĭs-ū'rē-ah)	painful urination
		hematuria (hĕm″ah-tū'rē-ah)	blood in the urine

Word Element Review Exercises

Name: _____ Date: _____

MEANINGS*
Give the meaning of the italicized words.

1. We'll be doing a *nephrectomy* tomorrow on Mr. Glover.

    _____

2. The patient complained of *dysuria*.

    _____

3. There is evidence of *ureterectasis*.

    _____

4. I have ordered a *pyelogram* for tomorrow.

    _____

5. The urologist performed a *meatotomy*.

    _____

IDENTIFICATION*
Identify the following by providing the correct terms for each definition. Underline the word element in each term.

1. inflammation of the membrane lining of the urinary bladder _____
2. pertaining to the ureter _____
3. bacteria-caused infection of the kidney and its pelvis _____
4. blood in the urine _____
5. pertaining to the urinary bladder and uretus _____
6. inflammation of the urethra _____
7. dilation of the calyx of the kidney _____
8. any change in the condition of the kidney without the occurrence of inflammation _____
9. involuntary discharge of urine _____
10. excision of a cyst _____
11. pertaining to urinary and reproductive organs _____
12. cyst containing urine _____
13. plural of glomerulus _____
14. cluster of capillaries within the kidney _____
15. reduced capacity of kidney to perform its function _____

_____

*Answers are in Appendix A.

MATCHING

Match the word elements to their meanings.

1. _____ ball, cluster
2. _____ urination
3. _____ urinary tract, urine
4. _____ kidney
5. _____ ureter
6. _____ sac
7. _____ medulla
8. _____ trough, basin, pelvis
9. _____ urethra
10. _____ bladder

a. cyst/o
b. pyel/o
c. glomerul/o
d. ur/o
e. -uria
f. medull/o
g. nephr/o, ren/o
h. ureter/o
i. urethr/o
j. vesic/o

WORD ELEMENTS

Give the meaning of each word element. Then use your dictionary to find a new word that contains each of the word elements. Specify whether the new word is a noun or an adjective by placing N or A in the last column.

Word Element	Meaning	Word	N or A
1. cali/o			
2. calic/o			
3. cyst/o			
4. glomerul/o			
5. meat/o			
6. medull/o			
7. nephr/o			
8. pyel/o			
9. ren/o			
10. ur/o			
11. -uresis			
12. ureter/o			
13. urethr/o			
14. -uria			
15. urin/o			
16. vesic/o			

Dictionary Exercises

Name: _____ Date: _____

DICTIONARY EXERCISE 1*

Use your dictionary to find the pronunciation and definition of each of the following words.

	Word	**Pronunciation**	**Definition**
1.	diuretic	_____	_____
2.	prolapsed	_____	_____
3.	oliguria	_____	_____
4.	urinary retention	_____	_____
5.	glycosuria	_____	_____
6.	ketosis	_____	_____
7.	anuria	_____	_____
8.	urinary casts	_____	_____
9.	edema	_____	_____
10.	azotemia	_____	_____

DICTIONARY EXERCISE 2*

Select the correct meaning and provide the pronunciation where indicated.

1. albuminuria (_____)
   a. painful urination
   b. frequent urination
   c. albumin in the urine
   d. pus in the urine

2. calculus (_____)
   a. stone found in a body part
   b. tube for insertion into a duct or a cavity that allows the escape of fluid
   c. warty, dry, cauliflowerlike lesions
   d. one of the layers surrounding the front and side of the testicle

3. catheter (_____)
   a. removal of waste products from blood
   b. tubular, flexible instrument passed through a body channel for withdrawal of fluids
   c. stone found in a body part
   d. tube for insertion into a duct or cavity that allows the escape of fluid

4. infundibulum (_____)
   a. triangular area, especially one at the floor of the bladder
   b. one of the layers surrounding the front and side of the testicle
   c. funnel-shaped opening
   d. retaining excessive amounts of urine in the bladder

5. trigone (_____)
   a. funnel-shaped opening
   b. stone found in a body part
   c. circular arrangement of muscles controlling the urinary bladder
   d. triangular area, especially one at the floor of the bladder

6. ureterolysis (_____)
   a. incision of the ureter
   b. stone in the ureter
   c. paralysis of the ureter
   d. suppurative inflammation within a ureter

7. stricture of ureter (_____)
   a. localized narrowing of the tubular ureter, often caused by inflammation
   b. triangular area near the floor of the bladder
   c. layer surrounding the front and side of the testicle
   d. circular arrangement of muscles controlling the urinary bladder

8. tunica vaginalis (_____)
   a. triangular area near the floor of the bladder
   b. narrowing of the tubular ureter
   c. funnel-shaped opening
   d. one of the layers surrounding the front and side of the testicle

---

*Answers are in Appendix A.

9. urinary retention
   a. albumin in the urine
   b. retaining excessive amounts of urine in the bladder
   c. painful urination
   d. blood in the urine

10. vesicoureteral (_____)
    a. pertaining to the connection between the ureter and the urinary bladder
    b. pertaining to the area where the ureter leads off from the pelvis of the kidney
    c. pertaining to the triangular area at the floor of the bladder
    d. pertaining to the bladder and ureter

DICTIONARY EXERCISE 3

Pronunciation of the words below is provided. Using your dictionary, find the correct spelling and definition of each word.

	Word	**Pronunciation**	**Definition**
1.	_____	sfĭngk'ter	_____
2.	_____	kăn'ū-lah	_____
3.	_____	mĭk-tū-rĭ'shŭn	_____
4.	_____	băk-tē"rē-ū'rē-ah	_____
5.	_____	tŭr'bĭd	_____
6.	_____	pī-ū'rē-ah	_____
7.	_____	trĭg"ō-nī'tĭs	_____
8.	_____	ū-rē"ter-ō-vĕs'ĭ-kăl	_____
9.	_____	ū-rē'ter-al kŏl'ĭk	_____
10.	_____	ur'jĕn-sē	_____

DICTIONARY EXERCISE 4

Rewrite each sentence in your own words. Provide the pronunciation for each italicized word.

1. There was evidence of *condyloma acuminatum* (_____).

   _____

2. The patient suffered from *urodynia* (_____).

   _____

3. The record indicated "*nocturia* (_____) × 2."

   _____

4. The patient indicated that one of the symptoms he experienced was *polydipsia* (_____).

   _____

5. The condition was marked by *polyuria* (_____).

   _____

6. He has an *autonomous* (_____) bladder.

   _____

Listening Exercise

Name   Date

INSTRUCTIONS

1. Review the spelling, pronunciation, and meaning of the words provided in the preview.
2. Listen to the audio CD and fill in the blank as the word is dictated.
3. At the end of the exercise, check your spelling against the preview words. They appear in the preview in the order in which they are encountered in the exercise.
4. Review and practice the words you missed.
5. Look up words that are not familiar.

PREVIEW OF WORDS FOR LISTENING EXERCISE 15-1

Word	Pronunciation	Meaning
tomograms	tō'mō-grăms	x-ray pictures designed to show detailed images of selected structures
creatinine	krē-ăt'ĭn-ĭn	alkaline, nonprotein constituent of urine and blood; increased quantities are found in advanced states of renal disease
angiography	an"jē-ŏg'ră-fē	x-ray of blood vessels after injection of radiopaque substance
nephrectomy	nĕ-frĕk-tō'mē	surgical procedure to remove a kidney
voiding		evacuating the bowels or bladder
catheterization	kăth"ĕ-tĕr-ĭ-zā'shŭn	use of a catheter or passage into a body cavity to withdraw or drain fluids

Listening Exercise 15-1

Discharge Summary

HISTORY:

This 34-year-old lady was admitted because of a lump in her right side, which had solid echoes and appeared solid on CT. It was associated with the right kidney.

LABORATORY DATA:

The chest _____ were negative. The electrocardiogram was normal. Urine pH 5, specific gravity 1.021, negative protein and glucose, 5–8 white cells, 0–2 red cells. White count 6,200, differential normal. Hemoglobin 13.1, hematocrit 38.8. Partial thromboplastin time and prothrombin time normal. Sodium 142, potassium 4.5, chlorides 105. On SMA 1260, all parameters are within normal limits. Postoperative _____ is 0.9.

HOSPITAL COURSE:

On 10-19-20—, a selective _____ confirmed vascular tumor of the right kidney. Therefore, on 10-20-20—, under general anesthesia, a radical right _____ was carried out. A 310-gram specimen revealed a 4.5 centimeter mass in the mid-portion of the right kidney with extensive hemorrhage in it and a cystic pattern was an extremely well differentiated renal cell carcinoma. There was no capsular invasion, no lymphatic invasion, and no venous invasion. She also had a fibrotic appendix removed.

Her postoperative course was benign; she never had significant fever. She did have a little difficulty _____, necessitating _____ until the fifth postoperative day. Cath was out; she voided all right and was discharged on the sixth postoperative day. On discharge she was given a prescription for Gantanol and Tylenol 3 and I'll see her in the office in about two weeks.

Marcus Sibilsky, MD

d: 10-26-20—

t: 10-29-20—

CHAPTER 16

The Female Reproductive System

Where did you come from, baby dear?
Out of the everywhere into here.

—GEORGE MACDONALD

OBJECTIVES

When you have completed this chapter on the female reproductive system, you should be able to

1. Spell and define major system components and explain how they work.
2. Identify the meanings of related word elements.
3. Spell and define diagnostic procedures, diagnoses, treatment procedures, and abbreviations.
4. Spell the names of commonly used medications.
5. Be familiar with terminology used in reports.

INTRODUCTION

Human reproduction is accomplished by a process called fertilization, requiring female ova and male spermatozoa. In addition to reproduction, hormones produced by both genders affect a variety of other bodily functions.

The female reproductive system is studied by a **gynecologist** (gī"nĭ-kŏl'ō-jĭst), who may also manage the childbirth process as an **obstetrician** (ŏb-stĕ-trĭsh'ăn). The female anatomy is discussed in this chapter. The male reproductive system is part of the urologist's specialty and will be discussed in Chapter 17, along with sexually transmitted diseases.

FEMALE REPRODUCTIVE SYSTEM

adnex/o	tie, connection
gynec/o	female

The female reproductive system consists of the ovaries, fallopian tubes, uterus, and vagina. These are all internal organs. The external organs, which are called the vulva, include the pubis, labia, clitoris, vestibule, and Bartholin's glands. A discussion of each of the components of the female reproductive system follows.

OVARIES

oophor/o	ovary
ovari/o	ovary
ov/i, ov/o, ovul/o	egg

The two **ovaries** (2), illustrated in Figure 16-1, respond to hormones produced by the pituitary gland and are held in position by several ligaments. The largest is a broad ligament that also supports the tubes, uterus, and vagina.

The outer layer of each ovary is made of epithelium, and it is here that the ova are produced. They go through a maturation process of about fourteen days in small sacs called **ovarian follicles**. When an ovum ripens, the follicle literally ruptures, and the ovum is discharged from the surface of the ovary in a process called **ovulation**.

At the time of birth there are 200,000 to 400,000 ova present in each ovary, but only 400 or so will mature. The rest reach various stages of development and then regress and degenerate.

Following ovulation the cells of the follicle increase in size, take on a yellowish color, and become known as a **corpus luteum** (kor'pŭs loo'tē-ŭm). If the ovum is not fertilized, the corpus luteum begins to degenerate after about two weeks. If the ovum is fertilized, the corpus luteum will remain for several months before it degenerates. During that time it provides the hormone **progesterone** (prō-jĕs'tĕ-rōn). Another hormone, **estrogen** (ĕs'trō-jĕn), is produced by other maturing follicles. Progesterone and estrogen help keep the lining of the uterus in a favorable condition for development of the fertilized egg, or **embryo**.

FALLOPIAN TUBES (OVIDUCTS)

salping/o	tube

After the ovum is released at ovulation, it makes its way to the duct connected to the uterus known as the **fallopian** (făl-lō'pē-ăn) **tube** (1). There is no direct connection between the ovary and the fallopian tubes. Ova are swept into the tubes by a current in the peritoneal fluid produced by small fringelike extensions from the edges of the abdominal opening of the tube. These small extensions are called **fimbriae** (fĭm'brē-ā) (3).

Once inside the tube, the ova are kept moving toward the uterus by the action of cilia in the lining of the tubes, as well as by peristalsis. This journey from the ovary to the uterus takes approximately five days. Fertilization takes place in the first third of the fallopian tube within twenty-four hours of ovulation. If for some reason a fertilized egg does not reach the uterus, a tubal or **ectopic** (ĕk-tŏp'ĭk) **pregnancy** develops.

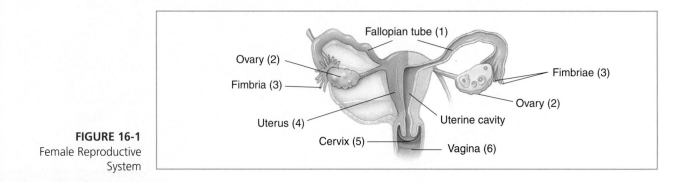

FIGURE 16-1
Female Reproductive System

UTERUS

cervic/o	neck, cervix
hyster/o	uterus
metr/o	uterus
uter/o	uterus

The **uterus** (4) is a muscular, pear-shaped organ located between the urinary bladder and the rectum. The larger upper portion is called the **corpus**. The small, rounded part above the level of the entrance to the fallopian tube is known as the **fundus**. The lower portion of the uterus is called the **cervix** (ser'vĭks) (5). The cervix leads to the vagina, which opens to the outside of the body.

The wall of the uterus has three layers: the endometrium, myometrium, and perimetrium. The innermost layer of the uterus is a specialized epithelium known as **endometrium** (ĕn-dō-mē'trē-ŭm). Each month this layer gradually thickens in preparation for a possible pregnancy. After ovulation, if the ovum is not fertilized while passing through the fallopian tube, it disintegrates upon reaching the uterus. The endometrium also begins to deteriorate. Small hemorrhages appear, producing bleeding known as menstrual flow. Even before the menstrual flow ceases (from one to five days), the endometrium begins to repair itself through the growth of new cells for the beginning of a new cycle. The muscular or middle layer, the **myometrium**, gives the uterus the ability to contract during the childbirth process. The uterus has an outer layer or membrane called the **uterine serosa** (ŭ'tĕr-ĭn sē-rō'sa) or perimetrium.

VAGINA

colp/o	vagina
vagin/o	vagina

The **vagina** (6) is a muscular tube about three inches long connecting the uterine cavity to the exterior of the body. The cervix of the uterus dips into the upper vagina, creating circular recesses and areas known as **fornices** (for'nĭ-sēz). The deepest of these spaces is behind the cervix and is called the posterior fornix. The lining of the vagina is similar to the mucous membrane found in the stomach. These rugae or folds permit enlargement of the vagina during childbirth. Near the vaginal canal opening to the outside, there is a foldlike membrane called the **hymen**.

EXTERNAL GENITALIA

episi/o	vulva
vulv/o	vulva

The collective external female genitalia are called the **vulva** (vŭl'vah) and provide protection for the genital area. Uppermost is the area called the **mons pubis** (mŏnz pū'bĭs), which is covered with pubic hair following puberty. Figure 16-2 shows the area below the mons pubis. There are two folds or lips called the **labia majora** (lā'bē-ah mah-jō'rah) (4). Medial to them are two smaller folds of tissue called the labia minora (mĭ-no'rah) (3). They surround a space called the vestibule into which the vagina (5) and urethra (2) open.

Just below and to each side of the vaginal opening are two mucous-producing **vulvovaginal** (vŭl"vō-văj'ĭ-năl) or **Bartholin's glands** (6). These glands lubricate the vestibule and facilitate sexual intercourse. The **clitoris** (klĭt'ō-rĭs) (1) is a small structure almost enclosed by the foreskin formed by the labia minora; the exposed portion is the glans. The tissue of the clitoris is similar to the penis in that it, too, is composed of erectile tissue.

Although the entire pelvic floor is properly called the **perineum** (pĕr"ĭ-nē'ŭm) in both males and females, health care specialists who care for pregnant women usually refer to the perineum as the limited area between the vaginal opening and the anus.

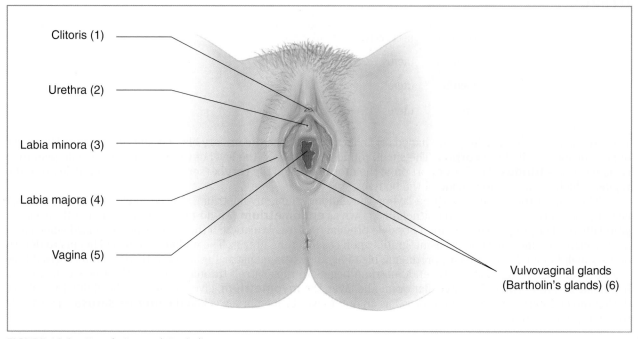

FIGURE 16-2   Female External Genitalia

BREASTS

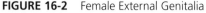

lact/o	milk
mamm/o	breast
mast/o	breast
papill/o	nipplelike
pect/o, pector/o	breast, chest
thel/o	nipple

The soft, hemispherical form of the **mamma** (măm'ah) or breast is due to the superficial fascia, which is heavily loaded with fat and surrounds the mammary gland. Technically, breasts are considered an appendage of the skin. In women, breasts are considered a secondary sex organ designed to produce milk after childbirth. In males, it is less common to refer to breasts because they neither function nor develop in the same way.

In a female, the tiny glands begin gradual development until just before the onset of menstruation (menarche). The mammary gland in the female then reflects and responds to the ovarian hormones and the pituitary gland, as does the endometrium (uterine lining).

In Figure 16-3, note that the center of the breast is the nipple (3), and its halo is called the **areola** (ah-rē'ō-lah) (2). The glandular tissue (5) of the breast is arranged in fifteen to twenty lobes. The duct (4) of each lobe branches and branches again into smaller ducts called ductules or lobules. The whole internal structure of the breast has been compared to a bunch of tiny grapes.

Milk secretion, which is controlled by the anterior pituitary lobe in humans, is carried to the nipple by sinuses (1). This happens during the lactation period of the birth process.

MENSTRUAL CYCLE

men/o	menses

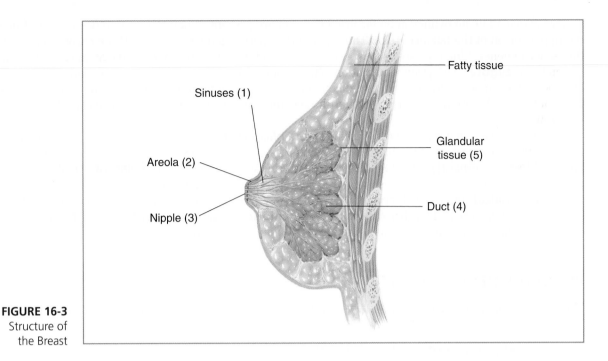

Fatty tissue

Sinuses (1)

Glandular tissue (5)

Areola (2)

Duct (4)

Nipple (3)

FIGURE 16-3
Structure of the Breast

The **menstrual cycle** refers to the monthly developmental changes that occur in the endometrium of the uterus. These changes result in a normal flow of blood called the **menses** (měn'sēz). The average length of the cycle is twenty-eight days, although this can vary among individuals. Usually the onset of menstrual cycles, or **menarche** (mě-năr'kē), occurs between the ages of nine and seventeen; the cessation, or **menopause** (měn'ō-pawz), generally occurs between the ages of forty-five and sixty.

Immediately after menstruation the endometrium is very thin; but during the postmenstrual period (from approximately the fifth to fourteenth day of the cycle), the endometrium becomes thicker. This is because of the presence of the hormone estrogen, which is contained in the fluid produced by the follicles on the surface of the ovaries.

Ovulation takes place when the follicle breaks open and the ovum is discharged. Then the cells that form the corpus luteum begin to secrete progesterone. This further develops the endometrium to provide a bed for a fertilized ovum. If the ovum is not fertilized, the corpus luteum ceases production of both hormones, the endometrium begins deterioration, menstrual discharge begins, and the cycle starts again.

The pituitary gland, located in the brain, is extremely important in the function of the reproductive system. It produces two principal gonadotropins that stimulate the ovary. One is the follicle-stimulating hormone (FSH), which stimulates the follicles during the first and second stages of the menstrual cycle. The other is the luteinizing hormone (LH), which is important in the third and fourth stages of the menstrual cycle (ovulation and secretion of progesterone). The release of the gonadotropic hormones by the pituitary is regulated by the hypothalamus, another specialized structure in the brain. If pregnancy occurs, another hormone, human chorionic gonadotropin (HCG), appears and acts on the corpus luteum. Essentially HCG tells the corpus luteum to continue producing estrogen and progesterone, which maintains the endometrium during pregnancy.

PREGNANCY AND BIRTH

amni/o	amnion
gravid/o	pregnancy
par-, part-	bear
prol-	offspring
umbilic/o	navel

Following ovulation, an ovum can be fertilized if sperm are present. When fertilization does occur, it happens in the upper region of the fallopian tube. The egg and the sperm each carry twenty-three chromosones containing thousands of genes. When the sperm penetrates to the center of the egg, sperm and egg merge to become a one-cell embryo (**zygote** [zī'gŏt]) and fertilization of the ovum is complete. Gender, eye color, and even texture of hair have been determined. Within 12 hours the new cell divides and continues to divide about every 12 hours, reaching about 500 cells within 4 to 5 days. The fertilized ovum then takes several days to travel to the uterus where it will grow.

By the time it reaches the uterus, it is known as a **blastocyst** (blăs'tō-sĭst), another stage in the development of the embryo. One section of the blastocyst contains the cells that will produce an embryo. The outermost layer (**trophoblast** [trŏf'ō-blăst]) will attach itself to the uterine wall and become the **placenta** (plah-sĕn'tah) and the membranes which will provide nourishment, respiration, and excretion for the developing fetus.

The **umbilical** (ŭm-bĭl'ĭ-kăl) **cord**, which contains two arteries and a vein, connects the fetus to the placenta. The fetus itself is encased in a structure called the **amniotic** (ăm"nē-ŏt'ĭk) **sac**. This sac is filled with a clear liquid called amniotic fluid and serves as a protective cushion for the fetus.

PRENATAL DEVELOPMENT

The average time from fertilization to delivery is 266 days, which is divided into three trimesters.

First Trimester (Conception to 13 Weeks)

All major organs of the body are formed during the first trimester. Rudiments of a spinal cord are evident almost immediately and the eyes and heart begin to form. By week 5, the placenta and umbilical cord are fully functioning. By week 6, the brain becomes more noticeable and by the end of the second month of the pregnancy, the baby looks like a miniature human with a large head. During week 10, the heart is beating and the embryo is now considered a **fetus** until it is born. At the end of this trimester the baby may be about 3 inches long and weigh about l ounce.

Second Trimester (Weeks 14 to 26)

All the organs formed in the first trimester continue to grow and mature. At the end of the fourth month, a heartbeat can be detected with a stethoscope. Soon movements of the fetus may become discernable by the mother. The fetus blinks, grasps, and moves the mouth. By the end of this trimester, the fetus is about 12 inches long and weighs about l pound. It has acquired the beginning of eyelashes, eyebrows, hair, and even fat deposits under the skin. Eyes are completely formed and the tongue actually has taste buds.

Third Trimester (Weeks 27 to 40)

During the last trimester, the fetus takes on most of its weight. By 28 weeks the baby's skin is covered with a thick, white protective coating called the **vernix caseosa** (vĕr'nĭks kā"sē-ō'sah). Eyes are open and the baby is capable of crying. At the end of this trimester, the average baby weighs about $7\frac{1}{2}$ pounds. (Figure 16-4.)

THE STAGES OF LABOR

At the end of the prenatal or pregnancy period (normally about 38 to 40 weeks), the process of giving birth, or **parturition** (pr"tū-rĭsh'ŭn), takes place. It is divided into three stages known as labor.

Stage One

Muscles of the uterus begin contractions, pushing the amniotic sac against the cervix, causing the cervix to dilate until it has opened about 10 centimeters (4 inches). While all women labor differently, there are some basic signposts that indicate progress. This first and longest stage is divided into three phases: early, active, and transition. The early phase lasts until the cervix has dilated 1–4 centimeters with light contractions about 20 minutes apart. During the active phase, the contractions become more intense, occurring 4–5 minutes apart and lasting up to 60 seconds. The cervix dilates to 4–8 centimeters. In the transition phase, contractions can be 2–3 minutes apart and

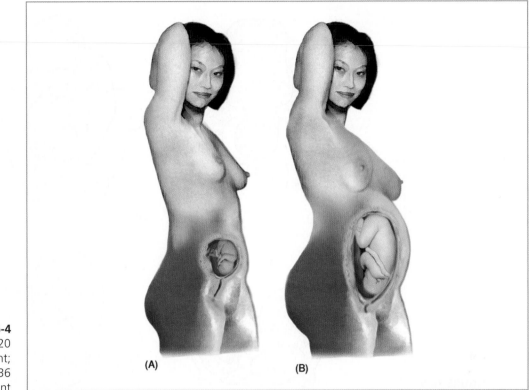

FIGURE 16-4
(A) Woman 20
weeks pregnant;
(B) Woman 36
weeks pregnant

(A)   (B)

last up to 90 seconds. At this point the cervix is completely dilated. After several hours of labor, the amniotic membranes usually rupture.

Stage Two

If the baby is positioned in the **occiput** (ŏk'sĭ-pŭt) **anterior position** with the head down and its face towards the mother's back (Figure 16-5A), the contractions will propel the baby downward, at which time the mother is instructed to assist by pushing. The vaginal opening becomes dilated and bulges. If the opening does not provide adequate room, the physician makes an incision called an **episiotomy** (ĕ-pĭs"ē-ŏt'ŏ-mē) at the opening of the vagina. About ninety-six percent of babies are born in this head-first, facing-back position.

Unfortunately, some babies are positioned in a way that is dangerous or that may require special measures. The abnormal fetal positions are breech, transverse, and occiput posterior.

The most common abnormal presentation is **breech**, where the baby's buttocks are positioned to emerge first instead of the head (Figure 16-5B). If the infant does not reposition before labor, most physicians will perform a cesarean section (C-section). A **cesarean** (sĭ-zăr'ē-ăn) **delivery** is birth through an incision made in the abdomen and into the uterus. The infant is lifted out, the placenta is removed, and the uterus and abdomen are stitched closed. This is considered major surgery and requires a longer period of recuperation.

The **transverse presentation** (Figure 16-5C) occurs when the baby is at right angles to the birth canal. Vaginal delivery is impossible from this position. Cesarean sections should begin before or just after active labor begins to minimize the risk to mother and child.

The **occiput posterior position** (Figure 16-5D) is when the infant's head is positioned near the cervix, but the baby's face is towards the mother's front. This position makes it difficult to travel down the birth canal and may require use of forceps, and less frequently, a cesarean delivery.

Once the physician clears the baby's airway and the baby is expelled, the baby's umbilical cord, which connects the baby to the placenta, is cut. The depressed scar on the infant's abdomen marks the point of attachment of the cord and is called the **umbilicus** (ŭm-bĭ-lī'kŭs) or navel. The baby is examined, weighed, and cleaned.

As soon as the baby is born, the **Apgar score** is taken at 1 and 5 minutes. It is a quick score to determine the physical condition of the newborn. The scale is based on a score of 1 to 10, with 10 indicating the healthiest infant and a score below 5 indicating the newborn needs immediate assistance.

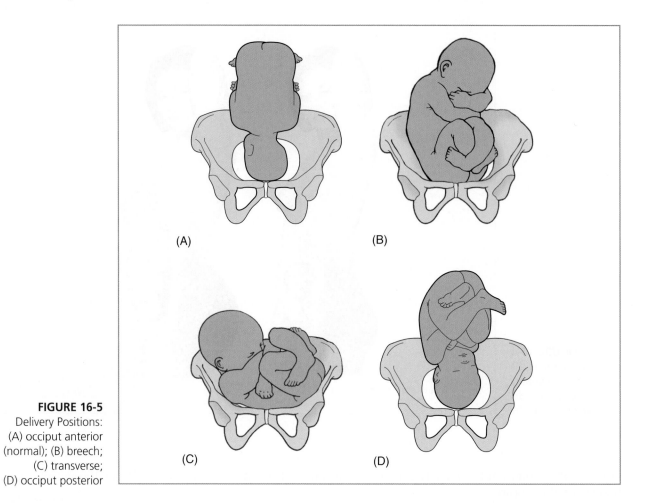

FIGURE 16-5
Delivery Positions:
(A) occiput anterior
(normal); (B) breech;
(C) transverse;
(D) occiput posterior

Five categories are assessed: heart rate, respiratory effort, muscle tone, reflex irritability, and color.

APGAR FACTORS	Score 0	Score 1	Score 2
Heart Rate (as evaluated by a stethoscope)			
There is no heartbeat	X		
Heartbeat is less than 100 beats per minute		X	
Heartbeat is greater than 100 beats per minutes			X
Respiratory Effort			
There are no respirations	X		
Respirations are slow or irregular		X	
There is good crying			X
Muscle Tone			
Muscle tone is flaccid	X		
There is some flexion of the extremities		X	
There is active motion			X

continues

APGAR FACTORS	Score 0	Score 1	Score 2
Reflex Irritability (the level of newborn irritation in response to stimuli such as a mild pinch)			
There is no reflex irritability	X		
There is grimacing		X	
There is a vigorous cry			X
Color			
The baby is pale blue	X		
The baby is pink and the extremities are blue		X	
The entire body is pink			X

Stage Three

The placenta, membranes of the amniotic sac, and the umbilical cord are expelled as the uterus continues to experience mild contractions during the third stage of labor. Once the placenta and other materials are expelled, the uterus should clamp down to prevent hemorrhage. This is within the first 30 minutes after the birth. Changes in the body include contracting of the uterus and shifting of the internal organs to pre-pregnancy places and sizes. The period after birth is referred to as **postpartum**.

POSTPARTUM PERIOD

During pregnancy the hormones estrogen, progesterone, and **prolactin** (prō-lăk'tĭn) are produced to promote the growth of special breast tissue designed to produce milk. Prolactin, produced by the pituitary gland, also stimulates the production of milk, but this process is suppressed during pregnancy. With the delivery of the placenta, the suppression ends and prolactin begins producing **colostrum** (kō-lŏs'trŭm), a thin, yellowish, milky fluid that fills the breast. The baby's suckling contributes to this process and also stimulates the production of the pituitary hormone oxytocin, which helps the uterus to contract. Colostrum contains a large number of proteins and calories as well as antibodies to resist viruses and bacteria to nourish and protect the baby until true **lactation**, the secretion of milk, begins following the marked decrease of estrogen and progesterone.

The huge hormonal change (by as much as ninety percent within 48 hours of delivery) and the external stresses that come with having a baby can trigger serious emotional problems. In about eighty percent of new mothers, a mild depression commonly referred to as the "**baby blues**" occurs within a few days or weeks of birth and typically lasts 2 to 3 weeks. Symptoms are crying, irritability, forgetfulness, insomnia, lethargy, anxiety, and appetite loss. In most cases, with support from family and friends, this remains a normal part of the lifestyle change that occurs with motherhood.

A more severe form of the blues, **postpartum depression**, occurs in ten to twenty percent of women, with symptoms more intense and lasting longer than the initial 2 to 3 weeks. Symptoms may include change in mood, sleep patterns, eating, and concentration; body preoccupations or phobias and fear of hurting herself or the baby; loss of interest in activities; and extreme irritability. It can occur anytime during the first year after childbirth and interferes with the mother's ability to function. Professional treatment is advisable. If not treated, the depression can last for years, resulting in long-term or permanent consequences for the child.

An even more severe form, called **postpartum psychosis**, is relatively rare. Symptoms include a break with reality, delusions, hallucinations, a feeling that the baby is either the devil or divine, and development of plans to harm the child. This condition may require others to intervene on behalf of the mother and child or children.

Six weeks after delivery, a postpartum checkup is performed to be sure organs have returned to the correct size and position. This is an opportunity to discuss any issues regarding the mother's health and to consider options for contraception.

Nonsurgical contraception options include the rhythm method or natural family planning that relies on the "safe" days in a woman's menstrual cycle; birth control pills, the most effective method of contraception with 1 pregnancy in 1,000 women per year; **intrauterine devices** (IUD), which are inserted in the uterine cavity by a physician; and **barrier methods**, which block the sperm from access to the egg. Barrier methods include the diaphragm, vaginal sponge, and male or female condoms. Success rates on these devices are eighty to ninety percent effective but vary considerably. **Contraceptive implants** are similar to progestin-only birth control pills and are implanted under the skin of the upper arm. They last about five years and are about ninety-five percent effective, although the initial cost is high. Another option is birth control shots every one to three months. Some of these are safe immediately after childbirth and while breast feeding.

Surgical options include tubal ligation, which is accomplished by interrupting the fallopian tubes so that the egg cannot travel down the tubes and the sperm cannot move upward. It is the most common method of female sterilization. A good time for a tubal ligation is immediately after giving birth, shortly thereafter, or at the time of a cesarean section.

FERTILITY

For some women, preventing unwanted pregnancies is a major concern. For others, the inability to become pregnant is devastating. **Infertility** occurs if a couple is unable to achieve pregnancy after a year of unprotected intercourse. At that point they are advised to seek specialized medical help. Infertility affects 6.1 million couples in the United States alone—about ten to fifteen percent of couples in the reproductive age population. Various factors in both men and women contribute to infertility. The cause may be either male or female, joint, or unexplained. About forty percent of couples have more than one cause for infertility.

The first step is a physical examination of both partners to determine their general state of health and to evaluate physical disorders that may be causing infertility. In most infertility cases, about eighty-five to ninety percent are treated with conventional therapies such as drug treatment or surgical repair of reproductive organs.

More recent medical advances also enable many couples to have their own biologic child with assisted reproductive technology (ART). The ART team includes physicians, psychologists, embryologists, laboratory technicians, nurses, and allied health professionals who work together to help infertile couples.

The most common ART is **in vitro fertilization** (IVF) where eggs are surgically removed from the ovary and mixed with sperm outside the body in a Petri dish. After 40 hours, the eggs are examined to see if they have become fertilized by the sperm and are dividing into cells. Some or all of the fertilized eggs (now called embryos) are then placed in the women's uterus, thus bypassing the fallopian tubes.

Other forms of ART include zygote intrafallopian transfer (ZIFT), in which an ova is mixed with sperm and the resulting zygote is placed into a fallopian tube the day after removal. With gamete intrafallopian transfer (GIFT), unfertilized ova and sperm are placed directly into a fallopian tube. Other options include electroejaculation, aspiration techniques, and intracytoplasmic sperm injection (ICSI). All options should be discussed thoroughly before embarking on fertility therapy.

INTERNET ASSIGNMENT

The American Medical Association (AMA) maintains a web site at **www.ama-assn.org**. AMA's work includes the development and promotion of standards in medical practice, research, and education; strong advocacy on behalf of patients and physicians; and the commitment to providing timely information on health matters. One of the aims of the AMA is to make patients active participants in their health care.

Information on the web site is presented separately for physicians and patients. Under Patients, the subsection entitled Atlas of the Body provides a collection of anatomy and medical illustrations. The Health Information subsection provides information to promote the art and science of medicine and provides links to the Medem web site and the AMA Library.

ACTIVITY

Visit the AMA site at **www.ama-assn.org**. Move your cursor to the Patients button and select Atlas of the Body from the drop down list. Click Female Reproduction—Pregnancy and view the illustrations provided. Compare the views at 6 months and 9 months and summarize the differences.

Move the cursor to Patients again and click on Health Information. This will take you to Medem's Medical Library site. Select Women's Health and Pregnancy and Fertility Issues. Then click on Bleeding During Pregnancy. Write a brief report on the information provided about ectopic pregnancies.

Submit your reports to your instructor.

Review: The Female Reproductive System

- In response to hormones, the ovaries cyclically produce ova, which travel to the fallopian tube where they may or may not be fertilized by male sperm.
- The internal layer of the uterus thickens each month in preparation for a fertilized ovum.
- The uterine lining deteriorates if the ovum has not been fertilized, which causes bleeding known as menstrual flow.
- The vagina leads to the exterior of the body and is surrounded by external genitalia for protection.
- The menstrual cycle is influenced by functions of the pituitary gland.
- When an ovum is fertilized, a pregnancy progresses for approximately 38 to 40 weeks and ends with parturition, or the birth process.
- The female breast produces milk after childbirth.
- The period after birth, postpartum, is marked by hormonal changes that produce the "baby blues" in eighty percent of new mothers.
- A postpartum checkup is performed six weeks after delivery and includes a medical examination as well as discussion of contraceptive options, if desired.

Review of Terminology Presented

Word	Definition
amniotic sac	sac filled with fluid that encloses the fetus and provides a protective cushion
Apgar score	assessment of baby's heart rate, respiratory effort, muscle tone, reflex irritability, and color at l and 5 minutes after birth
areola	darkened halo surrounding the nipple of the breast
baby blues	a mild form of depression occurring within a few days of childbirth that may last for about two weeks
barrier methods	contraceptive measures, including the diaphragm, vaginal sponge, cervical cap, and male and female condoms, that block the sperm from access to the egg
blastocyst	a stage in the development of an embryo
breech birth position	baby's buttocks presents first instead of the head
cervix	lower portion of the uterus
cesarean delivery	birth through an incision made in the abdomen and into the uterus
clitoris	small structure of the vagina made of erectile tissue
colostrum	a thin, yellowish, milky fluid that precedes the secretion of breast milk
contraceptive implant	a device implanted under the skin of the upper arm to prevent conception
corpus	large upper part of the uterus
corpus luteum	cells of the ruptured ovarian follicle that have increased in size and taken on color; they rapidly degenerate if the ovum has not been fertilized

continues

Word	Definition
ectopic pregnancy	condition in which a fertilized egg remains in the fallopian tube instead of reaching the uterus
embryo	name of a fertilized ovum from about the second through the tenth week
endometrium	innermost layer of the uterus
episiotomy	incision in the opening of the vagina to widen it for delivery of a baby
estrogen	hormone that aids in the development of female secondary sex characteristics and cyclic changes such as menstruation and pregnancy
fallopian tube	duct connected to the uterus; where fertilization of an ovum occurs
fetus	developing infant in the uterus after the embryonic period
fimbriae	fringelike extensions of the fallopian tube that help to sweep ova into the tubes
fornix, *pl.* fornices	circular recesses created by the cervix of the uterus dipping into the upper vagina
fundus	small, rounded part of the uterus above the level of the entrance to the fallopian tube
gynecologist	physician who specializes in diseases of the female reproductive system and the breasts
hymen	fold of membrane near the vaginal canal opening
in vitro fertilization	fertilization procedures whereby eggs are surgically removed from the ovary and mixed with sperm in a Petri dish; fertilized eggs are placed in the woman's uterus
infertility	inability of a couple to achieve pregnancy after a year of unprotected intercourse
intrauterine device (IUD)	birth control device inserted in the uterine cavity by a physician
labia majora	two folds or lips that are part of the external genitalia
labia minora	two small folds or lips medial to the labia majora
lactation	secretion of milk produced by the breast to nourish the baby
mamma	breast
menarche	onset of the first menstruation cycle
menopause	permanent cessation of menstrual activity
menses	normal flow of blood during the menstrual cycle
menstrual cycle	monthly developmental changes in the endometrium of the uterus resulting in menses
mons pubis	part of the external genitalia that is covered with hair after puberty
myometrium	muscular layer of the uterus that enables the walls to contract during childbirth
obstetrician	physician who treats women during pregnancy and childbirth
occiput anterior presentation	birth position where baby's head is down and facing mother's back; normal position
occiput posterior presentation	birth position where baby's head is down and facing mother's front
ovarian follicles	small sacs on the ovary in which ova mature
ovaries	female glands that produce eggs
ovulation	process that discharges an ovum from the ovarian follicle

continues

Word	Definition
parturition	process of giving birth
perineum	entire pelvic floor in both men and women; for pregnant women, health care specialists usually limit the perineum to the area between the vaginal opening and the anus
placenta	organ of nutrition, respiration, and excretion for the fetus during pregnancy
postpartum	after birth
postpartum depression	condition marked by continuation and deepening of symptoms exhibited in the baby blues
postpartum psychosis	serious form of depression that may lead to harm to the child or children
progesterone	hormone that keeps the uterine lining in a favorable condition for a fertilized egg
prolactin	hormone that stimulates the breasts to produce milk and colostrum
transverse presentation	birth position where baby lies across the abdomen making vaginal delivery impossible
trophoblast	outermost layer of a blastocyst, which will attach itself to the uterine wall and become the placenta
umbilical cord	structure that connects the fetus to the placenta
umbilicus	navel
uterine serosa	membrane covering the uterus
uterus	pear-shaped organ located between the urinary bladder and the rectum
vagina	muscular tube connecting the uterine cavity to the exterior of the body
vernix caseosa	layer of material that protects the skin of the fetus
vulva	collective female external genitalia
vulvovaginal (Bartholin's) glands	glands that lubricate the vaginal area
zygote	fertilized, one-cell embryo

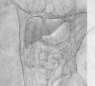

Terminology Review Exercises

Name: _____ Date: _____

COMPLETION*

Complete the following statements.

1. The ova from the female ovary mature in the _____.

2. After ovulation the cells of the ovarian follicle increase in size, take on a yellowish color, and become known as a _____.

3. The uterus has three portions: they are the _____, _____, and _____.

4. Circular recesses and areas created by the dip of the uterus into the upper vagina are called _____; the deepest of the areas is called the _____.

5. The organ of nutrition, respiration, and excretion for a developing fetus is called the _____.

6. Until about the tenth week, the fertilized ovum is called a(n) _____; after that it is called a(n) _____.

7. Onset of the first menstrual cycle is referred to as _____; permanent cessation of menstrual activity is called _____.

8. After ovulation the ovum is swept into tubes by fringelike extensions on the fallopian tube called _____.

9. The external female genitalia are called the _____.

10. A normal pregnancy lasts approximately _____ weeks.

11. _____ is the process of giving birth.

12. The three layers of the uterine wall are _____

13. Depression, ranging from mild _____ to _____ to a rare serious form, called _____, may occur within a few days to a year after a mother gives birth.

14. A one-cell embryo is a _____; it grows to become a _____ whose outer layer or _____ will become the placenta.

15. Two hormones that influence the menstrual cycle in preparation for a possible pregnancy are _____ and _____.

_____
*Answers are in Appendix A.

MATCHING

Match the terms to their meanings.

1.	halo surrounding the nipple of the breast	a.	amniotic sac
2.	flow of blood during menstruation	b.	Apgar score
3.	mucous-producing glands at vaginal opening	c.	areola
4.	connects fetus and placenta	d.	Bartholin's gland
5.	structure that encases a fetus	e.	breech
6.	process of giving birth	f.	clitoris
7.	baby is positioned to emerge buttocks first	g.	colostrum
8.	baby is at right angles to the birth canal	h.	ectopic pregnancy
9.	baby is head down, face to mother's back	i.	mamma
10.	baby is head down, face to mother's front	j.	menses
11.	test taken of infant at 1 and 5 minutes after delivery	k.	occiput anterior
12.	thin, sticky fluid that initially after birth is secreted by the breast	l.	occiput posterior
13.	hormone produced by the pituitary that triggers production of colostrum	m.	parturition
14.	after birth	n.	perineum
15.	thick, protective coating over fetus' skin	o.	postpartum
16.	a fertilized egg that does not reach the uterus	p.	prolactin
17.	small structure of the vagina that is composed of erectile tissue	q.	transverse
18.	pelvic floor, in gynecology, between vaginal opening and anus	r.	umbilical cord
19.	breast	s.	umbilicus
20.	navel	t.	vernix caseosa

DIAGNOSTIC PROCEDURES

Word	Pronunciation	Definition
General amniocentesis	ăm″nē-ō-sĕn-tē'sĭs	needle puncture of the amniotic sac to withdraw amniotic fluid for analysis in order to detect genetic disorders or maternal-fetal blood incompatibility or to determine fetal maturity (See Figure 16-6)
breast biopsy (aspiration)	bī'ŏp-sē	extraction of suspicious breast tissue to determine the presence of cancer or other conditions; biopsies may be (1) stereotaxic—uses mammograms taken from different angles to locate a suspicious area, aligns a needle with that area, and allows the radiologist to remove a small amount of tissue; (2) needle—withdraws fluid from a fluid-filled lesion; or (3) surgical—physician removes entire lump under local or general anesthesia
cervical biopsy	ser'vĭ-kăl	removal of tissue to evaluate the presence of abnormalities of the cervix; biopsy of tissue at 12, 3, 6, and 9 o'clock positions on the cervix is referred to as a *four-quadrant cervical biopsy*

continues

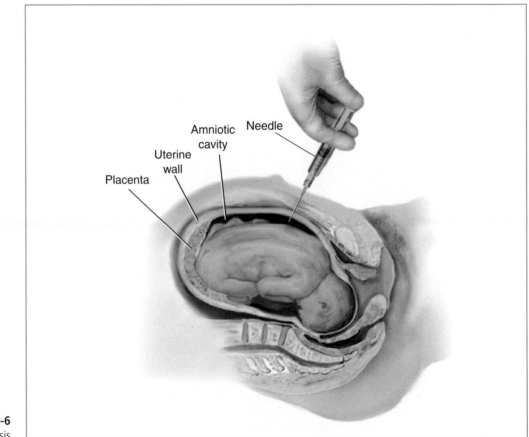

FIGURE 16-6
Amniocentesis

DIAGNOSTIC PROCEDURES

Word	Pronunciation	Definition
General *(continued)*		
colposcopy	kōl-pŏs'kō-pē	examination of the cervix with a scope to look for abnormalities
dilation and curettage (D&C)	dī-lā'shŭn kū"rĕ-tahzh'	surgical procedure that expands the cervix of the uterus (dilation) so that the uterine wall can be scraped (curettage)
fetal monitoring	fē'tăl	recording the fetal heart rate by a direct or indirect method
fetoscopy	fē-tŏs'kō-pē	visual examination of the fetus using a lighted instrument inserted through the abdominal and uterine walls into the amniotic sac
hysteroscopy	hĭs"tĕr-ŏs'kō-pē	inspection of the uterus by use of a special endoscope
laparoscopy	lăp"ah-rŏs'kō-pē	examination of the interior of the abdomen by inserting a laparascope through the abdominal wall (See Figure 16-7)
laparotomy	lăp-ah-rŏt'ō-mē	surgical incision through the abdominal wall
Nuclear Medicine		
beta human chorionic gonadotropin (beta-HCG)	bā'tah hū-măn kō"rē-ŏn'ik gŏn"ah-dō-trō'pĭn	pregnancy hormone produced by the placenta; used in the presence of a suspicious adnexal mass to identify the need for surgery and/or further treatment

continues

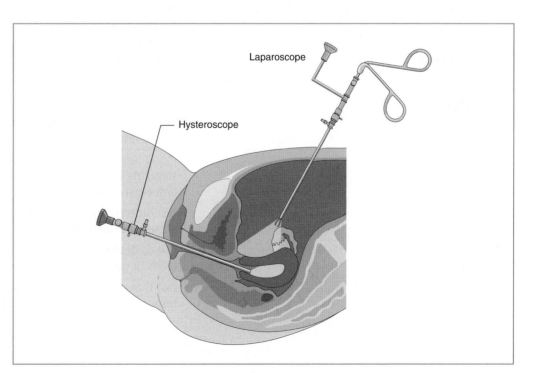

FIGURE 16-7
Laparoscopy Performed with a Hysteroscopy: allows visualizing both the inside and outside of the uterus at the same time

Laparoscope

Hysteroscope

DIAGNOSTIC PROCEDURES

Word	Pronunciation	Definition
Radiology		
chorionic villus sampling (CVS)	kō"rē-ŏn'ĭk	transcervical insertion of a catheter to obtain a sampling of placenta tissue (chorionic villi) to check for fetal abnormalities; procedure is ultrasound guided
endovaginal ultrasound	ĕn"dō-văj'ĭ-nal ŭl-trah-sownd	diagnostic procedure that uses a sound probe placed in the vagina for a closer, sharper look within the pelvis
hysterosalpingography	hĭs"ter-ō-săl"pĭng-gŏg'rah-fē	radiographic procedure using radiopaque material to provide a picture of the uterus and uterine tubes
mammography	ma-mŏg'ră-fē	special breast x-ray used to detect tumors in the breast
pelvimetry	pĕl-vĭm'ĕ-trē	measurement of the proportions of the pelvis using an x-ray to help determine whether normal vaginal delivery is possible
pelvic ultrasonography	pĕl'vĭk ŭl"trah-sŏn-ŏg'rah-fē	use of sound waves to produce a picture of the pelvic area to check on a pregnancy or mass
sonohysterogram (saline-infusion sonography)	sŏn"ō-hĭs-tĕr'ō-grăm	vaginal ultrasound placement of a catheter through the cervix into the uterus to infuse saline into the uterine cavity to look for abnormalities within the uterus
Laboratory Tests		
estrogen receptor test	es'trō-gĕn	test done on breast tissue from malignant breast tumor to help plan further treatment depending on whether the tumor responds to estrogen
Pap (Papanicolaou) smear	păp"ah-nĭk"ō-lā'oo	test that uses scrapings from the cervix and stain to detect tissue changes that may indicate cancer (See Figure 16-8)
pregnancy test		test used to determine whether a woman is pregnant
Blood Tests		
alpha-fetoprotein analysis		blood test that measures the level of protein produced by the fetus to detect spinal cord abnormalities
FSH and LH		blood test that measures pituitary hormones that stimulate the ovaries; ordered in fertility cases or for detection of menopause (FSH)
glucose	gloo'kōs	test ordered during pregnancy to check for gestational diabetes
percutaneous umbilical cord sampling	pĕr"kū-tā'nē-ŭs	test to determine oxygen and carbon dioxide levels or genetic disorders
prolactin level	prō-lăk'tĭn	test that measures the pituitary hormone, which is responsible for breast milk production

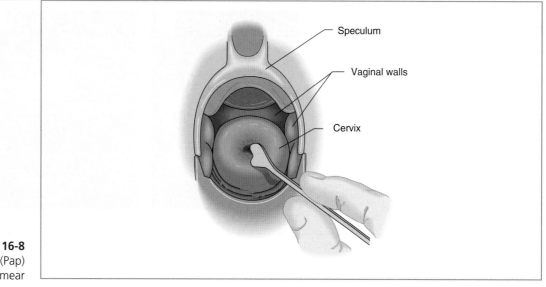

FIGURE 16-8
Papanicolaou (Pap) Smear

DIAGNOSES

Word	Pronunciation	Definition
Menses and Menstrual Disorders		
amenorrhea	ă-mĕn-ō-rē'ă	absence or abnormal cessation of the menses
dysmenorrhea	dis″mĕn-ō-rē'ah	painful or difficult menstruation
menopause	mĕn'ō-pawz	permanent cessation of the menses
menorrhagia, hypermenorrhea	men″ō-rā'jē-ah, hī″pĕr-mĕn″ō-rē'ah	heavy menstrual periods
metrorrhagia	mē″trō-rā'jē-ah	uterine bleeding at any time other than during the menstrual period
mittelschmerz	mĭt'ĕl-shmārts	pain that occurs at the time of ovulation
polymenorrhea	pŏl″ē-mĕn″ō-rē'ah	abnormally frequent menstruation
premenstrual syndrome (PMS)	prē-mĕn'stroo-ăl sĭn'drōm	predictable pattern of physical and emotional changes that occur just before menstruation
Problems of the Breast		
breast cancer		malignant tumor in the breast (See Figure 16-9)
fibrocystic disease	fī″brō-sĭs'tĭk	benign condition producing fibroglandular changes; sometimes called chronic cystic mastitis, mammary dysplasia, or benign breast disease
galactorrhea	gă-lăc″tō-rē'ah	condition marked by abnormal discharge of milk from the nipples
intraductal papilloma	ĭn-tră-dŭk'tăl păp-ĭ-lō'mah	tiny benign tumors in the milk ducts of the breast that may result in watery or blood discharge from the nipple
mastitis	măs-tī'tĭs	breast infections caused by bacteria that enter the breast; not uncommon to nursing mothers

continues

The Female Reproductive System ■ **431**

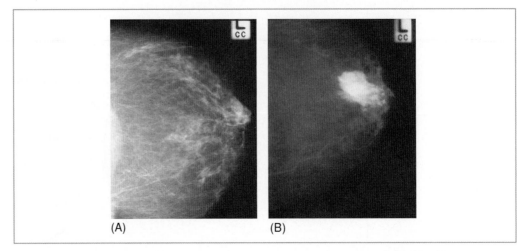

FIGURE 16-9
Mammograms: (A) normal breast; (B) breast with carcinoma

DIAGNOSES

Word	Pronunciation	Definition
Vaginal and Vulvar Disorders		
Bartholin's gland abscess	băr'tō-lĭnz	infection of the vulvovaginal gland (See Figure 16-10)
cystocele	sĭs'tō-sēl	weakness in the vaginal wall, allowing protrusion of the urinary bladder through the vaginal wall
dyspareunia	dĭs-pă-roo'nē-ah	painful sexual intercourse
enterocele	ĕn'tĕr-ō-sēl	hernia of the intestine through the vagina
Hemophilus vaginitis (bacterial vaginosis)	hē-mŏf'ĭ-lŭs văj"ĭ-nī'tĭs	inflammation of the vagina caused by a specific genus of bacteria
human papilloma virus	păp-ĭ-lō'mah	any number of strains that cause plantar and genital warts on skin or mucous membrane in humans; transmitted by direct or indirect contact

continues

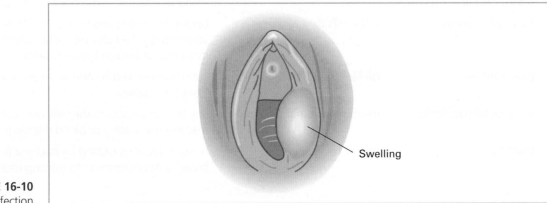

Swelling

FIGURE 16-10
Bartholin's Gland Infection

DIAGNOSES

Word	Pronunciation	Definition
Vaginal and Vulvar Disorders (*continued*)		
pruritus vulvae	proo-rī'tŭs vŭl'vă	intense itching, burning, or irritation in the genital area
pubic lice (crabs)	pū'bĭk	parasite that infects pubic and neighboring body parts
rectocele	rĕk'tō-sēl	weakness in the vaginal wall, allowing protrusion of part of the rectum into the vagina
sebaceous cyst	să-bā'shăs	painless, soft, smooth lump in the skin of the vulva
vaginitis	văj"ĭ-nī'tĭs	common treatable inflammation or sexually transmitted disease; may be *trichomoniasis, yeast infection* (See Figure 16-11), *nonspecific, atrophic* (caused by degeneration of vaginal tissue), or *postmenopausal* (caused by overall decrease in the estrogen level)
vulvitis	vŭl-vī'tĭs	inflammation of the external genitals
Cervix, Uterus, and Fallopian Tube Disorders		
adenomyosis	ăd"ĕ-nō-mī-ō'sĭs	growth of endometrial tissue (uterine lining) within the muscular walls of the uterus
carcinoma in situ	kăr"sĭ-no'mah ĭn sī'too	cancer confined to the original site
cervical cancer	sĕr'vĭ-kăl	common cancer affecting female reproductive organs; preceded by *cervical dysplasia* (precancerous) or *carcinoma in situ* (located on the surface of the cervix in the top layers of tissue)
cervical polyps	sĕr'vĭ-kăl pŏl'ĭps	bulging tissue mass on the cervix
cervicitis	sĕr"vĭ-sī'tĭs	inflammation of the cervix; may be caused by a local infection or a symptom of vaginal infections, some sexually transmitted diseases, or pelvic inflammatory disease
choriocarcinoma	kō"rē-ō-kăr-sĭ-nō'mah	highly malignant neoplasm frequently found in the vagina, pelvic organs or other body parts; may follow any type of pregnancy

continues

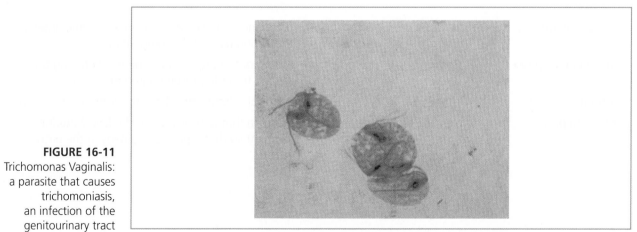

FIGURE 16-11
Trichomonas Vaginalis: a parasite that causes trichomoniasis, an infection of the genitourinary tract

DIAGNOSES

Word	Pronunciation	Definition
Cervix, Uterus, and Fallopian Tube Disorders *(continued)*		
dysplasia	dĭs-plā'zē-ah	abnormal tissue development
endocervicitis	ĕn"dō-sĕr"vĭ-sī'tĭs	inflammation of the inner mucous lining of the cervix
endometrial hyperplasia	ĕn"dō-mē'trē-ăl hī"pĕr-plā'zha	abnormal overgrowth of the endometrium
endometrial polyps	ĕn"dō-mē'trē-ăl pol'ĭps	small, sessile, benign projecting masses on endometrium composed of endometrous stroma containing cystically dilated glands
endometriosis	ĕn"dō-mē"trē-ō'sĭs	escape of endometrial tissue (tissue that lines the uterus) to become attached to other pelvic organs
fibroids	fī'broids	benign tumors in the uterus
nabothian cyst	nah-bō'thē-ăn	cyst that occurs when a mucus gland on the cervix is obstructed
pelvic inflammatory disease (PID)	pĕl'vĭk	inflammation and infection of pelvic tissue (uterus, tubes, and ovaries)
uterine cancer (endometrial cancer)	ū'tĕr-ĭn (ĕn"dō-mē'trē-ăl)	common, slow-growing cancer that starts in the lining of the uterus
uterine prolapse	ū'tĕr-ĭn prō'lăps	downward displacement of the uterus so that part or all of it is outside the vaginal orifice
Ovarian Disorders		
ovarian carcinoma	ō-vā'rē-ăn kăr"sĭ-nō'mah	hard-to-diagnose malignant tumor of the ovary
ovarian cyst	ō-vā'rē-ăn	sac filled with fluid on an ovary
polycystic ovary syndrome	pŏl"ē-sis'tĭk	sclerocystic disease of the ovary
Diseases Related to Pregnancy		
abruptio placentae	ăb-rŭp'shē-ō plă-sĕn'tē	premature detachment of normally situated placenta
eclampsia	ē-klamp'sē-ah	gravest form of toxemia, characterized by grand mal convulsions, coma hypertension, proteinuria, and edema
ectopic pregnancy	ĕk-tŏp'ĭk	pregnancy in which a fertilized egg is implanted in the wrong place; tubal pregnancy
incompetent cervix	sĕr'vĭks	mouth of the uterus opens generally during the second trimester, resulting in miscarriage
intrauterine death	ĭn"tră-ū'tĕr-ĭn	death of a fetus after the fifth month of gestation
placenta previa	plah-sĕn'tah prē'vē-ah	placenta that is implanted in the lower uterine segment so that it precedes a baby in the birth process

continues

DIAGNOSES

Word	Pronunciation	Definition
Diseases Related to Pregnancy (*continued*)		
preeclampsia	prē"ē-klamp'sē-ah	disorder of pregnancy characterized by hypertension, proteinuria, and edema; also called *toxemia of pregnancy*
spontaneous abortion (miscarriage)		a natural termination of the pregnancy before the fetus leaves on its own
toxemia	tŏk-sē'mē-ah	a condition appearing in the third trimester characterized by hypertension, proteinuria, edema, and sudden weight gain
Neonatal Terms		
Down syndrome		condition marked by mild to moderate mental retardation and certain physical characteristics
erythroblastosis fetalis	ĕ-rĭth"rō-blăs-tō'sĭs fē-tă'lĭs	hemolytic disease of newborn marked by anemia, jaundice, enlargement of liver and spleen, and generalized edema
hyaline membrane disease	hī'ă-lĭn	respiratory distress syndrome of the newborn
hydrocephalus	hī-drō-sĕf'ă-lŭs	accumulation of excessive amounts of cerebrospinal fluid within ventricles of the brain
kernicterus	kĕr-nĭk'tĕr-ŭs	form of jaundice occurring in a newborn during the second through eighth day after birth
pyloric stenosis	pī-lŏr'ĭk stē-nō'sĭs	narrowing of pyloric orifice, which in infants may require surgical division of the muscles of the pylorus

TREATMENT PROCEDURES

Word	Pronunciation	Definition
abortion	ah-bor'shŭn	premature termination of pregnancy, spontaneous or induced
adjuvant therapy	ăd'jŭ-vănt	giving cancer-killing drugs during the early stages of treatment to assist surgery or radiation procedures
breast reconstruction		procedure that uses saline-filled silicone implants in postmastectomy patients to reshape the breast
cauterization	kaw"tĕr-ĭ-zā'shŭn	destruction of abnormal tissue with chemicals or heat
conization	kŏn"ĭ-zā'shŭn	removal of a cone of tissue from the mouth of the cervix
cryosurgery	krī"ō-sŭr'jĕr-ē	use of cold to destroy tissue; cryocauterization
C-section (cesarean section)	sē-sā'rē-ăn	birth of an infant by surgical incision into the uterus

continues

TREATMENT PROCEDURES

Word	Pronunciation	Definition
episiotomy	ĕ-pĭs″ē-ŏt′ō-mē	incision made to widen the vagina for delivery of the infant
hormone replacement therapy (HRT)		prescription of estrogen and progestin to replace hormones lost during menopause and to slow down the rate of bone density loss
hysterectomy	hĭs′tĕ-rĕk′tō-mē	surgical removal of the uterus through the abdominal wall or through the vagina (See Figure 16-12)
Kegel exercises	kē′gŭl	simple exercises for strengthening pubococcygeal muscles
laparoscopic tubal coagulation and division	lăp″ah-rō-skŏp′ĭk	sterilization procedure specifically using cauterization and division of the fallopian tubes
mastectomy	măs-tĕk′tō-mē	surgical procedure for the treatment of breast cancer; may be (1) radical—removing the entire breast including a portion of skin containing the nipple and areola and the underlying chest wall muscles, as well as extensive removal of lymph nodes underneath the armpit; (2) modified radical—similar to radical, but the chest wall is spared and fewer lymph nodes are removed; (3) breast conservation therapy (lumpectomy)—removes the tumor and a small rim of normal breast tissue followed with a 4- to 6-week course of radiation; (4) simple mastectomy—similar to modified radical mastectomy, but the armpit lymph nodes are not removed; (5) subcutaneous mastectomy—removes only breast tissue and spares skin, nipple, areola, chest wall muscles, and lymph nodes
oophorectomy	ō″ŏf-ō-rĕk′tō-mē	excision of an ovary
pelvic exenteration	eks-ĕn″tĕr-ā′shŭn	complete and radical removal of all pelvic organs in treatment of certain cancers

continues

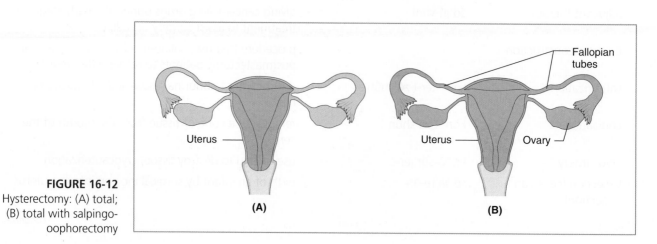

FIGURE 16-12
Hysterectomy: (A) total; (B) total with salpingo-oophorectomy

Fallopian tubes

Uterus

Uterus   Ovary

(A)   (B)

TREATMENT PROCEDURES

Word	Pronunciation	Definition
polypectomy	pŏl'ĭ-pĕk'tō-mē	excision of a polyp
salpingo-oophorectomy	săl-pĭng"gō-ō"ŏf-ō-rĕk'tō-mē	excision of a fallopian tube and an ovary
tubal ligation	lī-gā'shŭn	sterilization procedure that involves tying off (ligating) the fallopian tubes (See Figure 16-13)
uterine suspension	ū-ter-īn	surgical reinforcement of the supporting structure of the uterus

MEDICATIONS PRESCRIBED

Trade Name	Generic Name
General	
Ampicillin, Polycillin	ampicillin
Anaprox	naproxen sodium
Betadine Vaginal Suppositories	povidone iodine
Flagyl	metronidazole
Furadantin, Macrodantin	nitrofurantoin
Gyne-Lotrimin, Mycelex	clotrimazole
Monistat 7 Vaginal Cream	miconazole nitrate
Mycolog-II, Mycostatin, Nilstat	nystatin
Synalar	fluocinolone acetonide
Terazol Vaginal Cream	terconazole
Hormones	
Aygestin	norethindrone acetate
Cenestin	conjugated estrogens

continues

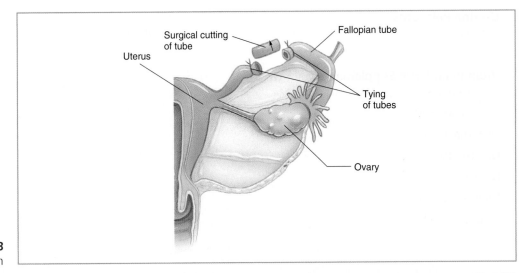

FIGURE 16-13
Tubal Ligation

MEDICATIONS PRESCRIBED

Trade Name	Generic Name
Hormones (continued)	
Depo-Provera, Provera	medroxyprogesterone acetate
Estrace	estradiol
Ogen	estropipate
Premarin	estrogens, conjugated
Ovulation Stimulants	
Clomid	clomiphene citrate
Gonadotropins	
Lupron	leuprolide acetate
Pergonal	menotropins
Profasi HP	chorionic gonadotropin
Synarel	nafarelin acetate

Birth Control Pills

Alesse	Mircette	Ortho-Novum
Demulen	Nordette	Ortho Tri-Cyclen
Desogen	Norinyl	Ovral
Loestrin	Norlestrin	Tri-Norinyl
Lo/Ovral	Ortho-Cyclen	Tri-Phasil

Trade Name	Generic Name
Labor Inducers	
Ergonovine	ergonovine
Methergine	methylergonovine maleate
Pitocin	oxytocin
Uterine Relaxants	
Yutopar	ritodrine

Vitamin and Iron Supplements

Ferro-Sequels

Iberet-Folic-500

Materna 1-60

Natabec Rx

Natalins

Niferex-PN Forte

Zenate

ABBREVIATIONS

AB	abortion
ART	assisted reproductive technology
beta-HCG	beta human chorionic gonadotropin
CIN	cervical intra-epithelial neoplasia (cervical dysplasia)
CIS	carcinoma in situ
C-section, CS	cesarean section
CVS	chorionic villus sampling
Cx	cervix
D&C	dilatation (dilation) and curettage
DES	diethylstilbestrol
DUB	dysfunctional uterine bleeding
ECC	endocervical curettage
ERT	estrogen replacement therapy
FHT	fetal heart tones
FSH	follicle-stimulating hormone
G	gravida (pregnant)
GIFT	gamete intrafallopian transfer
gyn	gynecology
HCG, hcg	human chorionic gonadotropin
HRT	hormone replacement therapy
HPV	human papillomavirus
ICSI	intracytoplasmic sperm injection
IUD	intrauterine device
IVF	in vitro fertilization
LMP	last menstrual period
NB	newborn
OB	obstetrics
Pap test	Papanicolaou test
PID	pelvic inflammatory disease
PMS	premenstrual syndrome
SIL	squamous intra-epithelial lesion (cervical dysplasia)
TSS	toxic shock syndrome
ZIFT	zygote intrafallopian transfer

Working Practice Review Exercises

Name: _____ Date: _____

CHOICES*

Circle the correct answer in each statement.

1. (Hysterosalpingography/ultrasonography) is a technique that uses sound waves to produce a picture.

2. (Dilation and curettage/cervical biopsy) is the procedure used to scrape the uterine wall.

3. A (laparotomy/laparoscopy) is an incision through the abdominal wall to look for gynecological problems.

4. (Prolactin level/LH) is a test used in fertility cases.

5. (Amniocentesis/pregnancy test) is ordered to determine whether any genetic disorders are present in a pregnancy.

6. (Galactorrhea/mastitis) is a condition marked by abnormal discharge of milk from the nipples.

7. Measurement of the proportions of the pelvis using an x-ray is (pelvimetry/pelvic ultrasoundography).

8. A (stereotaxic/needle/surgical) breast biopsy removes an entire lump under anesthesia.

9. Painful or difficult menstruation is (menorrhagia/metrorrhagia/dysmenorrhea).

10. Premature detachment of a normally situated placenta is (abruptio placentae/placenta previa).

11. Escape of endometrial tissue that then becomes attached to other pelvic organs is (adenomyosis/endometriosis).

12. Abnormal tissue development is (dysplasia/choriocarcinoma).

13. Predictable patterns of physical and emotional changes that occur before onset of monthly menstruation is (premenstrual syndrome/polycystic ovary syndrome).

IDENTIFICATION*

Identify the following surgical procedures.

1. surgically reinforcing the supporting structure of the uterus   _____

2. excision of an ovary   _____

3. removal of a cone of tissue from the mouth of the cervix   _____

4. sterilization procedure that involves tying off the fallopian tubes   _____

5. birth of an infant by a surgical incision into the uterus   _____

6. procedure that uses saline-filled silicone implants to reshape a breast   _____

7. surgical treatment of breast cancer that spares the chest wall and takes fewer lymph nodes   _____

8. complete removal of all pelvic organs   _____

9. use of cold to destroy tissue   _____

10. the surgical removal of a polyp   _____

_____

*Answers are in Appendix A.

MATCHING
Match the terms to their meanings.

1. _____ inflammation of the inner mucous lining of the cervix

2. _____ abnormally frequent menstruation

3. _____ gravest form of toxemia

4. _____ benign tumors in the uterus

5. _____ protrusion of the rectum into the vagina

6. _____ inflammation of pelvic tissue

7. _____ protrusion of the bladder through the vaginal wall

8. _____ cancer confined to the original site

9. _____ vaginitis caused by a specific bacteria

10. _____ test done on malignant tumor for receptivity to estrogen

11. _____ blood test that detects level of protein produced by the fetus

12. _____ test ordered to determine oxygen and CO_2 levels or genetic disease in fetus

a. fibroids

b. PID

c. carcinoma in situ

d. cystocele

e. polymenorrhea

f. eclampsia

g. endocervicitis

h. rectocele

i. Hemophilus vaginitis

j. percutaneous umbilical cord sampling

k. estrogen receptor test

l. alpha-fetoprotein analysis

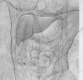

Word Element Review

Root	Meaning	Example	Definition
adnex/o	tie, connection	**adnexa** (ăd-nĕk′sah)	appendages
amni/o	amnion	**amniocentesis** (ăm″nē-ō-sĕn-tē′sĭs)	puncture of the amniotic sac to remove amniotic fluid for examination
cervic/o	neck, cervix	**cervix uteri** (ser′vĭks ū′ter-ī)	neck of the uterus
colp/o	vagina	**colpoperineorrhaphy** (kŏl″pō-pĕr″ĭ-nē-or′ah-fē)	operation for mending perineal tears in the vagina
episi/o	vulva	**episiotomy** (ĕ-pĭz″ē-ŏt′ō-mē)	incision of the perineum at the end of the second stage of labor to prevent tearing
gravid/o	pregnancy	**gravida** (grăv′ĭ-dah)	pregnant woman
gynec/o	female	**gynecologic** (gī″nĕ-kō-lŏj′ĭk)	pertaining to the female reproductive tract
hyster/o	uterus	**hysterectomy** (his″tĕ-rĕk′tō-mē)	excision of the uterus
lact/o	milk	**lactation** (lăk-tā′shŭn)	period of milk secretion
mamm/o	breast	**mammary** (măm′er-ē)	pertaining to the breast
mast/o	breast	**mastalgia** (măs-tăl-jē-ah)	pain in the breast
men/o	menses	**menorrhagia** (mĕn″ō-rā′jē-ah)	excessive bleeding during menstruation
metr/o	uterus	**metrorrhagia** (mē″trō-rā′jē-ah)	abnormal bleeding from the uterus, especially at a time other than menstruation
oophor/o	ovary	**oophorectomy** (ō″ŏf-ō-rĕk′tō-mē)	excision of one or both ovaries
ovari/o	ovary	**ovarian** (ō-vă′rē-ăn)	pertaining to or resembling an ovary
ov/i, ov/o, ovul/o	egg	**ovum, ova** (ō′vŭm), (ō′vah)	egg, eggs
papill/o	nipplelike	**papilla** (pah-pĭl′ah)	small, nipplelike elevation
pect/o, pector/o	breast, chest	**pectoral** (pĕk′tō-răl)	pertaining to the breast or chest
salping/o	tube	**salpingocele** (săl-pĭng′gō-sēl)	herniation of a fallopian tube
thel/o	nipple	**thelitis** (thē-lī′tĭs)	inflammation of the nipple
umbilic/o	navel	**umbilical** (ŭm-bĭl′ĭ-kăl)	pertaining to the naval (umbilicus)
uter/o	uterus	**uterocervical** (ū″ter-ō-ser′vĭ-kăl)	pertaining to the uterus and cervix
vagin/o	vagina	**vaginitis** (văj″ĭ-nī′tĭs)	inflammation of the vagina
vulv/o	vulva	**vulvovaginal** (vul″vō-văj′ĭ-năl)	pertaining to the vulva and vagina

Prefix	Meaning	Example	Definition
par-, part-	bear	**parturition** (păr″tū-rĭsh′ŭn)	process of giving birth
prol-	offspring	**proliferation** (prō-lĭf″ĕ-rā′shŭn)	reproduction of similar forms

Word Element Review Exercises

Name: _____ Date: _____

WORD ELEMENTS
Provide the correct word element to complete the following words.

1. process of giving birth   _____ turition
2. pertaining to the ovary   _____ an
3. excision of the uterus   _____ ectomy
4. suture of tears in the vagina and perineum   _____ rrhaphy
5. incision of the vulva for obstetric purposes   _____ otomy
6. abnormal bleeding from the uterus   _____ orrhagia
7. puncture of the amniotic sac to remove fluid for examination   _____ centesis
8. pertaining to the female reproductive tract   _____ logic
9. inflammation of the vagina   _____ itis
10. pertaining to the navel   _____ al
11. pain in the breast   _____ algia
12. inflammation of the nipple   _____ itis

MATCHING*
Match the meanings to their word elements.

1. _____ appendages
2. _____ neck of the uterus
3. _____ pregnant woman
4. _____ pertaining to vulva and vagina
5. _____ small nipplelike elevation
6. _____ reproduction of similar forms
7. _____ excision of one or both ovaries
8. _____ pertaining to the uterus and cervix
9. _____ period of milk secretion
10. _____ egg or eggs
11. _____ herniation of a fallopian tube
12. _____ pertaining to the breast
13. _____ pertaining to the breast or chest
14. _____ excessive bleeding during menstruation

a. cervix uteri
b. gravida
c. lactation
d. mammary
e. menorrhagia
f. adnexa
g. oophorectomy
h. ovum, ova
i. papilla
j. pectoral
k. proliferation
l. salpingocele
m. uterocervical
n. vulvovaginal

_____

*Answers are in Appendix A.

WORD ELEMENT MEANINGS

Give the meaning of each word element. Then use your dictionary to find a new word that contains each of the word elements. Specify whether the new word is a noun or an adjective by placing N or A in the last column.

Word Element	Meaning	Word	N or A
1. adnex/o			
2. amni/o			
3. cervic/o			
4. colp/o			
5. episi/o			
6. gravid/o			
7. gynec/o			
8. hyster/o			
9. lact/o			
10. mamm/o			
11. mast/o			
12. men/o			
13. metr/o			
14. oophor/o			
15. ovari/o			
16. ov/i			
17. ov/o			
18. ovul/o			
19. papill/o			
20. par-			
21. part-			
22. pect/o			
23. pector/o			
24. prol-			
25. salping/o			
26. thel/o			
27. umbilic/o			
28. uter/o			
29. vagin/o			
30. vulv/o			

Dictionary Exercises

Name: _____ Date: _____

DICTIONARY EXERCISE 1*

Use your dictionary to find the pronunciation and definition of the following words:

Word	Pronunciation	Definition
1. adenomatous	_____	_____
2. anteflexion	_____	_____
3. caput	_____	_____
4. climacteric	_____	_____
5. engagement	_____	_____
6. forceps	_____	_____
7. fourchette	_____	_____
8. hematocele	_____	_____
9. hematocolpos	_____	_____
10. hematosalpinx	_____	_____
11. mesothelioma	_____	_____
12. oligohydramnios	_____	_____
13. paraurethral	_____	_____
14. puerperium	_____	_____
15. toxic shock syndrome	_____	_____

DICTIONARY EXERCISE 2*

Provide the pronunciation and select the correct meaning of each term.

1. canal of Nuck (_____)
   a. structure in the female pelvis containing ovarian vessels and nerves
   b. opening to the vagina
   c. prolongation of peritoneal cavity between anterior surface of the rectum and posterior surface of the uterus
   d. persistent peritoneal pouch that accompanies the round ligament of the uterus through the inguinal canal

2. primigravida (_____)
   a. early weeks of a pregnancy
   b. woman's first pregnancy
   c. abdominal stretch marks during pregnancy
   d. woman who has given birth for the first time

3. cul-de-sac of Douglas (_____)
   a. pouch that accompanies the round ligament of the uterus through the inguinal canal
   b. prolongation of peritoneal cavity between anterior surface of the rectum and posterior surface of the uterus
   c. small cyst at the terminal end of the fallopian tube
   d. structure in the female pelvis containing the ovarian vessels and nerves

4. dystocia (_____)
   a. painful, difficult delivery or birth
   b. painful menses
   c. congenital absence of a normal body opening
   d. menstruation

---

*Answers are in Appendix A.

5. chorion (_____)
   a. head
   b. menstruation
   c. outer membrane around the fetus
   d. before the onset of labor

6. velamentous insertion (_____)
   a. umbilical cord attachment to membranes instead of to the placenta
   b. entrance to the vagina
   c. pouch that accompanies the round ligament of the uterus through the inguinal canal
   d. long grasping forceps used in vaginal hysterectomies

7. hydrosalpinx (_____)
   a. excessive accumulation of amniotic fluid
   b. distention of the fallopian tube by a clear fluid
   c. retained menstrual blood in the vagina
   d. malignant tumor of the ovary

8. uterine serosa (_____)
   a. near the urethra
   b. menstruation
   c. thin peritoneal covering of the uterus
   d. outer membrane around the fetus

9. antepartum (_____)
   a. time it takes the uterus to return to normal after delivery
   b. thin peritoneal covering of the uterus
   c. forward flexion of the body of the uterus upon the cervix
   d. before the onset of labor

10. oligomenorrhea (_____)
    a. painful or difficult menstruation
    b. fewer than normal number of menstrual periods in a year
    c. failure of menstruation
    d. heavy periods

11. amnion (_____)
    a. before the onset of menstruation
    b. outer membrane around the fetus
    c. bag of water holding the fetus
    d. thin peritoneal covering of the uterus

DICTIONARY EXERCISE 3

Provide the pronunciation for the italicized words and then rewrite the sentences in your own words.

1. The patient was *gravida* IV (_____), para II, and there was concern about *Couvelaire* (_____) uterus.

   _____

2. During her first delivery, *version* (_____) was necessary.

   _____

3. The physician saw that the patient had presented with a *prolapse* (_____) of the umbilical cord during labor.

   _____

4. The danger of *hyaline* (_____) membrane disease is present in many premature deliveries.

   _____

5. The patient was relieved that she had a *Brenner's* (_____) tumor rather than a malignant tumor.

_____

6. The physician suspected *hydatid of Morgagni* (_____).

_____

7. The nurse checked the baby's *fontanelles* (_____).

_____

8. The final diagnosis was *dysgerminoma* (_____).

_____

9. Her problem was caused by an *arrhenoblastoma* (_____).

_____

10. On Friday, the patient will undergo *colpoperineoplasty* (_____).

_____

11. The obstetrician administered a *pudendal block* (_____).

_____

12. Sometimes delivery requires a *vacuum extractor* (_____).

_____

DICTIONARY EXERCISE 4

Pronunciation of the words below is provided. Using your dictionary, find the correct spelling and definition of each word.

	Word	Pronunciation	Definition
1.	_____	ah-trē'zē-ah	_____
2.	_____	kăt"ah-mē'nē-ah	_____
3.	_____	kō'ĭ-tŭs	_____
4.	_____	hĕm"ah-tō-mē'trah	_____
5.	_____	hī-drăm'nē-ŏs	_____
6.	_____	ĭn"fŭn-dĭb"ū-lō-pĕl'vĭk	_____
7.	_____	ĭn-trō'ĭ-tŭs	_____
8.	_____	pī"ō-mē'trah	_____
9.	_____	vă'sah prē'vē-ah	_____
10.	_____	mŭl-tĭp'ah-rus	_____

MALE REPRODUCTIVE SYSTEM

The male reproductive system consists of several organs—the testes, epididymis, vas deferens (all of which are paired), the ejaculatory duct, urethra, and penis. The accessory organs are the seminal vesicles, prostate gland, and Cowper's or bulbourethral glands. Note each of the organs in Figure 17-1.

TESTES (TESTICLES)

orch/o, orchi/o, orchid/o	testis	sperm/o, spermat/o	spermatozoa
scrot/o	scrotum	test/o	testes, testicles

The male **testes** (tĕs'tēz) (8) are located outside the body in a sac of skin called the **scrotum** (skrō'tŭm) (7). The testes begin their development in the abdominopelvic cavity and later move or descend into the scrotum. This places the testes in an environment where the optimum temperature can be maintained for sperm production and maturation. **Spermatozoa** (sper"mah-tō-zō'ah) (sperm) development occurs in highly convoluted structures in

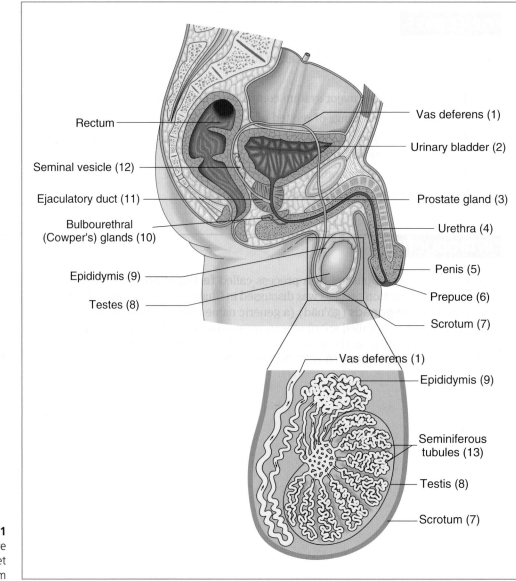

FIGURE 17-1
Male Reproductive System with Inset of Scrotum

the testes called **seminiferous tubules** (sě"mĭ-nĭf'er-ŭs too'būles) (13). A single sperm has a body and tail and is about one six hundredth of an inch long. The tail enables the sperm to move (See Figure 17-2).

Also produced in the testes is the male sex hormone **testosterone** (těs-tŏs'tě-rōn). This hormone is responsible for the growth of facial and body hair and for the deepening of the male voice, sexual drive, and the ability to have an erection.

EPIDIDYMIS

epididym/o	epididymis

Sperm need to mature after they are produced. Maturation begins to take place in the **epididymis** (ěp"ĭ-dĭd'ĭ-mĭs) (9) as shown in Figure 17-1. Sperm continue to mature as they move through the epididymis, which is a coiled tube 20 feet long. Eventually the spermatozoa reach the vas deferens.

VAS DEFERENS

vas/o	vessel, duct

The **vas deferens** (văs děf'er-ěnz) (1) is a tube or duct that is a continuation of the epididymis. There is one on each side of the midline. Its path is upward from the epididymis to the inferior portion of the urinary bladder (2). Here it is joined by ducts of the seminal vesicles.

SEMINAL VESICLES

semen, semin/o	seed	vesicul/o	seminal vesicles

There are two **seminal vesicles** (sěm'ĭ-năl věs'ĭ-k'ls) (12), or membranous pouches. The duct of each joins with a vas deferens to form an ejaculatory duct. Seminal vesicles produce a protective fluid that is added to spermatozoa at the time of ejaculation.

EJACULATORY DUCT

The union of both vas deferens and the seminal vesicle is called the **ejaculatory** (ē-jăk'ū-lah-tō"rē) **duct** (11). This duct passes through the prostate and enters the urethra just below where the urethra exits from the urinary bladder. Spermatozoa are propelled from the vas deferens into the urethra (4) by contraction of the ejaculatory duct. This occurs at the culmination of sexual arousal.

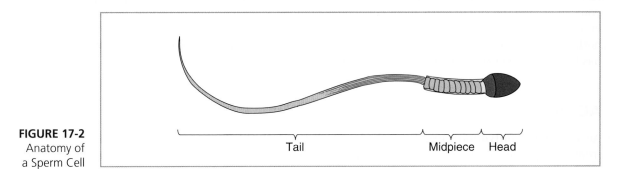

FIGURE 17-2
Anatomy of
a Sperm Cell

Tail   Midpiece   Head

DIAGNOSTIC PROCEDURES

Word	Pronunciation	Definition
General		
digital rectal examination (DRE)		examination of the prostate gland using finger palpation through the rectum
semen analysis		procedure in which sperm cells are counted and examined for motility and shape
Laboratory Tests		
prostate specific antigen (PSA)		blood test used to help identify prostrate carcinoma and monitor effectiveness of therapy for prostate cancer
prostatic acid phosphatase (PAP)	prŏs-tat'-ĭk as'ĭd fŏs'fah-tās"	blood test used to help identify prostate carcinomas or other conditions such as benign prostatic hypertrophy

DIAGNOSES

Word	Pronunciation	Definition
Testicles and Scrotum		
carcinoma of testes	kăr"sĭ-nō'mah; tĕs'tēz	malignant tumor of the testicles: seminoma is most common (See Figure 17-3)
cryptorchidism, cryptorchism	krĭpt-or'kĭ-dĭzm, krĭpt-or'kĭzm	failure of the testicle(s) to descend into the scrotum one month before birth; undescended testicle (See Figure 17-4)
epididymitis	ĕp"ĭ-dĭd"ĭ-mī'tĭs	inflammation of the epididymis (See Figure 17-5)
hydrocele	hī'drō-sēl	collection of fluid in the scrotum surrounding the testes (See Figure 17-6B)

continues

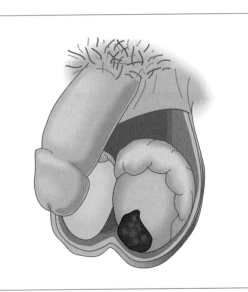

FIGURE 17-3   Carcinoma of the Testes

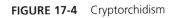

FIGURE 17-4   Cryptorchidism

Absent testicle

DIAGNOSES

Word	Pronunciation	Definition
Testicles and Scrotum (continued)		
orchitis	ōr-kī'tĭs	inflammation of a testicle
spermatocele	spĕr-măt'ō-sēl	cyst of the epididymis containing sperm
testicular torsion	tĕs-tĭk'ū-lăr tŏr'shŭn	rotation producing ischemia of the testes
varicocele	văr'ĭ-kō-sēl	enlarged, dilated veins near the testicle (See Figure 17-6C)
Penis, Urethra, Bladder		
balanitis	băl-ă-nī'tĭs	inflammation of the glans penis or glans clitoris
cystitis	sĭs-tī'tĭs	inflammation of the bladder
epispadias	ĕp-ĭ-spā'dē-ăs	malformation in which the urethra opens on the dorsum of the penis (See Figure 17-7)

continues

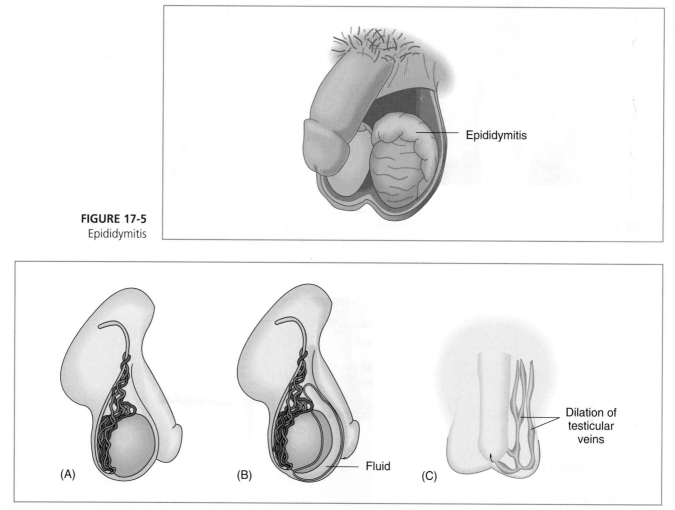

FIGURE 17-5
Epididymitis

FIGURE 17-6   Hydrocele and Varicocele: (A) normal; (B) hydrocele; (C) varicocele

The Male Reproductive System ■ **459**

DIAGNOSES		
Word	Pronunciation	Definition
Penis, Urethra, Bladder (continued)		
hypospadia, hypospadias	hī"pō-spā'dē-ah	developmental anomaly characterized by an abnormal urethral opening on the ventral side of the penis (See Figure 17-8)
paraphimosis	păr"ă-fī-mō'sĭs	painful swelling at the end of an uncircumcised penis due to failure to reduce (pull forward) the prepuce
phimosis	fī-mō'sĭs	narrowness of the opening of the prepuce preventing its withdrawal (See Figure 17-9)
urethral stricture	ū-rē'thral	narrowing lesion of the urethra

continues

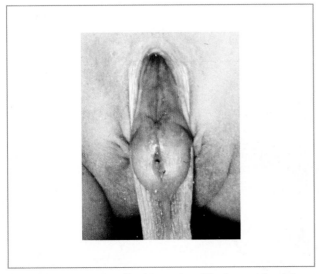

FIGURE 17-7   Epispadias (Courtesy of Dr. James Mandell, Children's Hospital, Boston)

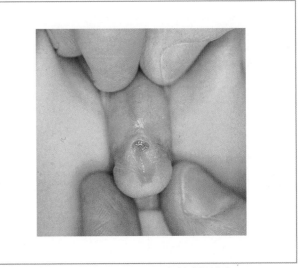

FIGURE 17-8   Hypospadias (Courtesy of Dr. James Mandell, Children's Hospital, Boston)

FIGURE 17-9
Phimosis
(Courtesy of Dr. James Mandell, Children's Hospital, Boston)

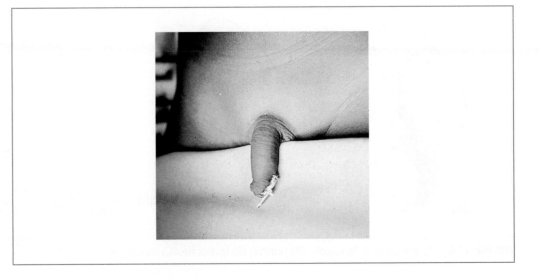

DIAGNOSES

Word	Pronunciation	Definition
Penis, Urethra, Bladder (*continued*)		
urethritis	ū"rē-thrī'tĭs	inflammation of the urethra
urinary incontinence	ū'rĭ-nār"ē	inability to control urination some of the time
Prostate Gland		
benign prostatic hypertrophy (BPH)	bē-nīn' prŏs-tăt'ĭk hī-per'trō-fē	benign overgrowth of the prostate gland; hyperplasia of the prostate
carcinoma of the prostate	kăr"sĭ-nō'mah; prŏs'tāt	malignant tumor of the prostate
prostatitis	prŏs"tah-tī'tĭs	inflammation of the prostate gland; may be acute or chronic
Sexual Dysfunction		
condyloma (genital warts)	kon"di-lo'mah	warts caused by papilloma virus
impotence	ĭm'pō-tĕnse	inability of male to achieve or maintain a penile erection
Peyronie's disease	pā-rŏn-ēz'	induration (hardening) of part of the penis
premature ejaculation	ē-jăk"ū-lā'shŭn	ejaculation too soon to satisfy the sexual partner
priapism	prī' ă-pĭzm	prolonged, painful erection of penis with no associated sexual excitement
retrograde ejaculation	rĕt'rō-grād ē-jăk"ū-lā'shŭn	little or no semen is ejaculated from the penis during sexual climax

TREATMENT PROCEDURES

Word	Pronunciation	Definition
circumcision	ser"kŭm-sĭzh'ŭn	removal of the end of the prepuce; usually performed on infant males in this culture as a hygienic measure; religious rite in the Hebrew culture
hydrocelectomy	hī"drō-sē-lĕk'tō-mē	excision of a hydrocele (sac containing watery fluid)
orchiectomy (castration)	or"kē-ĕk'tō-mē	excision of one or both testes
orchiopexy	or"kē-ō-pĕk'sē	surgical fixation of an undescended testis in the scrotum; brings testes into the scrotum
prostatectomy (perineal, suprapubic/ transvesical, or retropubic)	prŏs"tah-tĕk'tō-mē	removal of the prostate
transurethral incision of the prostate (TUIP)	trăns"ū-rē'thrăl; prŏs'tāt	surgical procedure that makes small cuts in the bladder neck to widen the urethra

continues

TREATMENT PROCEDURES

Word	Pronunciation	Definition
transurethral microwave thermotherapy (TUMT)	trăns"ū-rē'thrăl; thĕr"mō-thĕr'ă-pē	nonsurgical treatment for destruction of prostate tissue
transurethral needle ablation (TUNA)	trăns"ū-rē'thrăl; ăb-lā'shŭn	treatment using low-level radiofrequency energy through needles to burn away a defined region of an enlarged prostate
transurethral resection of the prostate (TURP)	trăns"ū-rē'thrăl	procedure in which an endoscope is passed through the urethra, and prostate tissue is removed by electrocautery, cryogenic, laser, or hyperthermia techniques (See Figure 17-10)
vasectomy	vah-sĕk'tō-mē	removal of all or a segment of the vas deferens to produce sterility in the male (See Figure 17–11)

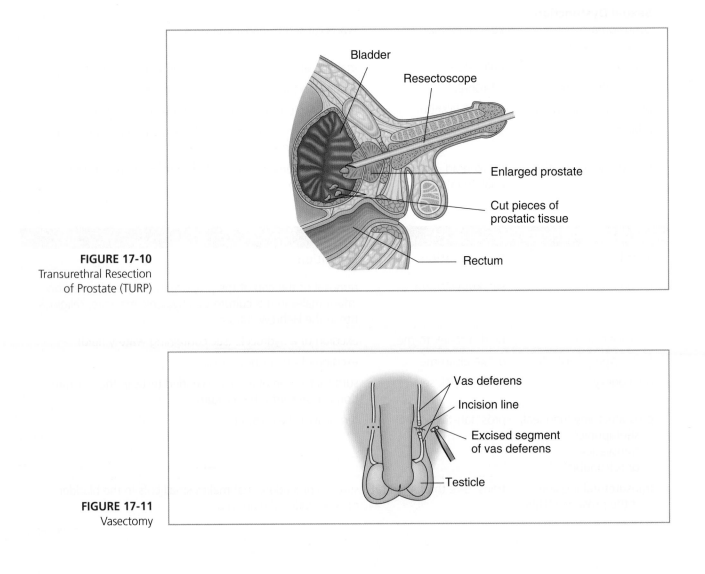

FIGURE 17-10
Transurethral Resection of Prostate (TURP)

Bladder

Resectoscope

Enlarged prostate

Cut pieces of prostatic tissue

Rectum

FIGURE 17-11
Vasectomy

Vas deferens

Incision line

Excised segment of vas deferens

Testicle

MEDICATIONS PRESCRIBED

Trade Name	Generic Name
Antibiotics	
Bactrim, Septra	sulfamethoxazole and trimethoprim
Cipro	ciprofloxacin
Noroxin	norfloxacin
Gonadotropins	
Pergonal	menotropins
For Impotence	
Viagra	sildenafil
Yocon	yohimbine

ABBREVIATIONS

BPH	benign prostatic hypertrophy
DRE	digital rectal examination
GU	genitourinary
NGU	nongonococcal urethritis
PAP	prostatic acid phosphatase
PSA	prostate specific antigen
TRUS	transrectal ultrasound
TUIP	transurethral incision of the prostate
TUMT	transurethral microwave thermotherapy
TUNA	transurethral needle ablation
TURP	transurethral resection of the prostate

MALE AND FEMALE SEXUALLY TRANSMITTED DISEASES (VENEREAL DISEASES)

Word	Pronunciation	Definition
Laboratory Tests		
cytomegalovirus test (CMV)	sī"tō-mĕg"ah-lo-vi'rus	test for the presence of cytomegalovirus
enzyme-linked immunosorbent assay (ELISA)*		blood test to detect for the presence of HIV antibodies
FTA-ABS test		test for syphilis
Gram stain/culture		test for gonorrhea or other bacterial infection

continues

---

*See Chapter 9 for additional information.

MALE AND FEMALE SEXUALLY TRANSMITTED DISEASES (VENEREAL DISEASES)

Word	Pronunciation	Definition
Laboratory Tests *(continued)*		
rapid plasma reagin (RPR)	rē'ah-jĭn	test for syphilis
TORCH test (toxoplasma, other infections, rubella, cyto-megalovirus, and herpes simplex virus)		test performed on the mother and newborn to determine exposure to any of the diseases caused by specific viruses
VDRL (Venereal Disease Research Laboratory) test		one of the screening tests for syphilis
Western blot		test to confirm the presence of the human immuno-deficiency virus (HIV)
Diagnoses		
acquired immune deficiency syndrome (AIDS)*		advanced stage of HIV infection, which is characterized by opportunistic infections, malignancies, and other disorders
chlamydia infection	klah-mĭd'ē-ah	genital infection in men and women caused by the bacteria *Chlamydia*; known as the "silent STD" because its symptoms may be mild
cytomegalic inclusion disease (CID)	sī"tō-mĕg"ăl'ĭk	viral infection that is transmitted in the uterus from the mother to the fetus
cytomegalovirus (CMV)	sī"tō-mĕg"ah-lo-vi'rus	herpes-type virus with a wide variety of disease effects
genital herpes, herpes genitalis	jĕn'ĭ-tăl hĕr'pēz; hĕr'pēz jĕn'ĭ-tăl-ĭs	infection of the skin and the mucosa of the genitals; caused by the herpes simplex virus (HSV)
gonorrhea	gŏn"ō-rē'ah	inflammation of the genital tract mucosa membrane caused by gonococcus
human immunodeficiency virus (HIV)*		viral infection that damages the body's natural immune defenses against disease; an infected individual may transmit the virus to another through the exchange of body fluids; this can be from sexual activity, sharing of contaminated needles and syringes, untested blood transfusion, or from mother to child during pregnancy or birth
syphilis	sĭf'ĭ-lĭs	chronic, infectious disease caused by spirochete bacterium, affecting any organ of the body
trichomoniasis	trĭk"ō-mō-nī'ah-sĭs	infection of the genitourinary tract caused by Trichomonas
venereal warts (genital warts)	vĕ-nē'rē-ăl	sexually transmitted condition caused by the human papillomavirus (HPV) that affects both men and women; may appear in men on the shaft or near the end of the penis or on the scrotum, and in women on the vaginal lips, inside the vagina, on the cervix, or around the anus

*See Chapter 9 for additional information.

MEDICATIONS PRESCRIBED FOR SEXUALLY TRANSMITTED DISEASES

Trade Name	Generic Name
Achromycin V	tetracycline
Ampicill, Ampicillin	ampicillin
Benemid	probenecid
Bicillin, Wycillin, Beepen-VK, Pen-Vee-K, Betapen-VK	penicillin
Flagyl	metronidazole
Gyne-Lotrimin, Mycelex	clotrimazole
Rocephin	ceftriaxone
Vibramycin	doxycycline
Zovirax	acyclovir

ABBREVIATIONS

CID	cytomegalic inclusion disease
CMV	cytomegalovirus
ELISA	enzyme-linked immunosorbent assay
HIV	human immunodeficiency virus
HSV	herpes simplex virus
RPR	rapid plasma reagin
STD	sexually transmitted disease
STI	sexually transmitted infection
VD	venereal disease
VDRL	Venereal Disease Research Laboratories

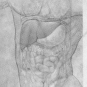

Working Practice Review Exercises

Name: _____ Date: _____

MATCHING
Match the terms to their meanings.

1. _____ a count and examination of spermatozoa
2. _____ excision of one or both testes
3. _____ inflammation of the prostate
4. _____ removal of prostate tissue by electrocautery or cryogenic techniques
5. _____ male sterilization procedure
6. _____ removal of the end of the prepuce
7. _____ surgical fixation of a testis
8. _____ an enlarged, swollen vein near the spermatic cord
9. _____ excision of the prostate gland
10. _____ testicle that has failed to drop into the scrotum
11. _____ rotation producing ischemia of the testes
12. _____ inflammation of the urinary bladder
13. _____ fluid in the scrotum or tubes leading from the testes
14. _____ abnormal urethral opening on the penis
15. _____ induration of part of the penis
16. _____ narrowing lesion of the urethra
17. _____ inflammation of the testicle
18. _____ inflammation of the urethra

a. circumcision
b. cryptorchidism
c. cystitis
d. hydrocele
e. hypospadia
f. orchiectomy
g. orchiopexy
h. orchitis
i. Peyronie's disease
j. prostatectomy
k. prostatitis
l. semen analysis
m. testicular torsion
n. transurethral resection of the prostate
o. urethritis
p. urethral stricture
q. variocele
r. vasectomy

MATCH ABBREVIATIONS
Match the meanings with their abbreviations.

1. _____ test for syphilis
2. _____ acquired immune deficiency syndrome
3. _____ venereal disease
4. _____ herpes simplex virus
5. _____ cytomegalovirus
6. _____ human immunodeficiency virus
7. _____ enzyme-linked immunosorbent assay
8. _____ rapid plasma reagin/test of syphilis
9. _____ cytomegalic inclusion disease
10. _____ sexually transmitted disease

a. AIDS
b. CID
c. CMV
d. ELISA
e. HIV
f. HSV
g. RPR
h. STD
i. VD
j. VDRL

COMPLETION*

Complete the following statements about sexually transmitted diseases.

1. An infection of the genitourinary tract is _____.

2. A test for gonorrhea is _____.

3. A test used to confirm the presence of HIV is the _____.

4. _____ is a bacterial infection found in both men and women and known as the "silent STD."

5. Infection of the skin and the mucosa of the genitals is called _____.

6. A _____ is performed on mother and newborn to determine exposure to any of several viral diseases.

7. Viral infection that is transmitted in the uterus from mother to fetus is called _____.

8. A test for syphilis is _____.

9. The advanced stage of HIV infection is known as _____.

10. _____ are a sexually transmitted condition caused by the human papillomavirus that affects both men and women.

ABBREVIATION MEANINGS*

Identify the following abbreviations. Specify whether it is a diagnosis (D), test (T), or procedure (P).

Abbreviation	Meaning	D, T, or P
1. BPH	_____	_____
2. DRE	_____	_____
3. PAP	_____	_____
4. TURP	_____	_____
5. PSA	_____	_____
6. TUIP	_____	_____

*Answers are in Appendix A.

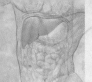

Word Element Review

Root	Meaning	Example	Definition
balan/o	glans penis	**balanitis** (băl"ah-nī'tĭs)	inflammation of the glans penis and mucous membrane beneath it
epididym/o	epididymis	**epididymotomy** (ĕp"ĭ-dĭd-ĭ-mŏt'ō-mē)	incision into the epididymis
orch/o, orchi/o orchid/o	testis	**orchiopathy** (ŏr"kē-ŏp'ah-thē)	any disease or condition of the testes
prostat/o	prostate gland	**prostatism** (prŏs'tah-tĭzm)	any condition of the prostate gland that causes retention of urine in the bladder
scrot/o	bag, pouch	**scrotum** (skrō'tŭm)	pouch containing the testes
semen, semin/o	seed	**seminal** (sĕm'ĭ-năl)	pertaining to the semen or to seed
sperm/o, spermat/o	spermatozoa	**spermatic** (spĕr-măt'ĭk)	pertaining to semen or spermatozoa
test/o	testes, testicles	**testicle** (tĕs'tĭ-k'l)	the testis; the male gonad
		testicular (tĕs'tĭk'ū-lăr)	pertaining to the male testes
vas/o	vessel, duct	**vasorrhaphy** (văs-ŏr'ah-fē)	suture of the vas deferens
vesicul/o	seminal vessels	**vesiculitis** (vĕ-sĭk"ū-lī'tĭs)	inflammation of a vessel, particularly the seminal vesicle

Word Element Review Exercises

Name: _____ Date: _____

WORD ELEMENTS*

Provide the correct word element to complete the following words.

1. any disease of the testes   _____ pathy
2. incision into the epididymis   _____ otomy
3. the male gonad   _____ icle
4. inflammation of the seminal vesicle   _____ itis
5. any condition of the prostate gland that causes retention of urine in the bladder   _____ ism
6. pertaining to semen or sperm   _____ ic
7. suture of the vas deferens   _____ rrhaphy
8. inflammation of glans penis and mucous membrane beneath it   _____ itis
9. pouch containing testicles   _____ um
10. pertaining to semen   _____ al

MATCHING

Match the word elements to their meanings.

1. _____ spermatozoa   a. orch/o, orchi/o, orchid/o
2. _____ testes   b. spermat/o
3. _____ epididymis   c. vas/o
4. _____ prostate gland   d. vesicul/o
5. _____ vessel   e. epididym/o
6. _____ glans penis   f. prostat/o
7. _____ seminal vessels   g. balan/o
8. _____ bag, pouch   h. scrot/o
9. _____ seed   i. semin/o
     j. test/o

_____

*Answers are in Appendix A.

WORD ELEMENT MEANINGS

Give the meaning of each word element. Then use your dictionary to find a new word that contains each of the word elements. Specify whether the new word is a noun or an adjective by placing N or A in the last column.

Word Element	Meaning	Word	N or A
1. balan/o			
2. epididym/o			
3. orch/o			
4. orchi/o			
5. orchid/o			
6. prostat/o			
7. scrot/o			
8. semen			
9. semin/o			
10. sperm/o			
11. spermat/o			
12. test/o			
13. vas/o			
14. vesicul/o			

Dictionary Exercises

Name: _____ Date: _____

DICTIONARY EXERCISE 1*

Provide the pronunciation and select the meaning of each term.

1. anorchism (_____)
   a. narrowing of the opening of the prepuce
   b. congenital absence of one or both testes
   c. male deprived of testes or external genitals
   d. absence of sperm in semen

2. ejaculation (_____)
   a. ejection of sperm and fluid from the male urethra
   b. a tube formed by union of vas deferens and duct of seminal vesicles
   c. secretion responsible for male sex characteristics
   d. formation of sperm

3. corpora cavernosa (_____)
   a. abnormal congenital opening on the underside of the penis
   b. deficient amount of sperm in the seminal fluid
   c. narrowing of the opening of the prepuce
   d. two columns of erectile tissue lying side by side that form the bulk of the penis

4. perineum (_____)
   a. pelvic floor
   b. area between anus and scrotum in the male
   c. tissue composed of the essential cells of any organ
   d. skin covering the tip of the penis

5. vasovasostomy (_____)
   a. removal of all or a segment of the vas deferens to produce male sterility
   b. excision of one or both testes
   c. surgical fixation of undescended testes in the scrotum
   d. reversal of a vasectomy by rejoining the cut ends of vas deferens

6. oligospermia (_____)
   a. deficient amount of sperm in the seminal fluid
   b. malignant tumor of the testes
   c. absence of sperm in the semen
   d. failure of testes to ejaculate semen

7. masturbation (_____)
   a. stimulation of the genital organs by some means other than sexual intercourse
   b. deficiency of the testes or their secretion with impaired sexual power and eunuchoid symptoms
   c. inability of the male to achieve an erection to perform sexual intercourse successfully
   d. sensitive tip of the penis

8. eunuchoidism (_____)
   a. male deprived of testes or external genitals
   b. inability of the male to achieve a sufficient erection
   c. stimulation of the genital organs by some means other than intercourse
   d. deficiency of the testes or their secretion with impaired sexual power and eunuchoid symptoms

---

*Answers are in Appendix A.

DICTIONARY EXERCISE 2

Pronunciation of the words below is provided. Using your dictionary, find the correct spelling and definition for each of these words.

Word	Pronunciation	Definition
1. _____	spĕr"măt-ō-jĕn'ĕ-sĭs	_____
2. _____	ah-spĕr'mē-ah	_____
3. _____	shăng'kĕr	_____
4. _____	spĕr"măt-ō-zō'ŏn	_____
5. _____	tĕr-ă-tō'mah	_____
6. _____	ū'nŭk	_____
7. _____	sĕm"ē-nō'mah	_____
8. _____	băl'ă-nō-plăs"tē	_____
9. _____	ă-zō"ō-spĕr'mē-ah	_____
10. _____	ăn'drō-jen	_____
11. _____	tĕs-tĭk'ū-lăr	_____
12. _____	ĭn"tĕr-stĭsh'ăl	_____
13. _____	kō'ĭ-tŭs ĭn-tĕr-rŭp'tŭs	_____
14. _____	ăn-ŏr'kĭz-ĕm	_____
15. _____	pō'tĕn-sē	_____
16. _____	spĕr-mō-lĭt'ĭk	_____
17. _____	flă-jĕl'ŭm	_____
18. _____	vĕ-nĕ'rē-ăl	_____
19. _____	stĕr"ĭl-ĭ-zā'shŭn	_____

Listening Exercise

INSTRUCTIONS

1. Review the spelling, pronunciation, and meaning of the words provided in the preview.

2. Listen to the audio CD and fill in the blank as the word is dictated.

3. At the end of the exercise, check your spelling against the preview words. They appear in the preview in the order in which they are encountered in the exercise.

4. Review and practice the words you missed.

5. Look up words that are not familiar.

PREVIEW OF WORDS FOR LISTENING EXERCISE 17-1

Word	Pronunciation	Meaning
nocturia	nŏk-tū'rē-ah	urination during the night
hematuria	hĕm"ah-tū'rē-ah	blood in the urine
pyelogram	pī'ĕ-lō-grăm	picture of the renal pelvis and ureter after the injection of a contrast material
meatus	mē-ā'tŭs	passage or opening on body surface through which urine is discharged
spermatocele	spĕr-măt'ō-sēl	cyst of the epididymis containing sperm
testicle	tĕs'tĭ-k'l	male sex gland located in the scrotum
benign prostatic hypertrophy	bē-nīn' prŏs-tăt'ĭk hī-pĕr'trō-fē	benign overgrowth of the prostate gland

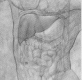

History and Physical Examination

HISTORY: This is an 81-year-old male referred by Dr. George with progressive symptoms of bladder outlet obstruction of approximately six to eight months' duration. He has experienced a decrease in the size of force of stream, strains to void, _____ × 2, and has some slight precipitant urgency. No history of urinary tract infection. About a month ago he noted _____ on several occasions with burning on urination and urgency. It cleared by forcing fluids. There is no history of calculus disease or previous retention. An intravenous _____ is being done on the day of admission.

PAST HISTORY: Surgery: He had an appendectomy in 1967 and a left inguinal hernia in 1942. He has never had cardiac symptoms, hypertension, myocardial infarction, or angina. He has not used cardiac medications. Allergies: No known drug allergies. No asthma or hay fever.

Review of Systems

RESPIRATORY: No hemoptysis or TB.

CARDIAC: Noncontributory at this time.

GASTROINTESTINAL: Denies ulcer, hematemesis, melena, jaundice, infectious mononucleosis, hepatitis, or diabetes.

GENITOURINARY: Symptoms and problems as described. No gross abnormalities present.

Physical Examination

GENERAL: This 81-year-old male is well developed, well nourished, alert, cooperative, and in no acute distress. Blood pressure is 160/80.

HEENT: Essentially negative. Mouth is clear.

NECK: Supple. Thyroid not enlarged.

CHEST: Symmetrical. Lungs are clear to auscultation and percussion.

HEART: No megaly, no murmurs.

ABDOMEN: Flat, no masses, with no flank pain or CVA pain. Bladder not distended.

GENITALIA: Penis has normal _____. Adequate scrotum and contents. He does seem to have a loculated _____ or hydrocele of the cord on the left. _____ itself is normal. Right scrotum and contents are normal.

RECTAL: About a 50-mm benign-feeling prostate. No other rectal masses.

EXTREMITIES: Negative.

IMPRESSION: 1. _____ _____ _____ with bladder outlet obstruction.

PLAN: Medical treatment will be initiated and tried for two weeks. Depending on progress, the patient will be advised as to the need for more aggressive intervention.

Pathology and Autopsies

> *Death should be distinguished from dying, with which it is often confounded.*
>
> —SYDNEY SMITH

When you have completed this chapter on pathology and autopsies, you should be able to

1. Identify and define components of surgical pathology and autopsy reports.
2. Identify the meanings of related word elements.
3. Spell the names of commonly used chemicals.
4. Identify abbreviations related to pathology and autopsy.
5. Be familiar with terminology that is dictated in reference to pathology reports and autopsies.

INTRODUCTION

Pathology (pă-thŏl'ō-jē) is a specialized branch of medicine that is concerned with disease-related deviations from normal anatomy and physiology. A **disease** usually refers to a condition in which there are abnormal symptoms occurring and a pathological state is present. A normal body is extraordinary in its ability to maintain **homeostasis** (hō"mē-ō-stā'sĭs), the state of normalcy; but when normalcy is not maintained, the body is said to be diseased. Two other terms are used interchangeably with disease, but they do not have exactly the same meaning. A **disorder** is often defined as an abnormality of function. A **syndrome** (sĭn'drōm) usually refers to a group of symptoms that may be caused by a specific disease or by several interrelated problems (e.g., Down syndrome).

    Pathologists (pă-thŏl'ō-jĭsts), who may be certified in clinical and/or anatomic pathology, are physicians who study disease. **Clinical pathology** is the study of blood and body fluids. Blood, urine, feces, and sputum are used in certain functional tests to determine the general working order of the body. These tests have been included with each system of the body.

    Anatomic (ăn"ă-tŏm'ĭk) **pathology** is the study of the effect of disease on the body structure as applied to both surgical pathology and autopsies. In either case, they take into account factors that are the cause or **etiology** (ē"tē-ŏl'ō-jē) of the disease; action of the disease; changes brought about in cells, tissues, organs, and the organism as a whole; any destructive forces; and the end result—healing.

In the study of disease, the pathologist uses a variety of terms to describe the disease or disease processes. Bacteria, viruses, fungi, protozoans, and helminth (worms) are **pathogens** (păth'ō-jĕnz) or agents that cause disease. **Pathogenesis** (păth"ō-jĕn'ĕ-sĭs) is a description of how a disease progresses. An acute disease is short term and includes problems such as pneumonia or a fracture. A chronic condition, such as hypertension or asthma, lasts for an extended period of time. If the cause or etiology is unknown, the term **idiopathic** (ĭd"ē-ō-păth'ĭk) is often used.

Surgical pathology is the study of body tissue removed by surgical means and seeks to identify and confirm the patient's disease or problem before, during, or after surgery. In doing so, prognosis and treatment will reflect the findings. Such tissue is placed in fixatives and chemical preparations to preserve it as close to its original state as possible. Samples are then sectioned, stained, placed upon a glass slide, and examined by means of a microscope.

Causes of disease are often divided into six categories.

1. *Hereditary diseases,* or congenital disorders, are caused by a genetic error and may be or may not be present at birth. They may also include problems during a pregnancy or a difficult delivery. Examples of hereditary diseases are cystic fibrosis, congenital heart anomalies, and Down syndrome.

2. *Traumatic diseases* are caused by physical injury from an external source. Motor vehicle accidents, falls, drowning, burns, ingesting or inhaling objects, poisoning, penetrating wounds, or physical abuse are responsible for most serious injury.

3. *Inflammation/infection* are the result of a protective immune response.

4. *Hyperplasias/neoplasms* are overgrowths of cells leading to an increase in tissue size. Hyperplasia is an overgrowth in response to a stimulus, while neoplasms are new growths (benign or malignant).

5. *Nutritional imbalance* may cause problems with physical growth, mental and intellectual retardation, and may even cause death. Malnutrition, obesity, and excessive or deficient vitamins or minerals are specific problems.

6. *Impaired immunity* occurs when part of the immune system breaks down, as in cases of allergy, autoimmunity, and immunodeficiency.

Certain factors predispose individuals to be more susceptible to disease—age, gender, environment, lifestyle, and heredity. Some factors cannot be controlled, such as age, but others, such as lifestyle, can be influenced by the individual.

Pathology specialists also generate autopsy reports. An **autopsy** (aw'tŏp-sē) is performed after the death of a patient. Chemical, bacteriologic, and analytic studies are performed on any part of the body. Tissue samples from all organs are eventually analyzed by microscope.

This chapter presents information about both surgical pathology and autopsy reports that will be encountered in the allied health field.

SURGICAL PATHOLOGY REPORT

During the course of an operation a surgeon must determine whether an inflammatory process or a malignancy is involved. This will often affect the extent of the surgery.

One method used to make the determination is to examine a quick-frozen tissue section. The procedure is simple. During surgery a small piece of tissue is given to the pathologist, who places it in an instrument that uses a quick-freezing technique. Freezing permits slicing thin sections of the sample for analysis under a microscope.

Other tests are applied to tissue samples that may require several days to complete. Therefore, the final report could be delayed until the additional information is made available.

All of this data is gathered in the Surgical Pathology Report. The Association of Directors of Anatomic and Surgical Pathology has recommended that all demographic information should be placed in the top portion of the report. This should include patient's name, location, gender, age and/or date of birth, and race; the requesting physician's name; the attending physician's name (if different from the requesting physician); and medical record or unit number.

The complete name and address of the laboratory should be presented at the top of the report, and the Surgical Pathology number should be in an easily identifiable location at the top of every page. A summary of pertinent Clinical History is also recommended.

Regardless of variations in reporting practices in individual institutions, a Surgical Pathology Report generally consists of three sections: the Gross Description, the Microscopic Description, and the Pathologic Diagnoses.

GROSS DESCRIPTION

The **Gross Description** of a specimen submitted for analysis includes the size, color, location, and any other descriptive data that are apparent to the naked eye. The following is an example of the Gross Description of a gallbladder removed from a patient.

> EXAMPLE
>
> GROSS: The specimen is a gallbladder weighing 46 gm and measuring 8.5 cm in length and 3.5 cm in diameter. It has been opened prior to this examination. The lumen contains numerous small stones, and the wall measures up to 7 mm in thickness. The cystic duct at the proximal portion measures 2 cm in length. The surface is dull and red and appears inflamed. The stones measure from 0.5 mm to 6 mm in diameter. Approximately eighty stones are present.

MICROSCOPIC DESCRIPTION

The second portion of the report, the **Microscopic Description**, details the microscopic examination of the specimen. Sometimes it is also referred to as either the *Micro* or the *Histology.* Listing each stain used and the results of that staining is recommended. When immunohistochemical stains are included, each antibody tested and the results of that testing should be included, as well as grading of tumors. This example continues describing the gallbladder being examined.

> EXAMPLE
>
> MICRO: The gallbladder mucosa has tall branching strands of connective tissue covered with a tall columnar epithelium. In focal areas, the connective tissue of the mucosa has collections of foam-filled macrophages. There are numerous acute and chronic inflammatory cells within the stroma. The muscle layer is thickened. The perimuscular layer has a marked increase in connective tissue and is infiltrated with numerous round cells and many eosinophils. Areas of erosion of the mucosa are present. There is no evidence of malignancy.

PATHOLOGIC DIAGNOSES

The final section of the pathology report is the **Pathologic Diagnoses**. The Diagnoses and Conclusions from the examination procedures are indicated in the same way as they are listed and/or numbered in a Physical and History or a Discharge Summary Report. This last example shows the diagnoses for the gallbladder being examined.

> EXAMPLE
>
> DIAGNOSES: 1. Cholelithiasis.
> 2. Chronic cholecystitis.

Standard practices vary from institution to institution, but all include gross microscopic descriptions and final diagnoses. See the web site (**www.panix.com**) of the Association of Directors of Anatomic and Surgical Pathology for the current recommendations. An example of a completed Pathology Report is presented in Figure 18-1.

AUTOPSY REPORT

A test performed on the body after death is called an autopsy or postmortem examination. The purpose of this examination, which requires written permission from the next of kin, is to ascertain the exact cause of death. The tests utilized may be chemical, bacteriologic, or analytical studies. Sections of tissues are taken from all representative organs, and apparent lesions are then analyzed. The branch of medicine that deals with criminal situations is called **forensic** (fo-rĕn'zĭk) **medicine**.

The Autopsy Committee of the College of American Pathologists (**www.autopsydb.org**) has the responsibility for setting guidelines for autopsy reporting. While they recognize that protocols will vary among institutions, they have identified common components that will appear in all reports: Autopsy Face Sheet, Clinical Summary, Objective Description of Gross Autopsy Observation, a Slide and Block Catalog, reports of Ancillary Studies, and a Clinicopathologic Interpretive Summary.

The Autopsy Face Sheet should include information arranged in two subsections: the public information and the private information. This provides a balance between patient confidentiality and the need for public investigation. Information provided should include

1. Name and address of the institution
2. Patient name, hospital number, or social security for verification of identity
3. Patient date of birth and date and time of death
4. Gender and race/ethnicity as indicated by patient in the medical record

HILLCREST Medical Center

NAME: Dorothy Martinez   HOSPITAL NO.: 608563

TISSUE: Left fallopian tube   ROOM NO.: 682A

DATE RECEIVED: August 15, 20—   PATHOLOGY REPORT NO.: 7809-10

DATE REPORTED: August 17, 20—

GROSS: The specimen is submitted as ectopic pregnancy and consists of fallopian tube measuring 7 cm in length. Near the isthmus there is a bulging which protrudes 2 mm. On dissection of the tube, it contains a hemorrhagic substance which is seen within the lumen of the tube. Representative pieces are submitted.

MICROSCOPIC: Two slides are examined. Sections are of fallopian tube. The tube is dilated, and in the lumen of the tube there is a large amount of hemorrhagic debris. The mucosa of the tube shows some local thickening, and lymphocytes are present in the wall. The vessels in the wall are dilated and congested. In another slide chorionic villi are seen associated with the hemorrhagic material. The chorionic villi are avascular, and they are lined with a double row of cells.

PATHOLOGICAL DIAGNOSIS: Ectopic gestation (tubal pregnancy).

FIGURE 18-1
A Pathology Report

5. Final admission date from hospital record
6. Place of death
7. Date and time of autopsy
8. If pertinent, designation as a forensic case, including permissions, restrictions, and responsible party
9. Prosecutor's name
10. Patient's address, occupation, list of ancillary studies, and patient's physicians of record
11. Cause of death statement

The autopsy procedure is similar to the procedure applied to surgically removed tissue. It is first examined by the naked eye (macroscopically) and then by the microscope. However, the autopsy is more extensive in scope, and the Autopsy Report includes some additional information. The sections of an Autopsy Report are: a History Summary (or Clinical History); a Gross (or Macroscopic) Examination and a Gross Diagnosis; a Microscopic Examination and a Final Diagnosis; and a Discussion or Summary Statement specifying the cause of death.

The examples used in the rest of this chapter represent each section of an Autopsy Report. Words commonly found in such reports are in bold and are pronounced and defined in the Review of Terminology Presented, pp. 569–571.

HISTORY SUMMARY

The first part of an autopsy report, the **History Summary** or Clinical History, *briefly* describes the patient's hospital stay or the circumstances of his or her death.

> EXAMPLE
>
> HISTORY SUMMARY: This patient had an apparent cardiac arrest at home where CPR was attempted by a daughter. An ambulance arrived at the scene to find the patient with constricted pupils and a pulse that was questionably present. On arrival at the emergency room, pupils were dilated and fixed, and there was no response. The patient had repeated defibrillation attempts with no response. Provisional diagnosis was cardiac arrest. The family requested an autopsy.

MACROSCOPIC (GROSS) EXAMINATION

The second part of the report is the **Macroscopic**, or **Gross**, **Examination**, which is examination by the *naked eye*. It usually contains the results of an external and internal examination and includes every major section of the body.

> EXAMPLE
>
> GROSS EXAMINATION:
>
> EXTERNAL EXAMINATION: The body is that of a 78-year-old white male measuring 64.5 inches in length and weighing approximately 145 pounds. The scalp is balding, and hair is light gray in color. There is a laceration with crusted blood present over the left midnose. This measures 10 mm in length and is horizontal. There is an **abrasion** (ah-brā′zhŭn) present over the left mideyebrow that also measures approximately 10 mm in length. The entire left eye, including both upper and lower lids and onto the cheek, is deep purple in color from **ecchymoses** (ĕk″ĭ-mō′sēz) and measures 5 cm from top to bottom and 7.5 cm from medial to lateral. A bluish-black raised firm lesion is present over the right cheek 23 mm below the outer portion over the right eye. The lesion measures 6 mm in diameter, is elevated 1.5 mm, and has a pearly border. The ears and mouth are not remarkable. A 5 cm incision in the right lower neck was for introduction of embalming fluid. The chest is not unusual. Breasts are flat. Abdomen is **scaphoid** (skăf′oid). Several needle marks are present in the anterior left chest. The external genitalia are male. The testicles are small. Extremities are well developed, and there is no peripheral edema. There is a grade 2 **lividity** (lĭ-vĭd′ĭ-tē) of the dependent portions of the back.
>
> INTERNAL EXAMINATION: There is hemorrhage into the tissues of the interior chest bilaterally with fractured ribs secondary to CPR. On opening the abdominal cavity, the right lobe of the

liver is 6 cm above the right **costal** (kŏs'tal) margin in the midclavicular line. The left lobe of the liver is at the base of the **xiphoid** (zīf'oid) **process**. The right diaphragm is in the region of the third interspace. The left diaphragm stands in the region of the fourth rib. **Musculature** (mŭs'kŭ-lah-chur) of the anterior chest is pink in color and somewhat thin. Bone marrow is a deep red-brown in color and juicy. The appendix is present in the right lower quadrant and **retrocecal** (rĕt"rō-sē'kăl) in position. Small and large bowels are not remarkable. Pleural spaces are moist, and there is no free fluid. The pericardial space contains approximately 10 cc of bloody fluid. The transpericardial diameter is 14 cm. Milk patches are noted over the anterior left ventricle. These areas measure up to 6 × 5 cm.

HEART: The heart weighs 550 gm. Four centimeters from its origin, the right coronary artery has a marked calcification of its wall, and the **lumen** (loo'mĕn) is narrowed to approximately 60%. The left anterior descending coronary artery also has **calcification** (kăl"sǐ-fǐ-kā'shŭn) of the wall with some thickening and a narrowing of the lumen of approximately 50%. There is some arteriosclerotic change also noted in the left circumflex coronary artery. All four chambers of the heart are dilated. The valve measurements are as follows: tricuspid 12 cm, pulmonary 8.5 cm, mitral 7 cm, aortic 6.5 cm. The valve edges are thin and not remarkable. The **chordae tendineae** (kor'dē tĕn-dǐn'ē-ē) are thin and delicate. The **trabeculae carneae** (trah-bĕk'ū-lĕ kăr'nē-ē) are flattened. The **foramen ovale** (fō-rā'mĕn ō-vā'lē) is closed. The myocardium is red-brown in color. The left ventricle measures 17 mm in thickness, and the right ventricle measures 4 mm in thickness.

LUNGS: The left lung weighs 350 gm. The right lung weighs 450 gm. The trachea and bronchi have a light pink-tan mucosa, which is moist. There is a small amount of foamy white material present. The lungs collapse readily on removal from the chest. Sections are **crepitant** (krĕp'ǐ-tănt). The lower lobes are **atelectatic** (ăt"ĕ-lĕk-tăt'ǐk). The upper lobes are **emphysematous** (ĕm"fǐ-sĕm'ah-tŭs).

GI TRACT: The esophagus is in its usual position and of equal caliber throughout. The mucosa is blue-gray in color, and longitudinal **striations** (strī-ā'shŭnz) are present. The stomach contains approximately 50 cm of watery fluid and mucous material. The mucosa is gray-tan in color; rugal folds are present and not remarkable. The duodenum contains greenish semifluid material; its muscle walls, mucosa, and serosa are not remarkable. On compression of the gallbladder, a green bile **exudes** (ĕks-ūdz') from the ampulla of Vater. The gallbladder contains approximately 20 cc of a green bile. The mucosa is soft and velvety. The extrahepatic bile ducts are patent, and the common duct measures 10 mm in circumference.

LIVER: The liver weighs 1530 gm. The surface is smooth and edges are sharp. On sectioning, the **parenchyma** (pah-rĕng'kǐ-mah) is light brown in color, and consistency is somewhat increased.

PANCREAS: The pancreas is light pink in color and coarsely lobular. It is of usual size, shape, and position. On sectioning, the duct is patent and not unusual. It has an appearance of **autolysis** (aw-tŏl'ǐ-sǐs).

SPLEEN: The spleen weighs 125 gm. Its surface is purple-gray in color and dull. On sectioning, the parenchyma is deep purple in color, and pulp scrapes with difficulty from the surface.

ADRENAL GLANDS: The adrenal glands are the usual size, shape, and position. On sectioning, the cortex is light yellow in color, and the medulla is light gray.

KIDNEYS: The left kidney weighs 157 gm; the right kidney weighs 160 gm. The capsules strip with ease. Surfaces are relatively smooth. On sectioning, the cortex measures 9 mm in thickness, and the **corticomedullary** (kor"tǐ-kō-mĕd'ū-lār"ē) **junction** is distinct. The pyramids stand out as dark purple, while the cortex is light tan. Ureters are of their usual position and size. The bladder is not remarkable. The prostate measures 3 × 2.5 × 3 cm. On sectioning, the parenchyma is firm and gray in color. The seminal vesicles contain their usual yellow gelatinous material. The rectum is not remarkable.

SPINE: The spine has a grade 1 bridging of the bodies of the vertebrae in the lower portion.

AORTA: The aorta has a minimal plaquing in the upper portion. In the lower portion there is calcium deposition within the wall. The superior mesenteric, celiac, and renal arteries are not remarkable.

HEAD: The scalp is not remarkable. The **calvarium** (kăl-vā'rē-ŭm) measures up to 6 mm in thickness. The dura is tough and not unusual. The cerebral spinal fluid is clear and colorless. The brain weighs 1,180 gm. The vessels at the base of the brain have their usual configuration. The **gyri** (jī'rī) and **sulci** (sŭl'sī) are not remarkable. Multiple sections through the cerebrum, midbrain, pons, medulla, and cerebellum are not remarkable.

GROSS DIAGNOSIS

The gross examination concludes with the **Gross Diagnoses** made on the basis of changes visible to the naked eye.

EXAMPLE

GROSS DIAGNOSES:

I.   Hypertrophy and dilatation of heart, consistent with hypertensive cardiovascular disease.
A.   Cardiac arrest with status after CPR.

II.   Coronary arteriosclerosis, grade 1.

III.   Osteoarthrosis of spine, grade 1.

MICROSCOPIC EXAMINATION

The **Microscopic Examination** is the next section of an autopsy report. Specimens from representative sections of the body are closely examined with the use of a microscope, as the following example shows.

EXAMPLE

MICROSCOPIC EXAMINATION:

CORONARY ARTERIES: The coronary arteries reveal severe arteriosclerosis with **atheroma** (ăth"er-ō'mah) showing **hyalinization** (hī"ah-lĭn"ĭ-zā'shŭn) and calcification. The lumena are narrowed up to 70%.

HEART: The myocardial fibers are hypertrophied. Cross striations are present. A few scattered inflammatory cells are seen.

LUNGS: The lungs have a grade 2 to 3 chronic passive congestion with pigmented macrophages in alveolar spaces and thickened alveolar walls. A pulmonary edema is present. Sections reveal a grade 3 pulmonary emphysema. Focal areas of atelectasis are noted. There is a congestion of large vessels.

LIVER: The liver has a grade 3 fatty **metamorphosis** (mĕt"ah-mor'fō-sĭs). An early portal cirrhosis is present. Pigment is present within **canaliculi** (kăn"ah-lĭk'ū-lĭ).

PANCREAS: The pancreas has a grade 4 autolysis with loss of nuclear staining. This includes islets of Langerhans.

SPLEEN: The splenic sinusoids are dilated and contain few red blood cells. Cords of billroth are prominent. Scattered neutrophils are seen within the parenchyma. **Malpighian corpuscles** (măl-pĭg'ĭ-ăn kor'pŭs'lz) are not remarkable.

ADRENAL GLANDS: There is a tubular formation of the cortex that is consistent with a loss of lipoid content. The medullae are not remarkable.

KIDNEYS: Glomerular capillaries contain few red blood cells. Subcapsular spaces contain small amounts of **amorphous** (ah-mor'fŭs) eosinophilic material. Convoluted tubules contain large amounts of eosinophilic material; they are dilated. Bowman's capsules of the glomeruli are thin. Small vessels through the kidney are not remarkable. A few hyalinized glomeruli are noted.

PROSTATE: Many **corpora amylacea** (kor'pō-rah ăm"ĭ-lā'sē-ah) are present within the lumens of the glands.

BRAIN: Neuron and glial cells are orderly. There is no evidence of congestion.

FINAL DIAGNOSES

The **Final Diagnoses** section lists the findings of the microscopic examination.

EXAMPLE

FINAL DIAGNOSES:

I.   Cardiomegaly consistent with hypertensive cardiovascular disease (550 gm).
   A. Dilatation of heart.
     1. Grade 3 chronic passive congestion of lungs.
     2. Pulmonary edema.
     3. Laceration of left midforehead and ecchymoses of left eye.

II.   Grade 2 coronary arteriosclerosis.

III. Grade 3 pulmonary emphysema.

IV.   Grade 3 fatty metamorphosis of liver.

V.   Early portal cirrhosis of liver.

VI.   Autolysis of pancreas (postmortem).

VII. Basal cell carcinoma of right cheek.

VIII. Grade 1 osteoarthrosis of spine.

DISCUSSION

The **Discussion**, or Clinicopathological Correlative Summary and Comments, is the final section of an autopsy report. It summarizes the cause of death in three parts. First is the *underlying cause*, which refers to the disease or injury that initiated events leading directly to death. Second, the *intermediate cause* presents the important diseases, complications, or conditions that occur sometime between the underlying and immediate cause of death. And finally, the *immediate cause* provides the final disease or complications leading to death.

EXAMPLE

DISCUSSION: This patient had an apparent cardiac arrest at home, and CPR was given. When the ambulance arrived, the pupils were constricted; however, when the patient arrived at the emergency room, the pupils were dilated and fixed, and there was no response. Defibrillation attempts had no response, and a medical examiner's autopsy was performed. The autopsy examination revealed a cardiomegaly, which is consistent with hypertensive cardiovascular disease. There was also a coronary arteriosclerosis present. Secondary to the myocardial **decompensation** (dē"kŏm-pĕn-sā'shŭn), a grade 3 chronic passive congestion of lungs was noted, and there was a pulmonary edema present. The body had already been embalmed; therefore, blood levels for alcohol could not be determined. A grade 3 fatty metamorphosis of the liver was present, and an early portal cirrhosis was noted. The cause of death was due to the hypertensive cardiovascular disease with cardiac arrest.

THE PATHOLOGIST'S PRACTICE

Chemicals, instruments, and stains used in the study of body tissues, as well as commonly used abbreviations, are listed in the following sections.

CHEMICALS

Word	Pronunciation	Definition
acetone	ăs'ĕ-tōn	dimethyl ketone, a colorless liquid that is a fat solvent
Bouin's solution	bwahz'	fixation solution for tissue using picric acid, formalin, and acetic acid
formaldehyde	fōr-mal'dĕ-hīd	colorless, water-soluble gas
formalin	fōr'mah-lĭn	aqueous solution of thirty-seven percent formaldehyde in distilled water used to fix tissues in preparation for sectioning and making microscopic slides
Zenker's fixative	zĕng'kerz	solution for fixing tissue

INSTRUMENTS

Word	Pronunciation	Definition
cryostat	krī'ō-stăt	microtome (instrument that is used to cut tissue in very thin slices) that is contained in a refrigerated chamber
tissue processor		instrument in which selected tissue sections are successively passed into different solutions by a timed mechanism in preparation for sectioning, staining, and mounting on microscopic slides

STAINS

Word	Pronunciation	Definition
eosin	ē'ō-sĭn	pink-orange stain used for cytoplasmic staining
Giemsa stain	gēm'sah	deep blue dye that stains bacteria and cellular details
Gomori's methenamine	gō-mor'ēz mĕth-ĕn'ah-mēn	stain specifically for melanin, iron, or urate crystals
Gram's stain	gramz	stain to differentiate gram-positive and gram-negative bacteria
hematoxylin stain	hēm"ah-tŏk'sĭ-lĭn	intense blue stain used for nuclear staining
iron stain		stain for hemosiderin
luxol fast blue	lŭk'sŏl	special stain for myelin sheaths, nerve cells, and fibers
mucicarmine stain	mū"sĭ-kăr'mĭn	reddish stain designed to show selectively the presence of mucinous material

continues

COMMONLY USED ABBREVIATIONS

ASCP	American Society of Clinical Pathologists
MT	medical technologist
MT (ASCP)	Registered Medical Technologist
Path	pathology
spec	specimen
stat	immediately
cc (cm³)	cubic centimeter
mm	millimeter
cm	centimeter
mg	milligram
mL or ml.	milliliter

INTERNET ASSIGNMENT

The mission of the College of American Pathologists (CAP), the principal organization of board-certified pathologists, is to represent the interests of patients, the public, and pathologists by fostering excellence in the practice of pathology and laboratory medicine worldwide. CAP serves in excess of 15,000 physician members and the laboratory community throughout the world. It is the world's largest association composed exclusively of pathologists.

Pathologists and other professionals in medicine and science have free access to Archives of Pathology & Laboratory Medicine at **www.cap.org**. It is also possible to link directly with Medline from this site.

ACTIVITY

Visit the College of American Pathologists site at **www.cap.org**. Explore the features of this web site and indicate which sections may be helpful to an individual who works with a pathologist. Report your findings to your instructor.

Review: Pathology and Autopsies

■ Pathology deals with deviations from normal anatomy or physiology.

■ Pathogens are agents that cause disease. Pathogenesis is a description of how a disease progresses.

■ Samples submitted to the pathologist during surgery can be quick-frozen for a rapid determination of the presence of malignancy or inflammation and/or submitted for a more detailed analysis taking several hours or days.

■ The Surgical Pathology Report made by the pathologist includes a Gross Description (apparent to the naked eye), a Microscopic Description (made after examination with a microscope), and a Diagnosis based on this examination.

■ An autopsy is a thorough pathological examination of the body after death.

■ The sections of an Autopsy Report are: a History Summary (or Clinical History); a Macroscopic (or gross) Examination and a Gross Diagnosis; a Microscopic Examination and a Final Diagnosis; and a Discussion or Summary Statement specifying the cause of death.

Review of Terminology Presented

Word	Definition
abrasion	injury resulting in the scraping away of a portion of the skin or mucous membrane
amorphous	without definite structure
anatomic pathology	study of the effect of disease on the body structure as applied in both surgical pathology and autopsies
atelectatic	pertaining to incomplete expansion or collapse of the lung
atheroma	fatty degeneration or thickening of the walls of the larger arteries
autolysis	self-digestion in tissues by enzymes from the cells, such as occurs after death
autopsy	tests performed on the body after death
calcification	process in which organic tissue becomes hardened by the deposit of lime salts in the tissue
calvarium	domelike superior portion of the cranium composed of the top portion of the frontal, parietal, and occipital bones; also called the skull cap
canaliculi	small channels or canals
chordae tendineae	small tendinous cords that connect the free edges of the atrioventricular valves to the papillary muscles
clinical pathology	study of blood and body fluids and fragments using laboratory methods
corpora amylacea	small masses of degenerate cells found in the prostate
corticomedullary junction	junction of the cortex and medulla of the kidneys
costal	pertaining to a rib
crepitant	crackling
decompensation	failure of the heart to maintain adequate circulation
Discussion	last part of the Autopsy Report where causes of death are summarized
disease	a condition marked by abnormal symptoms occurring and a pathological state is present
disorder	a function that is abnormal
ecchymoses	bruises; large purplish patches
emphysematous	affected with chronic pulmonary disease, characterized by larger than normal air sacs in the lungs
etiology	science dealing with the causes of disease
exude	to pass off slowly through the tissues
Final Diagnoses	part of the Autopsy Report that lists the findings of the microscopic examination
foramen ovale	opening between the two atria of the heart in the fetus
forensic medicine	branch of medicine dealing with criminal situations
Gross Description	part of the Surgical Pathology Report that provides a physical description of the specimen as determined by the naked eye
Gross Diagnoses	part of the Autopsy Report that lists the findings of the macroscopic examination by the naked eye
gyri	convolutions of the cerebral hemispheres of the brain

continues

Word	Definition
History Summary	first part of an Autopsy Report briefly describing the patient's hospital stay or circumstances of death; also called *Clinical History*
homeostasis	the body's normal state
hyalinization	conversion into a glasslike substance
idiopathic	describes a situation where the cause or etiology of a disease is unknown
lividity	skin discoloration, as from a bruise
lumen	space within an artery, vein, intestine, or tube
Macroscopic or Gross Examination	part of an autopsy reporting the results of the examination of the internal and external parts of the body by the naked eye
malpighian corpuscles	renal corpuscles that consist of a glomerulus and Bowman's capsule
metamorphosis	change in form or structure
microscopic description	part of a surgical pathology procedure that reports results of microscopic examination of specimens from representative sections of the body
Microscopic Examination	part of an Autopsy Report that indicates the result of microscope examination of representative sections of the body
musculature	arrangement of the muscles in a body part
parenchyma	essential part of an organ concerned with its function rather than its framework
pathogenesis	description of how a disease progresses
pathogens	agents that cause disease
Pathologic Diagnoses	part of a Surgical Pathology Report listing the various diagnoses or conclusions from the examination procedures
pathologist	physician who studies disease
pathology	specialized branch of medicine dealing with diseases causing deviations from normal anatomy or physiology
retrocecal	pertaining to the area in back of the cecum
scaphoid	boat-shaped
striations	series of streaks
sulci	depressions or grooves that separate convolutions of the brain
surgical pathology	study of body tissues removed by surgical means
syndrome	a group of symptoms caused by several interrelated problems
trabeculae carneae	thick, muscular tissue bands attached to the inner walls of the ventricles of the heart
xiphoid process	lowest portion of the sternum

Terminology Review Exercises

Name: _____ Date: _____

COMPLETION*

Complete the following statements.

1. The two areas classified under anatomic pathology are _____ and _____.

2. A _____ provides information about whether tissue is cancerous or inflammatory.

3. A brief description of the circumstances of a patient's hospital stay or death is the _____.

4. Diagnoses based on the macroscopic observation are called _____.

5. Descriptions of specimens examined under a microscope for an autopsy are found in the _____.

6. An instrument that prepares tissues for sectioning, staining, and mounting on microscopic slides is a _____.

7. Two solutions for fixing tissue are _____ and _____.

8. A function that is abnormal is a _____.

9. The body's normal state is _____.

10. A description of how a disease progresses is _____.

11. _____ describes a situation where cause or etiology of a disease is unknown.

MATCHING

Match the terms to their meanings.

1. _____ report section that details the examination by the naked eye

2. _____ very cold microtome used to cut very thin slices

3. _____ thirty-seven percent formaldehyde in distilled water used to fix tissue in preparation for sectioning and making slides

4. _____ a colorless liquid that is a fat solvent

5. _____ report section summarizing the cause of death that follows the final diagnoses

6. _____ a group of symptoms caused by several interrelated problems

7. _____ agents that cause disease

a. acetone

b. cryostat

c. discussion

d. formalin

e. Macroscopic or Gross Examination

f. pathogens

g. syndrome

_____

*Answers are in Appendix A.

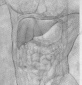

Word Element Review

Root	Meaning	Example	Definition
alg/o	pain, cold	**algor** (ăl'gor)	chill; coldness
ameb/o	change	**ameba, amoeba** (ah-mē'bah)	one-celled animal that moves by constantly changing its shape; causes infection
antr/o	chamber, cavity	**antrum** (ăn'trŭm)	cavity or sinus
astr/o	star-shaped	**astroblast** (ăs'trō-blăst)	star-shaped cell
		astroid (ăs'troid)	star-shaped
coll/o	gluelike	**collagen** (kŏl'ah-jĕn)	gelatin or sticky substance of skin, bone, cartilage, and connective tissue
		colloid (kŏl'oid)	gluelike substance
cry/o	cold	**cryobank** (krī'ō-bănk")	facility for storage of biological tissues at very low temperatures
dendr/o	branching	**dendroid** (dĕn'droid)	branching like a tree
ependym/o	wrapping	**ependyma** (ĕ-pĕn'dĭ-mah)	membrane lining the cavities of the brain and the canal in the spinal column
fibr/o	fiber	**fibrosarcoma** (fī"brō-săr-kō'mah)	spindle-cell sarcoma containing much connective tissue
hist/o	tissue	**histology** (hĭs-tŏl'ō-jē)	microscopic study of the structure, composition, and function of tissues
		histoma (hĭs-tō'mah)	tumor formed from fully developed tissue
hydr/o	water	**hydremia** (hī-drē'mē-ah)	excess of watery fluid in the blood
		hydrocyst (hī'drō-sĭst)	cyst filled with water
lei/o	smooth	**leiomyoma** (lī"ō-mī-ō'mah)	tumor composed of smooth muscle fibers
lip/o	fat	**lipoid** (lĭp'oid)	resembling fat
lob/o	section	**lobe** (lōb)	well-defined portion of an organ separated by boundaries
micr/o	small size, microscopic	**microsurgery** (mī'krō-ser"jer-ē)	dissection of small structures under a microscope

continues

Root	Meaning	Example	Definition
necr/o	death	**necrosis** (nĕ-krō'sĭs)	death of individual or groups of cells or localized areas of tissue
		radiculoneuritis (rah-dĭk"ū-lō-nū-rī'tĭs)	disease of nerve roots and nerves
oment/o	covering	**omentum** (ō-mĕn'tŭm)	fold of peritoneum extending from the stomach to adjacent abdominal organs
pariet/o	wall of an organ, cavity	**parietal** (pah-rī'ĕ-tăl)	pertaining to or forming the walls of a cavity
radic/o	root	**radical** (răd'ĭ-kăl)	directed to the cause, origin, or root
scirrh/o, scirr/o	hard	**scirrhous** (skĭr'rŭs)	hard, like a scirrhus
		scirrhus (skĭr'ŭs)	hard cancerous tumor due to an overgrowth of fibrous tissue
sphen/o	wedge	**sphenoid** (sfē-noid)	resembling a wedge
		sphenoid bone	wedge-shaped bone at the base of the cranium
spir/o	coil	**spirillum** (spī-rĭl'ŭm)	spiral-shaped bacterium
		spiroid (spī'roid)	resembling a coil
strept/o	twisted	**strep throat**	abbreviation for streptococcal infection of the throat
		streptococcus (strĕp"tō-kŏk'ŭs)	infectious, twisted-shaped microorganism
turbin/o	shaped like a top	**turbinal** (tur'bĭ-năl)	shaped like a top; one of the turbinates
vestibul/o	entrance	**vestibular** (vĕs-tĭb'ū-lăr)	pertaining to the entrance or beginning of a canal

Prefix	Meaning	Example	Definition
meta-	change	**metabolism** (mĕ-tăb'ō-lĭzm)	sum of all physical and chemical processes by which a living organized substance is produced and maintained
neo-	new, recent	**neonatal** (nē"ō-nā'tăl)	newborn
		neoplasm (nē'ō-plăzm)	any new, abnormal growth, such as a tumor

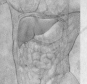

Word Element Review Exercises

Name: _____ Date: _____

IDENTIFY
Provide the term for the following definitions.

1. resembling fat _____

2. dissection of small structures with a microscope _____

3. shaped like a top _____

4. gluelike substance _____

5. spiral-shaped bacterium _____

6. directed to the cause _____

7. tumor of smooth muscle fibers _____

8. resembling a wedge _____

MATCHING*
Match the word elements to their meanings.

1. _____ excess fluid in the blood
2. _____ branching like a tree
3. _____ disease of nerve roots and nerves
4. _____ forming the walls of a cavity
5. _____ hard, cancerous tumor
6. _____ infectious, twisted-shaped microorganisms
7. _____ any new, abnormal growth
8. _____ chill, coldness
9. _____ cavity or sinus
10. _____ star-shaped cell
11. _____ membrane lining the cavities of the brain and the canal in the spinal column
12. _____ spindle-cell sarcoma containing much connective tissue
13. _____ tumor formed from fully developed tissue
14. _____ fold of peritoneum extending from stomach to adjacent abdominal organs
15. _____ facility for storage of biological tissues at very low temperatures
16. _____ well-defined portion of an organ separated by boundaries
17. _____ pertaining to the beginning of a canal

a. algor
b. antrum
c. astroblast
d. cryobank
e. dendroid
f. ependyma
g. fibrosarcoma
h. histoma
i. hydremia
j. lobe
k. neoplasm
l. omentum
m. parietal
n. radiculoneuritis
o. scirrhus
p. streptococcus
q. vestibular

*Answers are in Appendix A.

WORD ELEMENT MEANINGS

Give the meaning of each word element. Then use your dictionary to find a new word that contains each of the word elements. Specify whether the new word is a noun or an adjective by placing N or A in the last column.

Word Element	Meaning	Word	N or A
1. alg/o			
2. ameb/o			
3. antr/o			
4. astr/o			
5. coll/o			
6. cry/o			
7. dendr/o			
8. ependym/o			
9. fibr/o			
10. hist/o			
11. hydr/o			
12. lei/o			
13. lip/o			
14. lob/o			
15. meta-			
16. micr/o			
17. necr/o			
18. neo-			
19. oment/o			
20. pariet/o			
21. radic/o			
22. scirr/o			
23. scirrh/o			
24. sphen/o			
25. spir/o			
26. strept/o			
27. turbin/o			
28. vestibul/o			

Dictionary Exercises

Name: _____ Date: _____

DICTIONARY EXERCISE 1*

Use your dictionary to find the pronunciation and definition of the following words.

Word	Pronunciation	Definition
1. rigor mortis	_____	_____
2. livor mortis	_____	_____
3. putrefaction	_____	_____
4. patent	_____	_____
5. imperforate	_____	_____
6. incarcerated	_____	_____
7. pathognomonic	_____	_____
8. stroma	_____	_____
9. granulation	_____	_____
10. keloid	_____	_____
11. exudation	_____	_____
12. fibrosis	_____	_____
13. sloughing	_____	_____
14. chromatin	_____	_____
15. caseation	_____	_____
16. concretion	_____	_____
17. fasciculus	_____	_____
18. focus	_____	_____
19. syncytial	_____	_____
20. hyaline	_____	_____
21. mitosis	_____	_____
22. pyknosis	_____	_____

DICTIONARY EXERCISE 2

Select the correct meaning and provide the pronunciation of each term.

1. cavitation (_____)
   a. becoming like cheese
   b. a calculus or an inorganic mass
   c. to surround with a capsule
   d. formation of a cavity or an empty space

2. postmortem lividity (_____)
   a. cooling of the body after death
   b. rigidity of skeletal muscles developing 2–4 hours after death and lasting 3–4 days
   c. discoloration of dependent parts of the body after death
   d. degeneration of cells or tissues by endogenous enzymes

_____

*Answers are in Appendix A.

3. desquamation (_____)
    a. process of removing calcium and other elements from bone
    b. shedding of the epidermis
    c. broken-down cellular material
    d. to remove a natural surface

4. frond (_____)
    a. base of an organ
    b. point from which disease arises
    c. oval opening
    d. movable, branchlike structure

5. glairy (_____)
    a. smooth, glassy substance
    b. benign overgrowth of normal cellular elements
    c. sticky, gummy, gelatinlike
    d. like a fish scale

6. hyperemia (_____)
    a. presence of bacterial poisons in the blood
    b. unusual amount of blood in any part of the body
    c. benign overgrowth of normal cellular elements
    d. containing blood

7. panniculus (_____)
    a. clothlike layer of tissue
    b. fine net or network
    c. little beam or crossbar
    d. a covering membrane

8. stippling (_____)
    a. shedding
    b. surrounding a capsule
    c. like cheese
    d. a speckled condition

9. whorl (_____)
    a. fine net or network
    b. spiral arrangement of cells or tissues
    c. pear-shaped
    d. movable, branchlike structure

10. serosanguineous (_____)
    a. pertaining to blood
    b. presence of bacterial poisons in the blood
    c. containing serum and blood
    d. fibrous tissue left after healing of a wound

11. theca (_____)
    a. enclosing case or sheath
    b. covering membrane
    c. cellular structure lining major body cavities
    d. scar

12. proliferation (_____)
    a. physical makeup of a substance
    b. multiplication of similar forms
    c. conversion into a liquid form
    d. conversion of tissues into a dry, amorphous mass

13. trabecula (_____)
    a. a supporting structure
    b. tissue forming the supporting framework of an organ
    c. base of an organ
    d. small pit or hollow cavity

14. autolysis (_____)
    a. process of removing calcium and other elements from bone
    b. degeneration of cells or tissues by endogenous enzymes
    c. series of changes through which the muscles of a cell go in the course of division
    d. condensation and increased basophilic staining of a cell nucleus

15. vacuole (_____)
    a. fine net or network
    b. outgrowth from the surface of a part
    c. structure with open spaces that may be filled with fluid or the remains of ingested materials
    d. points from which a disease arises

DICTIONARY EXERCISE 3

Match the terms to their meanings. Provide the pronunciation for words where indicated.

1. _____ caseous (_____)
2. _____ denude
3. _____ exfoliation (_____)
4. _____ globoid (_____)
5. _____ hydatid (_____)
6. _____ infiltrate
7. _____ lacuna (_____)
8. _____ foramen ovale (_____)
9. _____ reticulum (_____)
10. _____ section
11. _____ stellate (_____)
12. _____ tenacious (_____)
13. _____ tunica (_____)
14. _____ daughter cyst
15. _____ parent cyst
16. _____ bulla (_____)
17. _____ fundus (_____)
18. _____ translucent (_____)
19. _____ septicemia (_____)
20. _____ serrated (_____)

a. scaling off dead tissue
b. to invade an area
c. thin slice of tissue
d. like cheese
e. covering membrane
f. fetal heart opening
g. arising from preexisting cyst
h. to remove a natural surface
i. fine net or network
j. primary cyst
k. cyst formed in the tissues
l. clinging or adhering to
m. small pit or hollow cavity
n. shaped like a star
o. resembling a globe
p. blister
q. base of an organ
r. bacterial poisons in blood
s. sawtoothlike borders
t. permitting passage of light

DICTIONARY EXERCISE 4*

Pronunciation of the words below is provided. Using your dictionary, find the correct spelling and definition of each word.

	Word	Pronunciation	Definition
1.	_____	kō"lē-sĭs-tī'tĭs	_____
2.	_____	dĕs'ĭ-kāt-ĕd	_____
3.	_____	ĕks-krĕs'ĕns	_____
4.	_____	flō'rah	_____
5.	_____	jĕm-ĭs"tō-sī'tĭk	_____
6.	_____	hē"mō-sĭd'er-ĭn	_____
7.	_____	kĕr'ah-tĭn-īzed	_____
8.	_____	loo'tē-ĭn	_____
9.	_____	pō"dō-rahnj'	_____
10.	_____	săng-gwĭn'ē-ŭs	_____

---

*Answers are in Appendix A.

11. _____ skwā'mŭs _____

12. _____ trah-bĕk'ū-lah _____

13. _____ lĭk"wĕ-făk'shŭn _____

14. _____ ăb'sĕs _____

15. _____ lŏb'ūl _____

16. _____ mĕs'en-kīm _____

17. _____ mĕs"ō-thē'lē-ŭm _____

18. _____ ŏs'tē-ŭm _____

19. _____ pah-rĕng'kĭ-mah _____

20. _____ prī-mor'dē-ăl _____

Listening Exercise

Name	Date

INSTRUCTIONS

1. Review the spelling, pronunciation, and meaning of the words provided in the preview.
2. Listen to the audio CD and fill in the blank as the word is dictated.
3. At the end of the exercise, check your spelling against the preview words. They appear in the preview in the order in which they are encountered in the exercise.
4. Review and practice the words you missed.
5. Look up words that are not familiar.

PREVIEW OF WORDS FOR LISTENING EXERCISE 18-1

Word	Pronunciation	Meaning
foci	fō'sī	chief centers of a morbid process (singular—focus)
paravesical	păr"ă-vĕs'ĭk-ăl	beside the bladder
endometrioid	ĕn"dō-mē'trē-oid	similar to the endometrium
perisigmoidal	pĕr"ĭ-sĭg"moy'dăl	pertaining to the peritoneum of the sigmoid curvature
cystadenoma	sĭst"ăd-ĕn-ō'mă	cystic tumor blended with an adenoma (benign epithelial tumor)
subserosal	sŭb-sē-rō'săl	pertaining to the area below membrane-producing or containing serum

Letter of Consultation

Dear Dr. Barton:

Mrs. Casandra Petaja was evaluated for increasing pelvic discomfort with a history of endometriosis. At exploration she was noted to have pelvic endometriosis, but in addition, had carcinoma which had arisen in _____ of endometriosis. Total abdominal hysterectomy, bilateral salpingo-oophorectomy, and cytoreductive surgery were performed. At the end of the procedure, there was no evidence of visible or palpable residual tumor.

The pathology was as follows: "Uterus (135 grams), left tube and ovary (95 grams), tissue from _____, cul-de-sac, and peritoneal regions, 25 cm of sigmoid colon and portion of omentum (12 × 7 × 2 cm). Grade 3 adenocarcinoma compatible with gynecologic origin is identified forming a mass, 1 × 1 × 0.9 cm, on the surface of the resected sigmoid colon. The tumor shows an _____ histologic pattern and is present forming a tumor mass in the cul-de-sac as well. Metastatic carcinoma is present in one of the eight _____ lymph nodes removed with the resected bowel. Foci of endometriosis are present in the peritoneum and paravesical tissues. Microscopic foci of carcinoma are also present in tissue submitted from paravesical region. A benign _____ (9 × 5.5 × 2 cm) is identified in the left ovary. The hysterectomy specimen shows inactive endometrium, mild chronic cervicitis, and multiple (12) intramural, _____, and submucosal leiomyomas ranging in size from 0.5 to 2 cm in greatest dimension. Right and left fallopian tube and omentum are negative for tumor. 07-13-20—ADDENDUM: Permanent sections show a microscopic foci of endometrioid adenocarcinoma in the left ovary."

I will send further plans for postoperative chemotherapy at her dismissal from Grandview Hospital. Thank you for the opportunity to share in her care.

Sincerely yours,

Duane Crookston, MD

chapter 19

The Endocrine System

> 66 *It would indeed be rash for a mere pathologist to venture forth on the uncharted sea of the endocrines, strewn as it is with the wrecks of shattered hypotheses, where even the most wary mariner may easily lose his way as he seeks to steer his bark amid the glandular temptations whose siren voices have proved the downfall of many who have gone before.* 99

—WILLIAM BOYD

OBJECTIVES

When you have completed this chapter on the endocrine system, you should be able to

1. Spell and define major system components and explain how they operate.
2. Identify the meaning of related word elements.
3. Spell and define diagnostic procedures, diagnoses, treatment procedures, and abbreviations.
4. Spell the names of commonly used medications.
5. Be familiar with terminology used in reports.

INTRODUCTION

Endocrinology (ĕn″dō-krĭ-nŏl′ō-jē) is a science concerned with the function of glands that secrete chemical compounds known as hormones into the bloodstream. Physicians who are trained to diagnose and treat endocrine disorders are called **endocrinologists**. Probably no other system of the anatomy has experienced so many shifts and changes in theory and thinking as has the endocrine system. While the anatomy of the system is fairly well known, all of its functions are not.

COMPOSITION OF THE SYSTEM

The glands that make up the endocrine system are the thyroid, parathyroids, pituitary, adrenals, pancreas, testes or ovaries, and the pineal gland. (Many texts also include the thymus as part of the endocrine system. However, its function is usually attributed to the immune system.) While each of these glands has one or more specific functions, they are all dependent upon other glands in the system for maintenance of a normal hormonal balance.

The glands of the endocrine system affect the activity of every cell in the body. Some of their specific effects are mental alertness, physical agility, body build and stature, bodily hair growth, voice pitch, and sexual behavior. They constantly modify the way we feel, think, behave, and react to all sorts of stimuli. For this reason, the endocrine system is closely linked to the nervous system.

Specifically, a **gland** is any organ that produces a secretion. This secretion is manufactured from blood constituents by specialized cells within the gland. Glandular secretions may be divided into two main groups. The first is secretions carried through a duct from glandular cells to a nearby organ or body surface. Examples are digestive juices and tears. These secretions come from **exocrine** (ĕk'sō-krĭn) **glands**. The second group of glands produces internal secretions, which are carried to all parts of the body by blood or lymph systems. These are called hormones and originate in the **endocrine glands**. These endocrine glands, which are ductless, make up the endocrine system. Note in the following table how many hormones there are.

MAJOR ENDOCRINE GLANDS AND THE HORMONES THEY PRODUCE

Endocrine Gland	Hormones Produced	Function
Adrenals		
cortex	aldosterone (mineralocorticoid)	regulates the amount of salts in the body and the body fluid volume
	cortisol (glucocorticoid)	regulates the quantities of sugars, fats, and proteins in cells
	androgens, estrogens, and progestins	maintains secondary sex characteristics
medulla	epinephrine (adrenaline)	sympathomimetic; constriction or dilatation of arterioles depending on type of vascular tissue involved; accelerates the heart rate
	norepinephrine (noradrenaline)	sympathomimetic; constriction of arterioles; neurotransmitter
Ovaries	estrogen	development and maintenance of secondary sex characteristics in the female
	progesterone	prepares the uterus for pregnancy and maintenance of pregnancy
Pancreas		
islets of Langerhans	insulin	regulates the transport and storage of glucose in the body
	glucagon	increases blood sugar by causing the conversion of glycogen to glucose
Parathyroids	parathyroid hormone (PTH)	regulates calcium in the blood
Pituitary (hypophysis)		
anterior lobe (adenohypophysis)	adrenocorticotropin (ACTH) (corticotropin)	stimulates the adrenal cortex to secrete cortisol and weak androgens, which control adrenal cortex development and functioning

continues

MAJOR ENDOCRINE GLANDS AND THE HORMONES THEY PRODUCE

Endocrine Gland	Hormones Produced	Function
Pituitary (hypophysis) *(continued)*		
	gonadotropins	
	• follicle-stimulating hormone (FSH)	stimulates ovarian follicles to grow and produce estrogen; stimulates spermatozoa development
	• gonadotropin-releasing hormone (GnRH) (also called luteinizing hormone-releasing hormone [LHRH])	increases synthesis of testosterone in males; stimulates the synthesis of androgens, estrogen, and progestin in the ovaries and the development of the corpus luteum in females
	• melanocyte-stimulating hormone (MSH)	causes pigmentation of the skin
	• prolactin	stimulates breast development during pregnancy and milk secretion after delivery of the baby; male function unknown
	• growth hormone (GH), (somatotropin), human growth hormone (HGH)	stimulates growth in bone and other tissues
	• thyroid-stimulating hormone (TSH) (thyrotropin)	regulates the structure and function of the thyroid gland and stimulates synthesis and release of the thyroid hormone thyroxine
posterior lobe (neurohypophysis)	antidiuretic hormone (ATH) (vasopressin)	produced by hypothalamus and stored here for release to stimulate the reabsorption of water by kidney tubules; also stimulates muscles of blood vessels to cause vasoconstriction
	oxytocin	produced by hypothalamus and stored here for release to stimulate contraction of the uterus during labor and childbirth; necessary for milk let-down during lactation
Testes	testosterone	promotes growth and maintenance of secondary sex characteristics in the male
Thyroid	calcitonin	secreted by the thyroid C cells; tends to lower plasma calcium concentration
	thyroxine (T_4), triiodothyronine (T_3)	increases the rate of metabolism in body cells

PITUITARY GLAND

The **pituitary** (pĭ-tū'ĭ-tār"ē) **gland**, or **hypophysis** (hī-pŏf'ĭ-sĭs) (1), as shown in Figure 19-1, is a small gland about the size of a raisin located behind the optic nerve crossing. It is surrounded by bone except for the area where it connects with the brain. The gland consists of two parts: the anterior lobe (or adenohypophysis) and the posterior lobe (or neurohypophysis). The anterior lobe is glandlike in nature while the posterior lobe is made up of neural tissue.

The pituitary gland is called the *master gland* because it regulates the functions of the other endocrine glands. In turn, the pituitary gets its direction from the hypothalamus region of the brain. These directions may be in the form of neurons to stimulate or inhibit hormone secretion by the anterior lobe or may be neurohormones

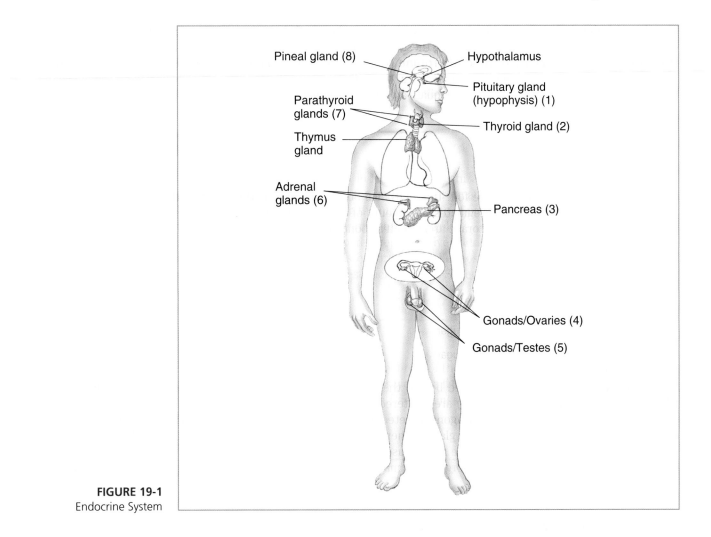

Pineal gland (8)

Hypothalamus

Parathyroid glands (7)

Pituitary gland (hypophysis) (1)

Thyroid gland (2)

Thymus gland

Adrenal glands (6)

Pancreas (3)

Gonads/Ovaries (4)

Gonads/Testes (5)

FIGURE 19-1
Endocrine System

sent to the posterior lobe for storage and later release. See the following list of hypothalamic neurohormones and their function.

Hypothalamic Neurohormone	Function
corticotropin-releasing hormone (CRH)	stimulates ACTH secretion
dopamine	inhibits prolactin, LH, FSH, and TSH secretion
gonadotropin-releasing hormone (GnRH) (luteinizing hormone-releasing hormone [LHRH])	stimulates LH and FSH secretion
growth hormone-releasing hormone (GHRH)	stimulates GH secretion
somatostatin	inhibits GH and TSH secretion
thyrotropin-releasing hormone (TRH)	stimulates prolactin and TSH secretion

THYROID GLAND

parathyroid/o	parathyroid glands	thyr/o, thyroid/o	thyroid gland

Word	Definition
adrenals	two small glands each composed of a medulla and a cortex
aldosterone	hormone from the adrenal cortex and gonads that controls reabsorption of sodium in kidney tubules and excretion of potassium
androgens	hormones from the adrenal cortex that influence secondary sexual characteristics
cortisol	hormone from the adrenal cortex that maintains carbohydrate reserves of the body
endocrine glands	glands that produce hormones that are carried to all parts of the body by blood or lymph systems
endocrinologist	physician who is trained to diagnose and treat endocrine disorders
endocrinology	science concerned with the function of glands that secrete chemical compounds known as hormones into the bloodstream
epinephrine (adrenaline)	hormone produced in the adrenal medulla that helps the body to respond to emergency situations
estrogens	hormones from the adrenal cortex and ovaries that influence secondary sexual characteristics
exocrine glands	glands that produce external secretions that are carried through a duct from glandular cells to a nearby organ or body surface
gland	any organ that produces a secretion
gonads	sex glands in males and females; produce the hormones testosterone in the male and estrogen and progesterone in the female
hypothalamus	part of the diencephalon that contains centers for control of various body functions; produces neurons and neurohormones that act on or are stored by the pituitary gland
islets or islands of Langerhans	small specialized collections of cells in the pancreas that manufacture insulin, glucagon, and other hormones
melatonin	hormone produced by the pineal gland; affects circadian rhythm
norepinephrine (nonadrenaline)	hormone produced in the adrenal medulla that helps the body to respond to emergency situations
pancreas	gland that produces insulin, which controls the normal use of glucose in the body
parathyroid glands	four tiny glands that regulate the amount of calcium and phosphorous stored and circulated in the body
pineal gland	gland that secretes melatonin
pituitary gland (hypophysis)	small gland composed of two lobes located in the brain; master gland
progestins	hormones from the adrenal cortex and ovaries that influence secondary sexual characteristics
steroids	hormones that are produced in the adrenal cortex
thyroid gland	gland that produces the hormones thyroxine (T_4) and triiodothyronine (T_3)
thyroxine (T_4)	hormone produced by the thyroid gland that regulates production of heat and energy in the body
triiodothyronine (T_3)	hormone produced by the thyroid gland that regulates production of heat and energy in the body

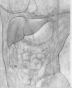

Terminology Review Exercises

Name: _____ Date: _____

SELECTION*

Select the correct word from the list below to complete each of the following statements.

adrenals   gonads   pancreas   parathyroids   pituitary   thyroid

1. The _____ gland is located in the neck just below the larynx.

2. The master gland is the _____.

3. Calcium is regulated by the _____.

4. The islets of Langerhans, located in the _____, produce insulin and glucagon.

5. The _____ is composed of two lobes called the adenohypophysis and neurohypophysis.

6. Another name for the sex glands is _____.

7. The _____ gland produces thyroxine and triiodothyronine.

8. Two glands made up of two parts called the medulla and cortex are the _____.

9. GH or HGH, TSH, ACTH, FSH, and LH are produced by the anterior lobe of the _____.

10. Oxytocin is produced by the hypothalamus and stored in the posterior lobe of the _____.

11. Estrogen, progesterone, and testosterone are produced by the _____.

12. Epinephrine and norepinephrine are produced by the medulla of the _____.

13. Aldosterone and cortisol are produced by the cortex of the _____.

SHORT ANSWER

Supply a short answer to the following.

1. Explain the overall function of hormones.

_____

_____

_____

_____

_____

2. State the difference between endocrine and exocrine glands.

_____

_____

_____

_____

_____

_____
*Answers are in Appendix A.

DIAGNOSTIC PROCEDURES

Laboratory Tests *(continued)*
Parathyroid Gland

- parathyroid hormone (PTH), parathormone
- calcium, total/ionized Ca++
- phosphorus

Adrenal Gland

- adrenocorticotropic hormone (ACTH) stimulation test, cortisol stimulation test, cosyntropin test
- cortisol
- dehydroepiandrosterone (DHEA)
- dexamethasone suppression test (DST), prolonged/rapid DST, cortisol suppression test, ACTH suppression test
- plasma renin assay, plasma renin activity (PRA)
- progesterone assay (17-hydroxyprogesterone)

Other Blood Tests

- serum thyroglobulin

The following tests are done on urine samples.

- 17-hydroxycorticosteroids (17-OHCS)
- 17-ketosteroids (17-KS)
- aldosterone assay
- calcium
- catecholamines: epinephrine, free catecholamines, metanephrines, norepinephrine, vanillylmandelic acid (VMA)
- cortisol, free cortisol
- creatinine clearance
- ketone
- potassium
- sodium
- specific gravity

DIAGNOSES

Word	Pronunciation	Definition
General		
multiple endocrine neoplasia (MEN) or multiple endocrine adenomatosis (MEA)	ĕn'dō-krīn nē"ō-plā'zē-ah ăd"ĕ-nō-mă-tō'sĭs	associated endocrine disorders that tend to run in families

continues

DIAGNOSES		
Word	Pronunciation	Definition
Adrenal		
congenital adrenal hyperplasia	kŏn-jĕn'ĭ-tăl ăd-rē'năl hī"pĕr-plā'zē-ah	genetic abnormality causing adrenal glands to produce a distorted pattern of steroid hormones
hypoadrenalism (Addison's disease)	hī"pō-ăd-rē'năl-ĭzm	decreased functioning of the adrenal cortex
hyperadrenalism	hī"pĕr-ăd-rē'năl-ĭzm	oversecretion of hormones; the hormone determines the specific form of the problem
• *Conn's syndrome (primary aldosteronism)*		overproduction of aldosterone
• *Cushing's syndrome*		abnormalities due to chronic exposure to excessive cortisol
• *gynecomastia*	jī"nĕ-kō-măs'tēah	excessive breast development in males
• *hirsutism*	hŭr'sūt'ĭzm	presence of an adult male pattern of hair distribution in women
• *precocious puberty*	prē-ko'shŭs pū'bĕr-tē	early development in children
• *virilism*	vĭr'ĭl-ĭzm	development of male secondary sex characteristics in a female
pheochromocytoma	fĕ-ō-krō"mō-sī-tō'mah	tumor of the adrenal medulla
Pancreas		
diabetes mellitus	dī-ă-bē'tēz mĕ-lī'tŭs	inability to oxidize and utilize carbohydrates because of a lack of insulin secretion or insulin resistance
• *Type 1 (IDDM)*		insulin-dependent
• *Type 2 (NIDDM)*		noninsulin-dependent
• *secondary diabetes*		diabetes secondary to other conditions or medicines
diabetic ketoacidosis (DKA)	dī-ă-bĕt'ĭk kē"tō-ă"sĭ-dō'sĭs	acute complication of Type1 diabetes
diabetic nephropathy	nĕ-frŏp'ă-thē	secondary complication of diabetes; renal insufficiency
diabetic retinopathy	rĕt"ĭ-nŏp'ă-thē	secondary complication of diabetes resulting in visual loss and blindness
hypoglycemia	hī"pō-glī-sē'mē-ah	low blood sugar that may be the result of excessive insulin production by the islet cells
hyperglycemic-hyperosmolar coma (syndrome) or non-ketotic hyperglycemic-hyperosmolar coma (syndrome) (NKHHC)	hī"pĕr-glī-sē'mē-ĭk hī"pĕr-ŏz'mō-lăr nŏn-kē-tō'tĭk	condition that occurs when there is insufficient insulin to prevent hyperglycemia

continues

DIAGNOSES

Word	Pronunciation	Definition
Pancreas (continued)		
impaired fasting glucose	gloo'kōs	evaluated fasting glucose not high enough to diagnose diabetes
impaired glucose tolerance		abnormally high glucose level after carbohydrate ingestion
Parathyroid		
hyperparathyroidism	hī"per-păr"ah-thī'royd-ĭzm	excessive production of the parathyroid hormone, resulting in hypercalcemia
hypoparathyroidism	hī"pō-păr"ah-thī'royd-ĭzm	underactivity of the parathyroid gland, which may result in hypocalcemia
Pituitary		
acromegaly	ăk"rō-mĕg'ah-lē	disorder characterized by enlargement of facial and extremity bones; caused by excessive growth hormone
diabetes insipidus	ĭn-sĭp'ĭ-dŭs	congenital disorder resulting from insufficient secretion of the antidiuretic hormone (ADH) from the posterior pituitary gland; should not be confused with diabetes mellitus
dwarfism		congenital disorder characterized by extreme shortness of stature; caused by growth hormone deficiency
gigantism	jī-găn'tĭzm	disorder resulting in excessive size and stature; caused by excessive secretion of growth hormone
hypopituitarism	hī"pō-pĭ-tū'ĭ-tă-rĭzm	disorder resulting from a deficiency of anterior pituitary hormones
panhypopituitarism	păn-hī"pō-pĭ-tū'ĭ-tăr-ĭzm	disorder resulting from the deficiency of all anterior pituitary hormones
pituitary incidentaloma	ĭn"sĭ-den"tă-lō'mă	nonfunctioning pituitary tumor discovered by chance
syndrome of inappropriate ADH secretion (SIADH)		disorder caused by excessive secretion of the antidiuretic hormone, resulting in excess water retention in the body and low serum sodium
Reproductive Gland Diseases		
erectile dysfunction		may be caused by testosterone deficiency
hypergonadism	hī"păr-gō'năd-ĭzm	increased sex hormone production
hypogonadism	hī"pō-gō'năd-ĭzm	decreased sex hormone production

continues

DIAGNOSES		
Word	Pronunciation	Definition
Thyroid		
euthyroid sick syndrome	ū-thī'royd	syndrome where abnormal thyroid function tests occur in euthyroid patients with severe nonthyroid illness
goiter (endemic, colloid, nodular, adenomatous, Hashimoto's, simple)	goi'ter	enlargement of the thyroid gland (See Figure 19-2)
Hashimoto's thyroiditis (autoimmune or chronic lymphocytic thyroiditis)	hăsh"ĭ-mō'tōz thī"royd-ī'tĭs	chronic inflamation of the thyroid; often a cause of hypothyroidism
hyperthyroidism (Graves' disease)	hī"per-thī'roy-dĭzm	overactivity of the thyroid gland; also called *thyrotoxicosis* (thī"rō-tŏk"sĭ-kō'sĭs); the crisis state of Graves' disease
hypothyroidism	hī"pō-thī'roy-dĭzm	underactivity of the thyroid gland
• *myxedema*	mĭks-ĕ-dē'mah	severe form of hypothyroidism
• *cretinism*	krē'tĭn-ĭzm	form of hypothyroidism found in youngsters
iodine-induced hyperthyroidism (Jod-Basedow phenomenon)		overactivity of the thyroid gland caused by excessive iodine intake
thyroid cancer		type of cancer; common varieties are papillary and follicular
thyroiditis	thī-roy-dī'tĭs	inflammation of the thyroid gland

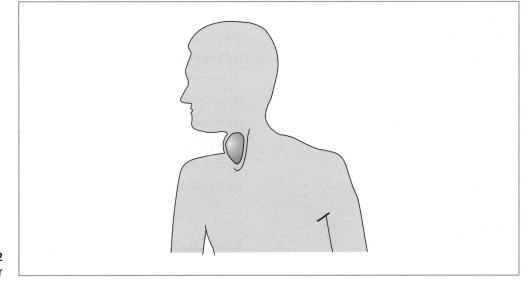

FIGURE 19-2
Goiter

TREATMENT PROCEDURES

Word	Pronunciation	Definition
adrenalectomy	ah-drē"năl-ĕk'tō-mē	surgical removal of the adrenal gland
oophorectomy	ō"ŏf-ō-rĕk'tō-mē	surgical removal of the female gonads
orchiectomy	or"kē-ĕk'tō-mē	surgical removal of the male gonads
pancreas transplantation		surgical procedure performed primarily on patients with Type 1 diabetes who also need kidney or other organ transplants
pancreatectomy	păn"krē-ah-tĕk'tō-mē	surgical removal of the pancreas
parathyroidectomy	par"ah-thi"roy-dek'tō-me	total or partial removal of the parathyroid glands
pituitary irradiation		method of treating pituitary tumors
thymectomy	thī-mĕk'tō-mē	surgical removal of the thymus
thyroidectomy	thī"roy-dĕk'tō-mē	total or partial removal of the thyroid gland
transsphenoidal hypophysectomy	trăns"sfē-noi'dăl hī-pŏf"ĭ-sĕk'tō-mē	removal of all or part of the pituitary gland through the sphenoid sinus

MEDICATIONS PRESCRIBED

Trade Name	Generic Name
Adrenal	
Acthar	corticotropin
Aldactone	spironolactone HCTZ
Cortrosyn	cosyntropin (synthetic corticotropin)
Mithracin	plicamycin
Adrenocortical Steroids	
Aristocort, Kenalog	triamcinolone acetonide
Celestone	betamethasone
Cortef, Solu-cortef, Hydrocortone	hydrocortisone
Decadron	dexamethasone
Deltasone, Orasone	prednisone
Florinef	fludrocortisone
Medrol	methylprednisolone
Pediapred, Prelone, Orapred	prednisolone
Androgens	
Halotestin	fluoxymesterone

continues

MEDICATIONS PRESCRIBED

Trade Name	Generic Name
Diabetes	
Actos	pioglitazone
Amaryl	glimepiride
Avandia	rosiglitazone
DiaBeta, Micronase, Glynase	glyburide
Diabinese	chlorpropamide
Glucagon, GlucaGen	glucagon
Glucotrol	glipizide
Glucophage	metformin
Glucovance	glyburide/metformin hydrochloride
Glyset	miglitol
Orinase	tolbutamide
Prandin	repaglinide
Precose	acarbose
Starlix	nateglinide
Tolinase	tolazamide
Insulins	
Humalog	insulin lispro
Humulin (L, N, R, U)	human insulin
Lantus	insulin glaring
Novolin (N, L or R)	human insulin
Novolog	insulin aspart
Pituitary Hormones	
Growth Hormones	
• Genotropin, Humatrope, Nutropin, Norditropin	somatropin
Antidiuretic Hormones	
• DDAVP, Desmopressin AC, Stimate	desmopressin acetate
• Pitressin	vasopressin
Labor Inducers	
• Ergonovine	ergonovine
• Methergine	methylergonovine maleate
• Pitocin	oxytocin
Uterine Relaxants	
• Yutopar	ritodrine

continues

MEDICATIONS PRESCRIBED

Trade Name	Generic Name
Pituitary Hormones *(continued)*	
Other	
• Parlodel	bromocriptine mesylate
• Sandostatin	octreotide acetate
Thyroid	
Cytomel	liothyronine sodium
Levothroid, Synthroid, Levoxyl	levothyroxine sodium
Lugol's Solution	iodine and potassium iodide
Proloid	thyroglobulin
P.T.U.	propylthiouracil
S.S.K.I.	potassium iodide saturated solution
Tapazole	methimazole
Thyrogen	thyrotropin
Thyroid, U.S.P.	desiccated thyroid
Thyrolar	liotrix
Treatment of Hyperlipidemia	
Atromid-S	clofibrate
Colestid	colestipol
Lescol	fluvastatin
Lipitor	atorvastatin
Lopid	gemfibrozil
Lorelco	probucol
Mevacor	lovastatin
Niaspan, Nicobid, Slo-Niacin, Nicolar	nicotinic acid
Pravachol	pravastatin sodium
Questran, Prevalite	cholestyramine
Tricor	fenofibrate
Welchol	colesevelam
Zocor	simvastatin
Treatment of Osteoporosis	
Actonel	risedronate sodium
Calciferol, DHT, Hytakesol, Rocaltrol	vitamin D preparations (calcitriol)
Caltrate, OSCal	oyster shell calcium
Citracal	calcium citrate

continues

MEDICATIONS PRESCRIBED

Trade Name	Generic Name
Treatment of Osteoporosis (continued)	
Climera, Estrace, Estraderm, Vivelle	estradiol
Evista	raloxifene hydrochloride
Fosamax	alendronate
Miacalcin Nasal Spray	calcitonin salmon
Ogen, Ortho-Est	estropipate
Premarin, Cenestin	conjugated estrogens
Prempro, Premphase	conjugated estrogen *and* medroxyprogesterone

ABBREVIATIONS

17-KS	17-ketosteroids
17-OHCS	17-hydroxycorticosteroids
2hPPG	2-hour postprandial glucose
ACTH	adrenocorticotropic hormone
ADH	antidiuretic hormone
anti-TPO	thyroid peroxide antibodies
CRH	corticotropin-releasing hormone
DHEA	dehydroepiandrosterone
DI	diabetes insipidus
DM	diabetes mellitus
DST	dexamethasone suppression test
FBS	fasting blood sugar
FSH	follicle-stimulating hormone
FT_3, Free T_3	triiodothyronine serum free
FT_I, FT_4 Index	thyroxine index free
FT_4, Free T_4	thyroxine serum free
GH	growth hormone
GnRH	gonadotropin-releasing hormone
GTT	glucose tolerance test
Hb A_{1C}	glycosylated hemoglobin
HGH	human growth hormone
IDDM	insulin-dependent diabetes mellitus
IGF-I	insulin-like growth factor I

continues

ABBREVIATIONS

ITT	insulin tolerance test
K	potassium
LH	luteinizing hormone
LHRH	luteinizing hormone-releasing hormone
MEA	multiple endocrine adenomatosis
MEN	multiple endocrine neoplasia
MSH	melanocyte-stimulating hormone
Na	sodium
NIDDM	noninsulin-dependent diabetes mellitus
NKHHC	nonketotic hyperglycemia-hyperosmolar coma (syndrome)
OCT	oxytocin challenge test
PRA	plasma renin activity
PRL	prolactin level
PTH	parathyroid hormone
RAIU	radioactive iodine uptake
RIA	radioimmunoassay
SH	somatotropin hormone
T_3	triiodothyronine
T_4	thyroxine
TBG	thyroid-binding globulin
TFT	thyroid function test
THBR	thyroid-hormone binding ratios
TRF	thyrotropic-releasing factor
TRH	thyrotropin-releasing hormone
TSH	thyroid-stimulating hormone
VMA	vanillylmandelic acid

Working Practice Review Exercises

Name: _____ Date: _____

IDENTIFICATION
Identify the following procedures.

1. measures the uptake of a dose of iodine by the thyroid gland

   _____

2. measures the extent of eyeball protrusion

   _____

3. measures hormone levels in plasma by using radioactively labeled molecules

   _____

4. removal of all or part of the pituitary gland through the sphenoid sinus

   _____

5. surgical removal of male gonads

   _____

6. total or partial removal of parathyroid glands

   _____

7. surgical removal of the thymus

   _____

8. partial or total removal of the thyroid gland

   _____

MATCHING*
Match the terms to their meanings.

1. _____ overactivity of the thyroid
2. _____ enlargement of the thyroid gland
3. _____ chronic exposure to excessive cortisol
4. _____ lack of insulin secretion
5. _____ inflammation of the thyroid gland
6. _____ deficiency of all anterior pituitary hormones
7. _____ abnormal growth of hair
8. _____ severe underactivity of the thyroid gland
9. _____ enlargement of facial and extremity bones
10. _____ tumor of the adrenal medulla

a. Cushing's syndrome
b. panhypopituitarism
c. diabetes mellitus
d. hirsutism
e. hyperthyroidism
f. goiter
g. myxedema
h. thyroiditis
i. acromegaly
j. pheochromocytoma

ABBREVIATIONS
Identify the following abbreviations.

1. ACTH _____
2. FSH _____
3. LH _____
4. ADH _____
5. TSH _____
6. RIA _____
7. T_3 _____
8. T_4 _____

_____
Answers are in Appendix A.

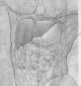

Word Element Review

Root	Meaning	Example	Definition
adrenal/o, adren/o	adrenal gland	**adrenopathy** (ăd"rĕn-ŏp'ah-thē)	any disease of the adrenal glands (also called adrenalopathy)
duct/o	carry	**ductule** (dŭkt'ūl)	very small duct
ect/o	outside	**ectopic** (ĕk-tŏp'ĭk)	located away from the normal position
gluc/o	sugar	**glucose** (gloo'kōs)	sugar
glyc/o	sugar	**glycosuria** (glī"kō-sū'rē-ah)	presence of glucose in urine (also called glucosuria)
pancreat/o	pancreas	**pancreatitis** (păn'krē-ah-tī'tĭs)	inflammation of the pancreas
parathyroid/o	parathyroid glands	**parathyroidectomy** (păr"ă-thī-royd-ĕk'tō-mē)	excision of one or more of the parathyroid glands
thyr/o, thyroid/o	thyroid gland	**hypothyroidism** (hī"pō-thī'roy-dĭzm)	deficiency of thyroid activity
		hyperthyroidism (hī"per-thī'roy-dĭzm)	excess activity of the thyroid gland

Prefix	Meaning	Example	Definition
crin-	secrete	**crinogenic** (krī"nō-jĕn'ĭk)	stimulating secretion

Suffix	Meaning	Example	Definition
-fusion	pour	**transfusion** (trăns-fū'zhŭn)	introduction of blood directly into the bloodstream
		effusion (ĕ-fū'zhŭn)	escape of fluid into a material

Word Element Review Exercises

Name: _____ Date: _____

WORD ELEMENTS*

Provide the correct word element to complete the following words.

1. deficiency of thyroid activity   hyp( ) _____ ism
2. stimulating secretion   _____ genic
3. a very small duct   _____ ule
4. escape of fluid into a material   ef _____
5. presence of glucose in urine   _____ uria
6. any disease of the adrenal glands   _____ opathy
7. excess activity of the thyroid   hyp( ) _____ ism
8. sugar   _____ ose

MATCHING

Match the word elements to their meanings.

1. _____ thyroid gland
2. _____ sugar
3. _____ secrete
4. _____ adrenal gland
5. _____ carry
6. _____ outside
7. _____ pour

a. gluc/o, glyc/o

b. adrenal/o, adren/o

c. thyr/o, thyroid/o

d. duct/o

e. crin-

f. ect/o

g. -fusion

WORD ELEMENT MEANINGS

Give the meaning of each word element. Then use your dictionary to find a new word that contains each of the word elements. Specify whether the new word is a noun or an adjective by placing N or A in the last column.

Word Element	Meaning	Word	N or A
1. adrenal/o	_____	_____	_____
2. adren/o	_____	_____	_____
3. crin-	_____	_____	_____
4. duct/o	_____	_____	_____
5. ect/o	_____	_____	_____
6. -fusion	_____	_____	_____
7. gluc/o	_____	_____	_____
8. glyc/o	_____	_____	_____
9. pancreat/o	_____	_____	_____
10. parathyroid/o	_____	_____	_____
11. thyr/o	_____	_____	_____
12. thyroid/o	_____	_____	_____

*Answers are in Appendix A.

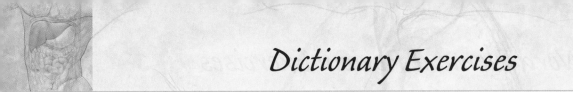

Dictionary Exercises

Name: _____ Date: _____

DICTIONARY EXERCISE 1*

Use your dictionary to find the pronunciation and definition of the following words.

	Word	**Pronunciation**	**Definition**
1.	metabolism	_____	_____
2.	tophus	_____	_____
3.	osmolarity	_____	_____
4.	osmolality	_____	_____
5.	aldosteronism	_____	_____
6.	alkalosis	_____	_____
7.	hypoplasia	_____	_____
8.	thyroglossal duct	_____	_____
9.	pressor effect	_____	_____

DICTIONARY EXERCISE 2

Pronunciation of the words below is provided. Using your dictionary, find the correct spelling and definition of each word.

	Word	**Pronunciation**	**Definition**
1.	_____	ăs"ĭ-dō'sĭs	_____
2.	_____	ĭk'ter-ŭs	_____
3.	_____	tĕt'ah-nē	_____
4.	_____	gloo'kă-gŏn	_____
5.	_____	hī"pĕr-plā'zē-ah	_____
6.	_____	kăt"ĕ-kŏl'ah-mēns	_____

DICTIONARY EXERCISE 3

Rewrite each sentence in your own words. Provide the pronunciation for each italicized word.

1. One of the patient's problems was *polyphagia* (_____).

   _____

2. The diagnosis included *thymoma* (_____).

   _____

3. She reported *polydipsia* (_____).

   _____

4. Blood tests revealed *hyperuricemia* (_____).

   _____

---

*Answers are in Appendix A.

Listening Exercise

Name	Date

INSTRUCTIONS

1. Review the spelling, pronunciation, and meaning of the words provided in the preview.
2. Listen to the audio CD and fill in the blank as the word is dictated.
3. At the end of the exercise, check your spelling against the preview words. They appear in the preview in the order in which they are encountered in the exercise.
4. Review and practice the words you missed.
5. Look up words that are not familiar.

PREVIEW OF WORDS FOR LISTENING EXERCISE 19-1

Word	Pronunciation	Meaning
hyperparathyroidism	hī"pĕr-păr"ă-thī'roy-dĭzm	excessive production of the parathyroid hormone, resulting in hypercalcemia
hypercalcemia	hī"pĕr-kăl-sē'mē-ah	excessive amount of calcium in the blood
triglycerides	trī-glĭs'ĕr-īds	combination of glycerol with three of five different fatty acids
hypertrophy	hī-pĕr'trō-fē	increase in the size of a body part that does not involve tumor formation
xerosis	zē-rō'sĭs	abnormal dryness of skin
hyperglycemia	hī"pĕr-glī-sē'mē-ah	increase of blood sugar

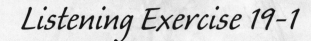

Discharge Summary

DISCHARGE SUMMARY

ADMITTED: 6/12/20—   DISCHARGED: 6/17/20—

CONSULTATIONS: Dr. Andres SanMiguel, cataract surgery

Dr. Herman Brunner, dermatology

SURGICAL PROCEDURES: Intracapsular cataract extraction of the left eye with peripheral iridectomy.

ADMITTING DIAGNOSIS: Rule out _____.

HISTORY: This 55-year-old woman exhibited symptoms of endocrine disturbance and other health problems during her office visit and consequently was admitted for further testing. A complete history and physical is in the patient's record.

LABORATORY DATA: Uric acid excretion was 296 mg/24 hours (normal from 400 to 800), calcium 61 mg/24 hours (30 to 150), phosphorus 278 mg/24 hours (340 to 1,000).

SMA–12 showed these abnormalities: _____ at 11.4, hyperglycemia at 112, hyperuricemia at 8.4, and total protein 8.2 with an albumin of 4.6. Several calcium determinations were elevated. Fasting glucose was 110. Fasting cholesterol was 291 mg%, and _____ were 152. Elevated parathyroid hormone levels have been found × 2 in the past when compared with calcium levels.

Hand x-rays showed degenerative arthritis. Chest, spine, and skull x-rays were normal. Electrocardiogram showed a possible left ventricular _____.

HOSPITAL COURSE: The patient was admitted at 182½ lb. and discharged at 178 lb. She was seen in consultation with Dr. Andres SanMiguel for cataract surgery and Dr. Herman Brunner, dermatologist. She was placed on a low-calcium diet and tolerated the above tests and procedures very well.

DISCHARGE DISPOSITION AND PLAN: Patient was improved at discharge. Instructions were to follow up with Dr. SanMiguel for her eyes, with me at the office in four to six weeks, and with Dr. Brunner in six to eight weeks. For her _____, she was given a dermatological ointment. She should follow a low-sodium, low-calcium diet for weight reduction.

DISCHARGE DIAGNOSES:

1. Hypercalcemia, probably primary hyperparathyroidism.
2. Intracapsular cataract, left eye.
3. Hypertension.
4. Hyperuricemia.
5. _____.
6. Xerosis.
7. Seborrheic dermatitis of the scalp.

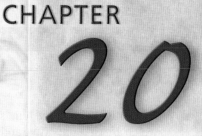

The Nervous System

> *The human brain is a world consisting of explored continents and great stretches of unknown territory.*
>
> —Santiago Ramón y Cajal

OBJECTIVES

When you have completed this chapter on the nervous system, you should be able to

1. Spell and define major system components and explain how they operate.
2. Identify the meaning of related word elements.
3. Spell and define diagnostic procedures, diagnoses, treatment procedures, and abbreviations.
4. Spell the names of commonly used medications.
5. Be familiar with terminology used in reports.

INTRODUCTION

The nervous system can most readily be described as the body's communication network. From the moment we are born to the moment we die, our every thought, emotion, movement, and impression is controlled by this communication network. Specialized communication cells create a network so intricate that nothing in the world can approach its complexity. A physician who specializes in the study of the nervous system is a **neurologist**. A surgeon who specializes in the surgical treatment of diseases of the nervous system is called a **neurosurgeon**.

COMPOSITION OF THE NERVOUS SYSTEM

neur/o	nerve, nervous system

The entire nervous system is composed of tissue made up of neurons interspersed with **neuroglia** (nū-rŏg'lē-ah), which are the supportive and connective cells of the nervous system. The basic unit of the nervous system, the **neuron** (nū'rŏn), is illustrated in Figure 20-1. It has the appearance of a drop of liquid that has splattered on the floor. The length of a neuron can be anywhere from a fraction of an inch to three or four feet, depending on its location.

The large part of the cell is referred to as the **cell body** (3), which is made up of cytoplasm and the nucleus. The **nucleus** (2) is the central controlling structure essential to the cell's life. Spraying out from the cell body are short, threadlike receptive fibers called **dendrites** (dĕn'drīts) (1). An **axon** (ăk'sŏn) (4), a long, straight fiber ending in a brushlike tip, conducts impulses away from the cell body. Many axons are covered by a sheath of white, fatty material called **myelin** (mī'ĕ-lĭn) (5).

Three general classes of neurons comprise more than ninety-nine percent of the approximately 12 billion neurons in the nervous system. They are grouped according to their function. **Sensory**, or **afferent** (ăf'ĕr-ĕnt), **neurons** carry signals or directives to the brain and spinal cord. **Motor**, or **efferent** (ĕf'ĕr-ĕnt), **neurons** stimulate the contraction or relaxation of muscles and spur the activity of glands. Finally, **interneurons** shuttle messages back and forth through the central nervous system pathways.

These neurons form a network for communicating messages through the body. For example, an axon transmits a signal to an adjacent neuron across a junction called a **synapse** (sĭn'ăps), where it is received by a dendrite. This transmission of neural impulses is chemical in nature, as there is no direct contact between the axon of one neuron and the dendrites of another.

Injury to neurons may result in temporary or permanent loss of function. If a neuron's nucleus is destroyed, it will not regenerate. On the other hand, if the nerve fiber is cut, it can eventually regrow. If enough related neurons are permanently destroyed, an entire bodily function may be impaired or lost.

The protection of the nervous system is very important because its continued operation is critical to so many body functions. For protection, major portions are located within the skull and the strong, flexible spinal column. Both the brain and spinal cord are also surrounded by cerebrospinal fluid, which acts as a shock absorber. Most of the other nerve trunks are protected by being buried deep in the body.

The parts of the nervous system are grouped according to structure and function: the **central nervous system**, which includes the brain and spinal cord as the two bases of operation; the **peripheral nervous system**, which is made up of cranial and spinal nerves; and the **autonomic** (aw"tō-nŏm'ĭk) **nervous system**, which applies to activities conducted automatically by certain peripheral nerves. A discussion of each subsystem follows.

CENTRAL NERVOUS SYSTEM

cephal/o	head	dur/o	dura mater
cerebell/o	cerebellum	encephal/o	brain
cerebr/o	brain	mening/o	meninges
cornu	horn-shaped	pont/o	pons
crani/o	head, skull	thalam/o	thalamus

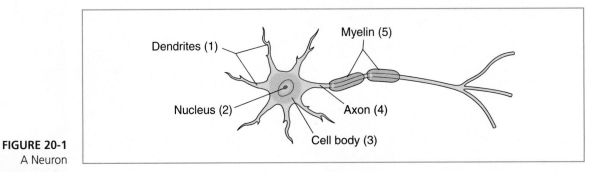

FIGURE 20-1
A Neuron

The central nervous system includes the brain and the spinal cord.

THE BRAIN

A physical description of the brain is unimpressive. It is pinkish-gray, furrowed, and weighs about three pounds. An estimated 12 billion nerve cells are present, each potentially linked to countless others.

The brain and its major components are illustrated in Figure 20-2. Both the brain and the spinal cord are covered by membranes called **meninges** (mĕ-nĭn'jēz) (2). The outer membrane is called the **dura mater** (dū'rah mā'ter) (3), which is tough connective tissue underlaid by a web of **arachnoid** (ah-răk'noid) **membrane** (4). The inner membrane follows the convolutions of the brain and is called the **pia mater** (pī'ah mā'ter) (5).

The largest part of the brain is the **cerebrum** (sĕr'ĕ-brŭm) (12). It has an outer surface of gray matter called the **cerebral cortex** (kor'tĕks), which is responsible for the generation of impulses. Figure 20-3 shows the location of some of the centers of the cerebral cortex.

Beneath the cerebral cortex is a white tissue that is responsible for the conduction of messages. As shown in Figure 20-2, the gray cortex is arranged in folds, forming elevated portions known as **gyri** (jī'rī) or **convolutions** (1). These are separated by depressions or grooves called **sulci** (sŭl'kī) or **fissures**. A deep vertical fissure divides the cerebrum into halves called hemispheres. Other fissures divide each hemisphere into lobes.

Although individual brains vary somewhat, the larger fissures in each hemisphere do remain constant enough to serve as surface landmarks by which each hemisphere can be divided. These lobes are the frontal (13), parietal (16), temporal (14), and occipital (15).

The **frontal lobe**, also known as the **somatic** (sō-măt'ĭk) **motor area**, controls voluntary muscles. The left side of the frontal lobe governs the right side of the body and the muscles involved in speech. The right side of the frontal lobe governs the left side of the body. The frontal lobe influences personality and is associated with mental activities such as planning, judgment, and conceptualizing.

The **parietal** (pah-rī'ĕ-tăl) **lobe** is the primary sensory area or **somatic sensory area**. It determines distance, size, shape, and taste, as well as the sensory aspects of speech.

The **temporal lobe** contains the auditory center for hearing impulses and determines the sense of smell. It also is involved with memory and learning. Choices about which thoughts to express are made here.

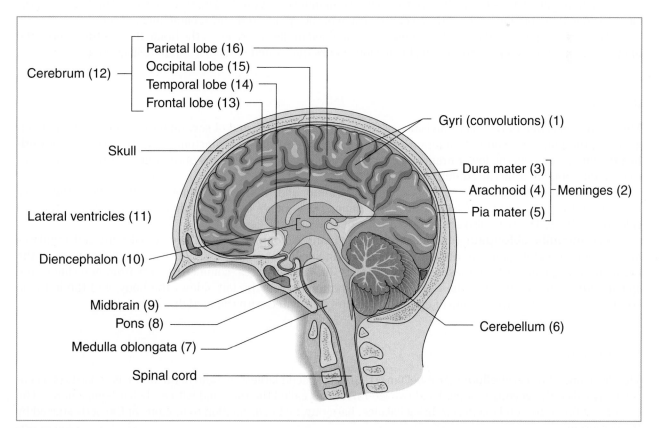

FIGURE 20-2   The Brain

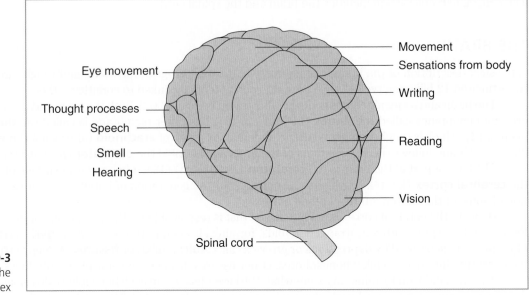

Eye movement

Thought processes

Speech

Smell

Hearing

Movement

Sensations from body

Writing

Reading

Vision

Spinal cord

FIGURE 20-3
Centers of the
Cerebral Cortex

The **occipital** (ŏk-sĭp'ĭ-tăl) **lobe** occupies a small area in the posterior portion of the cerebrum. Vision, one of the special senses, is governed by this lobe.

There are four ventricles, or cavities, in the brain. The two **lateral ventricles** (vĕn'trĭ-k'lz) (11), one located in each hemisphere, are the largest, extending from the frontal portion of the cerebral hemisphere to the posterior lobe. They have a hornlike projection, or **cornu** (kor'nū), that reaches into the frontal, occipital, and temporal lobes.

The third ventricle—the smallest of the four—communicates with the lateral ventricles. The fourth ventricle is the one that communicates with the central canal of the spinal cord and subarachnoid space.

The cerebrospinal fluid is a watery substance contained in the ventricles of the brain. It flows throughout the brain and around the spinal cord, serving to cushion shocks that would otherwise injure delicate organs.

Brainstem

The brainstem is one of the major divisions of the brain and is composed of several parts—the medulla oblongata (7), the pons (8), and the midbrain (9). At the upper part of the brainstem above the pons is the **midbrain**, which connects the lower brain centers to the higher centers, contains optic reflex centers, and serves to correlate optic and tactile (touch) impulses.

The **pons**, or bridge, is located between the midbrain and the medulla oblongata. It contains the nerve tracts from the right and left halves of the cerebellum. These nerve tracts coordinate the muscles on the two sides of the body. The pons also contains four pairs of cranial nerve centers.

The **medulla oblongata** (mĕ-dul'ah ŏb"lŏng-gā'tah) is continuous with the spinal cord and regulates heart action, breathing, and circulation. Nerve fibers establish communication between the higher parts of the brain and the spinal cord. As these nerve fibers pass through this area, some cross over from one side of the spinal cord to the other. Thus the right side of the brain controls the left side of the body, and the left side controls the right side. Eight pairs of cranial nerves are associated with the medulla oblongata.

Cerebellum

The "little brain," or **cerebellum** (sĕr"ĕ-bĕl'ŭm) (6), is the second largest division of the brain. It consists of a central body called the **vermis** (vĕr'mĭs) and two lateral masses called the right and left cerebellar hemispheres. The chief function of the cerebellum is to bring balance, harmony, and coordination to motions of the body started by the cerebrum.

Diencephalon

The section of the brain between the midbrain and the cerebrum is referred to as the **diencephalon** (dī"ĕn-sĕf'ah-lŏn) (10). It contains the thalamus, hypothalamus, and epithalamus. The third ventricle is also located in the diencephalon.

In the **thalamus** (thăl'ah-mŭs), the nerve fibers from the spinal cord and the lower part of the brain provide synaptic connection with neurons leading to the sensory areas of the cerebrum. The **hypothalamus** (hī'pō-thăl'ah-mŭs) contains centers for the control of body temperature, carbohydrate metabolism, fat metabolism, and emotions that affect heartbeat, blood pressure, appetite, and sexual reflexes. The **epithalamus** (ĕp"ĭ-thăl'ah-mŭs) contains the pineal body, which was discussed in Chapter 19.

THE SPINAL CORD

gangli/o	swelling	spondyl/o	vertebra
myel/o	marrow, spinal cord		

Below the medulla oblongata, the nervous system continues as the spinal cord. The cord performs the following two functions.

1. Reflex activities. This involves the translation of a sensory message entering the cord into a motor message as it leaves.
2. Pathway. The spinal cord serves as a pathway for conducting sensory impulses from the sensory nerve upward through the ascending tracts to the brain. It also serves as a pathway for motor impulses to move through the descending tracts from the brain to the nerve that will supply messages to muscles or glands.

Except for the twelve pairs of cranial nerves that connect directly with the brain, all spinal nerves enter or leave the spinal cord through openings in the vertebrae.

The spinal cord, as depicted in Figure 20-4, is divided into four parts: **cervical** (1), **thoracic** (2), **lumbar** (3), and **sacral** (4). It is comprised of an inner core of gray matter and an outer covering of white matter. The gray matter is composed of neuroglia and neuron networks of nerve fibers. The cord is covered with the meninges, the same three layers that cover the brain (dura mater, arachnoid, and pia mater). Injury of the spinal cord in any segment can endanger any or all of its functions.

PERIPHERAL NERVOUS SYSTEM

The peripheral nervous system is composed of spinal nerves and cranial nerves.

THE SPINAL NERVES

The thirty-one pairs of spinal nerves carry both voluntary and involuntary impulses, and all emerge from the spinal cord. At different levels of the cord, these spinal nerves regulate activities of different parts of the body. Each is named after its corresponding vertebra.

Figure 20-5 illustrates how each nerve is made up of all types of **sensory** (3) and **motor fibers** (4) of both the autonomic and voluntary nervous systems. Each spinal nerve divides into **dorsal** (7) and **ventral roots** (5), which enter the cord at different points.

The incoming nerve bulges into a **ganglion** (găng'glē-ŏn) (6) (a cluster of nerve cell bodies), enters the posterior section of the cord, and connects with one of the dorsal gray horns (1) of the H-shaped gray matter of the cord. Outgoing motor fibers connect with the corresponding ventral gray horn (2) at the front of the cord and send a direction or impulse to the effector in the muscle fiber.

In some areas of the body, these fibers form an interlocking network called a **plexus** (plĕk'sŭs), such as the brachial plexus in the shoulder. There is a cervical plexus (in the neck), a sacral plexus, a lumbar plexus, and a coccygeal plexus. As can be seen in Figure 20-6, many nerves are named after bones, organs, or the body regions in which they are located.

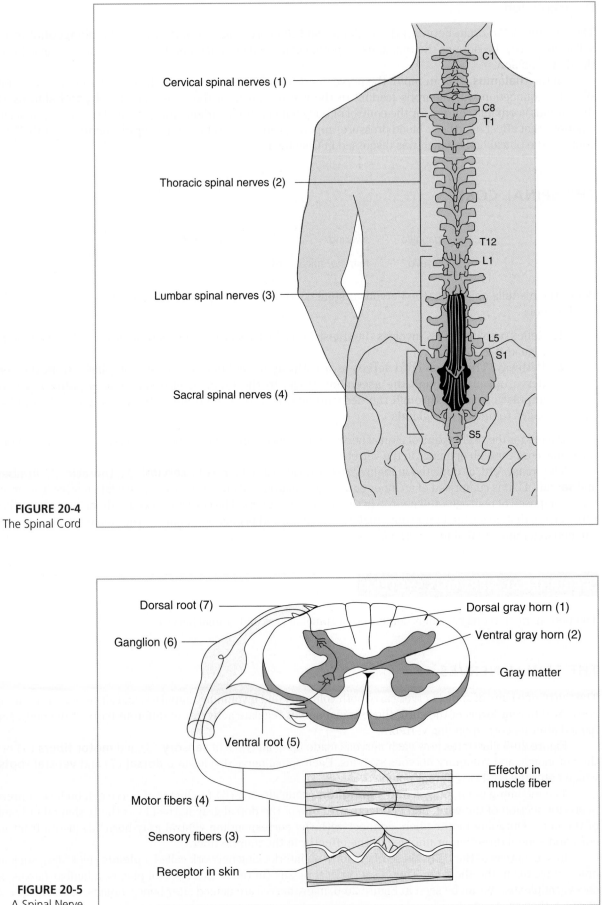

FIGURE 20-4
The Spinal Cord

Cervical spinal nerves (1)

Thoracic spinal nerves (2)

Lumbar spinal nerves (3)

Sacral spinal nerves (4)

C1

C8
T1

T12
L1

L5
S1

S5

FIGURE 20-5
A Spinal Nerve

Dorsal root (7)

Ganglion (6)

Dorsal gray horn (1)

Ventral gray horn (2)

Gray matter

Ventral root (5)

Effector in
muscle fiber

Motor fibers (4)

Sensory fibers (3)

Receptor in skin

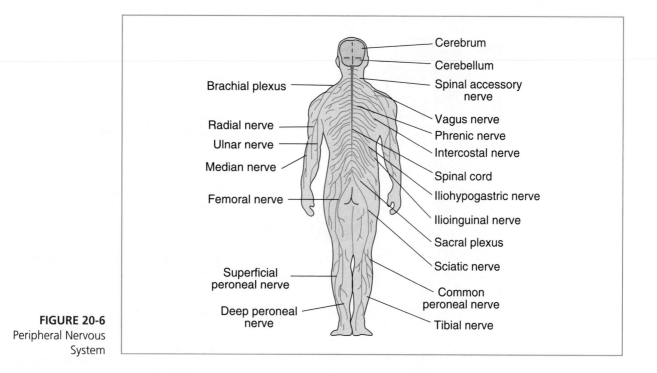

FIGURE 20-6
Peripheral Nervous System

THE CRANIAL NERVES

There are twelve pairs of cranial nerves. The first four are located in the front of the brain, the next four are related to the pons, and the last four are attached to the medulla. Ten of these pairs of nerves supply nerve fibers to structures of the head. Of the other two pairs, one extends to muscles in the neck and the other sends branches into the thoracic and abdominal organs.

From a functional point of view, these nerves handle messages of four types: special sense impulses; general sense impulses, such as pain and touch; voluntary muscle control; and involuntary control.

The twelve cranial nerves and their functions are listed below, including their Roman numeral reference. Physicians often refer to cranial nerves by Roman numeral reference.

	Nerve	Pronunciation	Function
I	olfactory	ŏl-făk'tō-rē	smell impulses to the brain
II	optic	op'tĭk	vision
III	oculomotor	ŏk"ū-lō-mō'tor	eye muscles and the pupil
IV	trochlear	trŏk'lē-ăr	one eyeball muscle on each side
V	trigeminal	trī-jĕm'ĭ-năl	sensory nerve of the face and head
VI	abducens	ăb-dū'sĕnz	eyeball muscle
VII	facial		largely motor to the face
VIII	acoustic	ah-kōōs'tĭk	balance and hearing
IX	glossopharyngeal	glŏs"ō-fah-rĭn'jē-ăl	taste, saliva secretion, swallowing
X	vagus	vā'gŭs	most organs in the thoracic and abdominal cavities
XI	accessory		two muscles of the neck
XII	hypoglossal	hī"pō-glŏs'ăl	muscles of the tongue

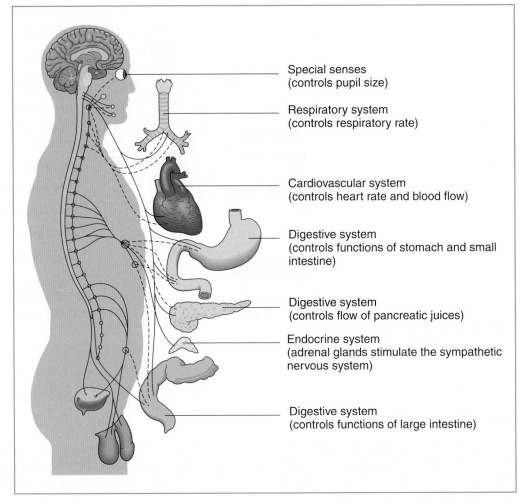

Special senses
(controls pupil size)

Respiratory system
(controls respiratory rate)

Cardiovascular system
(controls heart rate and blood flow)

Digestive system
(controls functions of stomach and small intestine)

Digestive system
(controls flow of pancreatic juices)

Endocrine system
(adrenal glands stimulate the sympathetic nervous system)

Digestive system
(controls functions of large intestine)

FIGURE 20-7
Autonomic Nervous System with Examples of Major Body Systems Involved

AUTONOMIC NERVOUS SYSTEM

The autonomic nervous system automatically controls various involuntary body functions and activities based on feedback from sensory nerves. Some of these are shown in Figure 20-7; they include the action of the glands, the smooth muscles of the hollow organs, and the heart.

This system has two divisions—the sympathetic and parasympathetic—both controlled by the hypothalamus, cerebral cortex, and medulla oblongata.

Essentially, the sympathetic system increases activity, while the arasympathetic system decreases activity. For instance, action of the heart would be quickened by the sympathetic system, whereas the parasympathetic system would slow it down. Interaction of these two systems normally keeps the body processes at a steady state of activity.

INTERNET ASSIGNMENT

The National Institute of Neurological Disorders and Stroke (NINDS) is part of the National Institutes of Health and is accessible at **www.ninds.nih.gov**. The mission of the NINDS is to reduce the burden of neurological disease in people all over the world. To accomplish this goal, the NINDS supports and conducts research, both basic and clinical, on the normal and diseased nervous systems; fosters the training of investigators in the basic and clinical neurosciences; and seeks better understanding, diagnosis, treatment, and prevention of neurological disorders.

This site covers a wide variety of neurological disorders that can be accessed by clicking on Disorders in the banner of the homepage. News and Events highlight current NINDS press releases.

ACTIVITY

Visit the National Institute of Neurological Disorders and Stroke (NINDS) at **www.ninds.nih.gov**. Check your text to find a condition about which you would like more information. Click on Disorders and either select the first letter of the condition in the A to Z choices or scroll through the links. Select the condition and submit a report to your instructor on the results of your investigation.

Review: The Nervous System

■ Neurons interspersed with neuroglia cells are the basic structural and functional components of the nervous system.

■ The three parts of the nervous system, grouped according to structure and function, are referred to as the central, peripheral, and autonomic nervous systems.

■ The central nervous system includes the brain and spinal cord, the two bases of operation.

■ The peripheral nervous system is composed of cranial and spinal nerves that carry messages to and from the brain and spinal column.

■ The autonomic nervous system functions automatically, responding and adjusting as necessary without the individual's help.

■ All parts of the nervous system are interdependent and interconnected.

Review of Terminology Presented

Word	Definition
arachnoid membrane	weblike membrane between the dura mater and the pia mater of the meninges
autonomic nervous system	system concerned with activities conducted automatically by certain peripheral nerves
axon	a long, straight fiber originating from a cell body and ending in a brushlike tip; its purpose is to conduct impulses away from the cell body
cell body	part of a cell that contains the nucleus and surrounding cytoplasm
central nervous system	brain and spinal cord
cerebellum	second largest division of the brain; "little brain"
cerebral cortex	outer surface of the cerebrum that is responsible for the generation of impulses
cerebrum	largest part of the brain
cervical, thoracic, lumbar, sacral	four sections of the spinal cord
cornu	hornlike projection of the lateral ventricle reaching into the frontal, occipital, and temporal lobes
dendrites	short fibers that branch out from a cell body

continues

Word	Definition
diencephalon	section of the brain between the midbrain and cerebrum
dorsal and ventral roots	divisions of the spinal nerve that enter the spinal cord at different points
dura mater	outer membrane of meninges
epithalamus	part of the diencephalon that contains the pineal body
frontal lobe	anterior lobe of the brain that controls voluntary muscles
ganglion	cluster of nerve cell bodies
gyri (convolutions)	folds of cortex forming elevated portions
hypothalamus	part of the diencephalon that contains centers for the control of body temperature, carbohydrate metabolism, fat metabolism, and emotions that affect heartbeat, blood pressure, appetite, and sexual reflexes
interneurons	neurons that shuttle messages back and forth through the pathways
lateral ventricle	cavity of the brain extending from the frontal portion of the cerebral hemisphere to the posterior lobe
medulla oblongata	one part of the brainstem that regulates heart action, breathing, and circulation
meninges	membranes that cover the brain and spinal cord
midbrain	upper part of the brainstem
motor (efferent) neurons	neurons that stimulate the contraction or relaxation of muscles and spur the activities of glands
myelin	white, fatty material that forms a sheath around most axons
neuroglia cells	supporting and connecting cells of the nervous system
neurologist	physician who specializes in the study of the nervous system
neuron	basic unit of the nervous system
neurosurgeon	surgeon who specializes in the surgical treatment of diseases of the nervous system
nucleus	central controlling structure within a living cell
occipital lobe	posterior lobe of the brain that governs vision
parietal lobe	lobe of the brain that contains the sensory areas and determines distance, size, shape, taste, and the sensory aspects of speech
peripheral nervous system	cranial and spinal nerves
pia mater	inner membrane of meninges
plexus	interlocking network of nerves
pons	part of the brainstem located between the midbrain and medulla oblongata
sensory and motor fibers	part of the composition of spinal nerves of both the autonomic and voluntary nervous systems
sensory (afferent) neurons	neurons that carry signals to the brain and spinal cord
somatic sensory area	parietal lobe
somatic motor area	frontal lobe
sulci (fissures)	depressions or grooves that separate convolutions
synapse	junction between neurons

continues

Word	Definition
temporal lobe	lobe of the brain that contains the auditory center for hearing impulses and determines the sense of smell
thalamus	part of the diencephalon where nerve fibers from the spinal cord and lower part of the brain synapse with neurons leading to the cerebrum
vermis	central portion of the cerebellum

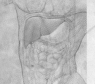

Terminology Review Exercises

Name: _____ Date: _____

MATCHING*

Match the cranial nerves to the functions they control.

1. _____ taste
2. _____ one eyeball muscle on each side
3. _____ smell impulses to the brain
4. _____ muscles of the tongue
5. _____ sensory nerve of the face and head
6. _____ largely motor to the face
7. _____ most organs in the thoracic and abdominal cavities
8. _____ two muscles of the neck
9. _____ vision
10. _____ balance and hearing
11. _____ eyeball muscle
12. _____ eye muscles controlling the pupil

a. hypoglossal
b. accessory
c. vagus
d. glossopharyngeal
e. acoustic
f. facial
g. abducens
h. trigeminal
i. trochlear
j. oculomotor
k. optic
l. olfactory

COMPLETION*

Complete the following statements.

1. The basic unit of the nervous system is the _____.
2. A _____ is a junction between one neuron and another.
3. There are more than _____ billion neurons in the nervous system.
4. The nervous system is made up of nerve cells interspersed with _____.
5. The hornlike projection of the lateral ventricle reaching into the frontal, occipital, and temporal lobes is called the _____.

SELECTION*

From the list at the right, select in which portion of the brain each of the following is located.

1. _____ vermis
2. _____ medulla oblongata
3. _____ cerebral cortex
4. _____ parietal lobe
5. _____ pons

a. cerebrum
b. brainstem
c. cerebellum

---

*Answers are in Appendix A.

DEFINITIONS
Define the following terms.

1. sulci

   _____

2. gyri

   _____

3. peripheral nervous system

   _____

4. central nervous system

   _____

5. meninges

   _____

6. dura mater

   _____

7. arachnoid membrane

   _____

8. plexus

   _____

SHORT ANSWERS
Supply a short answer to the following.

1. Name the four divisions of the spinal cord.

   _____

2. Name the four lobes of the cerebrum.

   _____

3. Describe the function of the spinal cord.

   _____

4. Identify the number of spinal and cranial nerves.

   _____

5. Define the autonomic nervous system, and name its two divisions.

   _____

   _____

   _____

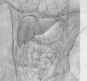

Working Practice

DIAGNOSTIC PROCEDURES		
Word	**Pronunciation**	**Definition**
General		
electroencepha-lography	ē-lĕk"trō-ĕn-sĕf"ah-lŏg'rah-fē	study of the electrical activity of the brain using electrodes attached to the scalp; produces an electroencephalogram (EEG)
electromyography	ē-lĕk"trō-mī'ŏg'rah-fē	study of the contraction of a muscle as a result of electrical stimulation; produces an electromyogram (EMG)
Glasgow Coma Scale		assessment tool that evaluates eye movement, verbal response, and motor response to describe the level of consciousness: may be semicomatose, stupor, lethargic, or comatose
lumbar puncture for cerebrospinal fluid (CSF) analysis	sĕr"ĕ-brō-spī'năl	procedure that detects abnormal substances and variations in the cerebrospinal fluid through extraction of fluid for examination, pressure recording, or injection
Nuclear Medicine		
brain scan		procedure using radioactive chemicals and special machines to record their passage and absorption into any brain lesions; brain barrier will not allow the radioactive chemical in normal brain tissue
positron emission tomography (PET scan)	pŏz'ĭ-trŏn, tō-mŏg'rah-fē	an agent is mixed with a radioactive substance and is injected into the blood to record and measure images of the target site
single-photon emission computer tomography (SPECT)	fō'tŏn, tō-mŏg'rah-fē	method for reconstructing sectional images of radiotracer distributions
Radiology		
arteriography (angiography)	ăr"tē-rē-ŏg'rah-fē (ăn"jē-ŏg'rah-fē)	x-ray using contrast material injected into arteries to diagnose blockages, tumors, and the like
cervical spine, thoracic spine, lumbosacral spine		x-ray of specific sections of the spinal column
computerized axial tomography (CAT)	tō-mŏg'rah-fē	computer-assisted x-ray technique used to distinguish pathological conditions such as tumors, abscesses, and hematomas
magnetic resonance imaging (MRI)		technique used to distinguish pathological lesions of the brain and spinal cord (See Figure 20-8)
myelography	mī"ĕ-lŏg'rah-fē	x-ray study of the spinal canal and cord after an injection of contrast material into the subarachnoid space
routine skull series		standard x-ray views of the skull

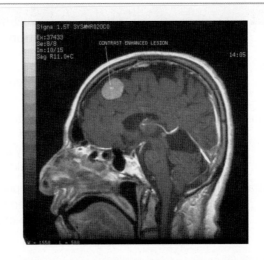

FIGURE 20-8
Tumor of the Brain
Visualized Through
Magnetic Resonance
Imaging (MRI)

DIAGNOSES		
Word	**Pronunciation**	**Definition**
Infections		
encephalitis	ĕn-sĕf"ă-lī'tĭs	inflammation of brain tissue
meningitis	mĕn-ĭn'jī'tĭs	inflammation of the meninges (membranes of the spinal cord or brain)
poliomyelitis	pōl"ē-ō-mī"ĕl-ī'tĭs	viral infection affecting brain and spinal cord
rabies	rā'bēz	often fatal encephalomyelitis caused by a virus transmitted to humans by an animal bite
shingles	shĭng'lz	viral disease affecting peripheral nerves (See Figure 20-9)
tetanus	tĕt'ă-nŭs	acute, often fatal infection of nerve tissue caused by the bacteria *Colstridium tetani*

continues

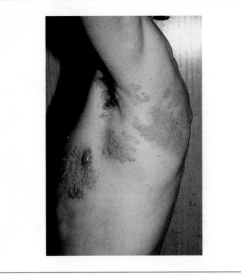

FIGURE 20-9
Shingles: vesicles
follow a nerve
pathway (Courtesy
of Robert A.
Silverman, M.D.,
Clinical Associate
Professor,
Department
of Pediatrics,
Georgetown
University)

DIAGNOSES

Word	Pronunciation	Definition
Vascular Disorders		
aneurysm	ăn'ū'rĭzm	sac formed by localized dilation of the walls of an artery or a vein
cerebrovascular accident (CVA)	sĕr-ē"brō-văs'kū-lăr	damage to the brain caused by a disorder of the blood vessels of the brain; also known as a stroke; may be caused by a *thrombus* (a blood clot), an *embolus* (a clot that breaks off), or a *hemorrhage*
transient ischemic attack (TIA)	trans'ē-ĕnt ĭs-kē'mĭk	sudden episode of temporary symptoms due to diminished blood flow through the brain; early warning symptom of stroke (See Figure 20-10)
Functional Disorders		
Bell's palsy	păl'zē	disease causing paralysis of one side of the face
cephalalgia (headache)	sĕf-ă-lăl'jē-ah	pain in various locations in the head or neck
• *cluster*		series of intense, short-term, recurring headaches felt near one eye; occur at night after falling asleep
• *migraine*	mī'grān	severe headache accompanied by nausea, vomiting, and vision problems; may be limited to one side
• *postlumbar puncture*	pōst-lŭm'băr	follows a lumbar puncture in forty percent of the cases
• *stress*		caused by stress, strain, tension of the face, neck, and scalp muscles

continues

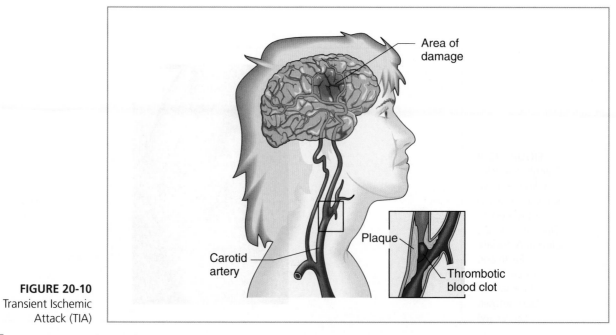

FIGURE 20-10
Transient Ischemic
Attack (TIA)

Area of damage

Carotid artery

Plaque

Thrombotic blood clot

DIAGNOSES

Word	Pronunciation	Definition
Functional Disorders (*continued*)		
cerebral palsy	sĕr'ĕ-brăl păl'zē	disorder discovered after birth, involving the brain
degenerative disc disease	dĭ-jĕ'nĕ-ră"tĭv	condition marked by wearing away of intervertebral disc causing spinal stenosis
dementia	dē-mĕn'shē-ah	decreased mental functioning
• *Alzheimer's disease*	ăltz'hī-mĕrz	irreversible senile dementia characterized by deteriorating intellectual capacities
• *head trauma*	trăw'mah	death of brain cells related to head trauma
• *substance induced*		death of brain cells caused by toxicity of drugs and toxins
• *vascular*	văs'cū-lăr	atrophy and death of brain cells due to decreased blood flow
epilepsy	ĕp'ĭ-lĕp"sē	recurrent disorder of neuronal function manifested by a variety of seizure types
hydrocephalus	hī-drō-sĕf'ah-lŭs	abnormal accumulation of excess spinal fluid within the ventricles of the brain
trigeminal neuralgia	trī-jĕm'ĭn-ăl nū-răl'jē-ah	severe, sharp pain along the fifth cranial nerve
Sleep Disorders		
insomnia	ĭn-sŏm'nē-ah	inability to fall or stay asleep
sleep apnea	ăp'nē-ah	sleep disorder characterized by periods of apnea or breathlessness
Tumors		
brain tumor		abnormal growth of brain tissue and meninges; may be *primary* (originating in brain tissue) or *secondary* (originating elsewhere and metastasizing to the brain)
Trauma		
concussion	kŏn-kŭsh'ŭn	posttraumatic syndrome, which can include severe headaches, memory loss, dizziness, and extreme breathing rates
contusion	kŏn-too'shŭn	injury to the brain causing bruising of the brain
hematoma		localized collection of blood within the cranium
• *subdural*	sŭb-dū'răl	blood collecting below the dura caused by a break in a blood vessel and often the result of a head injury
• *epidural*	ĕp"ĭ-dū'răl	blood collecting between the cranium and the dural matter
• *intracerebral*	ĭn"tră-sĕ-rē'brăl	blood collecting within the brain tissue itself (See Figure 20-11)

continues

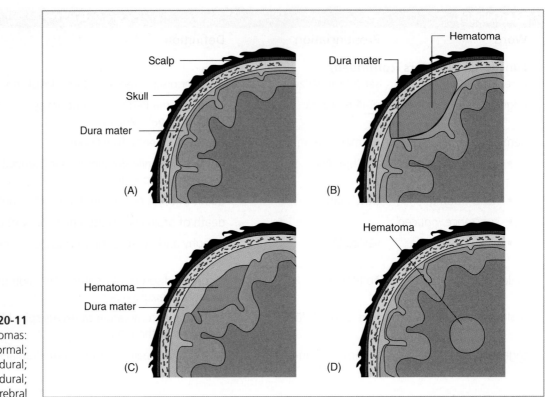

FIGURE 20-11
Cranial Hematomas:
(A) normal;
(B) epidural;
(C) subdural;
(D) intracerebral

DIAGNOSES

Word	Pronunciation	Definition
Trauma (continued)		
skull fractures		trauma causing bone fractures that may lead to permanent or temporary brain tissue damage
spinal cord injury		injury to spinal cord at any level; site, type, and degree of injury determine whether temporary or permanent paralysis will occur
• *hemiplegia*	hĕm-ē-plē'jē-ah	injury or paralysis to one side of the body
• *paraplegia*	păr-ă-plē'jē-ah	injury to thoracic or lumbar section of spinal cord, which leads to loss of movement and feeling either in both legs or both arms
• *quadriplegia*	kwod"rĭ-plē'jē-ah	injuries to cervical spine or neck area, C1 to C6; leads to loss of movement and feeling in all four extremities
Other Diseases		
amyotrophic lateral sclerosis (ALS)	ă-mī"ō-trŏf'ĭk lăt'ĕr-ăl sklē-rō'sĭs	destructive disease of motor or movement neurons; Lou Gehrig's disease
Guillain-Barré Syndrome	gē-yăn'băr-rā'	acute, progressive disease affecting the peripheral and spinal nerves

continues

DIAGNOSES

Word	Pronunciation	Definition
Huntington's chorea	kō-rē'ah	inherited disease that appears in middle age and is marked by progressive degeneration of the brain
multiple sclerosis (MS)	mŭl'tĭ-p'l sklē-rō'sĭs	disease that causes demyelination of nerves of the central nervous system
Parkinson's disease		slow, progressive brain degeneration with a deficiency of dopamine in the brain
spina bifida cystica	spī'nah bĭf'ĭ'dah sĭs'tĭ-kah	congenital defect in the walls of the spinal canal caused by a lack of union between the laminae of the vertebrae
spina bifida occulta	spī'nah bĭf'ĭ'dah ō-kŭl'tah	failure of the vertebrae to close, without protrusion of neural tissues (See Figure 20-12)

TREATMENT PROCEDURES

Word	Pronunciation	Definition
carotid endarterectomy	kah-rŏt'ĭd ĕnd"ăr-tĕr-ĕk'tō-mē	removal of plaque or thickened lining of a carotid artery to unclog the artery
cerebrospinal fluid shunts	sĕr"ĕ-brō-spī'năl	creation of channels to detour accumulated cerebrospinal fluid in the brain; the two most common are ventriculoatrial and ventriculoperitoneal
craniotomy	krā"nē-ŏt'ō-mē	any operation to open the cranium
decompression		surgical procedure to relieve intracranial pressure
halo traction		traction device for connecting the head and cervical area for neck stability
laminectomy	lăm"ĭ-něk'tō-mē	removal of a vertebral lesion or herniated disk

continues

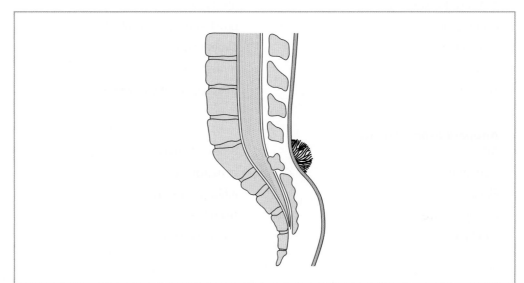

FIGURE 20-12
Spina Bifida Occulta

TREATMENT PROCEDURES

Word	Pronunciation	Definition
myelocele repair	mī'ĕ-lō-sēl	repair of an open spine or the cord components, which is usually congenital
percutaneous electrocoagulation	pĕr"kū-tā'nē-ŭs ē-lĕk"trō-kō-ăg"ū'lā'shŭn	procedure for longer-term pain relief affecting pain-sensory fibers
stereotaxic thalamotomy	stĕ"rē-ō-tăk'sĭk thăl-ă-mŏt'ō-mē	use of a stereotaxic instrument to locate a target and disrupt the transmission of motor impulses (tremors)
trephination	trĕf"ĭ-nā'shŭn	cutting a circular incision into the skull to make brain surgery possible
ulnar nerve transposition	ul'năr	transfer and decompression of the ulnar nerve at the elbow to relieve trauma to the nerve

MEDICATIONS PRESCRIBED

Trade Name	Generic Name
Anticonvulsants	
Depakene, Depakote	valproic acid
Diamox	acetazolamide
Dilantin	phenytoin
Klonopin	clonazepam
Mysoline	primidone
Phenobarbital	phenobarbital
Tegretol	carbamazepine
Tranxene	clorazepate dipotassium
Zarontin	ethosuximide
Antiemetic and Antivertigo	
Antivert, Bonine	meclizine
Compazine	prochlorperazine maleate
Dramamine	dimenhydrinate
Tigan	trimethobenzamide
Torecan	thiethylperazine maleate
Antiparkinson's Agents	
Artane	trihexyphenidyl
Cogentin	benztropine
Elavil	amitriptyline HCl
Eldepryl	selegiline
Pagitane	cycrimine HCl

continues

MEDICATIONS PRESCRIBED

Trade Name	Generic Name
Antiparkinson's Agents _(continued)_	
Parisdol	ethopropagine HCl
Parlodel	bromocriptine mesylate
Permax	pergolide mesylate
Sinemet	carbidopa, levodopa
Symmetrel	amantadine
Tofranil	imipramine HCl
CNS Stimulants	
Dexedrine	dextroamphetamine sulfate
Ritalin	methylphenidate
Edema control	
Decadron	dexamethasone
Mannitol	mannitol
Solu-Medrol	methylprednisolone
MS Agents	
ACTH	adrenocorticotropic steroid
Avonex, Betaseron	interferon beta
Capaxone	glatiramer acetate
Cytoxan	cyclophosphamide
Dantrium	dantrolene sodium
Deltasone	prednisone
Glatiramer acetate	copaxone
Imuran	azathioprine
Lioresal	baclofen
Pro-Banthine	propantheline bromide
Sandimmune	cyclosporine
Headache Agents	
Cafergot	ergotamine and caffeine
Catapres	clonidine HCl
Ergostat	ergotamine tartrate
Inderal	propranolol HCl
Phenergan	promethazine HCl
Sansert	methysergide maleate

ABBREVIATIONS

CAT	computerized axial tomography
CNS	central nervous system
CP	cerebral palsy
CSF	cerebrospinal fluid
CVA	cerebrovascular accident
EEG	electroencephalogram
EMG	electromyogram
LP	lumbar puncture
MRI	magnetic resonance imaging
MS	multiple sclerosis
TIA	transient ischemic attack

Working Practice Review Exercises

Name: _____ Date: _____

IDENTIFICATION*

Identify the following diagnostic procedures.

1. measures muscle contractions as a result of electrical stimulation   _____

2. extraction of cerebrospinal fluid for examination   _____

3. radioactive chemicals are given, and special machines record whether brain lesions are present   _____

4. injection of contrast material into arteries to diagnose blockages and tumors   _____

5. studies electrical activity of the brain by means of electrodes attached to the scalp   _____

6. x-ray study of spinal canal and cord after contrast material is injected into subarachnoid space   _____

MEANINGS

Give the meaning of the italicized words.

1. There is an *aneurysm* on the right middle cerebral artery.

   _____

2. The damage to the brainstem was caused by *hydrocephalus*.

   _____

3. The patient sustained a *subdural hematoma* as a result of the boating accident.

   _____

4. Miss Chenevey has *Parkinson's disease*.

   _____

5. Their son has a *contusion*.

   _____

6. After-surgery recovery was complicated by *meningitis*.

   _____

7. The patient suffered a *CVA* last year.

   _____

MATCHING*

Match the terms to their meanings.

1. _____ repair of an open spine or the cord components
2. _____ disc surgery
3. _____ removal of thickened lining of an artery
4. _____ an operation on the cranium
5. _____ creation of a channel to detour cerebrospinal fluid in the brain

a. carotid endarterectomy
b. craniotomy
c. laminectomy
d. cerebrospinal fluid shunt
e. myelocele repair

---

*Answers are in Appendix A.

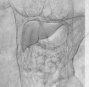

Word Element Review

Root	Meaning	Example	Definition
cephal/o	head	**cephalic** (sĕ-făl'ĭk)	pertaining to the head
cerebell/o	cerebellum	**cerebellitis** (sĕr"ĕ-bĕl-ī'tĭs)	inflammation of the cerebellum
cerebr/o	brain	**cerebrospinal** (sĕr"ĕ-brō-spī'năl)	pertaining to the brain and spinal cord
crani/o	head, skull	**craniotomy** (krā"nē-ŏt'ō-mē)	incision through the cranium
		cranium (krā'nē-ŭm)	that portion of the skull that encloses the brain
dur/o	dura mater	**duraplasty** (dŭ'ră-plăs"tē)	plastic repair of the dura mater
encephal/o	brain	**encephalon** (ĕn-sĕf'ah-lŏn)	the brain
		encephalopathy (ĕn-sĕf"ah-lŏp'ah-thē)	any disease of the brain
gangli/o	swelling	**ganglion** (găng'glē-ŏn)	mass of nerve tissue composed principally of nerve bodies and lying outside the brain or spinal cord
mening/o	meninges	**meningeal** (mĕ-nĭn'jē-ăl)	pertaining to the meninges
		meningitis (mĕn"ĭn-jī'tĭs)	inflammation of the membranes covering the brain and spinal cord
myel/o	marrow, spinal cord	**osteomyelitis** (ŏs"tē-ō-mī"ĕ-lī'tĭs)	inflammation of bone and bone marrow
neur/o	nerve, nervous system	**neuralgia** (nū-răl'jē-ah)	severe, sharp pain along the course of a nerve
pont/o	pons	**pontocerebellar** (pŏn"tō-sĕr"ĕ-bĕl-ăr)	pertaining to the pons and the cerebellum
spondyl/o	vertebra	**spondylosis** (spŏn"dĭ-lō'sĭs)	immobility or fixation of vertebrae
		spondylous (spŏn'dĭ-lŭs)	pertaining to the spinal column
thalam/o	thalamus	**thalamocele** (thal'ăm-ō-sēl")	third ventricle of the brain

Word Element Review Exercises

Name: _____ Date: _____

MATCHING*
Match the terms to their meanings.

1. _____ pertaining to the brain and spinal column
2. _____ pertaining to the spinal column
3. _____ any disease of the brain
4. _____ inflammation of the membranes covering the brain and spinal column
5. _____ severe, sharp pain along the course of a nerve
6. _____ plastic repair of dura mater
7. _____ pertaining to the pons and cerebellum
8. _____ third ventricle of the brain
9. _____ pertaining to the meninges
10. _____ the brain
11. _____ incision through the cranium
12. _____ pertaining to the head
13. _____ immobility or fixation of vertebrae
14. _____ inflammation of the cerebellum
15. _____ portion of the skull that encloses the brain
16. _____ inflammation of bone and bone marrow
17. _____ mass of nerve tissue composed principally of nerve bodies lying outside the brain or spinal cord

a. cephalic
b. cerebellitis
c. cerebrospinal
d. craniotomy
e. cranium
f. duraplasty
g. encephalon
h. encephalopathy
i. ganglion
j. meningeal
k. meningitis
l. neuralgia
m. osteomyelitis
n. pontocerebellar
o. spondylosis
p. spondylous
q. thalamocele

WORD ELEMENT MEANINGS
Give the meaning of each word element. Then use your dictionary to find a new word that contains each of the word elements. Specify whether the new word is a noun or an adjective by placing N or A in the last column.

Word Element	Meaning	Word	N or A
1. cephal/o	_____	_____	_____
2. cerebell/o	_____	_____	_____
3. cerebr/o	_____	_____	_____
4. crani/o	_____	_____	_____
5. dur/o	_____	_____	_____
6. encephal/o	_____	_____	_____
7. gangli/o	_____	_____	_____
8. mening/o	_____	_____	_____

Word Element	Meaning	Word	N or A
9. myel/o	_____	_____	_____
10. neur/o	_____	_____	_____
11. pont/o	_____	_____	_____
12. spondyl/o	_____	_____	_____
13. thalam/o	_____	_____	_____

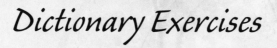

Dictionary Exercises

Name: _____ Date: _____

DICTIONARY EXERCISE 1*

Use your dictionary to find the pronunciation and definition of the following words.

	Word	**Pronunciation**	**Definition**
1.	cordotomy		
2.	disorientation		
3.	compression		
4.	neurotomy		
5.	polyneuritis		
6.	radiculoneuritis		
7.	tic douloureux		
8.	Babinski's reflex		
9.	Ménière's disease		
10.	meningoencephalo-myelitis		
11.	meningomyelitis		
12.	microcephaly		
13.	glioma		
14.	Hoffmann's reflex		
15.	jacksonian epilepsy		
16.	radiculitis		
17.	Romberg's sign		
18.	paraplegia		

*Answers are in Appendix A.

DICTIONARY EXERCISE 2*

Select the correct definition and provide the pronunciation where indicated.

1. anarthria (_____)
   a. inability to read
   b. inability to remember
   c. inability to speak
   d. inability to speak remembered words properly

2. anencephalus (_____)
   a. congenital absence of the brain and cranial space
   b. lack of memory
   c. loss of the power to recognize sensory stimuli even though sensory facilities are intact
   d. loss of sensation

3. astrocytoma (_____)
   a. tumor composed of neuroglial cells (astrocytes)
   b. tumor arising from specialized tissue found in the brain and spinal cord
   c. soft, infiltrating malignant tumor of the roof of the fourth ventricle and cerebellum
   d. rapidly growing malignant tumor composed of primitive glial cells

4. agnosia (_____)
   a. inability to read
   b. inability to fix the range of movement in muscular activity
   c. severe sharp pain
   d. loss of the power to recognize sensory stimuli even though sensory facilities are intact

5. dysmetria (_____)
   a. inability to read despite normal vision
   b. impairment of intellectual ability
   c. inability to fix the range of movement in muscular activity
   d. severe pain along the course of a nerve

6. paresthesia (_____)
   a. severe pain along the course of a nerve
   b. sensation of numbness, pricking, burning, crawling, or tingling
   c. disease marked by tingling, itching, and disturbing sensations
   d. impairment or lessening of sensitivity to touch

7. tabes dorsalis (_____)
   a. terminal portion of the spinal cord and roots of spinal nerves below first lumbar nerve
   b. proliferation of neuroglial tissue in CNS
   c. disease of CNS, usually caused by syphilis
   d. rare disease of nervous system; Guillain-Barré syndrome

8. encephalocele (_____)
   a. rapidly growing malignant tumor
   b. congenital hernia in which meninges protrude through an opening in the skull or spinal column
   c. abnormal smallness of the head
   d. protrusion of the brain through any opening in the skull

9. gliosis (_____)
   a. proliferation of neuroglial tissue in CNS
   b. impairment of sensitivity to touch
   c. inflammation of the spinal cord
   d. to and fro movement of the eyeballs as seen in brain damage

10. meralgia paresthetica (_____)
    a. sensitivity to pain
    b. severe pain along the course of a nerve
    c. disease marked by tingling, itching, and disturbing sensations in the thigh
    d. sharp pain along a nerve

---

*Answers are in Appendix A.

11. medulloblastoma (_____)
    a. soft, infiltrating malignant tumor of the roof of the fourth ventricle and cerebellum
    b. star-shaped tumor
    c. tumor arising from specialized tissue found in the brain and spinal cord
    d. tumor composed of glial cells in the cerebral hemisphere

12. retrogasserian neurotomy (_____)
    a. interruption of a nerve fiber tract within the spinal cord for relief of pain
    b. dissection of the posterior root of the trigeminal ganglion
    c. excision of a nerve
    d. suture of a nerve

13. convulsion (_____)
    a. injury resulting from a blow
    b. tremor
    c. violent involuntary muscular contractions and relaxations
    d. involuntary and quick repetitious spasms of a muscle

14. glioblastoma multiforme (_____)
    a. rapidly growing malignant tumor composed of primitive glial cells
    b. tumor arising from specialized tissue found in the brain and spinal cord
    c. tumor composed of glial cells in the cerebral hemisphere
    d. inflammation of the brain and spinal cord and their membranes

15. hypesthesia (_____)
    a. sensation of numbness, tingling, prickling, etc.
    b. lessening of sensitivity to touch
    c. decreased sensitivity to pain
    d. consciousness

DICTIONARY EXERCISE 3

Pronunciation of the words below is provided. Using your dictionary, find the spelling and definition of each word.

	Word	Pronunciation	Definition
1.	_____	dĕr'mă-tōm	_____
2.	_____	ă-grăf-ē-ah	_____
3.	_____	ă-lĕks'ē-ah	_____
4.	_____	ah-fă'zē-ah	_____
5.	_____	ăs-thē'nē-ah	_____
6.	_____	ah-tăk'sē-ah	_____
7.	_____	dĭs-lĕk'sē-ah	_____
8.	_____	ĕn-sĕf"ah-lŏp'ah-thē	_____
9.	_____	glī-ō'mah	_____
10.	_____	hĕm"ē-păr'ē-sĭs	_____
11.	_____	mī"ĕ-lī'tĭs	_____
12.	_____	năr'kō-lĕp"sē	_____
13.	_____	nĭs-tăg'mŭs	_____
14.	_____	sī-ăt'ĭ-kah	_____
15.	_____	tĭk	_____

DICTIONARY EXERCISE 4

Rewrite each sentence in your own words.

1. The patient displayed an *intention tremor* when attempting to remove the jar lid.

   _____

2. The first evidence of meningitis was *Brudzinski's sign*.

   _____

3. His wife experienced a *subarachnoid hemorrhage*.

   _____

4. On physical exam, there was no evidence of *neuropathy*.

   _____

5. The surgeon performed *neurorrhaphy* after his accident.

   _____

6. Cerebral *dysrhythmia* was evident.

   _____

7. Part of the reason for her problems in school was that she has *dyslexia*.

   _____

8. Her mother was confined to a wheelchair as a result of contracting *poliomyelitis* as a child.

   _____

DICTIONARY EXERCISE 5

Match the terms to their meanings.

1. _____ encephalitis
2. _____ encephalomalacia
3. _____ lethargy
4. _____ insomnia
5. _____ myelopathy
6. _____ neurectomy
7. _____ paresis
8. _____ sensorium
9. _____ tentorium
10. _____ tremor
11. _____ agraphia
12. _____ bulbar
13. _____ syncope
14. _____ polyneuropathy
15. _____ nuchal rigidity

a. softening of the brain

b. tentlike structure

c. any disease of the spinal cord

d. slight paralysis

e. loss of the ability to write

f. pertaining to the brainstem

g. excision of a nerve

h. inability to sleep

i. inflammation of the brain

j. shaking

k. fainting

l. roughly approximates consciousness

m. neck is resistant to flexion

n. state of being sluggish

o. disease involving many nerves at once

Listening Exercise

Name	Date

INSTRUCTIONS

1. Review the spelling, pronunciation, and meaning of the words provided in the preview.

2. Listen to the audio CD and fill in the blank as the word is dictated.

3. At the end of the exercise, check your spelling against the preview words. They appear in the preview in the order in which they are encountered in the exercise.

4. Review and practice the words you missed.

5. Look up words that are not familiar.

PREVIEW OF WORDS FOR LISTENING EXERCISE 20-1

Word	Pronunciation	Meaning
bradykinesia	brăd"ē-kĭ-nē'sē-ah	abnormal slowness of movement
facies	fā'shē-ēz	expression or appearance of the face
dysarthria	dĭs-ăr'thrē-ă	imperfect articulation of speech due to damage of the nervous system
pseudobulbar	sū"dō-bŭl'bĕr	apparently, but not really, due to a bulbar lesion
palsy	paul'zē	paralysis
extrapyramidal disorder	ĕks"tră-pĭ-răm'ĭ-dăl	disorder marked by abnormal involuntary movements such as Parkinsonism

Letter of Consultation

Dear Doctor Grimes:

Mr. Morton Herkimer recently returned for a recheck neurologic evaluation. Since leaving the hospital on the 7th of February, he has made considerable progress and has shown much improvement in his overall clinical condition. Of increasing concern has been tremor primarily involving the right upper extremity and _____.

On neurological examination at this time I found Morton to be alert, bright, and communicative. The major findings were a prominent rest tremor involving the right upper extremity as well as bradykinesia with masked _____, a mild hypokinetic _____ and associated postural change. In addition, he had signs of a _____ _____ with positive jaw jerk, suck and snout reflexes, brisk deep tendon reflexes, and bilateral extensor plantar responses. His tone was increased bilaterally. The clinical findings are, thus, those of a parkinsonian-like picture with superimposed pseudobulbar palsy.

The question of antiparkinson therapy was quite appropriately raised by yourself, and I believe this to be quite reasonable. On discussing this with him, I, however, felt that we might be able to hold off on this therapy in view of the way his clinical picture seems to be changing and perhaps improving. Therapy at this point, therefore, seems optional.

As I review his overall clinical picture, one wonders if his progressive dysfunction beginning in January was not an initial manifestation of what will subsequently become more typical of an _____ of the parkinsonian type.

I suggested a recheck neurologic examination in approximately two to three months.

Sincerely yours,

J. Michael Sandok, MD

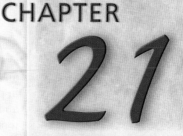

CHAPTER 21

Mental Health

> *The Brain—is wider than the sky—for—*
> *put them side by side—*
> *The one the other will contain with ease—*
> *and you—beside—*
>
> —EMILY DICKINSON

OBJECTIVES

When you have completed this chapter on mental health, you should be able to

1. Define classifications of mental disorders and the treatment process including the diagnostic interview, clinical tests, and psychotherapeutic techniques.
2. Spell the names of commonly used medications.
3. Identify the names of related word elements.
4. Identify abbreviations related to the mental health field.
5. Be familiar with terminology used in reports.

INTRODUCTION

iatr/o	treatment, physician
ment/o	mind
psych/o	mind

Mental health describes a relative state of mind in which individuals who are healthy are able to cope with and adjust to the events of life, good or bad, in a way that allows their personalities to remain intact and even to grow emotionally. **Psychiatry** (sī-kī'ă-trē) is the medical specialty that deals with the development and maintenance of good mental health by dealing with causes, treatment, and prevention of mental, emotional, and behavioral disorders.

Understanding the relationship of the body, including the brain and nervous system, and psychological factors requires the expertise of a **psychiatrist** (sī-kī'ă-trĭst), who is a medical doctor with several additional years of training in methods of psychotherapy, neurology, and pharmacology. A psychiatrist may also specialize. For instance, forensic psychiatrists deal with legal situations such as determining mental competence in criminal cases, while child psychiatrists treat children. Geropsychiatrists specialize in the treatment of older adults.

In addition to the psychiatrist, there are nonmedical persons trained in psychology. A **psychologist** (sī-kŏl'ō-jĭst) has a doctorate in psychology, is qualified to use many of the same treatments as a psychiatrist, but may not employ such techniques as electroconvulsive or drug therapies. A psychologist has training in psychotherapy and psychodiagnostic assessment through the use of various tests. Other specialties in psychology include *neuropsychology, educational psychology, geropsychology,* and *pediatric psychology.* All are directed at encouraging the development of good mental health.

Since psychiatry is not an anatomy-based specialty, this chapter will use a different format. It will look at the definition and classification of mental disorders, the types of treatment, the psychiatric interview, the clinical tests administered, and abbreviations commonly used.

MULTIAXIAL CLASSIFICATION OF MENTAL DISORDERS

The *Diagnostic and Statistical Manual of Mental Disorders* (DSM-IV-TR) (2000) is the principal guide for mental health professionals. This edition incorporates information found when a literature review was conducted of research published since the 1994 version was printed. The term used in the DSM-IV-TR for a mental disturbance is **mental disorder**, but the term historically has not had one distinct definition. In fact, the DSM-IV-TR conceptualizes each mental disorder as

a clinically significant behavioral or psychological syndrome or pattern that occurs in an individual and is associated with present distress or disability or with significantly increased risk of suffering death, pain, disability, or important loss of freedom. (p. xxii)

From the manual's perspective, categories of mental disorders are not limited by absolute boundaries dividing them from other mental disorders or, for that matter, from no mental disorder.

To help a mental health professional plan treatment for and predict outcomes of mental disorders, information from several domains, or axes, is useful. There are five axes included in the DSM-IV-TR. They are collectively referred to as the multiaxial assessment classification and are viewed as an efficient, effective way to organize and communicate information (see Table 21-1). These axes also closely coordinate with the *International Statistical Classification of Diseases and Related Health Problems* (ICD-9). The next version, ICD-10, expands the number of categories and will be available in the near future.

These five axes and some of their subcategories are discussed in the sections that follow.

TABLE 21-1   MULTIAXIAL ASSESSMENT CLASSIFICATIONS

Axis	Classification	Description
I	Clinical Disorders Other Conditions That May Be a Focus of Clinical Attention	Reports all various conditions or disorders in the classification except for personality disorders and mental retardation.
II	Personality Disorders Mental Retardation	Reports personality disorders and mental retardation.
III	General Medical Conditions	Reports current medical conditions that are potentially relevant to understanding or managing an individual's mental disorders.

continues

TABLE 21-1 MULTIAXIAL ASSESSMENT CLASSIFICATIONS		
Axis	Classification	Description
IV	Psychosocial and Environmental Problems	Reports psychosocial and environmental problems that may affect the diagnosis, treatment, and prognosis of mental disorder(s).
V	Global Assessment of Functioning	Reports the clinician's judgment of the individual's overall level of functioning and is useful in planning treatment, measuring its impact, and predicting its outcome.

AXIS I: CLINICAL DISORDERS AND OTHER CONSIDERATIONS THAT MAY BE A FOCUS OF CLINICAL ATTENTION

This is a list of some of the Axis I disorders included in the DSM-IV-TR.

Disorders first diagnosed in infancy, childhood, and adolescence
Delirium, dementia, and amnestic and other cognitive disorders
Substance-related disorders
Schizophrenia and other psychotic disorders
Mood disorders
Anxiety disorders
Somatoform disorders
Sexual and gender identity disorders
Sleep disorders
Impulse-control disorders

Disorders First Diagnosed in Infancy, Childhood, and Adolescence

Disorders First Diagnosed in Infancy, Childhood, and Adolescence include, among others, learning disorders, motor skills disorders, communication disorders, pervasive development disorders, and attention-deficit and disruptive behavior disorders.

Learning disorders may occur in children with normal health and intelligence but who have problems with the *ability* to learn. Usually such difficulties are limited to one particular academic skill such as reading, mathematics, or written expression. **Motor skills disorders** are characterized by motor coordination that is substantially below that expected for a person of a given age and intellectual level and includes developmental coordination disorder. **Communication disorders** are often characterized by failure to use speech sounds correctly, stuttering, or by slow speech development. **Pervasive development disorders** relate most specifically to social interaction with others as well as with family members. Behavior may include unreasonable insistence on routines, repetition of previously heard speech, or difficulty in naming objects. **Attention-deficit** and **disruptive behaviors** are separate problems despite the similarity of their names. An attention-deficit hyperactivity disorder (ADHD) is defined as the habitual inability of a child to pay attention for more than a minute or two. Medications can be used to help focus the child's attention and reduce overactivity. Disruptive behavior disorders violate the basic rights of others and include negative, hostile, and age-inappropriate behaviors.

Delirium, Dementia, and Amnestic and Other Cognitive Disorders

A significant drop in memory capacity is the one prominent symptom shared by delirium, dementia, amnestic, and other cognitive disorders. The cause may be either a general medical condition, injury, or a substance.

DIAGNOSTIC PROCEDURES

Word	Pronunciation	Definition
General		
corneal topography	kŏr'nē-ăl tō-pŏg'ră-fē	computer-aided examination of the curvature of the cornea
electroretinogram (ERG)	ē-lĕk"trō-rĕt'ĭ-nō-grăm	recording of changes in electrical potential of retina after stimulation with light
fluorescein staining	floo"ō-rĕs'ē-ĭn	procedure using fluorescein-stained sterile filter paper strips to visualize a corneal abrasion
fundoscopy	fŭn-dŏs'kō-pē	examination of fundus of eye with an ophthalmoscope
gonioscopy	gō"nē-ŏs'kō-pē	examination of the angle of the anterior chamber with a gonioscope
ocular motility evaluation	ŏk'ū-lăr mō-tĭl'ĭ-tē	determination of the ability of the eye muscles to move in various gaze positions
ophthalmoscopy	ŏf-thăl-mŏs'kō-pē	visual examination of the interior eye
refraction/visual acuity	ah-kū'ĭ-tē	determination of the amount of *nearsightedness (myopia), farsightedness (hyperopia),* or *astigmatism* for the prescription of corrective lenses; uses Snellen's chart
slit lamp biomicroscopy	bī"ō-mī-krŏs'kō-pē	test that uses light emitted through a slit; used in combination with a biomicroscope to study the cornea, conjunctiva, iris, lens, and vitreous humor
tonometry	tō-nŏm'ĕ-trē	measurement of intraocular tension; increased tension may indicate the presence of glaucoma
visual field examination		measurement of the area within which objects may be seen when the eye is looking straight ahead; Goldmann perimeter visual field examination
Nuclear Medicine		
^{32}P scan		test using radioactive phosphorus to diagnose tumors
Radiology		
anteroposterior and lateral (AP & LAT)	ăn"tĕr-ō-pŏs-tēr'ē-or	x-ray procedure used to determine the presence of an intraocular foreign body
computer-assisted tomography (CAT)	tō-mŏg'rah-fē	procedure used to evaluate the optic nerve and orbital pathology
fluorescein angiography	floo"ō-rĕs'ē-ĭn ăn"jē-ŏg'răh-fē	test that uses retinal photography and an intravenous dye to reveal lesions of the retina and choroid
magnetic resonance imaging (MRI)		use of magnetism to create images on a computer screen to distinguish between normal and abnormal tissue changes
ultrasound		test used to locate tumors when there are vitreous, corneal, or lenticular opacities

continues

DIAGNOSTIC PROCEDURES

Word	Pronunciation	Definition
Blood Tests		
erythrocyte sedimentation rate	ĕ-rĭth'rō-sīt sĕd"ĭ-mĕn-tā'shŭn	test used to determine the presence of temporal arteritis
white blood count and differential	dĭf"er-ĕn'shăl	test that counts the number of leukocytes and gives an estimation of the percentage of five types of white cells

DIAGNOSES

Word	Pronunciation	Definition
Inflammation and Infection		
blepharitis	blĕf"ah-rī'tĭs	infection involving eyelashes and inflammation of both eyelid edges
chalazion	cah-lā'zē-ŏn	small, hard mass on the eyelid resulting from a plugged and infected meibomian gland
conjunctivitis	kŏn-jŭnk"tĭ-vī'tĭs	inflammation of the conjunctiva; pinkeye
episcleritis	ĕp"ĭ-sklē-rī-tĭs	inflammation of the subconjunctival layers of the sclera
iritis	ĭ-rē'tĭs	inflammation of the iris
keratitis	kĕr-ah-tī'tĭs	inflammation of the cornea
papilledema	păp"ĭl-ĕ-dē'mah	edema and inflammation of the optic nerve
scleritis	sklē-rī'tĭs	superficial or deep inflammation of the sclera
sty, stye (hordeolum)	stī (hor-dē'ō-lŭm)	localized, inflammatory swelling of one of several sebaceous glands of the eyelid
uveitis	ŭ-vē-ī'tĭs	inflammation of all or parts of the uvea
Conditions of the Eye		
age-related macular degeneration (ARMD)	măk'ū-lăr	impaired vision due to scar tissue produced by blood vessels in the macular region
amblyopia	ăm"blē-ō'pē-ah	lazy eye; vision in nondominant eye is poor
cataract	kăt'ah-răkt	clouding of the lens, which causes decreased vision (See Figure 22-3)
color blindness		inherited disorder that affects the ability to distinguish between reds and greens
diabetic retinopathy	rĕt"ĭn-ŏp'ă-thē	disease of the retina caused by diabetes; may lead to blindness
diplopia	dĭp-lō'pē-ah	seeing two images of an object at the same time
ectropion	ĕk-trō'pē-ŏn	lower lid turns *outward* causing tears to run out instead of lubricating the eye
entropion	ĕn-trō'pē-ŏn	upper or lower lid turns *inward* and allows lashes to scratch the eyes

continues

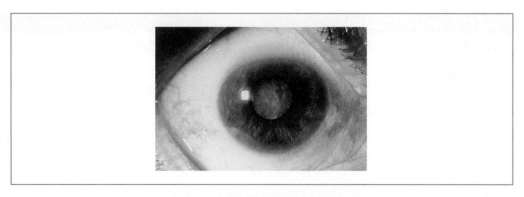

FIGURE 22-3
Cataract (Courtesy of the National Eye Institute, NIH)

DIAGNOSES		
Word	Pronunciation	Definition
Conditions of the Eye *(continued)*		
glaucoma	glaw-kō'mah	increased pressure in the eye; may be chronic or acute (See Figure 22-4)
nystagmus	nĭs-tăg'mŭs	rapid, jerky eye movements
pterygium	tĕ-rĭj'ē-ŭm	triangular overgrowth of the cornea, usually the inner side, by thickened and degenerative conjunctiva
ptosis	tō'sĭs	drooping of the upper eyelid (See Figure 22-5)

continues

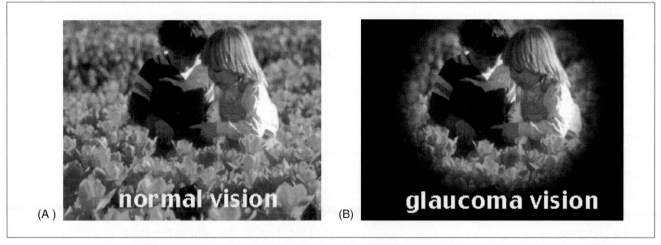

(A)   (B)

FIGURE 22-4   Decreased Vision with Glaucoma: (A) normal vision; (B) glaucoma vision

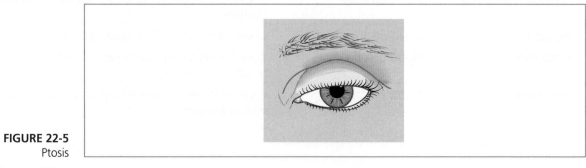

FIGURE 22-5
Ptosis

DIAGNOSES

Word	Pronunciation	Definition
Conditions of the Eye *(continued)*		
retinoblastoma	ret"ĭ-nō-blăs-to'mah	malignant tumor of the eye
scotoma	skō-tō'mah	blind spot in the field of vision
strabismus	strah-bĭz'mŭs	abnormal eye alignments; estropia, exotropia (See Figure 22-6)
Trauma		
corneal abrasion	kor'nē-ăl ă-brā'zhŭn	injury to cornea by foreign objects, poorly fitting contacts, extreme light, or physical injury
retinal detachment	rĕt'ĭ-năl	separation of the inner layer of the retina from the choroid

TREATMENT PROCEDURES

Word	Pronunciation	Definition
blepharoplasty	blĕf'ah-rō-plăs"tē	surgical repair of the eyelids
corneal transplantation	kor'nē-ăl	replacement of the cornea from one person to another
cryopexy	krī'ō-pĕks-ē	use of intense cold to produce scar tissue that holds retina to underlying tissue
cryotherapy	krī'ō-thĕr'ah-pē	very cold probe is applied to scleral surface directly over the hole in the retina
cyclocryotherapy	sī"klō-krī"ō-thĕr'ah-pē	freezing of the ciliary body for treatment of glaucoma

continues

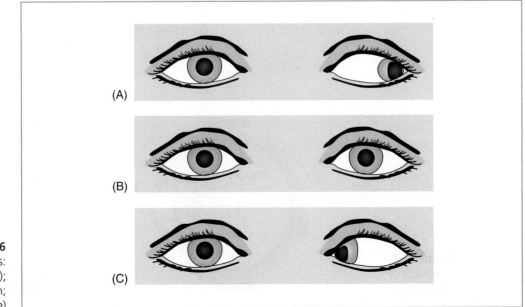

FIGURE 22-6
Strabismus:
(A) exotropia (walleye);
(B) normal pattern;
(C) esotropia (cross-eye)

TREATMENT PROCEDURES

Word	Pronunciation	Definition
dacryocystorhinostomy	dăk″rē-ō-sĭs″tō-rī-nŏs′tō-mē	surgical creation of an opening between the lacrimal sac and nasal cavity
ectropion correction	ĕk-trō′pē-ŏn	correction of an eversion, or outward turning, of the margin of the eyelid
entropion correction	ĕn-trō′pē-ŏn	correction of an inversion, or inward turning, of the margin of the eyelid
enucleation	ē-nū″klē-ā′shŭn	removal of the eye from its socket
evisceration	ē-vĭs″er-ā′shŭn	removal of the contents of the eyeball (viscera), leaving the sclera
extracapsular cataract extraction	ĕks″tră-căp′sū-lăr	removal of the anterior portion of the capsule and the whole lens; an intraocular lens (IOL) is implanted (See Figure 22-7)
glaucoma operation	glaw-kō′mah	procedure that relieves increased intraocular pressure that has not been relieved by medications
iridectomy	ĭr″ĭ-dĕk′tō-mē	excision of part of the iris; treats closed-angle glaucoma
keratoplasty	kĕr′ah-tō-plăs″tē	plastic surgery on the cornea; corneal grafting or transplant
laser-assisted in situ keratomileusis (LASIK)	kĕr″ă-tō-mĭ-loo′sĭs	corrects near- and farsightedness and other refractive errors by using a laser to sculpt corneal tissue after the creation of a corneal flap
laser iridotomy	ĭr″ĭ-dŏt′ō-mē	incision in the iris to relieve built-up pressure between the iris and lens
laser photocoagulation	fō″tō-kō-ăg″ū-lā′shŭn	use of a laser to treat a number of eye conditions such as diabetic retinopathy, acute and chronic simple glaucoma, retinal detachment, orbital and eyelid tumors, or secondary cataracts
nasolacrimal duct probing	nā″zō-lăk′rĭm-ăl	probing of the lacrimal drainage system
orbitotomy	or″bĭ-tŏt′ō-mē	orbital surgery

continues

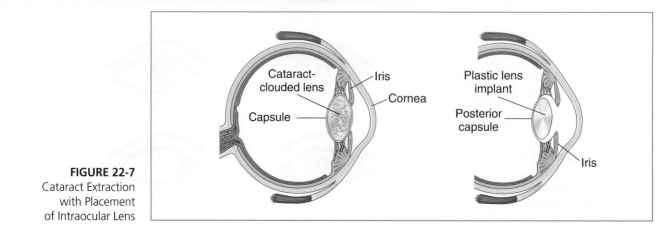

FIGURE 22-7
Cataract Extraction with Placement of Intraocular Lens

TREATMENT PROCEDURES

Word	Pronunciation	Definition
photorefractive keratectomy (PRK)	fō"tō-rĭ-frăk'tĭv kĕr-ă-tĕk'tō-mē	procedure to shave off a few layers of corneal surface cells to flatten cornea and reduce nearsightedness (myopia) without a flap
radial keratotomy	kĕr"ah-tŏt'ō-mē	surgical correction of mild to moderate myopia (See Figure 22-8)
scleral buckling	sklē'răl bŭk'lĭng	repair of retinal detachment
strabismus operation	strah-bĭz'mŭs	correction of squint or ocular misalignment; *resection* is strengthening of an ocular muscle; *recession* is weakening of an ocular muscle
trabeculectomy	tră-bĕk"ū-lĕk'tō-mē	surgical glaucoma diffusing procedure
trabeculoplasty	tră-bĕk"ū-lō-plăs"tē	laser glaucoma procedure
vitrectomy	vĭ-trĕk'tō-mē	removal of vitreous humor and its replacement with a clear solution

ERRORS OF REFRACTION

Word	Pronunciation	Definition
astigmatism	ah-stĭg'mah-tĭzm	defective curvature of the cornea, resulting in blurry vision (See Figure 22-9B)
hyperopia (hypermetropia)	hī"per-ō'pē-ah (hī"per-mē-trŏ'pē-ah)	farsightedness (See Figure 22-10B)

continues

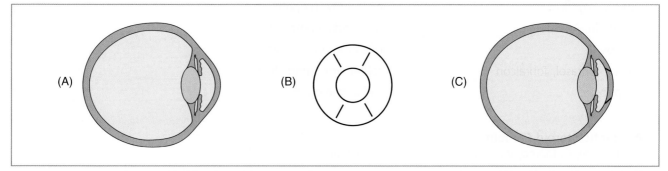

FIGURE 22-8 Radial Keratotomy: (A) cross section of eye prior to surgery; (B) small incisions are made in the cornea from the middle outward; (C) this causes the cornea to become flatter, improving vision

FIGURE 22-9
Presbyopia and Astigmatism:
(A) presbyopia (light rays focus behind the retina);
(B) astigmatism (light rays focus on multiple areas of the retina)

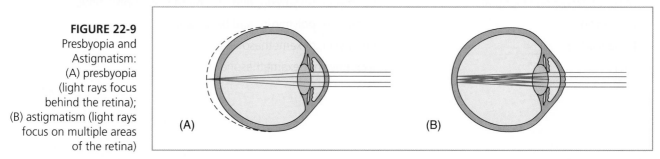

FIGURE 22-10
Myopia and Hyperopia:
(A) myopia
(nearsightedness), light
rays focus in front of the
retina; (B) hyperopia
(farsightedness),
light rays focus beyond
the retina

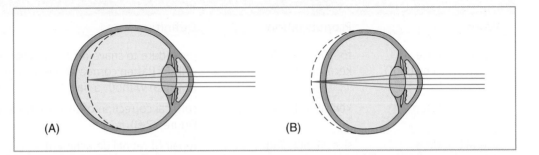

(A)   (B)

ERRORS OF REFRACTION

Word	Pronunciation	Definition
myopia	mī-ō'pē-ah	nearsightedness (See Figure 22-10A)
presbyopia	prĕs"bē-ō'pē-ah	impairment of near vision in old age, resulting from loss of elasticity of the lens or accommodation (See Figure 22-9A)

MEDICATIONS PRESCRIBED

Trade Name	Generic Name
Antibiotics/Antivirals	
AK-Tracin	bacitracin ophthalmic
Bleph-10	sulfacetamide ophthalmic
Ciloxan	ciprofloxacin ophthalmic
Genoptic, Garamycin, Gentak	gentamicin sulfate ophthalmic
Ilotycin, Roymicin	erythromycin ophthalmic
Neosporin, AK-Spore	gramicidin ophthalmic
Ocuflox	ofloxacin ophthalmic
Tobrex, Tobrasol, Tobralcon	tobramycin ophthalmic
Viroptic	trifluridine ophthalmic
Antibiotic/Steroid Combinations	
Blephamide, Cetapred, Vasocidin	sulfacetamide, prednisolone
Cortisporin Ophthalmic, Ocu-Cort, Neotricin HC	neomycin, polymyxin and hydrocortisone
Maxitrol, Neosporin Ophthalmic	neomycin, polymyxin, and dexamethasone ophthalmic
Mycitracin	neomycin, polymyxin, and bacitracin
Neodecadron	neomycin, dexamethasone
Tobradex	tobramycin, dexamethasone

continues

MEDICATIONS PRESCRIBED

Trade Name	Generic Name
Glaucoma Treatment	
Alphagan	brimonidine tartrate
Betagan	levobunolol ophthalmic
Betoptic	betaxolol ophthalmic
Diamox	acetazolamide
Epifrin, Epinal, Glaucon	epinephrine bitrate
Isopto Carpine, Pilocar, Akarpine	pilocarpine ophthalmic
Miostat, Carboptic, Carbachol, Isopto Carbachol	carbachol
Osmoglyn	glycerin
Propine, AK-Pro	dipivefrin ophthalmic
Timoptic Ocumeter, Betinol	timolol maleate ophthalmic
Trusopt	dorzolamide
Xalatan	latanoprost
Corticosteroids	
AD-DEX, Decadron Ocumeter, Dexasol, Maridex	dexamethasone ophthalmic
AK-Pred	prednisolone sodium phosphate ophthalmic
Econopred, Pred Mild	prednisolone acetate ophthalmic
FML, Eflone, Flarex, Fluor-Op	fluormetholone ophthalmic
HMS	medrysone ophthalmic
Vexol	rimexolone ophthalmic
Ophthalmic Agents	
AK-Con, Vasocon-A	naphazoline ophthalmic
Isopto Atropine, Atropine-1	atropine ophthalmic
Isopto Homatropine	homatropine ophthalmic
Anti-Inflammatory Drugs	
Acular	ketorolac ophthalmic
Ocufen	flurbiprofen
Voltaren	diclofenac sodium ophthalmic
Anti-Allergy Topicals	
Allerest	naphazoline ophthalmic
Patanol	olopatadine HCl
Zaditor	ketotifen fumarate

ABBREVIATIONS

accom	accommodation
ARMD	age-related macular degeneration
Em	emmetropia (normal vision)
EOM	extraocular movement
IOL	intraocular lens
IOP	intraocular pressure
LASIK	laser-assisted in situ keratomileusis
OD	*oculus dexter* (right eye)
ophth	ophthalmology
OS	*oculus sinister* (left eye)
OU	*oculi unitas* (both eyes)
PERRLA	pupils equal, round, reactive to light and accommodation
PRK	photorefractive keratectomy
VA	visual acuity
VF	visual field

Name: _____ Date: _____

IDENTIFICATION/DIAGNOSTIC PROCEDURES*

Identify the following definitions.

1. visual examination of the interior eye   _____

2. using radioactive phosphorus in the diagnosis of tumors of the eye   _____

3. dye is used intravenously with photography to reveal lesions of the retina and choroid   _____

4. examining the angle of the anterior chamber with a gonioscope   _____

5. determines the ability of the eye muscles to move in various gaze positions   _____

6. measurement of intraocular tension   _____

DEFINITIONS

Define and provide the pronunciation for the following surgical procedures.

1. blepharoplasty   _____

   _____

2. enucleation   _____

   _____

3. keratoplasty   _____

   _____

4. laser photocoagulation   _____

   _____

5. strabismus operation   _____

   _____

IDENTIFICATION/DIAGNOSIS

Identify the following diagnoses.

1. drooping of the upper eyelid   _____

2. rapid, jerky, side-to-side eye movements   _____

3. inflammation of the conjunctiva   _____

4. clouding of the lens   _____

5. a blind spot   _____

6. an enlarged meibomian gland on the eyelid   _____

7. abnormal alignment of the eye   _____

---

*Answers are in Appendix A.

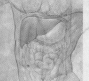

Word Element Review

Root	Meaning	Example	Definition
aque/o	water	**aqueous humor** (ā'kwē-ŭs)	clear, watery fluid circulating through the anterior and posterior chambers of the eye
blephar/o	eyelid	**blepharectomy** (blĕf"ah-rĕk'tō-mē)	excision of an eyelid
conjunctiv/o	conjunctiva	**conjunctivitis** (kŏn-jŭnk"tĭ-vī'tĭs)	inflammation of the conjunctiva
cor/o, core/o	pupil	**corectasis** (kōr-ĕk'tah-sĭs)	dilation of the pupil
corne/o	cornea	**corneal** (kor'nē-ăl)	pertaining to the cornea
dacry/o	tear, tear duct	**dacryocystitis** (dăk"rē-ō-sĭs-tī'tĭs)	inflammation of the lacrimal sac
ir/o, irid/o	iris	**iridectomy** (ĭr"ĭ-dĕk'tō-mē)	surgical removal of the iris
kerat/o	horny, cornea	**keratoid** (kĕr'ah-toid)	resembling horny or corneal tissue
lacrim/o	tear	**lacrimotomy** (lăk"rĭ-mŏt'ō-mē)	incision of the lacrimal duct
ocul/o	eye	**ocular** (ŏk'ū-lăr)	pertaining to the eye
ophthalm/o	eye	**ophthalmalgia** (ŏf"thăl-măl'jē-ah)	pain in the eye
		ophthalmic (ŏf-thăl'mĭk)	pertaining to the eye
opt/o, optic/o	eye, vision	**optic** (ŏp'tĭk)	pertaining to the eye
palpebr/o	eyelid	**palpebrate** (păl'pĕ-brāt)	to wink
pupill/o	pupil	**pupillary** (pū'pĭ-lĕr-ē)	pertaining to the pupil
retin/o	retina	**retinopathy** (rĕt"ĭ-nŏp'ah-thē)	any disease of the retina
scler/o	sclera	**scleritis** (sklē-rī'tĭs)	inflammation of the sclera
tars/o	eyelid	**tarsus** (tahr'sŭs)	dense, white fibrous tissue forming the supporting structure of the eyelid
vitre/o	glassy	**vitreous humor** (vĭt'rē-ŭs)	transparent, semi-gelatinous substance in the posterior chamber of the eye

Suffix	Meaning	Example	Definition
-opia, -opsia	vision	**presbyopia** (prĕs"bē-ō'pē-ah)	impaired vision because of age
-tropia	to turn	**isometropia** (ī"sō-mĕ-trō'pē-ă)	equality of refraction in both eyes

Word Element Review Exercises

Name: _____ Date: _____

CIRCLE AND DEFINE*

Circle and define the word element in the following terms.

1. dacryocystitis _____
2. corectasis _____
3. ophthalmalgia _____
4. blepharectomy _____
5. presbyopia _____
6. palpebrate _____
7. tarsus _____
8. retinopathy _____
9. scleritis _____
10. iridectomy _____
11. keratoid _____
12. ophthalmic _____

MATCHING

Match the word elements to their meanings.

1. _____ horny, cornea
2. _____ retina
3. _____ eyelid
4. _____ cornea
5. _____ eye, vision
6. _____ vision
7. _____ pupil
8. _____ eye
9. _____ sclera
10. _____ tear
11. _____ glassy
12. _____ iris
13. _____ conjunctiva
14. _____ water
15. _____ to turn

a. conjunctiv/o
b. dacry/o, lacrim/o
c. scler/o
d. cor/o, core/o, pupill/o
e. vitre/o
f. aque/o
g. corne/o
h. ir/o, irid/o
i. kerat/o
j. retin/o
k. opt/o, optic/o
l. -opia, -opsia
m. blephar/o, palpebr/o, tars/o
n. ocul/o, ophthalm/o
o. -tropia

_____

*Answers are in Appendix A.

SPELLING*

Rewrite the misspelled words.

1. isometropea _____

2. blepherectomy _____

3. corectasis _____

4. palpebraite _____

5. ocular _____

WORD ELEMENT MEANINGS

Give the meaning of each word element. Then use your dictionary to find a new word that contains each of the word elements. Specify whether the new word is a noun or an adjective by placing N or A in the last column.

Word Element	Meaning	Word	N or A
1. aque/o	_____	_____	_____
2. blephar/o	_____	_____	_____
3. conjunctiv/o	_____	_____	_____
4. cor/o	_____	_____	_____
5. core/o	_____	_____	_____
6. corne/o	_____	_____	_____
7. dacry/o	_____	_____	_____
8. ir/o	_____	_____	_____
9. irid/o	_____	_____	_____
10. kerat/o	_____	_____	_____
11. lacrim/o	_____	_____	_____
12. ocul/o	_____	_____	_____
13. ophthalm/o	_____	_____	_____
14. -opia	_____	_____	_____
15. -opsia	_____	_____	_____
16. opt/o	_____	_____	_____
17. optic/o	_____	_____	_____
18. palpebr/o	_____	_____	_____
19. pupill/o	_____	_____	_____
20. retin/o	_____	_____	_____
21. scler/o	_____	_____	_____
22. tars/o	_____	_____	_____
23. -tropia	_____	_____	_____
24. vitre/o	_____	_____	_____

*Answers are in Appendix A.

Dictionary Exercises

Name: _____ Date: _____

DICTIONARY EXERCISE 1*

Use your dictionary to find the pronunciation and definition of the following words.

Word	Pronunciation	Definition
1. canthus	_____	_____
2. choroiditis	_____	_____
3. corneal dystrophy	_____	_____
4. floaters	_____	_____
5. orbital cellulitis	_____	_____
6. meibomian gland	_____	_____
7. melanoma of the eye	_____	_____
8. retrolental fibroplasia	_____	_____
9. vitreous hemorrhage	_____	_____

DICTIONARY EXERCISE 2

Match the terms to their meanings.

1. _____ keratitis
2. _____ mydriasis
3. _____ optic neuritis
4. _____ corneal ulcer
5. _____ exophthalmos
6. _____ optic atrophy
7. _____ orbital cellulitis
8. _____ coloboma
9. _____ uveoplasty
10. _____ choroiditis

a. inflammation of the optic nerve

b. repair of the uvea

c. wasting away of the eye

d. inflammation of the cornea

e. acute infection of the eye socket

f. destructive lesion of the cornea

g. congenital defect in the development of the eye

h. abnormal protrusion of the eyeball

i. inflammation of the choroid

j. pronounced dilation of the pupil

---

*Answers are in Appendix A.

DICTIONARY EXERCISE 3

Pronunciation of the words below is provided. Using your dictionary, find the correct spelling and definition of each word.

	Word	**Pronunciation**	**Meaning**
1.	_____	ā'kwē-ŭs	_____
2.	_____	dī-ŏp'tĕr	_____
3.	_____	dăk"rē-ăd-ĕn-ăl'jē-ah	_____
4.	_____	rĕt-ĭ-nī'tĭs pĭg-mĕn-tō'sah	_____
5.	_____	lĭm'bŭs	_____
6.	_____	rĕt"ĭ-nō'sĭs	_____
7.	_____	tahr'sŭs	_____
8.	_____	ū'vē-ah	_____

DICTIONARY EXERCISE 4*

Rewrite each sentence in your own words.

1. The cornea of the 72-year-old patient was marked by *arcus senilis*.

   _____

   _____

2. The doctor performed *cyclodiathermy*.

   _____

   _____

3. The problem was diagnosed as *ambiopia*.

   _____

   _____

4. Unfortunately, *iridodialysis* has occurred.

   _____

   _____

5. *Ophthalmoplegia* was the final diagnosis.

   _____

   _____

---

*Answers are in Appendix A.

Listening Exercise

INSTRUCTIONS

1. Review the spelling, pronunciation, and meaning of the words provided in the preview.

2. Listen to the audio CD and fill in the blank as the word is dictated.

3. At the end of the exercise, check your spelling against the preview words. They appear in the preview in the order in which they are encountered in the exercise.

4. Review and practice the words you missed.

5. Look up words that are not familiar.

PREVIEW OF WORDS FOR LISTENING EXERCISE 22-1

Word	Pronunciation	Meaning
phacoemulsification	fak"ō-ē-mŭl'sĭ-fĭ-kā"shŭn	a technique of cataract extraction that uses high-frequency ultrasound vibrations, irrigation, and suction
retrobulbar	rĕt"rō-bŭl'băr	behind the eyeball
scleral	sklē'răl	concerning the tough, white fibrous tissue covering the "white" of the eye
limbus	lĭm'bŭs	an edge; in this case, the edge of the cornea where it joins the sclera
capsulotomy	kăp"sū-lŏt'ō-mē	incision into a lens
lenticular	len-tĭk'ū-lăr	pertaining to the lens of the eye

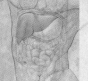

Operative Report

PREOPERATIVE DIAGNOSIS: Senile nuclear sclerotic cataract, right eye.

POSTOPERATIVE DIAGNOSIS: Senile nuclear sclerotic cataract, right eye.

PROCEDURE: _____ with posterior chamber intraocular lens implantation, right eye.

INDICATIONS: Decreased vision due to cataract, right eye, affecting the patient's functional activities.

INFORMED CONSENT: The patient is alert, oriented, and understands the risks, benefits, and indications of the above procedure, and consents to the same.

PROCEDURE: After achievement of satisfactory _____ anesthesia, the patient was prepped and draped in the routine sterile manner. A wire lid speculum was placed in the right eye. A superior limbal peritomy was performed. Cautery, as necessary, was achieved with bipolar cautery. A partial thickness _____ tunnel incision was advanced to the _____ through which the anterior chamber was entered with a 3.2 mm keratome. A separate stab incision was made at the six o'clock limbus. Under Amvisc Plus, an anterior _____ was performed with forceps. BSS was irrigated underneath the anterior capsule. Phacoemulsification was utilized to remove _____ nucleus. Remnant lenticular cortical material was removed with irrigation-aspiration device. The posterior capsule was polished with Graether collar button. A posterior chamber intraocular lens was implanted into the capsular bag. The intraocular lens utilized is the IOLAB model LI41U, power (-2) diopter. Remnant Amvisc Plus was removed with the irrigation-aspiration device.

The superior scleral wound was closed with a single interrupted 10-0 nylon suture. Cautery was utilized to reapproximate the conjunctiva. A subconjunctival injection with gentamicin was given in the inferior fornix. The eye was patched over Polysporin ointment and topical application of Iopidine.

The patient tolerated the procedure well. There were no operative complications. The patient left the operating suite in good condition.

_____   _____

Douglas R. Flannigan, MD   Date

The Ear, Nose, and Throat

Nature has given man one tongue, but two ears, that we may hear twice as much as we speak.

—EPICTETUS

OBJECTIVES

When you have completed this chapter on the ear, nose, and throat systems, you should be able to

1. Spell and define major system components and explain how they operate.
2. Identify the meaning of related word elements.
3. Spell and define diagnostic procedures, diagnoses, treatment procedures, and abbreviations.
4. Spell the names of commonly used medications.
5. Be familiar with terminology used in reports.

INTRODUCTION

The ear, nose, and throat contain receptor cells and structures that allow us to experience the senses of hearing, balance, smell, and taste. Physicians who specialize in the treatment of diseases and disorders of these organs and adjacent structures of the head and neck are called **otolaryngologists** (ō"tō-lăr"ĭn-gŏl'ō-jĭsts) (or otorhino-laryngologists). Head and neck surgery has recently been added to this specialty.

THE EAR

acous/o	hearing	-cusis	hearing
audi/o, audit/o	hearing, sound	myring/o	eardrum
auri/o, auricul/o	ear	ot/o	ear
cochle/o	cochlea	tympan/o	eardrum

The ear is divided into three parts—the external ear, the middle ear, and the inner (internal) ear.

EXTERNAL EAR

As you will note in Figure 23-1, the external ear has two parts—the auricle and the **orifice** (or'ĭ-fĭs), or opening that leads into the auditory canal. The **auricle** (aw'rĕ-kl), or **pinna** (2) is the outermost portion of the ear. It is composed of an elastic cartilage that is covered with skin and a lobe (3) that extends from the lower portion of the auricle.

The external portion of the ear directs sound waves into the **external auditory canal** (4). This canal serves a double purpose. First, it guides sound waves to the **tympanic** (tĭm-păn'ĭk) **membrane** (eardrum) (1); second,

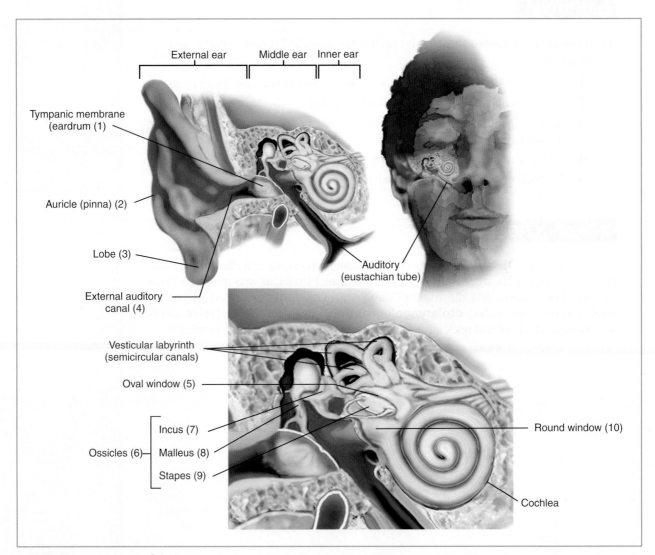

Tympanic membrane (eardrum (1)

Auricle (pinna) (2)

Lobe (3)

External auditory canal (4)

External ear   Middle ear   Inner ear

Auditory (eustachian tube)

Vesticular labyrinth (semicircular canals)

Oval window (5)

Incus (7)

Ossicles (6)— Malleus (8)

Stapes (9)

Round window (10)

Cochlea

FIGURE 23-1   Structure of the Ear

it protects the internal structure of the ear. The fine hairs and cerumen in the canal assist in the protective function. **Cerumen** (sĕ-roo'mĕn) (referred to as earwax) is secreted by modified sebaceous glands. When sound waves reach the eardrum through the auditory canal, they are picked up by the tympanic membrane and the bones of the middle ear and transmitted to the inner ear.

MIDDLE EAR

The **middle ear** is an irregularly shaped, air-filled cavity within the temporal bone and is lined with mucous membranes. These mucous membranes are continuous with those that line the throat, which is why infections spread so readily to the middle ear. The air in the cavity comes from the nasal part of the pharynx through the auditory or **eustachian** (ū-stā'kē-ăn) **tube**. In this way, air pressure on both sides of the eardrum is equalized.

At one end of the cavity is the tympanic membrane (eardrum), and on the other end is a bone wall. This bone wall has two small membrane-covered openings called the **oval window** (5) and **round window** (10).

There are also three small bones or ossicles (ŏs'sĭ-k'lz) (6) in the middle ear. These are the **malleus** (măl'ē-ŭs) (hammer) (8), **incus** (ĭng'kŭs) (anvil) (7), and **stapes** (stā'pēz) (stirrup) (9). These three ossicles form a flexible bridge across the middle ear chamber and transmit sound waves to the internal ear in the following way. Since the malleus and the eardrum are in contact, a sound that sets the eardrum into motion is immediately transferred to the malleus. The motion of the malleus then moves the incus, which in turn moves the stapes. The vibrations of the footplate of the stapes are transmitted to the flexible membrane covering the oval window opening to the inner ear.

INNER EAR

The **inner ear**, shown in Figure 23-2, is the most complex structure of the ear. This structure, also called the **labyrinth** (lăb'ĭ-rĭnth), is divided into three fluid-filled areas—the **cochlea** (kŏk'lē-ah) (2), the **semicircular canals** (10), and the **vestibule** (6).

Delicate membranes lining the inner ear enable us to hear and maintain our balance. As was stated above, when the ear receives a sound, the stapes strikes against the oval window (8), which creates vibrations. The vibrations set off wavelike movements in the fluid of the inner ear. These fluid waves are cushioned and dampened by the round window (7). Waves in the inner ear travel through the cochlea (a snail-shaped structure), where the **organ of Corti** is located. The organ of Corti contains the receptors for hearing—more than 20,000 sensory hair cells with additional supporting cells. As the waves travel through the cochlea, the hair cells vibrate. This stimulates the sensory fibers of the vestibulocochlear (vĕs-tĭb"ū-lō-kŏk'lē-ăr) nerve, which transmits the information to the brain.

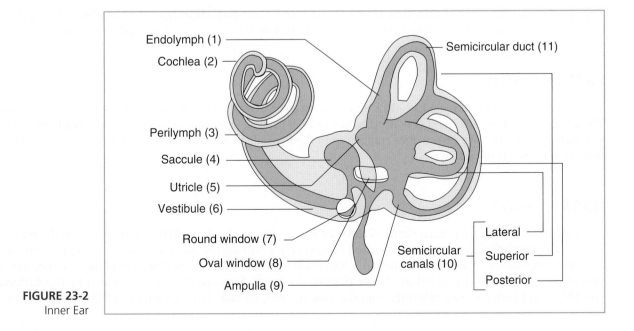

FIGURE 23-2
Inner Ear

The inner ear also controls the body's equilibrium. Near the cochlea are three semicircular canals, each containing a semicircular duct (11). Each duct contains an enlargement called an **ampulla** (ăm-pul'lah) (9), which in turn contains sensory cells that provide directional information about the body's position. For example, as the head is turned, the fluid in the ducts flows to or from the ampulla, stimulating the sensory cells and telling the brain which way the head is moving.

The vestibule is a chamber between the cochlea and semicircular canals and separated from the middle ear by the oval window. This chamber is filled with a fluid called **perilymph** (pĕr'ĭ-lĭmf) (3) and separates the walls of the membranous labyrinth and the osseous labyrinth. The vestibule contains two membranous labyrinth enlargements called the **saccule** (săk'ūl) (4) and **utricle** (ū'trē-k'l) (5). These, along with the semicircular canals, are structures of equilibrium. The membranous labyrinth is filled with a fluid called **endolymph** (ĕn'dō-lĭmf) (1). This entire complicated structure called the ear gives us the ability to hear sounds and to maintain our balance and equilibrium.

Review: The Ear

- ■ The ear is a delicate instrument of hearing composed of the external, middle, and inner ears.
- ■ The external ear conducts sound to the eardrum, which activates the three ossicles of the middle ear.
- ■ Vibrations on the oval window leading to the inner ear stimulate the cochlea.
- ■ The inner ear transmits sound wave information to the brain and senses movement and position to aid in the control of the body's equilibrium.

THE NOSE AND THROAT

gingiv/o	gum	or/o	mouth
gloss/o	tongue	-osmia	smell
lingu/o	tongue	phon/o	sound
mastoid/o	mastoid process	sial/o	salivary
odont/o	tooth		

The closely related senses of **olfaction** (ŏl-făk'shŭn) (smell) and **gustation** (gŭs-tā'shŭn) (taste) are located in the nasal and mouth area. The nose is composed of an external nose, a nasal cavity, and nasal sinuses.

EXTERNAL NOSE

The nose takes outside air as cold as −30°F and warms it to 98°F by the time it reaches the upper part of the throat. The bridge of the nose is formed of bone; the tip is built of cartilage and connective tissue. The **septum** (sĕp'tŭm) separates the nostrils into two cavities running from the floor of the skull to the base of the nasal cavity. The septum is made mostly of cartilage.

NASAL CAVITY

In Figure 23-3, note that the main cavity of the nose rests between the floor of the brain cavity and the roof of the mouth. The **conchae** (kŏn'chē) are three scroll-shaped bones forming the nasal sidewall. The conchae are covered with moist membranes forming the turbinates. Essentially, these are the air conditioners of the nose because they provide moisture and warmth before the air reaches the lungs. Beneath the shelves formed by the **turbinates** (tŭr'bĭ-nāts) (1) are recesses called the superior (not shown), middle (13), and inferior (12) **meatus** (mē-ā'tŭs).

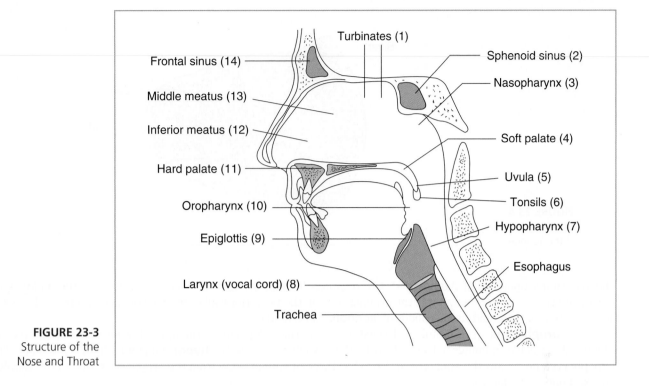

FIGURE 23-3
Structure of the
Nose and Throat

The floor of the nasal cavity is formed by the bony **hard palate** (păl'ăt) (11) anteriorly and the muscular **soft palate** (4) posteriorly. Together the hard and soft palates separate the nasal cavity from the mouth.

The membranes in the nasal passage continuously secrete mucus and fluids. Coarse and fine hairs inside the nasal vestibule trap foreign particles, as does the sticky mucus of the internal nose.

NASAL SINUSES

Surrounding the nasal cavity within the skull are a series of air-filled spaces called **sinuses**. There are four major pairs of sinuses—frontal (14), sphenoid (2), maxillary (not shown), and ethmoidal (not shown). There is one of each pair on either side of the face.

MOUTH

The tongue forms the floor of the mouth and is covered with numerous tiny projections called **papillae** (pah-pĭl'ē). These are often referred to as taste buds. Four tastes (sweet, salty, bitter, and sour) are identified in specific regions of the tongue, as shown in Figure 23-4. The receptor cells of the taste buds are in contact with the sensory nerve fibers, which run to the brain through the facial, glossopharyngeal, and vagus nerves.

Posterior and inferior to the mouth, the pharynx and larynx provide passages for food and air.

PHARYNX

The hard palate, or roof of the mouth, merges with the soft palate and a small peninsula of tissue called the **uvula** (ū'vū-lah) (5), as shown in Figure 23-3. If the **tonsils** (6) are still intact, they can be seen as small rounded masses of lymphoid tissue on either side of the passageway into the throat. Saclike cavities called **crypts** (krĭpts) are present on the mucous membrane covering of the exposed surface of the tonsil.

Technically the **pharynx** extends from the base of the skull to the larynx (8). The pharynx is a common passageway for food from the mouth and for air from the nose. It consists of three sections—the nasopharynx, oropharynx, and hypopharynx (laryngopharynx). The **nasopharynx** (nā"zō-făr'ĭnks) (3) is the area that lies above the level of the soft palate and is covered by mucous membrane. It has five openings: two posterior nares or

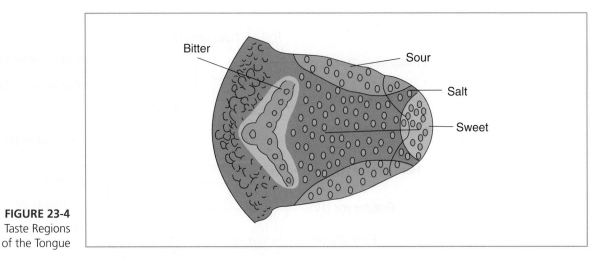

FIGURE 23-4
Taste Regions
of the Tongue

choanae (inner openings of the nostrils), two openings leading through the eustachian tubes to the middle ears (tori), and the downward opening to the oropharynx. On the posterior wall of the nasopharynx there is a localized accumulation of lymphoid tissue called the **adenoid** (ăd'ĕ-noid).

The **oropharynx** (ō"rō-făr'ĭnks) (10) extends from the soft palate to the upper border of the epiglottis (9). The oropharynx has openings to the oral cavity, the nasopharynx, and the **hypopharynx** (hī"pō-făr'ĭnks) (7). The hypopharynx lies below the epiglottis and also has three openings—one from the oropharynx, one to the esophagus, and one to the larynx.

LARYNX

The **larynx** (lăr'ĭnks), or vocal cord, (8) connects the laryngopharyngeal section with the trachea and is used for conduction of air to and from the lungs. It is framed by nine cartilages—three paired and three unpaired. The cartilages are held together by ligaments and muscles. The most familiar one is the **epiglottis** (ĕp"ĭ-glŏt'ĭs) (9). It acts as a lid to prevent solids and fluids from entering the larynx, directing them instead to the esophagus. The opening through which air enters the larynx is the **glottis** (glŏt'ĭs). Air passing through the glottis causes the vocal cords to vibrate and produce sounds, which become the voice. If the mucous membrane of the glottis becomes irritated or inflamed, the ability of the vocal cords to vibrate is inhibited, and hoarseness may result.

INTERNET ASSIGNMENT

Combined Health Information Database (CHID) Online at **www.chid.nih.gov** is a bibliographic data base that leads health professionals, patients, and the general public to thousands of journal articles and patient education materials that contain information about different health topics.

CHID has 16 database topics which are updated four times a year in January, April, July, and October. Each of these topics is a rich source of hard-to-find literature that is not often referenced in other data bases. Examples of items listed include booklets produced by federal health agencies and brochures and newsletters produced by patient-advocacy organizations. Health literature and educational resources for special populations are other examples of items cited in CHID. Of particular interest to this chapter is the Deafness and Communication Disorders topic of CHID, which contains citations to more than 4,000 publications.

ACTIVITY

Access the Combined Health Information Database Online at **www.chid.nih.gov**. Select Simple Search and then Database Topics. Choose the topic Deafness and Communication Disorders. From the Working Practice section of this chapter select one of the diagnoses and enter it as the search argument and press enter. Prepare a brief report for your instructor of what you found.

Review: The Nose and Throat

- ■ To reach the lungs, air first passes through a bone and cartilaginous structure composed of two nostrils and a nasal cavity lined with mucous membrane and protective hairs.

- ■ Air continues on its journey through the pharynx, which consists of the nasopharynx, oropharynx, and hypopharynx.

- ■ The larynx connects the laryngopharyngeal section with the trachea to conduct air to and from the lungs.

Review of Terminology Presented

Word	Definition
adenoid	localized accumulation of lymphoid tissue on the nasopharynx
ampulla	enlargement of the semicircular canal that contains sensory cells that provide directional information about the body's position
auricle (pinna)	outermost portion of the external ear
cerumen	substance, also called earwax, that is secreted from the ear canal
cochlea	snail-shaped structure of the inner ear
concha, *pl.* conchae	bony projections of the lateral nasal sidewall
crypts	saclike cavities contained in the mucous membrane covering of the exposed surface of the tonsil
endolymph	fluid that fills the membranous labyrinth
epiglottis	lid that prevents solids and fluids from entering the larynx, directing them to the esophagus instead
eustachian tube	auditory tube; ventilation pathway between the nasopharynx and the middle ear
external auditory canal	part of the ear that guides sound waves into the eardrum and protects the internal structure of the ear
glottis	opening through which air enters the larynx
gustation	sense of taste
hard palate	roof of the mouth, which separates the mouth from the nasal cavity
hypopharynx	portion of the pharynx that lies below the epiglottis; laryngopharynx
incus	one of three ossicles of the middle ear
inner ear (labyrinth)	complex structure of the ear that transmits sound waves to the brain and controls equilibrium
larynx	structure that connects the laryngopharyngeal region with the trachea and is used for air conduction to and from the lungs
malleus	one of three ossicles of the middle ear

continues

Word	Definition
meatus	recesses formed by the turbinate through which the sinuses drain and ventilate; called the superior, middle, and inferior meatus
middle ear	irregularly shaped, air-filled cavity lined with mucous membranes
nasopharynx	space that lies above the level of the soft palate in the back of the nose
olfaction	sense of smell
organ of Corti	organ that contains the receptors for hearing and is located within the cochlea
orifice	opening to the auditory canal
oropharynx	division of the pharynx that extends from the soft palate to the upper border of the epiglottis
otolaryngologist	physician who specializes in the treatment of diseases and disorders of the ear, nose, throat, and adjacent structures of the head and neck
oval window	small membrane-covered opening in the bone wall between the middle ear and inner ear through which sound is transmitted
papilla, *pl.* papillae	small projections on the tongue that are also known as taste buds
perilymph	fluid in the vestibule that separates the membranous labyrinth and the osseous labyrinth
pharynx	passageway for food and air
round window	small, membrane-covered opening in the bone wall between the middle and inner ears
saccule	structures of equilibrium located in the vestibule
semicircular canals	structures of the inner ear that contain the fluid and sensory cells that provide information about equilibrium and movement
septum	bone and cartilage partition separating the nose into two nostrils
sinuses	series of air spaces surrounding the nasal cavity; major pairs are frontal, sphenoid, maxillary, and ethmoidal
soft palate	posterior portion of the floor of the nasal cavity that is involved in speech and swallowing functions
stapes	one of the three ossicles of the middle ear
tonsils	small, rounded masses of lymphoid tissue on either side of the passageway into the throat
turbinates	three scroll-shaped bones that form the sidewall of the nasal cavity; covered by mucous membrane
tympanic membrane	eardrum
utricle	structure of equilibrium located in the vestibule
uvula	small peninsula of tissue at the back of the mouth
vestibule	perilymph-filled chamber connected to the oval window that leads to the middle ear

Terminology Review Exercises

Name: _____ Date: _____

COMPLETION
Complete the following statements.

1. The three parts of the ear are the _____, _____, and _____.

2. The outermost portion of the ear is the _____.

3. The canal leading to the eardrum is lined with _____ and _____ glands.

4. The bone wall in the middle ear has two windows; they are the _____ and _____.

5. The three ossicles in the middle ear are the _____, _____, and _____.

6. The three areas of the labyrinth are the _____, _____, and _____.

7. The part of the ear that controls equilibrium is the _____.

8. The secretion of modified sebaceous glands is _____.

9. The _____ directs air so pressure is equalized on both sides of the eardrum.

10. The vestibule of the ear is filled with a fluid called _____.

IDENTIFICATION*
From the list below, select the correct term to identify the definitions.

adenoid   concha   epiglottis   glottis   gustation   labyrinth
olfaction   organ of Corti   papillae   sinuses   soft palate   tympanic membrane

1. eardrum _____

2. inner ear _____

3. organ that contains receptors for hearing in the inner ear _____

4. sense of smell _____

5. sense of taste _____

6. small projections on the tongue _____

7. lid on the larynx _____

8. bony projections of the lateral nasal sidewall _____

9. separates the nasal cavity from the mouth _____

10. series of air-filled spaces surrounding the nasal cavity _____

11. localized accumulation of lymphoid tissue on the nasopharynx _____

12. opening through which air enters larynx _____

_____

*Answers are in Appendix A.

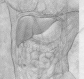

Working Practice

DIAGNOSTIC PROCEDURES		
Word	Pronunciation	Definition
General		
audiometry	aw″dē-ŏm′ĕ-trē	use of an electronic device that delivers specific sound frequencies to determine a patient's hearing threshold
impedance audiometry	ĭm-pēd′ăns ăw″dē-ŏm′ĕ-trē	evaluation of the middle ear function by measurement of the movement of the tympanic membrane and pressure in the middle ear
laryngoscopy	lăr″ĭng-gŏs′kō-pē	visual examination of the larynx with a laryngoscope or a mirror (See Figure 23-5)
myringotomy	mĭr″ĭn-gŏt′ō-mē	incision into the tympanic membrane for diagnostic evaluation (See Treatment Procedures)
otoscopy	ō-tŏs′kō-pē	visual examination of the ear with an otoscope
pneumatic otoscopy	nū-măt′ĭk	air insufflation during an otoscopy to detect tympanic membrane movement; best way to diagnose middle ear effusion or infection
tuning fork test		test in which a tuning fork is placed near the ear to test for air conduction and in contact with the skull to test for bone conduction (Weber and Rinne tests) (See Figure 23-6)
Laboratory		
throat cultures (swabs or washings)		test in which secretions from inflamed areas are analyzed for presence of various pathogens by removing samples from these areas
nasal cultures (swab)		test in which secretions from the nares or meatus of the nose are checked for various pathogens

continues

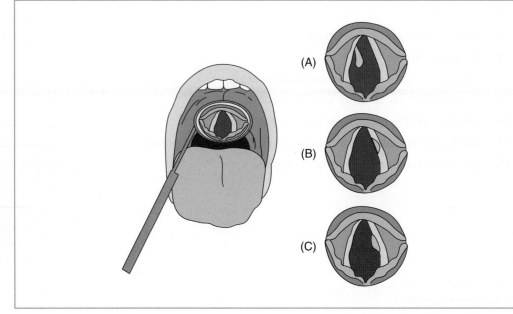

FIGURE 23-5
Laryngoscopy with Polyp: An indirect laryngoscopy is performed by using a small angled mirror, which provides a direct view of the vocal cords. (A) vocal cord polyp, (B) contact ulcer; (C) vocal cord cancer

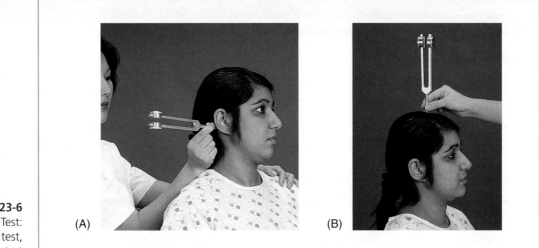

FIGURE 23-6
Tuning Fork Test:
(A) Rinne test,
(B) Weber test

(A)   (B)

DIAGNOSTIC PROCEDURES

Word	Pronunciation	Definition
Radiology		
computer-assisted tomography (CAT) of the skull	tō-mŏg'-rah-fē	computer-reconstructed x-ray of a body section to look for abnormalities in the brain that may be causing visual, hearing, or other problems
magnetic resonant imagery (MRI)		use of radio waves and a strong magnetic field to make cross-sectional images of the body to reveal lesions and changes in organs and tissues
x-ray studies of the skull, mastoids, sinuses, and chest		standard views of the specific parts

DIAGNOSES

Word	Pronunciation	Definition
The Ear		
acoustic neuroma	ah-koos'tĭk nŭ-rō'mah	slow-growing benign tumor of the eighth cranial nerve
auditory canal obstruction		limited hearing because of cerumen obstruction, foreign bodies, or infections that occlude the ear canal
benign paroxysmal positional vertigo (BPPV)	bē-nīn' păr"ŏk-sĭz'măl	recurrent episodes of brief vertigo occurring when the head is placed in certain positions and resolved when the head returns to normal position
choleseatoma	kŏ"lĕ-stē"ah-tō'mah	destructive cyst of the middle ear and mastoid formed from chronic disease of the tympanic membrane

continues

DIAGNOSES

Word	Pronunciation	Definition
The Ear (continued)		
hearing loss		condition of reduced ability to perceive sound at its normal levels; may be *conductive, presbycusis,* or *sensorineural*
• *conductive*		inability to conduct sound waves through the external ear canal to the tympanic membrane of the middle ear
• *presbycusis*	prĕz-bĭ-kū'sĭs	loss due to the normal aging process
• *sensorineural*	sĕn"sō-rē-nŭ'răl	loss due to nerve transmission failure within the inner ear or auditory nerve
labyrinthitis	lăb"ĭ-rĭn-thī'tĭs	inflammation of the inner ear causing hearing loss and vertigo (rare)
mastoiditis	măs"toyd-ī'tĭs	inflammation of the mastoid bone
vestibular neuritis	vĕs-tĭb'ū-lăr nū-rī'tŭs	inflammation of the vestibular nerve causing vertigo (common)
Meniere's disease	mēn"ē-ārz'	episodic vertigo with hearing loss, nausea, and tinnitus; may lead to progressive deafness
motion sickness		sensation of dysequilibrium that occurs when riding in autos, planes, boats, or amusement rides
otitis externa	ō-tī'tĭs ĕks-tĕr'nah	infection of the external ear canal; swimmer's ear
otitis media	ō'tī'tĭs mē'dē-ah	acute or chronic infection or inflammation of the middle ear occurring in the following two forms
• *serous otitis media*	sēr'ŭs	fluid in the middle ear following an infectious or inflammatory process (See Figure 23-7A)
• *suppurative otitis media*	sūp'ŭ-rā"tĭv	purulent fluid accumulation and infection build up in middle ear; may result in a ruptured eardrum (See Figure 23-7B)
otosclerosis	ō"tō-sklē-rō'sĭs	abnormal growth of bone at the stapes causing conductive hearing loss

continues

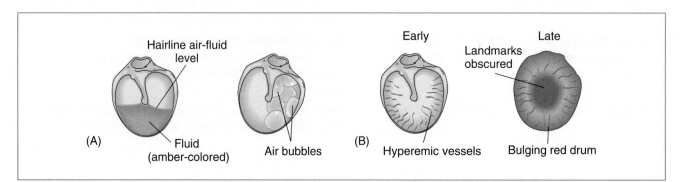

FIGURE 23-7   Otitis Media: (A) serous; (B) acute purulent (suppurative)

DIAGNOSES

Word	Pronunciation	Definition
The Ear (continued)		
ruptured eardrum		hole in the eardrum due to injury or infection
tinnitus	tĭn-ī'tŭs	perception of sound in the absence of stimuli
vertigo	vĕr'tĭ-gō	sensation of rotation or movement resulting from disease of the inner ear or disturbances of the vestibular centers or pathways in the central nervous system
The Nose and Sense of Smell		
adenoid hyperplasia	ăd'ĕ-noyd hī"pĕr-plā'zē-ah	condition characterized by enlargement of the adenoidal structure due to lymphoid hyperplasia
epistaxis	ĕp"ĭ-stăk'sĭs	bleeding from the nose
nasal polyp	pŏl'ĭp	growth or mass protruding from a mucous membrane in the nose
rhinitis: allergic, vasomotor, medicamentosus, viral	rī-nī'tĭs, văs-ō-mŏ'tor, mĕd"ĭ-kah-mĕn-tō'sŭs	inflammation and obstruction of the nose due to allergy, irritant, overuse of decongestant spray, or viral infection, respectively (See Figure 23-8)
septal deviation	sĕp'tăl	condition when the partition between the two sides of the nose is out of alignment due to developmental abnormalities or trauma; may cause airway obstruction
sinusitis	sī-nŭs-ī'tĭs	inflammation of a sinus cavity; may be acute or chronic
The Tongue and Sense of Taste		
contact ulcers		traumatic ulcers that appear on vocal cords where larynx cartilages are in contact with each other on the endotracheal tube (See Figure 23-5B)
epiglottitis	ĕp"ĭ-glŏt-tī'tĭs	inflammation, most common in very young children, of lidlike cartilage covering the windpipe

continues

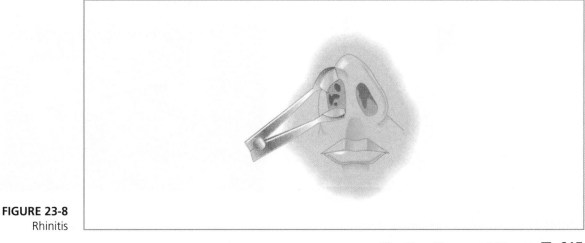

FIGURE 23-8
Rhinitis

DIAGNOSES

Word	Pronunciation	Definition
The Tongue and Sense of Taste (*continued*)		
laryngitis	lăr"ĭn-jī'tĭs	inflammation of the larynx
peritonsillar abscess	pĕr"ĭ-tŏn'sĭ-lăr	abscess formed between an infected tonsil and the surrounding soft tissue; known as quinsy
pharyngitis	făr"ĭn-jī'tĭs	inflammation of the pharynx
throat cancer		tumors on the vocal cords or in and around the larynx (See Figure 23-5C)
throat polyps	pŏl'ĭp	growth or mass protruding from a mucous membrane covering of the vocal cord (See Figure 23-5A)
tonsillitis	tŏn"sĭ-lī'tĭs	acute inflammation of the tonsils

TREATMENT PROCEDURES

Word	Pronunciation	Definition
adenoidectomy	ăd"ĕ-noid-ĕk'tō-mē	surgical excision of the adenoids
antral window (antrostomy)	ăn'trăl, ăn-trŏs'tō-mē	creation of an opening into the maxillary sinus or antrum
cochlear implant	kŏk'lē-ăr	device implanted in the cochlea that improves hearing when a regular hearing aid is of no benefit
endoscopic sinus surgery	ĕn"dō-skŏp'ĭk	use of endoscope to perform surgery on a sinus cavity
laryngectomy	lăr"ĭn-jĕk'tō-mē	excision of the larynx (voice box), following which speech can be facilitated by using esophageal speech or an artificial voice aid—either neck type or an intra-oral device (See Figure 23-9)

continues

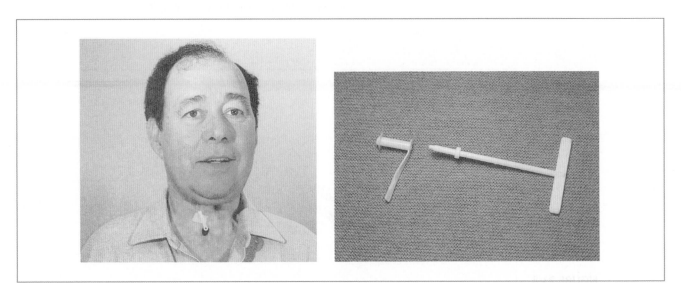

FIGURE 23-9   Voice Aids after Laryngectomy

TREATMENT PROCEDURES

Word	Pronunciation	Definition
mastoidectomy	măs"toi-děk'tō-mē	surgical removal of mastoid cells
myringoplasty (tympanoplasty)	mĭr-ĭn'gō-plăs"tē (tĭm"păn-ō-plăs'tē)	surgical repair of the tympanic membrane (eardrum) with a tissue graft
myringotomy (tympanostomy, tympanotomy)	mĭr"ĭn'gō"tō-mē (tĭm"păn-ŏs'tō-mē) (tĭm"păn-ŏt'ō-mē)	incision into the eardrum to relieve pressure or release fluid from the middle ear (See Diagnostic Procedures)
myringotomy with tubes		incision into the eardrum with the placing of a ventilation tube (See Figure 23-10)
otoplasty	ō'tō-plăs"tē	removal of a portion of the ear cartilage to bring the pinna or auricle nearer the head
polypectomy	pŏl"ĭ-pěk'tō-mē	excision of polyps
rhinoplasty	rī'nō-plăs"tē	plastic surgery or reconstruction of the nose
septoplasty	sěp"tō-plăs'tē	surgical procedure to realign the septum
stapedectomy	stā"pě-děk'tō-mē	surgical removal of the stapes and replacement with a prosthetic device (See Figure 23-11)
tonsillectomy	tŏn"sĭ-lěk'tō-mē	surgical excision of the tonsils
tracheostomy neck	trā"kē-ŏs'tō-mē	creation of an opening into the trachea through the
tympanoplasty	tĭm"pah-nō-plăs'tē	plastic reconstruction of the bones of the middle ear and eardrum

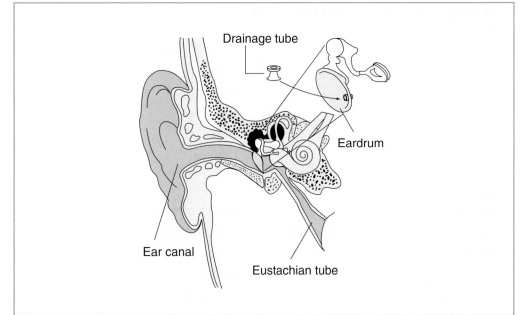

FIGURE 23-10
Myringotomy with Tubes

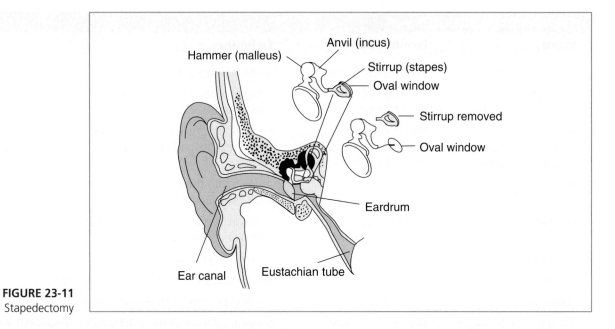

FIGURE 23-11
Stapedectomy

MEDICATIONS PRESCRIBED

Trade Name	Generic Name
Mouth and Throat	
Mycelex Troches	clotrimazole
Nilstat, Mycostatin, Bio-Statin	nystatin
Peridex, Periogard	chlorhexidine gluconate
Oral Antibiotics for ENT Disorders	
Amoxil, Biomox, Trimox	amoxicillin
Augmentin	amoxicillin and potassium clavulanate
Ceftin	cefuroxime axetil
E.E.S., Eryc, E-Mycin	erythromycin
Keflex, Keftab, Zartron	cephalexin
Omnipen, Principen, Totacillin	ampicillin
Suprax	cefixime
Otics	
Cerumenex	triethanolamine
Cortisporin Otic, Bacticort, Cortomycin	hydrocortisone, neomycin, polymyxin
Debrox	carbamide peroxide
Floxin Otic	ofloxacin
VoSol Otic	hydrocortisone, acetic acid

continues

MEDICATIONS PRESCRIBED

Trade Name	Generic Name
Antihistamines	
Allegra	fexofenadine HCl
Astelin	azelastine HCl
Atarax	hydroxyzine HCl
Claritin	loratadine
Deconamine SR	pseudoephedrine and chlorpheniramine
Optimine	azatadine maleate
Periactin	cyproheptadine HCl
Phenergan	promethazine HCl
Semprex-D	pseudoephedrine and acrivastine
Vistaril	hydroxyzine pamoate
Zyrtec	cetirizine HCl
Corticosteroids	
Beconase AQ, Vancenase	beclomethasone dipropionate
Flonase	fluticasone propionate
Nasacort	triamcinolone acetonide
Nasalide, Nasarel	flunisolide
Nasonex	mometasone furoate
Rhinocort	budesonide

ABBREVIATIONS

AC	air conduction
AD	*auris dextra* (right ear)
AS	*auris sinistra* (left ear)
AU	*aures unitas* (both ears)
BC	bone conduction
BOM	bilateral otitis media
dB	decibel
ENT	ear, nose, and throat
ETD	eustachian tube dysfunction
Oto	otology
PE tube	pressure equalization tube
PTS	permanent threshold shift
T & A	tonsillectomy and adenoidectomy
TM	tympanic membrane
TTS	temporary threshold shift

Name: _____ Date: _____

MATCHING*

Match the diagnoses to their meanings.

1. _____ episodic vertigo with hearing loss, nausea, and tinnitus; may lead to progressive deafness

2. _____ nosebleed

3. _____ growth protruding from a mucous membrane of the nose

4. _____ sensory hearing loss due to aging

5. _____ inflammation of air cells of the mastoid bone

6. _____ perception of sound in the absence of stimuli

7. _____ acute or chronic infection of the middle ear

a. mastoiditis

b. epistaxis

c. presbycusis

d. Ménière's disease

e. otitis media

f. nasal polyp

g. tinnitus

MEANING

Give the meaning of each of the italicized treatment procedures.

1. Ms. Macrino's hearing problem will be solved by a *stapedectomy*.

   _____

2. A *myringotomy* is commonly performed on little children.

   _____

3. Mr. Weber is scheduled for a *laryngectomy* tomorrow.

   _____

4. We do *antral windows* on Ms. Baxter tomorrow.

   _____

SELECTION

From the list below, select the correct term to identify each diagnostic procedure.

audiometry   impedance audiometry   otoscopy   pneumatic otoscopy   tuning fork test

1. use of sounds to test a patient's hearing   _____

2. detection of middle ear effusion or infection   _____

3. visual examination of the ears   _____

4. Rinne test or Weber test   _____

5. detects tympanic membrane movement   _____

*Answers are in Appendix A.

Word Element Review

Root	Meaning	Example	Definition
acous/o	hearing	**acousma** (a-kooz'mah)	buzzing or ringing sound
audi/o, audit/o	hearing, sound	**audiogram** (aw'dē-ō-grăm")	graphic record of a test of hearing
		audiometer (aw"dē-ŏm'ĕ-ter)	apparatus for measuring hearing at different sound frequencies
auri/o, auricul/o	ear	**auricle** (aw'rĕ-kl)	projecting part of the ear outside the head
cochle/o	cochlea	**cochlitis** (kōk-lī-tĭs)	inflammation of the cochlea
gingiv/o	gum	**gingivitis** (jĭn"jĭ-vī'tĭs)	inflammation of the gums
		gingivosis (jĭn"jĭ-vō'sĭs)	condition or disease of the gums of the mouth
gloss/o	tongue	**glossal** (glŏs'ăl)	pertaining to the tongue
		hypoglossal (hī"pō-glŏs'ăl)	underneath the tongue
lingu/o	tongue	**lingual** (lĭng'gwăl)	pertaining to the tongue
		lingually (lĭng'gwăl-lē)	toward the tongue
mastoid/o	mastoid process	**mastoidectomy** (măs"toy-děk'tō-mē)	hollowing out of the mastoid process by various means to remove bony partitions forming mastoid cells
myring/o	eardrum	**myringoplasty** (mĭ-rĭng'gō-plăs"tē)	surgical repair of defects of the eardrum
odont/o	tooth	**odontogenic** (ō-dŏn"tō-jĕn'ĭk)	originating in the teeth
or/o	mouth	**circumoral** (ser"kŭm-ō'răl)	around the mouth
		oral (ō'răl)	pertaining to the mouth
ot/o	ear	**otogenic** (ō"tō-jĕn'ĭk)	originating in the ear
phon/o	sound	**phonic** (fŏn'ĭk)	pertaining to the sound of the voice
		phonogram (fō'nō-grăm)	record of any sound
sial/o	salivary	**sialolith** (sī-ăl'ō-lĭth)	stone in the salivary duct
tympan/o	eardrum	**tympanic membrane** (tĭm-păn'ĭk)	eardrum

continues

Suffixes	Meaning	Example	Definition
-cusis	hearing	**presbycusis** (prĕs″bē-kū′sĭs)	sensory hearing loss due to aging
-osmia	smell	**anosmia** (ăn-ōz′mē-ah)	absence of the sense of smell

Word Element Review Exercises

Name: _____ Date: _____

WORD ELEMENTS
Provide the correct word element to complete the following words.

1. pertaining to the tongue _____ al
2. pertaining to the mouth _____ al
3. record of a sound _____ gram
4. originating in the teeth _____ genic
5. surgical repair of defects of the eardrum _____ plasty
6. graphic record of a test of hearing _____ gram
7. pertaining to sound of voice _____ ic
8. originating in the ear _____ genic
9. condition or disease of the gums _____ osis
10. inflammation of cochlea _____ itis

IDENTIFICATION*
Identify the following definitions.

1. apparatus for measuring hearing at different sound frequencies _____
2. eardrum _____
3. stone in the salivary duct _____
4. toward the tongue _____
5. inflammation of the gums _____
6. originating in the ear _____
7. sensory hearing loss due to aging _____
8. absence of sense of smell _____
9. part of ear projecting outside head _____
10. buzzing or ringing sound _____
11. underneath the tongue _____
12. around the mouth _____
13. hollowing out mastoid process to remove bony partitions _____

_____
*Answers are in Appendix A.

WORD ELEMENT MEANINGS

Give the meaning of each word element. Then use your dictionary to find a new word that contains each of the word elements. Specify whether the new word is a noun or an adjective by placing N or A in the last column.

Word Element	Meaning	Word	N or A
1. acous/o			
2. audi/o			
3. audit/o			
4. auricul/o			
5. auri/o			
6. cochle/o			
7. -cusis			
8. gingiv/o			
9 gloss/o			
10. lingu/o			
11. mastoid/o			
12. myring/o			
13. odont/o			
14. or/o			
15. -osmia			
16. ot/o			
17. phon/o			
18. sial/o			
19. tympan/o			

Dictionary Exercises

Name: _____ Date: _____

DICTIONARY EXERCISE 1

Use your dictionary to find the pronunciation and definition of each of the following words.

Word	Pronunciation	Definition
1. acoustic	_____	_____
2. anthelix	_____	_____
3. arytenoid	_____	_____
4. cleft palate	_____	_____
5. otomycosis	_____	_____
6. ossiculotomy	_____	_____
7. rhinophyma	_____	_____
8. torus palatinus	_____	_____

DICTIONARY EXERCISE 2*

Match the terms to their meanings.

1. _____ located or performed behind the auricle of the ear
2. _____ benign tumor of the nose in puberty
3. _____ main division of the auditory nerve
4. _____ abnormal sound made by the larynx in spasm
5. _____ principal duct of the parotid gland
6. _____ bleeding from the ear
7. _____ differences in pressure on both sides of the eardrum
8. _____ dizziness due to disease of the ear

a. auditory vertigo
b. barotrauma
c. juvenile angiofibroma
d. laryngeal stridor
e. otorrhagia
f. postauricular
g. Stensen's duct
h. vestibular nerve

DICTIONARY EXERCISE 3

Pronunciation of the words below is provided. Using your dictionary, find the correct spelling and definition of each word.

Word	Pronunciation	Definition
1. _____	fĕn"ĕs-trā'shŭn	_____
2. _____	hī"pō-ă-kū'sĭs	_____
3. _____	ō-tăl'jē-ah	_____
4. _____	rī"nō-rē'ah	_____
5. _____	nā"zō-mĕn'tăl	_____
6. _____	kald'wĕl-lŭk' operation	_____

_____

*Answers are in Appendix A.

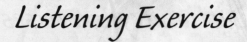

Listening Exercise

Name	Date

INSTRUCTIONS

1. Review the spelling, pronunciation, and meaning of the words provided in the preview.

2. Listen to the audio CD and fill in the blank as the word is dictated.

3. At the end of the exercise, check your spelling against the preview words. They appear in the preview in the order in which they are encountered in the exercise.

4. Review and practice the words you missed.

5. Look up words that are not familiar.

PREVIEW OF WORDS FOR LISTENING EXERCISE 23-1		
Word	**Pronunciation**	**Meaning**
sinusitis	sī-nŭs-ī'tŭs	inflammation of a sinus cavity
mucosal	mū-kō'săl	pertaining to mucous membrane
opacified	ō-păs'ĭ-fīd	made opaque—not penetrable by radiant energy
artifact	ăr'tĭ-făkt	a product produced by an external agent or action
nasopharynx	nā"zō-făr'ĭnks	the part of the pharynx above the soft palate
coronal	kō-rō'năl	pertaining to a crownlike structure

Computed Tomograph of the Sinuses

History is that of a chronic _____ with previous surgical intervention. A neo-synephrine study was performed.

FINDINGS:

Maxillary sinuses have some _____ thickening and air-fluid levels. Front sinuses, ethmoid sinuses, right sphenoid sinuses, and portions of the left sphenoid sinus are nearly completely _____ by soft tissue without definite evidence for expansion or erosion. A small fluid level is seen within the sphenoid sinuses. Dental amalgam creates what I believe to be significant _____ along the posterior lateral walls of the maxillary sinuses, but certainly a subtle erosion there cannot be excluded as a result of that. Axial sections may be necessary if that is important to delineate clinically. I believe previous surgery involving the medial walls of both maxillary sinuses into the _____ accounts for the lack of bony confines there. The osteomeatal complex certainly is compromised. Rather prominent frontal sinuses are seen with respect to the capacity but they are completely occupied by soft tissue. The integrity of the posterior wall of the front sinuses is not able to be evaluated in the _____ projection.

Appendix A
Answers to Selected Exercises

Answers for review exercises with an asterisk (*) are included in this Appendix. Answers are included for approximately half of the exercises in each chapter. Answers for all exercises are included in the Instructor's Manual.

CHAPTER 1

ANSWERS TO TERMINOLOGY REVIEW EXERCISES

Completion

1. Greek; Latin	4. prefix	7. retained	10. dropped
2. root	5. combining form	8. eponym	11. first
3. suffix	6. adjective	9. homonyms	12. re'; mat'

Plurals

1. viscera	4. lumina	7. criteria	10. ampullae
2. bacteria	5. diagnoses	8. cornua	
3. epididymides	6. stigmata	9. bronchi	

ANSWERS TO WORD ELEMENT REVIEW EXERCISES

Root, Prefix, Suffix, or Combining Form

1. cardio-; -logy	5. bas-	9. gastro-; -logist	13. cyano-
2. gastro-; -logy	6. cyan-; -osis	10. cardio-; a-	14. cardio-; -gen
3. physio-; logy	7. -gen	11. gran-	15. cardio-; -gram
4. pharmaco-; -logy	8. top-	12. acr-; cyan-; -osis	16. gastro-; -scopy

Word Ending—Noun or Adjective

1. -ac A	3. -is N	5. -y N	7. -um N
2. -al A	4. -al A	6. -ic A	8. -ule N

ANSWERS TO DICTIONARY EXERCISES

	Word	**Definition**
1.	cord	long, flexible structure of cells or fibers
	chord	combination of three or more different musical tones
2.	gait	manner of walking
	gate	movable barrier closing an opening
3.	humerus	name of a bone
	humorous	funny
4.	facet	small plane surface on a hard body, such as on a bone
	faucet	device for controlling flow of liquid from a pipe
5.	colic	acute abdominal pain
	choleic	pertaining to bile

Word	Definition
6. wen	sebaceous cyst
when	at the time
7. acidic	acid-forming
acetic	sour, pertaining to vinegar or its acid
acinic	pertaining to the smallest portion of a gland
8. form	configuration or shape
forum	a public meeting
9. shocky	in shock or showing signs suggestive of shock
shotty	nodes; lumpy, resembling buckshot
shoddy	anything of inferior quality
10. radical	directed to the root or cause
radicle	one of the smallest branches of a vessel or nerve
11. profusion	abundance
perfusion	passage of a fluid through vessels of a specific organ
12. casual	happens by chance; informal
causal	pertaining to cause

CHAPTER 2

ANSWERS TO TERMINOLOGY REVIEW EXERCISES

Choices
1. vertical
2. transverse
3. sagittal
4. median
5. epithelial
6. connective
7. muscular
8. nervous

Completion
1. abdominal; pelvic; thoracic
2. organs
3. viscera
4. pelvic
5. dorsal
6. diaphragm
7. pleural, mediastinum
8. nine
9. epigastrium, umbilical, hypogastrium
10. hypochondrium, lumbar, inguinal
11. differentiated cells cannot grow again; undifferentiated cells can
12. stem

Definitions
1. farthest from the source
2. closest to the source
3. lower, away-from-the-head end
4. farthest from the median
5. toward the front

ANSWERS TO WORD ELEMENT REVIEW EXERCISES

Root or Combining Form
1. dorso-, later-
2. cyto-
3. later-
4. somat-
5. viscer-
6. endo-, cardi-

Prefix
1. retro-
2. trans-
3. inter-
4. contra-
5. sub-
6. ex-
7. peri-
8. intra-

Word Endings—Noun or Adjective
1. -al   A
2. -ic   A
3. -ous   A
4. -al   A
5. -al   A
6. -um   N

ANSWERS TO DICTIONARY EXERCISES

Dictionary Exercise 2 (Definitions may vary.)

Word	Definition
1. endocarditis	inflammation of the endothelial lining of the heart
2. lateroversion	abnormal turning to one side
3. transthoracic	across the chest wall
4. retroaction	action in a reverse direction
5. subphrenic	under the diaphragm
6. viserogenic	originating in the viscera
7. cytopathology	study of the cellular changes in disease
8. dorsoventral	concerning the back and frontal surfaces of the body
9. somatogenic	originating in the body
10. intermediary	situated between two bodies
11. intravenous	within or into a vein
12. express	to squeeze out

CHAPTER 3

ANSWERS TO TERMINOLOGY REVIEW EXERCISES

Definitions

1. auscultation
2. palpation
3. visualization
4. percussion
5. vital signs
6. rubs
7. thrills
8. edema
9. hepatosplenomegaly
10. tympanic membrane
11. history

Short Answer

1. diplopia — perception of two images of a single object; double vision
2. extraocular — outside of the eye
3. fundi — back portion of the interior of the eyeball
4. lacrimation — secretion and discharge of tears

Sign, Symptom, or Diagnosis

1. diagnosis
2. sign
3. symptom
4. sign
5. symptom
6. sign
7. sign
8. diagnosis

Spelling

1. carotid
2. correct
3. femoral
4. correct
5. correct
6. correct
7. trachea
8. correct
9. cholesterol
10. murmur
11. septal

Matching

1. c
2. a
3. e
4. b
5. d

Identifications/Abbreviations

1. Chief Complaint — CC
2. Present Illness — PI
3. Past History or Past Medical History — PH or PMH
4. Family History — FH
5. Social History — SH
6. Review of Systems — ROS
7. Physical Examination — PX (PE)
8. Impressions/Diagnoses — —
9. Plan — —

ANSWERS TO WORD ELEMENT REVIEW EXERCISES

Meanings

1.	dys-	labored breathing
2.	in-	not able to cure
3.	path/o	any disease of the heart
4.	-algia	pain in a joint
5.	-rrhage	excessive flow of blood
6.	-malacia	softening of the muscular tissue of the heart
7.	-itis	inflammation of the stomach
8.	ect-	situated outside of the usual location
9.	-osis	condition of forming fibrous tissue
10.	epi-	above the stomach
11.	-emesis	vomiting of blood
12.	-iasis	condition marked by the formation of stones
13.	-ptosis	downward displacement of the kidney
14.	infra-	beneath the axilla
15.	-trophy	wasting away; without growth

ANSWERS TO DICTIONARY EXERCISES

Dictionary Exercise 2

1.	atypical	deviation from normal
2.	bilateral	having two sides; pertaining to both sides
3.	congestion	abnormal accumulation of blood in a part; engorgement of fluid
4.	dehydration	condition resulting from the excessive loss of body water; removal of water
5.	inflammation	protective response to injury or destruction characterized by pain, heat, swelling, and redness
6.	insomnia	inability to sleep
7.	migraine	sudden, severe attacks of head pain
8.	obstruction	abnormal blockage; state of being blocked
9.	supple	freely moveable; limber; readily bent
10.	unilateral	affecting only one side
11.	arrhythmia	loss of rhythm of the heartbeat
12.	serous	thin, watery liquid
13.	accommodation	adjustment or adaption

CHAPTER 4

ANSWERS TO TERMINOLOGY REVIEW EXERCISES

Fill in the Blank

1. generic	5. *Drug Information*	9. prescription	13. placebo
2. chemical name	6. toxicity	10. drug	14. prophylactic
3. pharmacology	7. topical administration	11. gastrointestinal tract	15. therapeutic
4. toxicologist	8. GI tract; parenteral	12. palliative	16. inhalation

ANSWERS TO WORD ELEMENT REVIEW EXERCISES

Circle and Define Combining Forms

1.	<u>pharmac</u>eutical	drug	6. <u>chemo</u>receptor	chemical
2.	<u>toxic</u>ant	poison	7. <u>derma</u>tologic	skin
3.	<u>cutane</u>ous	skin	8. <u>hypn</u>otic	sleep
4.	<u>narc</u>osis	stupor	9. <u>toxic</u>	poison
5.	<u>bucc</u>al	cheek	10. <u>lingu</u>al	tongue

Completion

1. chemo	3. contra	5. anti	7. bucc
2. narco	4. toxic	6. sub	8. tox

ANSWERS TO DICTIONARY EXERCISES

Dictionary Exercise 2 (Sentences may vary.)
1. (emetic) In the Emergency Room, the physician ordered a drug to make the child vomit.
2. (placebo) The control group took an imitation drug for the entire year.
3. (anticoagulant) The patient has been taking a drug to prevent clotting of the blood.
4. (hypersensitivity) The infant has an allergy to penicillin.
5. (anaphylactic) The patient was having a very serious allergic response.
6. (teratogenic) A drug taken by a pregnant woman may cause physical defects in a fetus.
7. (barbiturate) She was taking a drug to calm her.
8. (placebo effect) Her positive attitude affected the results.
9. (analgesic) He asked the doctor for a pain reliever.
10. (antibiotic) A drug that slowed the growth of bacteria, fungi, or parasites was prescribed to help her.
11. (allergic) The adverse response to the drug was severe.
12. (anthelmintic) The drug will get rid of worms.
13. (diuretic) She experienced minor inconvenience because the drug increased the amount of urine she produced.
14. (lipid) The substance was obtained from a plant or animal source and was insoluble in water.
15. (narcotic) A drug was used that had a sedative action, which did not help the situation.
16. (resistance) The antibiotic no longer worked for the patient's pneumonia.
17. (tincture) Physicians frequently write prescriptions for alcoholic or hydroalcoholic solutions.
18. (uricosuric) He prescribed a drug that increases the excretion of uric acid in the urine.
19. (anticonvulsant) The physician prescribed a drug that reduced the severity of the seizures the patient was experiencing.
20. (antidepressant) The patient is taking a medication to elevate his mood.

CHAPTER 5

ANSWERS TO TERMINOLOGY REVIEW EXERCISES

Completion
1. melanin
2. 2 million
3. apocrine; eccrine
4. papilla
5. dermatologist
6. epidermis; dermis; subcutaneous tissue
7. keratin
8. skin
9. stratum corneum
10. fat

ANSWERS TO WORKING PRACTICE REVIEW EXERCISES

Identification
1. cryosurgery
2. curettage
3. psoriasis
4. pemphigus
5. tinea
6. scratch test
7. punch or incisional biopsy
8. pediculosis
9. decubitus ulcer
10. nevus
11. varicella
12. alopecia
13. ephelis
14. hyperhidrosis
15. macule
16. purpura
17. wheal
18. pustule
19. papule
20. cheilitis
21. diaphoresis
22. full thickness burns
23. rosacea
24. UVB
25. hirsutism

ANSWERS TO WORD ELEMENT REVIEW EXERCISES

Completion
1. hidr/o; sud/o or sudor/o
2. cutane/o or cut/o; dermat/o or derm/o
3. pil/o; trich/o

Identify
1. fascicular
2. corneous
3. cutaneous
4. squamous
5. acrohyperhidrosis
6. sebum
7. macula
8. onychitis
9. keratosis
10. dermatitis
11. sudoriferous
12. pilose

ANSWERS TO DICTIONARY EXERCISES

Dictionary Exercise 1

Pronunciation	Definition
1. ăk"rō-kor'dŏn	a pedunculated skin tag; a small outgrowth of epidermal and dermal tissues
2. bŭl'ah	a blister
3. mĕl"ah-nō-dĕr'mah	an abnormal amount of the pigment melanin in the skin
4. kŏl'ah-jĕn	a protein substance found in the skin and connective tissue
5. băl"ah-nī'tĭs zē-rŏt'ĭ-kah ŏb-lĭt'er-ăns	inflammation of the glans penis
6. strawberry hē-măn"jē-ō'mah	dark red to purple birthmark, usually on the face
7. der"mah-tī'tĭs hĕr-pĕt"ĭ-for'mĭs	chronic inflammation of the skin characterized by itching and burning
8. kăn'dĭ-dah	a genus of yeastlike fungi that is commonly part of the normal flora of the mouth, skin, intestinal tract, and vagina
9. dĕr-mŏg'rah-fĭzm	a pale, raised welt that appears when the skin is scratched with a dull instrument
10. fō"tō-sĕn"sĭ-tĭv'ĭ-tē	abnormal sensitivity to light
11. noo"rō-der"mah-tī'tĭs	cutaneous inflammation with itching that is frequently associated with emotional disturbances
12. mī-kō'sĭs fung'gō-ĭ'dĕs	a chronic, malignant, lymphoreticular neoplasm of the skin and, in late stages, lymph nodes and viscera, with development of large, painful, ulcerating tumors

Dictionary Exercise 2

Word	Definition
1. cicatrix	a scar left by a healed wound
2. excoriation	destruction and removal of the surface of the skin or the covering of an organ due to scratching
3. purulent	containing or forming pus
4. tinea pedis	athlete's foot, fungal nail infection
5. condyloma	a wartlike growth of the skin, usually seen on external genitalia or near the anus
6. comedo	plugged pore, either whitehead or blackhead
7. cilia	eyelashes; hairlike processes
8. molluscum	any of various skin diseases marked by the formation of soft, rounded, cutaneous tumors
9. steatoma	a cyst occurring in the skin, resulting from local dilatation of either a sebaceous gland or its duct
10. telogen effluvium	shedding hair
11. pityriasis rosea	a skin disease marked by scaly eruptions on the back, legs, arms, and thighs

CHAPTER 6

ANSWERS TO TERMINOLOGY REVIEW EXERCISES

Completion

1. massage therapy
2. processes
3. osseous
4. compact (cortical); cancellous (spongy)
5. periosteum
6. L5
7. physiatrist
8. cervical; thoracic; lumbar; sacral; coccygeal
9. 40; 50
10. goniometry

ANSWERS TO WORKING PRACTICE REVIEW EXERCISES

Spelling

1. capsulorrhaphy
2. fasciectomy
3. lupus erythematosus
4. correct
5. meniscectomy

Definitions

1. entering a joint with an endoscope to examine that joint
2. study of joints after injection of opaque contrast material
3. removal of synovial fluid from a joint space for analysis
4. testing for the presence of an antibody found in people who have rheumatoid arthritis
5. records the strength of a muscle contraction as a result of electrical stimulation
6. a plain x-ray of a body part
7. a test that indicates an inflammatory process in the body
8. uses computers and magnetism to obtain detailed pictures of internal structures
9. measurement of the amount of creatine kinase present in the blood
10. rate at which erythrocytes settle out of solution when an anticoagulant is added
11. scan that tracks white cells (infection)
12. study of the spinal column after injection of opaque contrast material

ANSWERS TO WORD ELEMENT REVIEW EXERCISES

Word Elements

1. cephal/o; crani/o
2. cheir/o or chir/o; dactyl/o; digit/o
3. dactyl/o; digit/o; ped/o or pod/o; tars/o
4. caud/o; lumb/o; sacr/o; spondyl/o; vertebr/o

Matching

1. c	4. e	7. d	9. f
2. h	5. j	8. a	10. g
3. b	6. i		

Pronunciation and Definition

1. ĭn"ter-kŏs'tăl — situated between the ribs
2. ar"thrō-sĕn-tē'sĭs — puncture of a joint cavity with a needle to remove fluid
3. ber-sī'tĭs — inflammation of a bursa
4. mī"ō-kăr-dī'tĭs — inflammation of the myocardium, the middle layer of the heart wall
5. ŏs"tē-ō-ăr-thrī'tĭs — a chronic disease involving the joints
6. spŏn"di-lŏl'ĭ-sĭs — degenerative changes in the spine
7. tĕn'sor — any muscle that stretches or makes a body part tense

ANSWERS TO DICTIONARY EXERCISES

Dictionary Exercise 1

Pronunciation	**Definition**
1. ah-nŏm'ah-lē	marked deviation from the normal standard
2. kăl-sĭf'ĭk	forming lime
3. kō-lăt'er-ăl lĭg'ah-mĕnts	supportive ligaments at the medial and lateral sides of some joints
4. kŏs"tō-kŏn'drăl	pertaining to a rib and its cartilage
5. kŏk'sah	the hip or hip joint
6. dē'kăr-văns dĭ-zēz'	tenosynovitis due to relative narrowness of the tendon sheath of two muscles
7. flăl joint	a joint with excessive mobility, usually due to paralysis of the muscle that controls it
8. jē'nū	the knee or any structure bent like a knee
9. lĕg-kăl-vā'pĕr'tēz dĭ-zēz'	bone destruction of the head of the femur
10. pĕs plā'nŭs	flatfoot
11. ŏs"tē-ō-plăs"tē	plastic surgery of the bones
12. ŏs"ĭ-fĭ-kā'shŭn	conversion of another tissue into bone
13. ĭn"tĕr-trō"kăn-ter'ĭk	between the two trochanters of the femur; refers to a fracture
14. ŏs'tē-ō-klăst	large cells that function to reabsorb or digest bony tissue

Dictionary Exercise 2

1. kah-pĭt'ū-lŭm	a	11. ŏs-tĕk'tō-mē	b	
2. dī-ăf'ĭ-sĭs	b	12. ŏs"tē-ō'mah	b	
3. giant cell tumor	b	13. ŏs'tē-ō-fīt"	a	
4. glē'noid	a	14. roo"mă-tŏl'ō-gĭst	a	
5. glē'noid kăv'ĭ-tē	b	15. pŏl"ē-mī"ō-sī'tĭs	b	
6. hĕm"ăr-thrō'sĭs	a	16. saw"sĕr-ī-zā'shŭn	a	
7. lăm'ĭ-nah	b	17. sē"kwĕs-trĕk'tō-mē	a	
8. mĕ-tăf'ĭ-sĭs	b	18. sĕs'ah-moid	a	
9. noo'klē-ŭs pŭl-pō'sŭs	a	19. soo'dĕks ăt'rō-fē	b	
10. ō-lĕk'rah-nŏn	b	20. sĭn-dăk'tĭ-lĭzm	b	

CHAPTER 7

ANSWERS TO TERMINOLOGY REVIEW EXERCISES

Short Answer

1. preoperative diagnosis, postoperative diagnosis, name of the procedure (operation), indications, description of findings and technique, and signature block. (Students may include various subcategories, i.e., type of anesthesia, position, closure, sponge count, etc.)
2. endobronchial, endotracheal, inhalation, insufflation, intravenous
3. block, epidural block, intercostal block, saddle block, spinal block
4. infiltration, any of the regional methods

Completion

1. indications	4. findings and technique	7. continuous	9. laser
2. surgical position	5. suture materials	8. interrupted	10. sponge count
3. incision	6. suture techniques		

ANSWERS TO WORD ELEMENT REVIEW EXERCISES

Matching

1. o	6. m	11. n	15. d
2. f	7. j	12. p	16. c
3. l	8. a	13. g	17. b
4. h	9. r	14. k	18. i
5. q	10. e		

Word Elements and Definitions

1. -otomy	surgical incision into the stomach
2. -plasty	surgical repair of a joint
3. pro-	forward displacement or bulging
4. -desis	surgical fusion or immobilization of a joint
5. hyper-	excess blood in a part
6. anti-	medication that prevents or alleviates vomiting
7. -oma	malignant new growth or tumor

ANSWERS TO DICTIONARY EXERCISES

Dictionary Exercise 3

Answers will vary. Definitions of italicized terms are given below.

Pronunciation	Definition
1. clamped and lī'gāt-ĕd	surgical technique for compressing a part and then tying off the vessel
2. krī"ō-thēr'ah-pē	therapeutic use of cold
3. ĕn blŏk	to remove as a lump or as a whole
4. freely movable mass	not bound to surrounding structures
5. frī'ah-b'l	easily crumbled

	Pronunciation	Definition
6.	hē"mō-stā'sĭs	stop of the flow of blood
7.	blunt dissection	separation of tissue along natural cleavage lines without cutting
	sharp dissection	separation of tissue by means of the sharp edge of a knife, scalpel, or scissor
8.	skŭl-tē'tŭs bandage	a many-tailed bandage
9.	lĭg'ah-tŭrz	any material used to tie off blood or other vessels
10.	kū"rĕ-tahzh'	scraping or removal of growths or other materials from the wall of a cavity with an instrument called a curet/curette

CHAPTER 8

ANSWERS TO TERMINOLOGY REVIEW EXERCISES

Completion

1. septum
2. tricuspid; pulmonary; mitral; aortic
3. murmurs
4. systole; diastole
5. functional; organic
6. 60; 100
7. conduction
8. pacemaker
9. venules
10. right innominate; left carotid; left subclavian
11. sphygmomanometer
12. superior vena cava; inferior vena cava
13. aorta
14. aorta
15. abdominal aorta

ANSWERS TO WORKING PRACTICE REVIEW EXERCISES

Matching

1. g
2. e
3. a
4. d
5. b
6. k
7. l
8. j
9. f
10. h
11. c
12. i

Spelling

1. electrolytes
2. enzymes
3. correct
4. triglycerides
5. correct
6. correct
7. correct
8. prothrombin
9. correct
10. stent
11. transluminal

ANSWERS TO WORD ELEMENT REVIEW EXERCISES

Completion

1. tachycardia
2. coronary
3. myocardial infarction
4. stethoscope
5. aortorraphy; arteriorraphy
6. valvular
7. thrombus; thrombosis
8. cardiomyopathy
9. atriomegaly
10. pericardiectomy
11. furcal

Spellings and Definitions

1. correct; an enlarged heart; N
2. bradycardia; a slow heartbeat; N
3. tachycardia; a fast heart rate; N
4. ventriculotomy; incision into the ventricle of the heart; N
5. venous; pertaining to a vein; A

Definitions

1. arterioplasty
2. bifurcation
3. phlebitis
4. phlebostenosis
5. vascular
6. vasodilator

ANSWERS TO DICTIONARY EXERCISES

Dictionary Exercise 1

Pronunciation	Definition
1. prē-kŏr'dē-ŭm	area of the chest covering the heart and lower part of the thorax
2. ăt'rō-fē	a wasting away or decrease in size of a cell, a tissue, or an organ
3. aw'rĭ-k'l	the small, ear-shaped appendage of each atrium of the heart
4. bī-jĕm'ĭ-năl	occurring in twos
5. bundle branch block	obstruction of the impulse flow to neuromuscular fibers, interrupting normal beating of the heart
6. pŭr-kĭn'jē fī'bĕrz	cardiac muscle cells under the endocardium of the heart ventricles that form the last part of the cardiac conduction system
7. cardiac massage	closed-chest cardiac massage is external massage to restore the heartbeat; open-chest cardiac massage is internal compression after the chest is quickly opened
8. kăr"dē-ō-mō-tĭl'ĭ-tē	ability of the heart to move
9. kor pŭl"mō-nā'lē	a disease state that involves both the right side of the heart and the blood vessels of the lungs
10. dĭl-ah-tā'shŭn	stretching of a hollow structure or opening beyond its normal size
11. kŭsp	any one of the small flaps or valves of the heart
12. loo'mēn	space within an artery, vein, intestine, or tube
13. ŏ-kloo'zhŭn	closure of; state of being closed
14. noo"mō-pĕr"ĭ-kăr'dē-ŭm	air in the pericardial cavity of the heart
15. sinus arrest	stopping of the contractions of the heart caused by failure of the pacemaker (sinoatrial node) to function
16. vĕn-trĭk'ū-lăr septal defect	an abnormal opening in the septum, which separates the right and left ventricles of the heart
17. ah-trē'zē-ah	congenital absence or closure of a normal body orifice
18. dŭk'tŭs ăr-tē"rē-ō'sŭs	a channel from the pulmonary artery to the aorta in the fetus
19. pā'tĕnt dŭk'tŭs ăr-tē"rē-ō'sŭs	persistence after birth of the ductus arteriosus, a small vessel through which blood bypasses the lungs in the embryo
20. trăns"pō-zĭsh'ŭn	change in position of a structure to the opposite side
21. hē"mō-dī-năm'ĭks	study of blood circulation and blood pressure
22. broot	a sound or murmur heard in auscultation
23. kō"ărk-tā'shŭn	stricture or narrowing
24. păl'or	lack of color; paleness

CHAPTER 9

ANSWERS TO TERMINOLOGY REVIEW EXERCISES

Short Answer
1. Erythrocytes carry oxygen from the lungs to the tissues; leukocytes protect against infection; platelets are essential for coagulation.
2. thoracic and right lymphatic
3. A, B, AB, O; the presence or absence of protein substances

ANSWERS TO WORKING PRACTICE REVIEW EXERCISES

Definitions
1. an abnormally high number of white blood cells
2. growth of malignant tissue originating in the lymphatic system
3. tumor characterized by uncontrolled multiplication of plasma cells in the bone marrow
4. enlargement of the lymph nodes
5. multiple pinpoint hemorrhages and an accumulation of blood under the skin

ANSWERS TO WORD ELEMENT REVIEW EXERCISES

Completion

1. hemat/o, hem/o; sangui/o
2. blast/o; cyt/o
3. eosin/o; erythr/o; leuk/o
4. immun/o; lymph/o; splen/o; thym/o
5. agglutin/o
6. blast/o; -blast

Matching

1. k	5. i	9. b	13. a
2. o	6. m	10. l	14. j
3. f	7. e	11. h	15. n
4. c	8. d	12. g	

DICTIONARY EXERCISES

Dictionary Exercise 1

1. ah-grăn"ū-lō-sī-tō'sĭs — absence or severely reduced numbers of white blood cells in the bloodstream and bone marrow
2. ăn'tĭ-bŏd"ē — a protein substance developed in response to and interacting specifically with an antigen; this antigen-antibody reaction forms the basis of immunity
3. ē-lĭp"tō-sī-tō'sĭs — a hereditary disorder in which red cells are elliptical in shape
4. ĕ-rĭth"rō-poi-ē'sĭs — production of red blood cells
5. grăn"ū-lō-poi-ē'sĭs — formation of granulocytes
6. ĕ-rĭth'rō-blăst — an immature blood cell
7. vĭs"kŏs'ĭ-tē — thickness of blood as compared to water
8. măk"rō-sīt'ĭk ă-nē'mē-ă — anemia in which the red cells tend to be larger than normal
9. mĕt"ah-mī'ĕ-lō-sīt" — a transitional cell intermediate in development between a megalocyte and a mature granular leukocyte
10. pel-ĕb'stīn fever — fever in which the temperature rises by steps over several days and then goes down in steps in the same way
11. poi"kĭ-lō-sō-tī'sĭs — presence of red blood cells of a variety of shapes—elongated, round, or oval
12. hē-mŏl'ĭ-sĭs — breakdown of red blood cells and release of hemoglobin
13. thrŏm"bō-sī'tō-pē'nĭk pŭr'pū-rah — bleeding into the skin and mucous membranes occasioned by a decrease in the number of thrombocytes

---

CHAPTER 10

ANSWERS TO TERMINOLOGY REVIEW EXERCISES

Matching

1. n	6. a	11. r	16. s
2. f	7. k	12. o	17. i
3. c	8. g	13. h	18. d
4. e	9. m	14. p	19. b
5. q	10. j	15. l	20. t

Completion

1. metastasis
2. stage; grade
3. mixed-tissue
4. squamous; adenocarcinoma
5. carcinomas; sarcomas
6. acquired or somatic; germline
7. oncology
8. alkylates, antibiotics, antimetabolites, antimitotics, hormonal
9. chromosomes
10. genes
11. nucleus
12. internal radiation
13. immunotherapy
14. protocol
15. palliative therapy
16. radiosensitizers
17. treatment port

ANSWERS TO WORD ELEMENT REVIEW EXERCISES

Identify Word Roots

1. adeno-   gland
2. papillo-   papillary
3. scirrh-   hard
4. sarc-   flesh
5. blast-   immature

6. immuno-   immune
7. medullo-   soft inner part
8. cysto-   sac of fluid
9. fibro-   fibers

Identify Definitions

1. carcinogenic
2. radiotherapy
3. metastasis
4. polypoid

5. transmutation
6. mutagenesis
7. oncogenic
8. plasma

9. electrochemistry
10. carcinomatous
11. neoplasia

12. medulloblast
13. neoplasm
14. chemotherapy

ANSWERS TO DICTIONARY EXERCISES

Dictionary Exercise 1 (Examples will vary.)

1. Three types of transplantation: syngeneic, autologous, and allogenic.
2. Colony-stimulating factors stimulate development of cells in bone marrow, and growth factor is an agent that stimulates growth of cells.
3. NK (natural killers) cells and purging relate to getting rid of tumor cells.
4. SCID (severe combined immunodeficiency disease) and germ cell tumors refer to abnormal conditions.
5. Antithymocyte globulin and immunosuppression engraftment refer to the transplantation process and what it accomplishes.
6. Determining similarity of tissue before transplant by the use of human leukocyte antigens assists the transplant process.
7. All the terms relate to bone marrow transplant.
8. Allogenic transplantation, autologous transplantation, marrow harvest, engraftment, human leukocyte antigen, and syngeneic transplantation are all words about transplants.
9. Immunosuppression and severe combined immunodeficiency disease have to do with suppressing the immune system.
10. Antithymocyte and immunosuppression have to do with graft-versus-host and/or transplant rejection activity.
11. Germ cell tumor and growth factor have to do with tumor growth.

CHAPTER 11

ANSWERS TO TERMINOLOGY REVIEW EXERCISES

Completion

1. roentgen rays
2. alpha; beta; gamma
3. gamma
4. x-rays; sound waves; magnetism
5. in vivo

6. tomography (laminography)
7. barium sulfate
8. radiopharmaceutical or labeled compound
9. linear accelerator, betatron

Circle

1. Lateral   2. Posteroanterior   3. Oblique   4. Anteroposterior

Abbreviations

1. Ba   3. CAT   5. IVP   7. MRI   9. PET
2. AP   4. ^{131}I   6. PA   8. DVI

ANSWERS TO WORD ELEMENT REVIEW EXERCISES

Matching

1. k   6. q   11. h   16. v   21. o
2. a   7. d   12. b   17. j   22. r
3. s   8. c   13. x   18. m   23. e
4. i   9. f   14. n   19. y   24. l
5. w   10. u   15. p   20. g   25. t

ANSWERS TO DICTIONARY EXERCISES

Dictionary Exercise 1

Pronunciation	Definition
1. ah-koos'tĭk ĭm-pē'dans	resistance to the transmission of sound waves
2. ĕrg	one unit of work
3. prō'tŏn	a positively charged particle present in the nucleus of all elements
4. kwŏn'tŭm number	set of real numbers assigned to a physical system that characterizes the properties and the state of a particle or of the system
5. răd	radiation absorbed dose; measure of radiation absorbed
6. rā'dŏn	a radioactive, gaseous element resulting from the decaying of radium
7. rĕk"tĭ-lĭn'ē-ăr	moving in or forming into a straight line
8. tagging	a trace amount of a radioisotope added to a compound and introduced into the body so that the compound's path through the body can be tracked
9. atomic weight	weight of an atom of a chemical element as compared to the weight of an atom of carbon-12
10. half-life valve	time required for the radiation level of a radioactive particle to decay by one-half
11. cassette	a small box; in radiology, the lightproof film holder
12. tracer studies	name applied to the process of tagging radionuclides and following them through the body
13. dŏp'lĕr ĕ-fĕkt'	change in frequency of sound or light waves emitted by a source as it moves from or toward an observer
14. ĭ-ō-nĭ-zā'shŭn	process in which a neutral atom or molecule gains or loses electrons, acquiring a positive or negative charge
15. ĭ-rā"ē-ā'shŭn	exposure to any form of radiant energy such as heat, light, x-ray

Dictionary Exercise 2 (Answers will vary.)

1. Blood-brain barrier (BBB)	barrier membrane between circulating blood and the brain, preventing certain damaging substances from reaching brain tissue and cerebrospinal fluid
2. radioactive contamination	presence of radioactive material in any place where it is not desired
3. gī'gĕr-mĭl'ĕr counter	amplifying device for measuring the presence of radiation
4. lĭm-făn"jē-ŏg'rah-fē	x-ray study of the lymphatic system after the injection of a contrast medium
5. măm-ŏg'rah-fē	radiographic study of the breast
6. plā'nĭ-grăm	an x-ray; a photograph of a layer of a section of the body
7. radiation sickness	illness often associated with diarrhea, blood cell loss, vomiting, and hair loss resulting from over-exposure to electromagnetic waves, usually x-rays or gamma waves
8. spot film	radiograph of a small, isolated area taken during fluoroscopy
9. stopcock	a valve that regulates the flow of fluid from a container
10. ū-rŏg'rah-fē	method of studying the urinary tract by roentgenography after the injection of a contrast material
11. vē'nō-grăm	phlebogram; radiograph of a vein filled with contrast medium
12. lethal	capable of causing death
13. transducer	hand-held device that sends and receives a soundwave signal
14. multiple-gated acquisitions scan	test that studies the motion of the left ventricular walls and the ventricle's ability to eject blood

CHAPTER 12

ANSWERS TO TERMINOLOGY REVIEW EXERCISES

Selection

1. septum	5. epiglottis	9. hilum	13. bronchioles
2. palate	6. bronchi	10. alveoli	14. carina
3. pharynx	7. pleura	11. expiration	15. lobes
4. trachea	8. diaphragm	12. inspiration	

ANSWERS TO WORKING PRACTICE REVIEW EXERCISES

Identification/Procedures

1. pulmonary angiography
2. arterial blood gasses
3. pulmonary function test
4. thoracentesis
5. bronchoscopy

Identification/Abbreviations

1. acute respiratory distress syndrome
2. chronic obstructive pulmonary disease
3. intermittent positive pressure breathing
4. pulmonary function test

ANSWERS TO WORD ELEMENT REVIEW EXERCISES

Circle and Define

1. pnea	to breathe	5. pharyng	pharynx, throat	9. aer	air
2. phren	diaphragm	6. naso	nose	10. pulmon	lung
3. bronch	bronchus	7. laryng	larynx	11. thorax	chest
4. epiglott	epiglottis	8. trache	windpipe	12. spir	to breathe

ANSWERS TO DICTIONARY EXERCISES

Dictionary Exercise 1

	Pronunciation	**Definition**
1.	blăs"tō-mī-kō'sĭs	any infection caused by a yeast-like organism
2.	ăn"thră-kō'sĭs	accumulation of carbon deposits in the lungs due to inhalation of coal dust or smoke; black lung disease
3.	kŏk-sĭd"ē-oi"dō-mī-kō'sĭs	a disease caused by a fungus
4.	kŏn-sŏl"ĭ-dā'shŭn	solidification, such as is caused by the airlessness of the area of a lung affected with pneumonia
5.	fī-brō'sĭs	growth of fibrous connective tissue
6.	hē"mō-nū"mō-thō'răks	blood and air in the pleural cavity
7.	rahlz	abnormal sounds heard in the bronchi upon auscultation of the chest at inspiration or expiration
8.	sĭl"ĭ-kō'sĭs	an occupational disease due to the inhalation of silica (quartz) dust; it is a type of pneumoconiosis
9.	ĕm"fĭ-sĕm'ah-tŭs bŭl'ē	walled, cystlike structures that form in the lung from an overdistention of the air sacs (alveoli)
10.	acid-fast bah-sĭl'ŭs	a type of rod-shaped bacterial microorganism not readily decolorized after staining
11.	hī"drō-nū"mō-thō'răks	collection of fluid and air within the pleural cavity
12.	rŏng'kī	dry, rattling sounds in the bronchi due to obstruction of the airways
13.	ăs"pĕr-jĭl-lō'sĭs	disease caused by species of fungus and marked by inflammatory granulomatous lesions in the skin, ear, orbit, nasal sinuses, lungs, and sometimes bones and meninges

Dictionary Exercise 2

1. brŏng'kē-ăl brushing; b
2. a
3. d
4. b
5. ūp-nē'ah; c
6. a
7. ĭn"ter-stĭsh'ăl tissue; d
8. pūr'roo-lĕnt; b
9. krĭp"tō-kŏk-ō'sĭs; b
10. allergic ăl"vē-ō-lī'tĭs; c

CHAPTER 13

ANSWERS TO TERMINOLOGY REVIEW EXERCISES

Completion

1. thirty-six
2. small intestine
3. small intestine
4. esophagus
5. bile
6. liver
7. lesser omentum
8. lower esophageal sphincter; pyloric sphincter
9. duodenum; jejunum; ileum
10. liver
11. parotid; submandibular or submaxillary; sublingual
12. colon
13. ascending; transverse; descending; rectosigmoid; rectum
14. saliva
15. sphincters
16. pharynx
17. mucosa
18. villi
19. ileocecal valve
20. cecum

ANSWERS TO WORKING PRACTICE REVIEW EXERCISES

Matching

1. e	3. d	5. g	7. f	9. h
2. c	4. i	6. a	8. b	10. j

Word Elements

1. cholecyst	3. hemorrhoid	5. fistul	7. append	9. ile
2. col	4. jejun	6. fissur	8. gastr	10. vag

ANSWERS TO WORD ELEMENT REVIEW EXERCISES

Word Elements

1. proct	4. lapar	7. entero	9. phag
2. glossal	5. gingiv	8. cel	10. choledocho
3. phago	6. esophag		

Spelling

1. correct	4. appendectomy	7. gastrophyloric	9. correct
2. anus	5. cholecyctitis	8. ileocecostomy	10. choledochojejunostomy
3. correct	6. jujunorrhaphy		

ANSWERS TO DICTIONARY EXERCISES

Dictionary Exercise 1

Pronunciation	Definition
1. ah"klŏr-hī'drē-ah	absence of hydrochloric acid in the gastric juices
2. ăn-ō-rĕk'sē-ah	loss of appetite
3. ā-sī'tēz	abnormal accumulation of fluid in the abdomen
4. ĕ-sŏf"ah-gō-dū"ō-dē-nŏs'tō-mē	surgical formation of an artificial opening between the esophagus and duodenum
5. fŭn'dŭs of the stomach	the portion of the stomach that bulges upward and to the left of the entrance of the esophagus into it
6. ĕ-rŭk-tā'shŭn	belching
7. ī'lĕts of lahng'er-hănz	small accumulations of cells in the pancreas, which secrete insulin directly into the bloodstream
8. dī"vĕr-tĭk'ū-lŭm	occasional outpouching of the ileum derived from an unobliterated yolk stalk
9. vĭs'er-ah	internal organs of any of the four great cavities of the body, especially the large abdominal organs
10. trĭk"ō-bē'zōr	a mass of material composed of hair and mucoid material in the stomach; a hairball
11. ĕ-sŏf"ah-jī'tĭs	inflammation of the esophagus
12. hĕp"ah-tō-rē'năl	pertaining to the liver and kidneys
13. jawn'dĭs	high level of bilirubin in blood causing yellow-orange skin color
14. kō-lĕs"ter-ō'sĭs	a condition in which cholesterol materials are deposited in tissues
15. flā'tŭs	gas expelled through the anus
16. lăc'tōs intolerance	occurs when the lining of the walls of the small intestine does not produce normal amounts of lactose

Dictionary Exercise 4

1. ă-fā'zē-ah   The patient had difficulty swallowing.
2. bō'lŭs   An undigested mass of food was blocking the alimentary tract.
3. kō-lăn"jē-ō'mah   The tumor found in the bile duct proved to be benign.
4. kō-lĕd"ō-kō-lĭ-thŏt'ō-mē   Surgery was performed to remove the stone from the bile duct.
5. pŏl"ē-dĭp'sē-ah;   The woman complained of frequent thirst, gaseous burps, and difficulty in swallowing.
   ĕ"rŭk-tā'shŭn;
   dĕg"loo-tĭsh'ŭn
6. păl'măr ĕr'ĭ-thē'mah   The redness of skin on the patient's palms indicated the possibility of cirrhosis of the liver.
7. ĭk'ter-ŭs; ăs"ter-ĭk'sĭs   The man was jaundiced and exhibited neurologic signs of liver failure.
8. dĕf-ē-kāt'ing   The patient had trouble passing her bowel movements.
9. fē'tor hĕ-păt'ĭ-kŭs   The characteristic foul odor of breath suggested to the physician a possibility of a disease of the liver.
10. ĕn"ter-ī'tĭs   The patient was suffering from an inflammation of the intestine.
11. ē-mŭl"sĭ-fĭ-kā'shŭn   Her digestive problem is the result of her inability to digest fats.
12. găs"trō-dū-ŏd"ē-nī'tĭs   Her complaints and symptoms indicated an inflammation of the stomach and duodenum.
13. flăt'ŭs; kŏn"stĭ-pā'shŭn;   The patient's symptoms were passing gas and periods of difficulty on passing stools.
    ē-sŏf"ah-jē'ăl rē'flŭks
14. hī"pĕr-bĭl"ĭ-roo-   The physician noted that her skin, whites of her eyes, and mucous membranes were all yellow.
    bĭn-ē'mē-ah

CHAPTER 14

ANSWERS TO TERMINOLOGY REVIEW EXERCISES

Matching

1. b	3. a	5. f	7. g
2. d	4. c	6. e	

ANSWERS TO WORD ELEMENT REVIEW EXERCISES

Circle and Define

1. asthenia; weakness	3. malign; bad	5. pan; all	7. poly; many
2. mal; bad	4. penia; decrease, deficiency	6. hypo; under	8. macro; large

Matching

1. b	3. d	5. h	7. g	9. c
2. e	4. j	6. a	8. i	10. f

ANSWERS TO DICTIONARY EXERCISES

Dictionary Exercise 3 (Examples will vary.)

1. băk-tē'rē-ah   Some diseases can be caused by certain rod-shaped organisms.
2. kăn'ū-lah   A tube inserted into a duct or cavity can be used by physicians when they provide care to a patient.
3. dĭs-sĕm'ĭ-nāt"ĕd   Once the infection had spread over a larger area, several medications were required to control it.
4. sĕp'sĭs   Everyone involved in health care must be careful not to spread infection.
5. sē-kwē'lah   Sometimes the aftereffects of a disease are harder on the patient than the disease itself.

CHAPTER 15

ANSWERS TO TERMINOLOGY REVIEW EXERCISES

Completion

1. filtration of blood, excretion of waste products, maintenance of salt and water balance, regulation of acid-base balance
2. renal papilla
3. Bowman's capsule
4. peristalsis
5. urethra

Spelling
1. correct
2. calyx
3. glomeruli
4. tubule
5. correct
6. urethral meatus

ANSWERS TO WORKING PRACTICE REVIEW EXERCISES

Identification/Procedures
1. renal ultrasound
2. voiding cystourethrography
3. nephrotomography
4. intravenous pyelography
5. cystography
6. cystoscopy
7. renal biopsy
8. cystometrogram

Matching
1. f
2. h
3. e
4. g
5. a
6. c
7. b
8. d
9. j
10. k
11. l
12. i

ANSWERS TO WORD ELEMENT REVIEW EXERCISES

Meanings
1. excision of the kidney
2. painful urination
3. dilation of the ureter
4. radiography of the renal pelvis and ureter
5. incision to enlarge urinary meatus

Identification
1. endocystitis	cyst
2. ureteral	ureter
3. pyelonephritis	pyel
4. hematuria	-uria
5. vesicouterine	vesic
6. urethritis	urethr
7. calicectasis	calic
8. nephrosis	nephr
9. enuresis	-uresis
10. cystectomy	cyst
11. urogenital	uro
12. urinoma	urin
13. glomeruli	glomerul
14. glomerulus	glomerul
15. renal insufficiency	ren

ANSWERS TO DICTIONARY EXERCISES

Dictionary Exercise 1

Pronunciation	Definition
1. dī"ū-rĕt'ĭk	increasing urine excretion; an agent that promotes urine secretion
2. prō'lăpsd	falling down of a part or viscus
3. ŏl"ĭ-gū'rē-ah	diminished urine secretion relative to fluid intake
4. ū'rĭ-nār"ē retention	high urethral pressure that inhibits voiding and causes excessive urine to remain in the bladder
5. glī"kō-sū'rē-ah	abnormally high presence of glucose in the urine
6. kē-tō'sĭs	accumulation of large quantities of ketone bodies (acids and acetone) in the blood and tissues; also referred to as ketoacidosis
7. ah-nū'rē-ah	total suppression of urine formation in the kidney
8. ū'rĭ-nār"ē kăsts	substances that accumulate in the renal tubules and are found in the urine; indication of various abnormal conditions
9. ě-dē'mah	excess accumulation of fluid in a fluid cavity
10. ăz"ō-tē'mē-ah	presence of nitrogen-containing compounds in the blood

Dictionary Exercise 2

1. c	ăl-bū"mĭ-nū'rē-ah	5. d	trī'gōn	9. b		
2. a	kăl'kū-lŭs	6. c	ū-rē"tĕr-ŏl'ĭ-sĭs	10. d	vĕs"ĭ-kō-ū-rē'ter-ăl	
3. b	kăth'ĕ-ter	7. a	strĭk'chur of ureter			
4. c	ĭn"fŭn-dĭb'ū-lŭm	8. d	too'nĭ-kah văj"ĭ-nā'lĭs			

CHAPTER 16

ANSWERS TO TERMINOLOGY REVIEW EXERCISES

Completion

1. ovarian follicles
2. corpus luteum
3. corpus; cervix, fundus
4. fornices; posterior fornix
5. placenta
6. embryo; fetus
7. menarche; menopause
8. fimbriate
9. vulva
10. 38 to 40 weeks
11. parturition
12. endometrium; myometrium; uterine serosa
13. baby blues; postpartum depression; postpartum psychosis
14. zygote, blastocyst, trophoblast
15. progesterone, estrogen

ANSWERS TO WORKING PRACTICE EXERCISES

Choices

1. ultrasonography
2. dilation and curettage
3. laparotomy
4. LH
5. amniocentesis
6. galactorrhea
7. pelvimetry
8. surgical
9. dysmenorrhea
10. abruptio placentae
11. endometriosis
12. dysplasia
13. premenstrual syndrome

Identification

1. uterine suspension
2. oophorectomy
3. conization
4. tubal ligation
5. C-section
6. breast reconstruction
7. modified radical mastectomy
8. pelvic exenteration
9. cryosurgery
10. polypectomy

ANSWERS TO WORD ELEMENT REVIEW EXERCISES

Matching

1. f
2. a
3. b
4. n
5. i
6. k
7. g
8. m
9. c
10. h
11. l
12. d
13. j
14. e

ANSWERS TO DICTIONARY EXERCISES

Dictionary Exercise 1

1. ăd"ĕn-nō'mah-tŭs — pertaining to an adenoma; a tumor of the glandular epithelium
2. ăn"tē-flĕk'shŭn — forward flexion of the body of the uterus upon the cervix
3. kăp'ŭt — general term applied to the expanded or chief extremity of an organ or part; the head of an organ
4. klī-măk'tĕr-ĭk — menopause
5. ĕn-gāj'mĕnt — entrance of the fetal head or part being presented into the superior pelvic strait
6. for'sĕps — instrument for holding, seizing, or extracting
7. foor-shĕt — the raised ridge where the labia majora meet posteriorly
8. hē'mă-tō-sēl — a blood cyst; swelling due to effusion of blood
9. hĕm"ah-tō-kŏl'pŏs — accumulation of menstrual blood in the vagina due to an imperforate hymen
10. hē"mă-tō-sl'pĭnks — retained menstrual blood in the fallopian tube
11. mĕs"ō-thē"lē-ō'mah — a malignant tumor of the mesothelium
12. ōl"ig-ō-hī-drăm'nē-ŏs — abnormally small amount of amniotic fluid
13. păr"ah-ŭ-rē'thrăl — near the urethra
14. pū"ĕr-pē'rē-ŭm — the period of about six weeks from termination of labor to the return of the uterus to its normal non-pregnant size
15. tŏx'ĭk shock sĭn'drōm — rare disorder associated most often with the use of tampons or contraceptive sponges

Dictionary Exercise 2

1.	d	kă-năl' of nŭk	5.	c	kō'rē-ŏn	8.	c	ū'tĕr-ĭn sĕr-ō'sah
2.	b	prī-mĭ-grăv'ĭ-dah	6.	a	vĕl"ah-mĕn'tŭs	9.	d	ăn"tē-păr'tŭm
3.	b	kŭl'dĕ-săk' of Douglas			ĭn-sĕr'shŭn	10.	b	ōl"ĭ-gō-mĕn"ō-rē'ah
4.	a	dĭs-tō'sē-ah	7.	b	hī"drō-săl'pĭnks	11.	c	ăm'nē-ŏn

CHAPTER 17

ANSWERS TO TERMINOLOGY REVIEW EXERCISES

Completion

1. testes
2. scrotum
3. spermatozoa
4. epididymis
5. seminal vesicles
6. prostate; bulbourethral or Cowper's
7. urethra
8. penis
9. semen
10. prepuce
11. vas deferens

ANSWERS TO WORKING PRACTICE REVIEW EXERCISES

Completion

1. trichomoniasis
2. Gram stain
3. Western blot
4. Chlamydia
5. genital herpes
6. TORCH test
7. cytomegalic inclusion disease
8. FTA-ABS test
9. AIDS
10. venereal warts

Abbreviation Meanings

1. benign prostatic hypertrophy D
2. digital rectal exam P
3. prostatic acid phosphate T
4. transurethral resection of the prostate P
5. prostate specific antigen T
6. transurethral incision of the prostate P

ANSWERS TO WORD ELEMENT REVIEW EXERCISES

Word Elements

1. orchio
2. epididym
3. test
4. vesicul
5. prostat
6. spermat
7. vaso
8. balan
9. scrot
10. semen

ANSWERS TO DICTIONARY EXERCISES

Dictionary Exercise 1

1.	b	ăn-or'kĭzm	4.	b	pĕr"ĭ-nē'ŭm	7.	a	măs"tŭr-bā'shŭn
2.	a	ē-jăk"ū-lā'shŭn	5.	d	văs"ō-vă-sŏs'tō-mē	8.	d	ū'nŭk-oyd-ĭzm"
3.	d	kor'pō-rah kăv'ĕr-nō'sah	6.	a	ōl"ĭ-gō-spĕr'mē-ah			

CHAPTER 18

ANSWERS TO TERMINOLOGY REVIEW EXERCISES

Completion

1. surgical pathology; autopsies
2. quick-frozen section
3. history summary
4. gross diagnoses
5. microscopic examination
6. tissue processor
7. Bouin's solution; Zenker's fixation
8. disorder
9. homeostasis
10. pathogenesis
11. idiopathic

ANSWERS TO WORD ELEMENT REVIEW EXERCISES

Matching

1. i	5. o	9. b	12. g	15. d
2. e	6. p	10. c	13. h	16. j
3. n	7. k	11. f	14. l	17. q
4. m	8. a			

ANSWERS TO DICTIONARY EXERCISES

Dictionary Exercise 1

Pronunciation	**Definition**
1. rĭg′ŏr mŏr′tĭs	rigidity of skeletal muscles developing 6–10 hours after death and lasting for 3 or 4 days
2. lĭ′vŏr mŏr′tĭs	discoloration of dependent parts of the body after death due to pooling of blood
3. pū″trĕ-făk′shŭn	decomposition of animal or vegetable matter, due largely to action of microorganisms
4. păt′ĕnt	open, unobstructed
5. ĭm-pĕr′fō-rāt	abnormally closed
6. ĭn-kăr′sĕ-rā-tĕd	abnormally confined or constricted
7. păth″ŏg-nō-mŏn′ĭk	a lesion or characteristic, which is specific to only one disease or pathological condition
8. strō′mah	tissue that forms the supporting framework of an organ
9. grăn″ū-lā′shŭn	division of a hard substance into small particles
10. kē′loid	sharply elevated, irregularly shaped, progressively enlarging scar due to excessive collagen formation in the corium during connective tissue repair
11. ĕks″ū-dā′shŭn	escape of fluid, cells, or cellular debris from blood vessels
12. fī-brō′sĭs	formation of fibrous tissue
13. slŭf′ing	casting off or shedding
14. krō′mah-tĭn	the stainable, netlike substance of the nucleus of the cell
15. kā″sē-ā′shŭn	conversion of tissue into a dry, amorphous, cheeselike mass
16. kŏn-krē′shŭn	a calculus or an inorganic mass in tissue or a cavity
17. fah-sĭk′ū-lŭs	a small bundle or cluster, especially of nerve or muscle fiber
18. fō′kŭs	point from which a disease arises or where it is
19. sĭn-sĭsh′ăl	formed of a mass of protoplasm containing many nuclei but without apparent division into cells
20. hī′ah-lĭn	a smooth, glassy substance derived from degenerating collagen
21. mī-tō′sĭs	series of changes through which the nucleus of a cell goes in the course of division
22. pĭk-nō′sĭs	degeneration of a cell in which the nucleus and chromation condenses to a solid mass

Dictionary Exercise 4

Word	**Definition**
1. cholecystitis	inflammation of the gallbladder
2. desiccated	thoroughly dried out
3. excrescence	any abnormal outgrowth from the surface of a part
4. flora	in medicine, referring to kinds of bacteria or bacterial growth
5. gemistocytic	pertaining to an astrocyte in which the cell body swells considerably
6. hemosiderin	a form of stored iron
7. keratinized	cells have become hard or horny
8. lutein	lipochrome from the corpus luteum, fat cells, and egg yolk
9. peau d'orange	skin that is thickened and dimpled like an orange skin
10. sanguineous	containing blood
11. squamous	scaly or platelike
12. trabecula	supporting or anchoring strand of connective tissue
13. liquefaction	conversion into a liquid form
14. abscess	localized collection of pus in a body part
15. lobule	a small segment of a lobe
16. mesenchyme	a network of cells giving rise to connective tissue
17. mesothelium	the cellular structure lining the major body cavities
18. ostium	a small opening, especially one into a tubular organ
19. parenchyma	the part of an organ that is concerned with its function
20. primordial	existing in a primitive or early form

CHAPTER 19

ANSWERS TO TERMINOLOGY REVIEW EXERCISES

Selection

1. thyroid
2. pituitary
3. parathyroids
4. pancreas
5. pituitary
6. gonads
7. thyroid
8. adrenals
9. pituitary
10. pituitary
11. gonads
12. adrenals
13. adrenals

ANSWERS TO WORKING PRACTICE REVIEW EXERCISES

Matching

1. e
2. f
3. a
4. c
5. h
6. b
7. d
8. g
9. i
10. j

ANSWERS TO WORD ELEMENT REVIEW EXERCISES

Word Elements

1. (o)thyroid
2. crino
3. duct
4. fusion
5. glycos
6. adren
7. (er)thyroid
8. gluc

ANSWERS TO DICTIONARY EXERCISES

Dictionary Exercise 1

Pronunciation	Definition
1. mĕ-tăb'ō-lĭzm	all life processes of cells
2. tō'fŭs	a chalky mass of sodium biurate occurring in patients with gout
3. ŏz"mō-lār'ĭ-tē	property of a solution that is dependent on the amount of dissolved substance in the total volume
4. ŏz"mō-lăl'ĭ-tē	property of a solution that is dependent on the amount of the dissolved substance in it per unit of volume
5. ăl"dō-ster'ōn-ĭzm"	an abnormality of electrolyte metabolism caused by excessive secretion of aldosterone; also called hyperaldosteronism
6. ăl"kah-lō'sĭs	excessive alkalinity of body fluids due to the accumulation of alkalines or the reduction of acids
7. hī"pō-plā'zē-ah	defective development of tissue
8. thī"rō-glŏs'ăl	exists in the embryo between the pharynx and the thyroid gland
9. prĕs'or	some condition or substance that causes an increase in blood pressure

CHAPTER 20

ANSWERS TO TERMINOLOGY REVIEW EXERCISES

Matching

1. d
2. i
3. l
4. a
5. h
6. f
7. c
8. b
9. k
10. e
11. g
12. j

Completion

1. neuron
2. synapse
3. 12
4. neuroglia cells
5. cornu

Selection

1. c
2. b
3. a
4. a
5. b

ANSWERS TO WORKING PRACTICE REVIEW EXERCISES

Identification

1. electromyography
2. lumbar puncture
3. brain scan
4. arteriography
5. electroencephalography
6. myelography

Matching

1. e
2. c
3. a
4. b
5. d

ANSWERS TO WORD ELEMENT REVIEW EXERCISES

Matching

1. c
2. p
3. h
4. k
5. l
6. f
7. n
8. q
9. j
10. g
11. d
12. a
13. o
14. b
15. e
16. m
17. i

ANSWERS TO DICTIONARY EXERCISES

Dictionary Exercise 1

	Pronunciation	Definition
1.	kor-dŏt'ō-mē	interruption of a nerve fiber tract within the spinal cord for relief of pain
2.	dĭs-ō"rē-ĕn-tā'shŭn	loss of awareness of the position of oneself in relation to space, time, and persons
3.	kŏm-prĕsh'ŭn	squeezing together
4.	nū-rŏt'ō-mē	cutting, dividing, or transecting a nerve
5.	pŏl"ē-nū-rī'tĭs	inflammation of many nerves at one time
6.	rah-dĭk"ū-lō-nū-rī'tĭs	inflammation of the roots of spinal nerves
7.	tĭk doo-loo-roo'	degeneration of or pressure on the trigeminal nerve
8.	bah-bĭn'skēz	extension instead of flexion of the toes upon stimulation of the sole of the foot
9.	mĕn"ē-ārz'	recurrent and usually progressive group of symptoms, including deafness, tinnitus (ringing in the ears), and vertigo (dizziness)
10.	mĕ-ning"gō-ĕn-sĕf"ah-lō-mī"ĕ-lī'tĭs	inflammation of the brain and spinal cord and their membranes
11.	mĕ-ning"gō-mī"ĕ-lī'tĭs	inflammation of the spinal cord and its enveloping arachnoid and pia mater
12.	mī"krō-sĕf'ah-lē	congenital, abnormal smallness of the head
13.	glī-ō'mah	tumor composed of neuroglia cells
14.	hŏf'mănz	reflex bending of the thumb when the examiner flicks the terminal phalanx of the three middle fingers
15.	jăk-sō'nē-ăn ĕp'ĭ-lĕp"sē	recurrent episodes of localized convulsive seizures or spasms without loss of consciousness; limited to a part or region of the body
16.	rah-dĭk"ū-lī'tĭs	inflammation of a spinal nerve accompanied by pain and hyperesthesia
17.	rŏm'bĕrgz	inability to maintain body balance when eyes are shut and feet are close together
18.	păr"ah-plē'jē-ah	paralysis of the legs and lower part of the body

Dictionary Exercise 2

1.	d	ăn-ăr'thrē-ah	6.	b	păr"ĕs-thē'zē-ah	11.	a	mĕ-dŭl"ō-blăs-tō'mah
2.	a	ăn"ĕn-sĕf'ah-lŭs	7.	c	tā'bēz dor-sā'lĭs	12.	b	rĕt"rō-găs-sē'rē-ăn noo-rŏt'ō-mē
3.	a	ăs"trō-sī-tō'mah	8.	d	ĕn-sĕf'ah-lō-sēl	13.	c	kŏn-vŭl'shŭns
4.	d	ăg-nō'zē-ah	9.	a	glī-ō'sĭs	14.	a	glī"ō-blăs-tō'mah mŭl-tĭ-for'mē
5.	c	dĭs-mē'trē-ah	10.	c	mē-răl'jē-ah păr"ĕs-thĕ'tĭ-kah	15.	b	hīp"ĕs-thē'zē-ah

CHAPTER 21

ANSWERS TO TERMINOLOGY REVIEW EXERCISES

Completion

1. *Diagnostic and Statistical Manual of Mental Disorders* (DSM-IV-TR)
2. multiaxial assessment classification
3. *International Statistical Classification of Diseases and Related Health Problems*
4. personality
5. mental health
6. schizophrenia
7. personality, intelligence, neuropsychological, and projective
8. psychotherapy, psychotherapeutic medications, and electroconvulsive therapy
9. passive-aggressive personality disorder

Matching/Tests

1. h	3. a	5. j	7. c	9. g
2. f	4. e	6. d	8. b	10. i

Abbreviations

1. attention deficit hyperactivity disorder
2. chronological age
3. delirium tremens
4. electroconvulsive therapy
5. intelligence quotient
6. mental age
7. obsessive-compulsive disorder
8. seasonal affective disorder
9. Thematic Appreciation Test
10. Wechsler Adult Intelligence Scale—Revised

ANSWERS TO WORD ELEMENT REVIEW EXERCISES

Short Answers

1. ment/o, phren/o, psych/o
2. somat/o
3. anxi/o, phil/o, -mania, -phobia, -phoria
4. iatr/o
5. mania, phobia

Matching

1. d	3. a	5. c	7. b
2. g	4. f	6. e	

Word Elements

1. schiz	2. phobia	3. phoria	4. ment	5. phoria

ANSWERS TO DICTIONARY EXERCISES

Dictionary Exercise 1

	Pronunciation	Definition
1.	dĭs-sō"sē-ā'shŭn	situation occurring when some thoughts, feelings, or behaviors are removed from conscious awareness and control
2.	kăt-ah-tō'nē-ah	a form of schizophrenia in which the patient is unresponsive
3.	kŏn'făb-ū-lā'shŭn	the more or less unconscious filling in of actual memory gaps by imaginary or fantastic experiences
4.	sī"klō-thī'mē-ah	a mild psychosis of the manic-depressive type, which may be so mild as to be almost normal
5.	sī"klō-thī'mĭk	personality characterized by alternating moods of elation and sadness; mood swings are out of proportion to apparent stimuli
6.	dĭs-thī'mē-ah	depressive episodes, but not of same intensity or duration as major depression
7.	hah-lū"sĭ-nā'shŭn	false perception having no relation to reality or accounting for anything in the environment
8.	hĭp-nō'sĭs	altered state of conscious awareness induced by suggestion
9.	ĭd	part of the personality structure that harbors the unconscious, instinctive desires and strivings of the individual
10.	mā'nē-ah	a mental disorder characterized by excessive excitement
11.	ĕn"ū-rē'sĭs	involuntary urination usually while sleeping
12.	ē'gō	executive, coordinating aspect of the mind
13.	ĕn-kō-prē'sĭs	incontinence of feces not due to an organic problem
14.	năr'kō-lĕp"sē	recurrent uncontrollable desire for sleep

Dictionary Exercise 3

1. e	4. j	7. c	10. i	13. m
2. a	5. f	8. d	11. k	
3. h	6. b	9. g	12. l	

CHAPTER 22

ANSWERS TO TERMINOLOGY REVIEW EXERCISES

Completion

1. sclera; cornea
2. choroid; ciliary body; iris
3. accommodation
4. iris
5. ciliary muscles
6. vitreous humor
7. brain
8. conjunctiva
9. six
10. retina

ANSWERS TO WORKING PRACTICE REVIEW EXERCISES

Identification/Diagnostic Procedures

1. ophthalmoscopy
2. ^{32}P scan
3. fluorescein angiography
4. gonioscopy
5. ocular motility evaluation
6. tonometry

ANSWERS TO WORD ELEMENT REVIEW EXERCISES

Circle and Define

1. dacryo	tear, tear duct	5. opia	vision	9. scler	sclera
2. core	pupil	6. palpebr	eyelid	10. irid	iris
3. ophthalm	eye	7. tars	eyelid	11. kerat	horny, cornea
4. blephar	eyelid	8. retino	retina	12. ophthal	eye

Spelling

1. isometropia
2. blepharectomy
3. correct
4. palpebrate
5. correct

ANSWERS TO DICTIONARY EXERCISES

Dictionary Exercise 1

Word	Definition
1. kăn'thŭs	the angle at either end of the slit between the eyelids
2. kō"roid-ī'tĭs	inflammation of the choroid
3. kor'nē-ăl dĭs'trō-fē	primary fatty degeneration of the cornea
4. flō'terz	small bits of proteins or cells floating in the vitreous of the eye
5. or'bĭt-ăl sĕl-ū-lī'tĭs	acute inflammation of the eye socket
6. mī-bō'mē-ăn	the small, mucoserous gland in the lid of the eye that produces material to keep the conjunctiva moist
7. mĕl"ah-nō'mah	malignant brown or black spot on iris or conjunctiva
8. rĕ"trō-lĕn'tăl fī"brō-plā'sē-ah	growth of fibrous connective tissue behind the lens of the eye
9. vĭt're-ŭs hĕm'or-ĭj	blood in the vitreous humor

Dictionary Exercise 4

1. There was an opaque white ring at the periphery of the cornea.
2. The doctor destroyed part of the ciliary body of the eye by diathermy.
3. The patient was seeing double.
4. The iris has loosened from its attachment to the rest of the eye.
5. The eye could not move.

CHAPTER 23

ANSWERS TO TERMINOLOGY REVIEW EXERCISES

Identification

1. tympanic membrane
2. labyrinth
3. organ of Corti
4. olfaction
5. gustation
6. papillae
7. epiglottis
8. concha
9. soft palate
10. sinuses
11. adenoid
12. glottis

ANSWERS TO WORKING PRACTICE REVIEW EXERCISES

Matching

1. d
2. b
3. f
4. c
5. a
6. g
7. e

ANSWERS TO WORD ELEMENT REVIEW EXERCISES

Identification

1. audiometer
2. tympanic membrane
3. sialolith
4. lingually
5. gingivitis
6. otogenic
7. presbycusis
8. anosmia
9. auricle
10. acousma
11. hypoglossal
12. circumoral
13. mastoidectomy

ANSWERS TO DICTIONARY EXERCISES

Dictionary Exercise 2

1. f
2. c
3. h
4. d
5. g
6. e
7. b
8. a

Word Elements to Meanings

Word Element	Meaning
a-	no, not, without
ab-	away from, not
-ac	pertaining to
acous/o	hearing
acr/o	extremities
aden/o	gland
adip/o	fat
adnex/o	tie, connection
adren/o	adrenal gland
adrenal/o	adrenal gland
aer/o	air
agglutin/o	clumping, sticking
-agon	assemble, collect
-al	pertaining to
albin/o	white
albumin/o	albumin
alg/o	pain, cold
alges/o	excessive, sensitivity to pain
-algia	pain
alveol/o	alveolus, air sac
ambly/o	dim, dull
ameb/o	change
ameb-	change
amni/o	amnion
amyl/o	starch
an/o	anal
an-	no, not, without
ana-	again, backward, up
andr/o	male
angi/o	blood vessel
ankyl/o	crooked, bent
ant-	against
ante-	before, forward
anthrac/o	black
anti-	against
antr/o	chamber, cavity
anxi/o	anxious, uneasy
aort/o	aorta
append/o	appendix
appendic/o	appendix
aque/o	water
-ar	pertaining to
-arche	beginning
arter/o	artery
arteri/o	artery
arthr/o	joint
articul/o	joint
-ary	pertaining to
-asthenia	lack of strength, weakness
astr/o	star-shaped

Word Element	Meaning
astr-	star
ather/o	yellowish plaque, fatty substance
atri/o	atrium
audi/o	hearing, sound
audit/o	hearing, sound
auri/o	ear
auricul/o	ear
auto-	self
azot/o	nitrogen
bacteri/o	bacteria
balan/o	glans penis
bas/o	base, pertaining to a base
bi-	two
bili/o	bile
bilirubin/o	bilirubin
blast/o	embryonic, immature, primitive cell
-blast	immature
blast-	immature
blephar/o	eyelid
blephar-	eyelid
brachy-	short distance
brady-	slow
bronch/o	bronchus
bronchi/o	bronchus
bronchiol/o	bronchiole
bucc/o	cheek
burs/o	sac
calc/o	calcium
calci/o	calcium
cali/o	calyx
calic/o	calyx
capn/o	carbon dioxide
carcin/o	cancerous
carcin-	cancerous
cardi/o	heart
cardi-	heart
carp/o	wrist
cata-	down
caud/o	tail
cec/o	cecum
cel/o	abdomen
-cele	hernia
celi/o	abdomen
-centesis	puncture and aspiration of
cephal/o	head
cerebell/o	cerebellum
cerebr/o	brain
cervic/o	neck, cervix
cheil/o	lip

Word Element	Meaning
cheir/o	hand
chem/o	chemical, drug
chil/o	lip
chir/o	hand
chlor/o	green
chol/e	bile
chol/o	bile
cholangi/o	bile or hepatic duct
cholecyst/o	gallbladder
choledoch/o	bile duct
chondr/o	cartilage
cili/o	eyelid
cili-	eyelid
cine/o	movement
cirrh/o	tawny yellow
cleid/o	clavicle
coagul/o	clotting
-coccus	berry-shaped organism
cochle/o	cochlea
col/o	colon
coll/o	gluelike
colon/o	colon
colp/o	vagina
comat/o	deep sleep
cone/o	dust
conjunctiv/o	conjunctiva
contra-	against, opposite
cor/o	pupil
core/o	pupil
corne/o	cornea, horny
coron/o	heart
cost/o	rib
crani/o	head, skull
crin/o	secrete, separate
crin-	secrete
-crine	secrete, separate
-crit	separate
cry/o	cold
crypt/o	hidden
-cusis	hearing
cusis-	hearing
cut/o	skin
cutane/o	skin
cyan/o	blue
cyan-	blue
-cyesis	pregnancy
cyst/o	bladder, sac of fluid
cyt/o	cell
-cyte	cell
-cytosis	abnormal condition of cells
dacry/o	tear, tear duct
dactyl/o	finger, toe
dendr/o	branching
dendr-	branching
derm/o	skin
dermat/o	skin
-desis	binding, fixation
diaphor/o	profuse sweating
digit/o	finger, toe
dipl/o	double

Word Element	Meaning
dips/o	chest
dors/o	back
duct/o	carry
duoden/o	duodenum
dur/o	dura mater
dura-	hard
dynam/o	power
-dynia	pain
dys-	bad, labored
-eal	pertaining to
echo-	repeated sound
ect/o	outside
ect-	out, outside
-ectasia	dilation, expansion, stretching
-ectasis	dilation, expansion, stretching
-ectomy	excision, surgical removal
-ema	condition
-emesis	vomiting
-emia	blood condition
en-	in
encephal/o	brain
end/o	inside
endo-	within
enter/o	intestine
eosin/o	red
ependym/o	wrapping
epi-	above, upon
epididym/o	epididymis
epiglott/o	epiglottis
episi/o	vulva
eryth/o	red
erythr/o	red
esophag/o	esophagus
esthes/o	feeling, sensation
esthesi/o	feeling, sensation
eu-	good, normal
ex-	out, away from
fasci/o	sheet, band
fibr/o	fiber
fistul-	narrow opening
fluor/o	luminous
furc/o	division
-fusion	pour
gangli/o	swelling
gastr/o	stomach
gastr-	stomach
gemin-	two, twin
-gen	originate, produce
-genesis	formation
-genic	produced by
gingiv/o	gum
glauc/o	gray
gli/o	glue
-globin	protein
-globulin	protein
glomerul/o	ball, cluster
gloss/o	tongue
glott/o	glottis
gluc/o	sugar
glyc/o	sugar

Word Element	Meaning
gon/o	seed
-gram	record, picture, tracing
gran-	grain
granul/o	granule
-graph	instrument for recording
-graphy	processing of recording
gravid/o	pregnancy
-gravida	pregnant female
gynec/o	female
hallucin/o	hallucination
hem/o	blood
hemat/o	blood
hemi-	half
hemoglobin/o	hemoglobin
hepat/o	liver
hepatic/o	liver
hidr/o	sweat
hist/o	tissue
hydr/o	water, fluid
hydro-	water
hype-	deficient, less than, below
hyper-	above, more than
hypn/o	sleep
hypo-	below, deficient, under
hyster/o	uterus
-ia	condition, formation
-iac	pertaining to
-iasis	condition, formation
iatr/o	physician, treatment
-ic	pertaining to
-ical	pertaining to
ichthy/o	dry, scaly
ile/o	ileum
ili/o	ilium
immun/o	immune, immunity, protection
-in	substance
in-	into, not
-ine	substance
infra-	beneath
inter-	between
intra-	within
ir/o	iris
irid/o	iris
is/o	equal, same
ischi/o	hip
iso-	equal, same
-itis	inflammation
jaund/o	yellow
jejun/o	jejunum
kary/o	nucleus
kerat/o	cornea, horny
ket/o	ketone bodies
keton/o	ketone bodies
kines/o	movement
-kinesia	movement
-kinetic	movement
kyph/o	humpback
lacrim/o	tear
lact/o	milk
lamin/o	lamina

Word Element	Meaning
lapar/o	abdomen, abdominal wall
laryng/o	larynx
later/o	side
lei/o	smooth
leiomy/o	smooth or nonstriated muscle
lept/o	slender, thin
-leptic	to seize hold of
leuk/o	white
leuk-	white
ligament/o	ligament
lingu/o	tongue
lip/o	fat
lith/o	stone
lob/o	lobe, section
-logist	specialist in the study of
-logy	study of
lord/o	swayback
-lucent	shine
lumb/o	loin, lower back
lute/o	yellow
lymph/o	lymph
lymphaden/o	lymph nodes
lymphangi/o	lymph vessel
-lysis	loosening, setting free, destruction
-lytic	pertaining to destruction or loosening of
macro-	large
macul/o	spot
mal-	bad
-malacia	softening
malign-	bad
mamm/o	breast
-mania	excessive preoccupation
mast/o	breast
mastoid/o	mastoid process
maxill/o	upper jaw bone
meat/o	meatus
medull/o	soft inner part, medulla
mega-	large
-megaly	enlargement
melan/o	black
men/o	menses
mening/o	meninges, membranes around the central nervous system
ment/o	mind
meso-	middle
meta-	beyond, change
metr/o	uterus
mi/o	smaller, less
micr/o	small size, microscopic
micro-	small
mon/o	single
morph/o	form, shape
multi-	many
muscul/o	muscle
mut/a	genetic change
mutagen/o	causing genetic change

Word Element	Meaning
my/o	muscle
myc/o	fungus
mydr/o	widen, enlarge
myel/o	bone marrow, spinal cord
myring/o	eardrum
narc/o	stupor
nas/o	nose
necr/o	death
neo-	new, recent
nephr/o	kidney
neur/o	nerve, nervous system
neutr/o	neutral
noct/i	night
nulli-	no, none, not
nyct/o	night
ocul/o	eye
odont/o	tooth
-oid	like, resembling
-ologist	specialist in the study of
-ology	study of
-oma	tumor
oment/o	covering
onc/o	tumor
-one	hormone
onych/o	nail
oophor/o	ovary
-opaque	obscure
ophthalm/o	eye
-opia	vision
-opsia	vision
opt/o	eye, vision
optic/o	eye, vision
or/o	mouth
orch/o	testis
orchi/o	testis
orchid/o	testis
-ose	pertaining to, sugar
-osis	condition
-osmia	smell
ossicul/o	ossicle
oste/o	bone
-ostomy	creation of a new opening
ot/o	ear
-otio	ear condition
-otomy	incision into
-ous	pertaining to
ov/i	egg
ov/o	egg
ovari/o	ovary
ovul/o	egg
oxy-	rapid, sharp, acid
palpebr/o	eyelid
pan-	all
pancreat/o	pancreas
papill/o	papillary, nipplelike, optic disc
-par	birth, labor
par-	other than
para-	abnormal, beside
-para	to bear, birth, labor
parathyroid/o	parathyroid glands

Word Element	Meaning
-paresis	slight paralysis
pariet/o	wall of an organ, cavity
-parous	to bring forth
-part	birth, labor
part-	bear
-partum	birth, labor
path/o	disease
-pathy	disease
pect/o	breast, chest
pector/o	breast, chest
ped/o	foot
-penia	decrease, deficiency
-pepsia	digestion
peri-	about, around, surrounding
pericardi/o	pericardium
peritone/o	peritoneum
-pexy	surgical fixation
phac/o, phak/o	lens of the eye
phag/o	eat, swallow
-phagia	eating, swallowing
pharmac/o	drug, medicine
pharyng/o	pharynx, throat
-phasia	speech
phil/o	attracted to, love
-philia	attraction for
phleb/o	vein
-phobia	fear
phon/o	sound
-phonia	voice, sound
-phoresis	carrying
-phoria	feeling
phot/o	light
phren/o	diaphragm, mind
physi/o	nature
pil/o	hair
plas/o	formation
-plasia	development, growth, formation
-plasm	growth, formation
-plasty	surgical correction
-plegia	paralysis
pleur/o	pleura, rib, side
-pnea	to breathe
pneum/o	lung, air
pneumon/o	lung, air
pod/o	foot
-poiesis	formation
-poietin	substance that forms pus
poli/o	gray
poly-	many
polyp/o	polyp
pont/o	pons
post-	after, behind
-praxia	action
pre-	before, in front of
presby/o	old age
primi-	first
pro-	in front of, before
proct/o	anus and rectum
prol-	offspring
prostat/o	prostate gland

Word Element	Meaning
psych/o	mind
-ptosis	prolapse, downward
-ptysis	spitting
pulmon/o	lung
pupill/o	pupil
py/o	pus
pyel/o	trough, basin, pelvis
pyl/o	pylorus
pylor/o	pylorus
radi/o	ray, x-ray
radic/o	root
radicul/o	nerve root
rect/o	rectum
ren/o	kidney
retin/o	retina
retro-	backward
rhabdomy/o	skeletal or striated muscle
rhin/o	nose
roentgen/o	x-ray
-(r)rhage	bursting forth, excessive flow
-(r)rhagia	bursting forth, excessive flow
-(r)rhaphy	suture of
-(r)rhea	flow, discharge
-(r)rhexis	break, burst, rupture
sacr/o	sacrum
salping/o	tube
-salpinx	uterine tube
sangui/o	blood
sarc/o	flesh
schiz/o	split
scintill/o	spark
scirr/o	hard
scirr-	hard
scirrh/o	hard
scler/o	sclera
-sclerosis	hardening
scoli/o	crooked, bent
-scop	look
-scope	instrument for visual examination
-scopy	visual examination
scot/o	darkness
scrot/o	bag, pouch
seb/o	sebum
sem-	half
semen	seed
semi-	half
semin/o	seed
sial/o	salivary
sigmoid/o	sigmoid colon
somat/o	body
-somnia	sleep
spas/o	draw, pull
spas-	to draw or pull tight
-spasm	sudden, involuntary muscular contraction
sperm/o	spermatozoa
spermat/o	spermatozoa
sphen/o	wedge
-sphyhia	pulse
spir/o	to breathe, breathing, coil

Word Element	Meaning
splen/o	spleen
splen-	spleen
spondyl/o	vertebra
squam/o	scale
staped/o	stapes
-stasis	stop, control
steat/o	fat, lipid
-stenosis	tightening, structure
steth/o	chest
-sthenia	strength
stom/o	mouth
stomat/o	mouth
-stomy	creation of a new opening
strept/o	twisted
strict/o	drawing tight, narrowing
sub-	under, below
sud/o	sweat
sudor/o	sweat
super-	above, in the upper part of
supra-	above, over
-supression	to stop
sym-	together
syn-	together, with
syncop/o	to cut off, cut short
synov/o	synovial membrane
syring/o	tube
tachy-	fast, rapid
tars/o	of or pertaining to the foot, eyelid
tax/o	order, coordination
tele/o	distant
tele-	distant
teli/o	complete
ten/o	tendon
tend/o	tendon
tendin/o	tendon
tens/o	stretch
test/o	testes, testicles
thalam/o	thalamus
thec/o	sheath
thel/o	nipple
therap/o	treatment, therapy
-therapy	treatment
therm/o	heat
thorac/o	chest
-thorax	chest
thromb/o	clot, lump
thym/o	thymus
-thymia	mind
thyr/o	thyroid gland
thyroid/o	thyroid gland
-tic	pertaining to
-tocia	labor, birth
tom/o	cut
-tome	instrument to cut
top/o	place
tox/o	poison
toxic/o	poison
trache/o	windpipe
trans-	through, across
traumat/o	wound, injury

Word Element	Meaning
-tresia	opening
tri-	three
trich/o	hair
-tripsy	crushing, friction
-trophy	development, growth
trophy-	development
-tropia	to turn
-tropin	growth, development, nourish, stimulate
turbin/o	shaped like a top
tympan/o	eardrum
ultra-	beyond
umbilic/o	navel
ungul/o	nail
uni-	one
ur/o	urinary tract, urine
-uresis	urination
uret/o	urinary tract, urine
ureter/o	ureter
urethr/o	urethra
-uria	condition of the urine, urination
urin/o	urinary tract, urine

Word Element	Meaning
uter/o	uterus
uve/o	uvea, vascular layer of the eye
vag/o	vagus nerve
vagin/o	vagina
valv/o	valve
valvul/o	valve
vas/o	vessel, duct
vascul/o	vessel
ven/o	vein
ventricul/o	ventricle
-version	act of turning
vertebr/o	vertebra
vesic/o	bladder
vesicul/o	seminal vesicles
vestibul/o	entrance
viscer/o	internal organ
vitr/o	glass
vitre/o	glassy
viv/o	life
vulv/o	vulva
xanth/o	yellow
xer/o	dry

Appendix C
Meanings to Word Elements

Meaning	Word Element
abdomen	cel/o, celi/o, lapar/o
abnormal	para-
abnormal condition of cells	-cytosis
abdominal wall	lapar/o
about	peri-
above	epi-, hyper-, super-, supra-
acid	oxy-
across	trans-
act of turning	-version
action	-praxia
adrenal gland	adren/o, adrenal/o
after	post-
again	ana-
against	ant-, anti-, cantra-
air	aer/o, pneum/o, pneumon/o
air sac	alveol/o
albumin	albumin/o
all	pan-
alveolus	alveol/o
amnion	amni/o
anal	an/o
anus and rectum	proct/o
anxious	anxi/o
aorta	aort/o
appendix	append/o, appendic/o
around	peri-
artery	arter/o, arteri/o
assemble	-agon
atrium	atri/o
attraction for	-philia
attraction to	phil/o
away from	ab-, ex-
backward	ana-, retro-
bacteria	bacteri/o
bad	dys-, mal-, malign-
bag	scrot/o
ball	glomerul/o
band	fasci/o
base	bas/o
basin	pyel/o
(to) bear	-para
before	ante-, pre-, pro-
beginning	-arche
behind	post-
below	sub-, hype-
beneath	infra-
bent	ankyl/o, scoli/o
berry-shaped organism	-coccus
beside	para-
between	inter-

Meaning	Word Element
beyond	meta-, ultra-
bile	bili/o, chol/e, chol/o
bile duct	cholangi/o, choledoch/o
bilirubin	bolirubin/o
binding	-desis
birth	-par, -para, -tocia
black	anthrac/o, melan/o
bladder	cyst/o, vesic/o
blood	hem/o, hemat/o, sangui/o
blood condition	-emia
blood vessel	angi/o
blue	cyan/o, cyan-
body	somat/o
bone marrow	myel/o
bone	oste/o
brain	cerebr/o, encephal/o
branching	dendr/o, dendr-
break	-rrhexis
breast	mamm/o, mast/o
breast (chest)	pect/o, pector/o
(to) breathe	-pnea, spir/o
breathing	spir/o
bring forth	-parous
bronchiole	bronchiol/o
bronchus	bronch/o, bronchi/o
burst	-rrhexis
bursting forth	-(r)rhage, -(r)rhagia
calcium	calc/o, calci/o
calyx	cali/o, calic/o
cancerous	carcin/o, carcin-
carbon dioxide	capn/o
carry	duct/o
carrying	-phoresis
cartilage	chondr/o
causing genetic change	mutagen/o
cavity	antr/o, pariet/o
cecum	cec/o
cell	cyt/o, -cyte
cerebellum	cerebell/o
cervix	cervic/o
chamber	antr/o
change	ameb/o, ameb-, meta-
cheek	bucc/o
chest (breast)	dips/o, pect/o, pector/o, steth/o, thorac/o, -thorax
clavicle	cleid/o
clot	thromb/o
clotting	coagul/o
clumping	agglutin/o
cluster	glomerul/o

Meaning	Word Element
cochlea	cochle/o
coil	spir/o
cold	cry/o
collect	-agon
colon	col/o, colon/o
complete	teli/o
condition	-ema, -iasis, -osis
condition of the urine	-uria
conjunctiva	conjunctiv/o
connection	adnex/o
control	-stasis
coordination	tax/o
cornea	corne/o, kerat/o
covering	oment/o
creation of a new opening	-ostomy, -stomy
crooked	ankyl/o, scoli/o
(to) crush	-tripsy
crushing	-tripsy
(to) cut	tom/o
(to) cut off	syncop/o
cut short	syncop/o
darkness	scot/o
death	necr/o
decrease	-penia
deep sleep	comat/o
deficiency	-penia
deficient	hype-, hypo-
destruction	-lysis
development	-plasia, -trophy, -tropin
diaphragm	phren/o
digestion	-pepsia
dilation	-ectasia, -ectasis
dim	ambly/o
discharge	-rrhea
disease	path/o, -pathy
distant	tele/o, tele-
division	furc/o
double	dipl/o
down	cata-
downward	-ptosis
draw	pas/o
drawing tight	spas-, strict/o
drug	pharmac/o
dry	ichthy/o, xer/o
duct	vas/o
dull	ambly/o
duodenum	duoden/o
dura mater	dur/o
dust	cone/o
ear	auri/o, auricul/o, uri/o, ot/o
ear condition	-otio
eardrum	myring/o, tympan/o
eat	phag/o
eating	-phagia
egg	ov/i, ov/o, ovul/o
embryonic	blast/o
enlarge	mydr/o
enlargement	-megaly
entrance	vestibul/o
epididymis	epididym/o

Meaning	Word Element
epiglottis	epiglott/o
equal	is/o, iso-
esophagus	esophag/o
excessive	alges/o
excessive flow	-rrhage, -rrhagia
excessive preoccupation	-mania
excision	-ectomy
expansion	-ectasia, -ectasis
extremities	acr/o
eye	ocul/o, ophthalm/o, opt/o, optic/o
eyelid	blephar/o, blephar-, cili/o, cili-, palpebr/o, tars/o
fallopian tube	salping/o
fast	tachy-
fat	adip/o, lip/o, steat/o
fatty substance	ather/o
fear	-phobia
feeling	esthes/o, esthesi/o, -phoria
female	gynec/o
fiber	fibr/o
finger	dactyl/o, digit/o
first	primi-
fixation	-desis
flesh	sarc/o
flow	-rrhea
fluid	hydr/o
foot	ped/o, pod/o
foot, of or pertaining to	tars/o
form	morph/o
formation	-ia, -iasis, -genesis, plas/o, -plasia, -plasm-, -poiesis
forward	ante-
friction	-tripsy
fungus	myc/o
gallbladder	cholecyst/o
genetic change	mut/a
gland	aden/o
glans penis	balan/o
glass	vitr/o
glassy	vitre/o
glottis	glott/o
glue	gli/o
gluelike	coll/o
good	eu-
grain	gran-
granule	granul/o
gray	glauc/o, poli/o
green	chlor/o
growth	-plasia, -plasm, -trophy, -tropin
gum	gingiv/o
hair	pil/o, trich/o
half	hemi-, sem-, semi-
hallucination	hallucin/o
hand	cheir/o
hard	dura-, scirr/o, scirrh/o, scirr-
hardening	-sclerosis
head	cephal/o, crani/o
hearing	acous/o, audi/o, audit/o, -cusis, cusis-

Meaning	Word Element
heart	cardi/o, cardi-, coron/o
heat	therm/o
hemoglobin	hemoglobin/o
hepatic duct	cholangi/o
hernia	-cele
hip	ischi/o
hormone	-one
horny	corne/o, kerat/o
humpback	kyph/o
ileum	ile/o
ilium	ili/o
immature	blast/o, -blast, blast-
immune	immun/o
immunity	immun/o
in	en-
in front of	pre-, pro-
in the upper part of	super-
incision into	-otomy
inflammation	-itis
injury	traumat/o
inside	end/o
instrument for recording	-graph
instrument for visual exam	-scope
instrument to cut	-tome
intestine	enter/o
into	in-
iris	ir/o, irid/o
jejunum	jejun/o
joint	articul/o, arthr/o
ketone bodies	ket/o, keton/o
kidney	nephr/o, ren/o
labor	-par, -part, -partum, -tocia
labored	dys-
lack of strength	-asthenia
lamina	lamin/o
large	macro-, mega-
larynx	laryng/o
lens of the eye	phac/o, phak/o
less	mi/o
less than	hype-
life	viv/o
ligament	ligament/o
light	phot/o
like	-oid
lip	cheil/o
lipid	steat/o
liver	hepat/o, hepatic/o
lobe	lob/o
loin	lumb/o
look	-scop
loosening	-lysis
love	phil/o
lower back	lumb/o
luminous	fluor/o
lump	thromb/o
lung	pneum/o, pneumon/o, pulmon/o
lymph	lymph/o
lymph nodes	lymphaden/o
lymph vessel	lymphangi/o

Meaning	Word Element
male	andr/o
many	multi-, poly-
mastoid process	mastoid/o
meatus	meat/o
medicine	pharmac/o
medulla	medull/o
membranes around the central nervous system	mening/o
meninges	mening/o
menses	men/o
microscopic	micr/o
middle	meso-
milk	lact/o
mind	ment/o, phren/o, psych/o, -thymia
more than	hyper-
mouth	or/o, stom/o, stomat/o
movement	cine/o, kines/o, -kinesia, -kinetic
muscle	muscul/o, my/o
muscle, nonstriated or smooth	leiomy/o
muscle, striated or skeletal	rhabdomy/o
nail	onych/o, ungul/o
narrow opening	fistul-
narrowing	strict/o
nature	physi/o
navel	umbilic/o
neck	cervic/o
nerve	neur/o
nerve root	radicul/o
nervous system	neur/o
neutral	neutr/o
new	neo-
night	noct/i, nyct/o
nipple	thel/o
nipple-like	papill/o
nitrogen	azot/o
no	a-, an-; nulli-
none	nulli-
nonstriated muscle	leiomy/o
normal	eu-
nose	nas/o, rhin/o
not	a-, ab-, an-, in-, nulli-
nourish	-tropin
nucleus	kary/o
obscure	-opaque
of or pertaining to the foot	tars/o
offspring	prol-
old age	presby/o
one	uni-
opening	-tresia
opposite	contra-
order	tax/o
originate	-gen
ossicle	ossicul/o
other than	par-
out	ect-, ex-
outside	ect/o, ect-
ovary	oophor/o, ovari/o

Meaning	Word Element
over	supra-
pain	-algia, -dynia
pancreas	pancreat/o
papillary	papill/o
paralysis	-plegia
paralysis, slight	-paresis
parathyroid glands	parathyroid/o
pelvis	pyel/o
pericardium	pericardi/o
peritoneum	peritone/o
pertaining to	-ac, -al, -ar, -ary, -eal, -iac, -ic, -ical, ose, -ous, -tic
pertaining to a base	bas/o
pertaining to destruction or loosening of	-lytic
pharynx	pharyng/o
physician	iatr/o
picture	-gram
place	top/o
pleura	pleur/o
poison	tox/o, toxic/o
polyp	polyp/o
pons	pont/o
pouch	scrot/o
pour	-fusion
power	dynam/o
pregnancy	gravid/o, -cyesis
pregnant female	-gravida
primitive cell	blast/o
process of recording	-graphy
produce	-gen
produced by	-genic
profuse sweating	diaphor/o
prolapse	-ptosis
prostate gland	prostat/o
protection	immun/o
protein	-globin, -globulin
pull	spas/o, spas-
pulse	-sphyhia
puncture and aspiration of	-centesis
pupil	cor/o, core/o, pupill/o
pus	py/o
pylorus	pyl/o, pylor/o
rapid	oxy-, tachy-
ray	radi/o
recent	neo-
(a) record	-gram
rectum	rect/o
red	eryth/o, erythr/o
repeated sound	echo
resembling	-oid
retina	retin/o
rib	cost/o, pleur/o
root	radic/o
rosy	eosin/o
rupture	-(r)rhexis
sac	burs/o, cyst/o
sacrum	sacr/o
salivary	sial/o
same	is/o, iso-

Meaning	Word Element
scale	squam/o
scaly	ichthy/o
sclera	scler/o
sebum	lob/o, seb/o
secrete	-crine
section	lob/o
seed	gon/o, semen, semin/o
seize hold of	-leptic
self	auto-
seminal vesicles	vesicul/o
sensation	esthes/o, esthesi/o
sensitivity to pain	algesi/o
separate	-crit
setting free	-lysis
shape	morph/o
shaped like a top	turbin/o
sharp	oxy-
sheath	thec/o
sheet	fasci/o
(to) shine	-lucent
short distance	brachy-
side	later/o, pleur/o
sigmoid colon	sigmoid/o
single	mon/o
skeletal muscle	rhabdomy/o
skin	cut/o, cutane/o, derm/o, dermat/o
skull	crani/o
sleep	hypn/o, -somnia
slender	lept/o
slight paralysis	-paresis
slow	brady-
small	micro-
small size	micr/o
smaller	mi/o
smell	-osmia
smooth	lei/o
smooth muscle	leiomy/o
soft inner part	medull/o
softening	-malacia
sound	audi/o, audit/o, phon/o, -phonia
spark	scintill/o
specialist in the study of	-logist, -ologist
speech	-phasia
spermatozoa	sperm/o, spermat/o
spinal cord	myel/o
spleen	splen/o, splen-
split	schiz/o
splitting	-ptysis
spot	macul/o
stapes	staped/o
star	astr-
star-shaped	astr/o
starch	amyl/o
sticking	agglutin/o
stimulate	-tropin
stomach	gastr/o, gastr-
stone	lith/o
stop	-stasis, -suppression

Meaning	Word Element
strength	-sthenia
stretch	tens/o
stretching	-ectasia, -ectasis
striated muscle	rhabdomy/o
structure	-stenosis
study of	-logy, -ology
stupor	narc/o
substance	-in, -ine
substance that forms pus	-poietin
sudden involuntary muscle contraction	-spasm
sugar	gluc/o, glyc/o, -ose
surgical correction	-plasty
surgical fixation	-pexy
surgical removal	-ectomy
surrounding	peri-
suture of	-rrhaphy
swallow	phag/o
swallowing	-phagia
swayback	lord/o
sweat	hidr/o, sud/o, sudor/o
swelling	gangli/o
synovial membrane	synov/o
tail	caud/o
tawny yellow	cirrh/o
tear	dacry/o, lacrim/o
tear (to rip)	-spadia
tear duct	dacry/o
tendon	ten/o, tend/o, tendin/o
testes	test/o
testicles	test/o
testis	orch/o, orchi/o, orchid/o
thalamus	thalam/o
therapy	therap/o
thin	lept/o
three	tri-
throat	pharyng/o
through	trans-
thymus	thym/o
thyroid gland	thyr/o, thyroid/o
tie	adnex/o
tightening	-stenosis
tissue	hist/o
toe	dactyl/o, digit/o
together	sym-, syn-
tongue	gloss/o, lingu/o
tooth	odont/o
tracing	-gram
treatment	iatr/o, therap/o, -therapy
trough	pyel/o

Meaning	Word Element
tube	salping/o, syring/o
tumor	-oma, onc/o
(to) turn	-tropia
(act of) turning	-version
twin	gemin-
twisted	strept/o
two	bi-, gemin-
under	hype-, hypo-, sub-
uneasy	anxi/o
up	ana-
upon	epi-
upper jaw bone	maxill/o
ureter	ureter/o
urethra	urethr/o
urinary tract	ur/o, uret/o, urin/o
urination	-uresis, -uria
urine	ur/o, uret/o, urin/o
uterine tube	-salpinx
uterus	hyster/o, metr/o, uter/o
uvea	uve/o
vagina	colp/o, vagin/o
vagus nerve	vag/o
valve	valv/o, valvul/o
vascular layer of the eye	uve/o
vein	ven/o, phleb/o
ventricle	ventricul/o
vertebra	spondyl/o
vessel	vas/o, vascul/o, vertebr/o
vision	-opia, -opsia, opt/o, optic/o
visual examination	-scopy
voice	-phonia
vomiting	-emesis
vulva	episi/o, vulv/o
wall of an organ	pariet/o
water	aque/o, hydr/o, hydro-
weakness	-asthenia
wedge	sphen/o
white	albin/o, leuk/o
widen	mydr/o
windpipe	trache/o
with	syn-
within	intra-
without	a-, an-
wound	traumat/o
wrapping	ependym/o
wrist	carp/o
x-ray	radi/o, roentgen/o
yellow	jaund/o, lute/o, xanth/o
yellowish plaque	ather/o

Abbreviations

These abbreviations are used in this textbook. Italicized words and phrases are Latin.

17-KS	17-ketosteroids
17-OHCS	17-hydroxycorticosteroids
2hPPG	2-hour postprandial glucose
^{67}Ga	radioactive isotope of gallium
^{99m}Tc	radioactive isotope of technetium
^{99m}Th	radioactive isotope of thallium
^{131}I	radioactive isotope of iodine
^{201}Th	radioactive isotope of thallium
μm^3	cubic micrometers
A&P, P&A	auscultation and percussion
AB, ab	abortion
ABG, ABGs	arterial blood gas(es)
a.c.	*ante cibum* (before meals)
AC	air conduction
ACAT	automated computerized axial tomography
accom	accommodation
ACL	anterior cruciate ligament
ACTH	adrenocorticotropic hormone
AD	*auris dextra* (right ear)
ad lib	*ad libitum* (at pleasure)
ADH	antidiuretic hormone
ADHD	attention-deficit hyperactivity disorder
A/G	albumin globulin ration
AI	aortic insufficiency
AIDS	acquired immune deficiency; acquired immunodeficiency syndrome
alb	serum albumin
alk phos	alkaline phosphatase
ALL	acute lymphocytic leukemia
ALS	amylotrophic lateral sclerosis
ALT	alanine aminotransferase
AMA	American Medical Association
AML	acute myelogenous leukemia
ANA	antinuclear antibody
anti-TPO	thyroid peroxide antibodies
AP	anteroposterior
APAP	acetaminophen
ARB	angiotensin receptor blocker
ARC	AIDS-related complex
ARDS	acute respiratory distress syndrome
ARF	acute renal failure; acute respiratory failure
ARMD	age-related macular degeneration
ART	assisted reproductive technology
AS	*auris sinistra* (left ear); aortic stenosis
ASA	acetylsalicylic acid
ASCP	American Society of Clinical Pathologists
ASD	atrial septal defect
ASHD	arteriosclerotic heart disease
AST	aspartate aminotransferase

ATH	antidiuretic hormone
AU	*aures unitas* (both ears)
AV, A-V	atrioventricular (node)
Ba	barium
baso	basophil(s)
beta-HCG	beta human chronic gonadotropin
BBB	blood-brain barrier
BC	bone conduction
BE	barium enema
b.i.d.	*bis in die* (twice a day)
BMT	bone marrow transplantation
BOM	bilateral otitis media
BP	blood pressure
BPH	benign prostatic hypertrophy
BPPV	benign paroxysmal positional vertigo
Bronch	bronchoscopy
BSS	balanced salt solution
BUN	blood urea nitrogen
bx, BX	biopsy
c	with
C	Celsius
C-section, CS	cesarean section
C-spine	cervical spine film
C&S	culture and sensitivity
C1, C2, etc.	cervical vertebrae
Ca	calcium
CA	chronological age
CABG	coronary artery bypass graft
CAD	coronary artery disease
CAE	cyclophosphamide, doxorubicin, etoposide
CAMP	cyclophosphamide, doxorubicin, methotrexate, procarbazine
CAPD	continuous ambulatory peritoneal dialysis
cap(s)	capsule(s)
CAT	computerized axial tomography
cath	catheter; catheterization
CBC	complete blood count
CC	Chief Complaint
cc (cm^3)	cubic centimeter
CCU	coronary care unit
CEA	carcinoembryonic antigen
CGL	chronic granulocytic leukemia
cGy	centiGray
CHD	coronary heart disease
CHF	congestive heart failure
Chol	cholesterol
CID	cytomegalic inclusion disease
CIN	cervical intraepithelial neoplasia (cervical dysplasia)

CIS . . . . carcinoma in situ
CK . . . . creatine kinase
CLL . . . . chronic lymphocytic leukemia
cm. . . . . centimeter
CMF±P . . . . cyclophosphamide, methotrexate, fluo-
                       rouracil, prednisone
CML . . . . chronic myelogenous leukemia
CMV test . . . . cytomegalovirus test
CNS . . . . central nervous system
COLD. . . . . chronic obstructive lung disease
COPD. . . . . chronic obstructive pulmonary disease
CP. . . . . cerebral palsy
CPK . . . . creatine phosphakinase
CPR . . . . cardiopulmonary resuscitation
creat. . . . . creatinine
CRF . . . . chronic renal failure
CRH . . . . corticotropin-releasing hormone
CSF . . . . cerebrospinal fluid; colony-stimulating
                       factor
CT. . . . . computed tomography
CTS . . . . carpal tunnel syndrome
CTT . . . . computerized transaxial tomogram
CVA . . . . cerebrovascular accident; costovertebral
                       angle
CVD . . . . cardiovascular disease
CVP . . . . cyclophosphamide, vincristine, prednisone
CVS . . . . chorionic villus sampling
Cx. . . . . cervix
cysto. . . . . cystoscopic examination
D&C . . . . dilatation (dilation) and curettage
dB. . . . . decibel
DEA . . . . Drug Enforcement Administration
decub. . . . . decubitus ulcer (bed sore)
derm. . . . . dermatology
DES . . . . diethylstilbestrol
DEXA. . . . . dual-energy x-ray absorptiometry
DHEA . . . . dehydroepiandrosterone
DI . . . . diabetes insipidus
DIC. . . . . disseminated intravascular coagulation
diff . . . . differential blood count
disp. . . . . dispense
DKA . . . . diabetic ketoacidosis
DM . . . . diabetes mellitus
DNA . . . . deoxyribonucleic acid
D.O. . . . . Doctor of Osteopathy
DOE . . . . dyspnea on exertion
dr . . . . dram
DRE . . . . digital rectal examination
DSA . . . . digital subtraction angiography
DSM-IV-TR . . . . . *Diagnostic and Statistical Manual of*
                       Mental Disorders
DST . . . . dexamethasone suppression test
DT, DTs. . . . . delirium tremens
DTR . . . . deep tendon reflex
DUB . . . . dysfunctional uterine bleeding
DVI. . . . . digital vascular imaging
DVT . . . . deep vein thrombosis
DX, Dx. . . . . diagnosis
ECC . . . . extracorporeal circulation; endocervical
                       curettage
ECG . . . . electrocardiogram
ECHO. . . . . echocardiography

ECT . . . . electroconvulsive therapy
EEG . . . . electroencephalogram
EGD . . . . esophagogastroduodenoscopy
EKG . . . . electrocardiogram
ELISA . . . . enzyme-linked immunosorbent assay
Em . . . . emmetropia (normal vision)
EMG. . . . . electromyography; electromyogram
ENT . . . . ear, nose, and throat
EOM. . . . . extraocular movement
eos, eosins. . . . . . eosinophil(s)
ERCP . . . . endoscopic retrograde cholangiopancre-
                       atography
ERG . . . . electroretinogram
ERT . . . . estrogen replacement therapy
ESR . . . . erythrocyte sedimentation rate (Sed rate)
ESRD. . . . . end-stage renal disease
ESWL. . . . . extracorporeal shock wave lithotripsy
ETD . . . . eustachian tube dysfunction
ETT . . . . exercise tolerance test
F . . . . Fahrenheit
FAC . . . . fluorouracil, doxorubicin,
                       cyclophosphamide
FANA. . . . . fluorescent antinuclear antibody
FBS . . . . fasting blood sugar
FDA . . . . Food and Drug Administration
Fe . . . . iron
FH . . . . family history
FHT . . . . fetal heart tones
fl. oz.. . . . . fluid ounce
fl. dr . . . . fluid dram
FS. . . . . frozen section
FSH . . . . follicle-stimulating hormone
FT_3, Free T_3 . . . . triiodothyronine serum free
FT_4, Free T_4 . . . . thyroxine serum free
FTA-ABS test. . . test for syphilis
FTI, FT_4 Index . . thyroxine index free
FTI . . . . free thyroxine index
g . . . . gram
G . . . . gravida (pregnant)
g/dl . . . . grams per deciliter
Ga. . . . . gallium
GAD . . . . generalized anxiety disorder
GFR . . . . glomerular filtration rate
GGT . . . . gamma-glutamyl transpeptidase
GH . . . . growth hormone
GHRH . . . . growth hormone-releasing hormone
GI . . . . gastrointestinal
GIFT. . . . . gamete intrafallopian transfer
GIT. . . . . gastrointestinal tract
glu. . . . . glucose
gm . . . . gram
gm%. . . . . grams percent
GnRH. . . . . gonadotropin-releasing hormone
gr. . . . . grain
gt. . . . . *gutta* (drop)
gtt. . . . . *guttae* (drops)
GTT . . . . glucose tolerance test
GU . . . . genitourinary
gyn . . . . gynecology
H&P . . . . History and Physical
Hb. . . . . hemoglobin
Hb A^{1C} . . . . glycosylated hemoglobin

HCG, hcg....... human chorionic gonadotropin
HCl........... hydrochloride; hydrochloric acid
Hct........... hematocrit
HCTz......... hydrochlorothiazide
HD........... hemodialysis
HDL........... high-density lipoprotein
HEENT....... head, eyes, ears, nose, throat
Hgb........... hemoglobin
HGH........... human growth hormone
HIV........... human immunodeficiency virus
HJR........... hepato-jugular relex
HLA........... human leukocyte antigen
HMO........... health maintenance organization
HNP........... herniated nucleus pulposus
HPF........... high-power field
HPI........... History of Present Illness
HPV........... human papillomavirus
HRT........... hormone replacement therapy
h.s........... hor somni (at bedtime)
HSV........... herpes simplex virus
Hx........... History
I........... iodine
I&D........... incision and drainage
I/A........... irrigation/aspiration
IABP........... intra-aortic balloon pump
IBC........... iron-binding capacity
IBD........... inflammatory bowel disease
IBS........... irritable bowel syndrome
ICD........... internal cardioverter-defibrillator
ICD-9........... *International Statistical Classification of Diseases and Related Health Problems*
ICSI........... intracytoplasmic sperm injection
ID........... intradermal
IDDM........... insulin-dependent diabetes mellitus
IgA, IgD, IgE, IgG, IgM...... immunoglobulins
IGF-I........... insulinlike growth factor I
IL-2........... interleukin-2
IM........... intramuscular(ly)
inj........... injection
IOL........... intraocular lens
IOP........... intraocular pressure
IPD........... intermittent peritoneal dialysis
IPPB........... intermittent positive pressure breathing
IQ........... intelligence quotient
ITP........... idiopathic thrombocytopenia
ITT........... insulin tolerance test
IU/L........... international units per liter
IUD........... intrauterine device
IV........... intravenous(ly)
IVF........... *in vitro* fertilization
IVP........... intravenous pyelogram
JVD........... jugular vein distention
K........... potassium
kg........... kilogram
KOH........... potassium hydroxide
KUB........... kidney, ureter, and bladder
L........... liter
L1, L2, etc...... lumbar vertebrae
LASIK........... laser-assisted *in situ* keratomileusis

LDH........... lactic dehydrogenase; lactate dehydrogenase
LDL........... low-density lipoprotein
LE........... lower extremity
LE cell........... lupus erythematosus cell
LES........... lower esophageal sphincter
LH........... luteinizing hormone
LHRH........... luteinizing hormone-releasing hormone
LMP........... last menstrual period
LP........... lumbar puncture
LPF........... low-power field
LSD........... lysergic acid diethylamide
LTH........... prolactin (lactogenic hormone)
LVAD........... left ventricular assist device
lymph........... lymphocyte
MA........... mental age
MACI........... Millon Adolescent Clinical Inventory
MAO........... monoamine oxidase
MAOI........... monoamine oxidase inhibitor
MCH........... mean corpuscular hemoglobin
MCHC........... mean corpuscular hemoglobin concentration
MCMI-III........... Millon Clinical Mutiaxial Inventory-III
MCV........... mean corpuscular volume
M.D........... Doctor of Medicine
MDD........... major depressive disorder
MEA........... multiple endocrine adenomatosis
MEN........... multiple endocrine neoplasia
mEq........... milliequivalent
mEq/L........... milliequivalent per liter
mg........... milligram
mg%........... milligrams percent
MI........... mitral insufficiency; myocardial infarction
ml, mL........... milliliter
mm........... millimeters
mm^3........... millimeters cubed
mm/Hg........... millimeters of mercury
mMol, mMole... millimole
MMPI-2........... Minnesota Multiphasic Personality Inventory-2
MMPI-A........... Minnesota Multiphasic Personality Inventory-Adolescent
MMSE........... Mini-Mental Status Examination; Mini-Mental State Examination
mono........... monocyte
MOPP........... mechlorethamine, vincristine, procarbazine, prednisone
MR........... mitral regurgitation
MRI........... magnetic resonance imaging
MS........... multiple sclerosis; mitral stenosis
MSH........... melanocyte-stimulating hormone
MT........... medical technologist
MT (ASCP)........... Registered Medical Technologist
MUGA........... multiple-gated acquisition scan
MVP........... mitral valve prolapse
Na........... sodium
NSAID........... nonsteroidal anti-inflammatory drug
NB........... newborn
NF........... *National Formulary*
NGT........... nasogastric tube
NGU........... nongonococcal urethritis
NHL........... non-Hodgkin's lymphoma

NIDDM	noninsulin-dependent diabetes mellitus
NK	natural killer
NKHHC	nonketotic hyperglycemia-hyperosmolar coma (syndrome)
NMR	nuclear magnetic resonance
noc., noct.	*nocte* (night)
NPO	nothing by mouth
NSAID	nonsteroidal anti-inflammatory drug
O&P	ova and parasite (test)
OB	obstetrics
OCD	obsessive-compulsive disorder
OCT	oxytocin challenge test
OD	*oculus dexter* (right eye)
ophth	ophthalmology
ortho	orthopedics
OS	*oculus sinister* (left eye)
OTC	over the counter
Oto	otology
OU	*oculi unitas* (both eyes)
oz.	ounce
P	phosphorus
PA	posteroanterior
PAC	premature atrial contraction
Pap test	Papanicolaou test
PAP	prostatic acid phosphatase
Para 2-0-1-2	2 full-term infants, 0 premature, 1 abortion, 2 live births
PAT	paroxysmal atrial tachycardia
Path	pathology
p.c.	*post cibum* (after meals)
PCD	pacemaker cardiac defibrillator
PCP	phencyclidine
PD	peritoneal dialysis
PDR	*Physicians' Desk Reference*
PE tube	pressure equalization tube placed in the eardrum
PERRLA	pupils equal, round, react to light and accommodation
PET	positron emission tomography
PFT	pulmonary function test
pg	picogram
PH	Past History
Pharm.D.	Doctor of Pharmacy
phos	phosphorus
PI	Present Illness
PID	pelvic inflammatory disease
PKD	polycystic kidney disease
PMH	Past Medical History
PMN	polymorphonuclear neutrophil
PMNL, Poly, polys.	polymorphonuclear neutrophil leukocyte
PMS	premenstrual syndrome
PND	paroxysmal nocturnal dyspnea
p.o., po.	orally
POR (POMR)	problem oriented (medical) record
PPD	purified protein derivative
PPM	permanent pacemaker
PR	rectally
PRA	plasma renin activity
PRK	photorefractive keratectomy
PRL	prolactin level
p.r.n., PRN	*pro re nata* (as required)

ProTime	prothrombin time
PSA	prostate specific antigen
PSCT	peripheral stem cell transplantation
Pt	patient
PT	prothrombin time; protime
PTA	percutaneous transluminal angioplasty
PTC	percutaneous transhepatic cholangiography
PTCA	percutaneous transluminal coronary angioplasty
PTH	parathyroid hormone; parathormone
PTHC	percutaneous transhepatic cholangiography
PTS	permanent threshold shift
PTT	partial thromboplastin time
PUVA	psorafen ultraviolet A-range
PVC	premature ventricular contraction
PVD	peripheral vascular disease
PX, PE	physical examination
q.4h	*quaque quarta hora; quaque 4 hora* (every 4 hours)
q.d.	*quaque die* (everyday)
q.h.	*quaque hora* (every hour)
q.i.d.	*quater in die* (4 times/day)
q.n., q.noc.	*quaque nocte* (every night)
q.o.d.	every other day
RA	rheumatoid arthritis
rad	radiation absorbed dose
RAI	radioimmunoassay
RAIU	radioactive iodine uptake
RBC	red blood cell; red blood cell count
RDS	respiratory distress syndrome
RF	rheumatoid factor
Rh	Rhesus factor
RIA	radioimmunoassay
ROM	range of motion
ROS	review of systems
R.Ph.	registered pharmacist
RPR	rapid plasma regin
RTOG	radiation therapy oncology group
RX, Rx	treatment; prescription
$\bar{s}$	without
SA, S-A	sinoatrial (node)
SAD	seasonal affective disorder
SBFT	small bowel follow-through
SBS	small bowel series
SC	subcutaneous
SCID	severe combined immuno-deficiency disease
SH	Social History; somatotropin hormone
sig., Sig.	let it be labeled
SIL	squamous intra-epithelial lesion (cervical dysplasia)
SL	sublingual(ly)
SLE	systemic lupus erythematosus
SOAP	subjective; objective; assessment; plan
SOB	shortness of breath
sol, soln	solution
SOR	source oriented record
spec	specimen
SPECT	single-photon emission computed tomography

SPEP	serum protein electrophoresis
SPF	sun protection factor
SQ	subcutaneous(ly)
SSRI	selective serotonin reuptake inhibitor; serotonin serum reuptake inhibitor
stat., STAT	*statim* (immediately)
STD	sexually transmitted disease
STI	sexually transmitted infection
subcu, subq, SC, SQ	subcutaneous(ly)
supp	suppository
susp	suspension
syr.	syrup
T&A	tonsillectomy and adenoidectomy
T1, T2, etc.	thoracic vertebrae
T_3, T3	triiodothyronine
T_4, T4	thyroxine
T_7, T7	free thyroxin index
tabs.	tablets
TAT	Thematic Apperception Test
TB	tuberculosis
TBG	thyroid-binding globulin
T bili	total bilirubin
Tc	technetium
TENS	transcutaneous electrical nerve stimulation
TFT	thyroid function test
Th	thallium
THBR	thyroid-hormone binding ratios
TIA	transient ischemic attack
t.i.d.	*ter in die* (3 times/day)
tinct	tincture
TIPS	transjugular intrahepatic portosystemic shunt
TM	tympanic membrane
TMJ	temporomandibular joint
top	topically
TORCH test	toxoplasma, other infections, rubella, cytomegalovirus, and herpes simplex virus test
TP	serum total proteins
TPN	total parenteral nutrition
TPR	temperature; pulse; respirations

tr	tincture
TRF test	thyrotoxic-releasing factor test
TRH	thyrotropin-releasing hormone
TRUS	transrectal ultrasound
TSH	thyroid-stimulating hormone
TSS	toxic shock syndrome
TTS	temporary threshold shift
TUIP	transurethral incision of the prostate
TUMT	transurethral microwave thermotherapy
TUNA	transurethral needle ablation
TURP	transurethral resection of the prostate
UA	urinalysis
UC	urine culture
UE	upper extremity
UGI	upper gastrointestinal (series)
ung.	ointment
unst.	ointment
URI	upper respiratory infection
US, U/S	ultrasound
USP	*United States Pharmacopeia*
UTI	urinary tract infection
UV	ultraviolet
V/Q scan	ventilation-perfusion scan
VA	visual acuity
vag	vaginally
VCUG	voiding cystourethrogram
VD	venereal diseases
VDRL	Venereal Disease Research Laboratory
VF	visual field
VMA	vanillylmandelic acid
VSD	ventricular septal defect
W/D	well-developed
W/N	well-nourished
WAIS-III	Wechsler Adult Intelligence Scale-III
WBC	white blood cell; white blood cell count
WBST	Wonderlic Basic Skills Test
WISC	Wechsler Intelligence Scale for Children
WPPSI-R	Wechsler Preschool and Primary Scale of Intelligence-Revised
x	times, multiplied by
ZIFT	zygote intrafallopian transfer

Trade Name	Generic
—.....................	colchicine
—.....................	heparin
—.....................	morphine
—.....................	nitrous oxide (N_2O)
—.....................	oxaliplatin
—.....................	propranolol
5-FU	fluorouracil
6-MP	6-mercaptopurine
A/T/S	topical erythromycin
A-Hydrocort............	hydrocortisone topical
Abbokinase	urokinase
Accupril	quinapril
Accutane	isotretinoin
Achromycin V	tetracycline
Acthar.................	corticotropin
Acticin	permathrin
Actigall	ursodiol
Activase	alteplase
Actonel...............	risedronate sodium
Actos.................	pioglitazone
Acular	ketorolac ophthalmic
AD-DEX	dexamethasone ophthalmic
Adderall	amphetamine mixed salts
Adipex	phentermine
Adipost...............	phendimetrazine
Adrenalin	epinephrine
Adriamycin	doxorubicin hydrochloride
Adrucil	fluorouracil
Advil	ibuprofen
Afrin	pseudoephedrine
AK-Con................	naphazoline ophthalmic
AK-Pred	prednisolone sodium phosphate ophthalmic
AK-Pro	dipivefrin ophthalmic
AK-Spore	gramicidin ophthalmic
AK-Tracin.............	bacitracin ophthalmic
Akarpine...............	pilocarpine ophthalmic
Albuterol	albuterol
Aldactazide	spironolactone and HCTZ
Aldactone.............	spironolactone HCTZ
Aldomet	methyldopa
Alesse	levonorgestrel
Aleve.................	naproxen
Alfenta	alfentanil hydrocholoride
Alkeran	melphalan
Allegra	fexofenadine hydrochloride
Allerest	naphazoline ophthalmic
Alpha Keri	—
Alphagan	brimonidine tartrate
Alternagel.............	aluminum hydroxide

Trade Name	Generic
Alupent...............	metaproterenol sulfate
Amaryl	glimepiride
Ambien...............	zolpidem tartrate
Amcil.................	ampicillin
Amicar	aminocaproic acid
Amidate	etomidate
Aminophylline..........	aminophylline
Amoxil	amoxicillin
Amphogel.............	aluminum hydroxide gel
Ampicill	ampicillin
Ampicillin.............	ampicillin
Anacin................	acetaminophen and APAP
Anafranil..............	clomipramine
Anaprox	naproxen sodium
Anaspaz	hyoscyamine sulfate
Anexsia...............	hydrocodone with acetaminophen
Ansaid................	flurbiprofen
Antepar...............	piperazine citrate
Antiminth.............	pyrantel pamoate
Antivert	meclizine
Anturane	sulfinpyrazone
Anzemet..............	dolasetron
Apresoline	hydralazine hydrochloride
Arimidex..............	anastrozole
Aristocort.............	triamcinolone acetonide
Artane................	trihexyphenidyl
Asendin	amoxapine
aspirin................	acetylsalicylic acid and ASA
Astelin................	azelastine hydrochloride
Atacand	candesartan cilexetil
Atarax................	hydroxyzine hydrochloride
Ativan	lorazepam
Atromid-S.............	clofibrate
Atropine-1	atropine ophthalmic
Atrovent...............	ipratropium
ATS Theramycin 2; A/T/S................	topical erythromycin
Augmentin............	amoxicillin and potassium clavulanate
Avandia................	rosiglitazone
Aveeno Bath	—
Avita	tretinoin
Avonex	interferon beta
Axid..................	nizatidine
Aygestin	norethindrone acetate
Azelex................	azelek acid
Azmacort	triamcinolone
Azo Gantrisin...........	sulfisoxazole and phenazopyridine

Trade Name	Generic
Azulfidine	sulfasalazine
Bacid	lactobacillus
Baciguent	bacitracin
Bacticort	neomycin, polymyxin, hydrocortisone
Bactrim	trimethoprim and sulfamethoxazole
Bactroban	mupirocin topical
Balnetar oil	—
Bancap-HC	hydrocodone w/acetaminophen
Banophen	diphenhydramine
Baridium	phenazopyridine hydrochloride
BCNU	carmustine
Beclovent	beclomethasone
Beconase	beclomethasone dipropionate
Beconase AQ	beclomethasone dipropionate monohydrate
Beepen-VK	penicillin V and potassium
Benadryl	diphenhydramine
Benemid	probenecid
Bentyl	dicyclomine hydrochloride
Betaderm	betamethasone
Betadine	povidone iodine
Betadine Vaginal Suppositories	povidone iodine
Betagan	levobunolol ophthalmic
Betapen-VK	penicillin V and potassium
Betaseron	interferon beta
Betinol	timolol maleate ophthalmic
Betoptic	betaxolol ophthalmic
Biaxin	clarithromycin
Bicillin	penicillin G and benzathine
Bicitra	sodium citrate, citric acid
BiCNU	carmustine
Bio-Statin	nystatin
Biomox	amoxicillin
Blenoxane	bleomycin sulfate
Bleph-10	sulfacetamide ophthalmic
Blephamide	sulfacetamide, prednisolone
Blocadren	timolol
Bonine	meclizine
Brethine	terbutaline
Brevitol	methohexital sodium
Bronkaid	epinephrine
Brycanyl	terbutaline
Bumex	bumetanide
BuSpar	buspirone
Cafergot	ergotamine and caffeine
Calan	verapamil
Calciferol	vitamin D preparations
Calcimar	calcitonin
Calderol	calcifedial
Caltrate	oyster shell calcium
Camptosar	irinoteca
Capaxone	glatiramer acetate
Capoten	captopril
Carafate	sucralfate
Carbachol	carbachol
Carbocaine	mepivacaine hydrocholoride
Carboptic	carbachol

Trade Name	Generic
Cardene	nicardipine
Cardizem	diltiazem hydrochloride
Cardura	doxazosin mesylate
Cascara Sagrada	—
Casodex	bicalutamide
Catapres	clonidine hydrochloride
CCNU	lomustine
Ceclor	cefaclor
CeeNu	lomustine
Ceftin	cefuroxime axetil
Cefzil	cefprozil monohydrate
Celebrex	celecoxib
Celestone	betamethasone
Celexa	citalopram
Cenestin	conjugated estrogens
Cerubidine	daunorubicin
Cerumenex	triethanolamine
Cetacaine	tetracaine
Cetapred	sulfacetamide, prednisolone
Chronulac	lactulose
Ciloxan	ciprofloxacin ophthalmic
Ciobrevate	clobetasol topical
Cipro	ciprofloxacin
Citracal	calcium citrate
Citrucel	methyl cellulose
Claritin D	loratadine and pseudoephedrine sulfate
Claritin	loratadine
Cleocin	clindamycin
Climera	estradiol
Clindex	clidinium and chlordiazepoxide
Clinoril	sulindac
Clinoxide	clidinium and chlordiazepoxide
Clomid	clomiphene citrate
Clozaril	clozapine
Cogentin	benztropine
Colace	docusate sodium
Colestid	colestipol
Colyte	—
Compazine	prochlorperazine maleate
Cordarone	amiodarone hydrochloride
Cordran	flurandrenolide topical
Cordrol	prednisone
Cormax	clobetasol topical
Cort-Dome	hydrocortisone acetate
Cortaid	hydrocortisone topical
Cortef	hydrocortisone
Cortisporin Ophthalmic	neomycin, polymyxin, hydrocortisone
Cortisporin Otic	hydrocortisone, neomycin
Cortomycin	neomycin, polymyxin, hydrocortisone
Cortone	cortisone
Cortrosyn	cosyntropin (synthetic corticotropin)
Cosmegen	dactinomycin
Cotrim	trimethoprim and sulfamethoxazole
Coumadin	warfarin sodium
Cozaar	losartan

Trade Name	Generic
Creon	pancreatin
Crixivan	indinavir sulfate
Cutivate	fluticasone propionate
Cycloflex	cyclobenzaprine hydrochloride
Cyklokapron	tranexamic acid
Cylert	pemoline
Cystospas	hyoscyamine sulfate
Cytomel	liothyronine sodium
Cytosar-U	cytarabine
Cytotec	misoprostol
Cytoxan	cyclophosphamide
Dantrium	dantrolene sodium
Darvon	propoxyphene
Daypro	oxaprozin
DDAVP	desmopressin acetate (vasopressin)
Debrox	carbamide peroxide
Decadron	dexamethasone
Decadron Ocumeter	dexamethasone ophthalmic
Deconamine SR	pseudoephedrine and chlorpheniramine
Deltasone	prednisone
Demerol	meperidine
Demulen	ethynodiol diacetate/ ethinyl estradiol
Depakene	valproic acid
Depakote	valproic acid
Depo-Provera	medroxyprogesterone acetate
Deramycin	topical erythromycin
Dermacin	fluocinonide topical
Dermatop	prednicarbate topical
DES	diethylstilbestrol
Desmopressin acetate	vasopressin
Desogen	desogestrel/ethinyl estradiol
Desyrel	trazodone
Detrol	tolterodine tarte
Dexasol	dexamethasone ophthalmic
Dexedrine	dextroamphetamine sulfate
DHT	vitamin D preparations
DiaBeta	glyburide
Diabinese	chlorpropamide
Diamox	acetazolamide
Diapid	vasopressin
Didronel	etidronate
Differin	adapalene
Diflucan	fluconazole
Dilantin	phenytoin
Diprivan	propofol
Diprolene	betamethasone dipropionate
Diprosone	betamethasone dipropionate
Ditropan	oxybutynin chloride
Diuril	chlorothiazide
Dolacet	hydrocodone and APAP
Donnatal	atropine, scopolamine, hyoscyamine, phenobarbital
Donnazyme	pancreatin
Dovonex	calcipotriene
Dramamine	dimenhydrinate
DTIC-Dome	dacarbazine
Dulcolax	bisacodyl
Duphalac	lactulose
Duranest	etidocaine
Duricef	cefadroxil
Duvoid	bethanechol
Dyazide	triamterene/HCTz
Dyrenium	triamterene
E.E.S.	erythromycin
E-Mycin	erythromycin
Econopred	prednisolone acetate ophthalmic
Eflone	fluormetholone ophthalmic
Elamite	permathrin
Elavil	amitriptyline hydrochloride
Eldepryl	selegiline
Elimite	permathrin
Elspar	asparaginase
Emcyt	estramustine
Emgel	topical erythromycin
EMLA cream	prilocaine
Enbrel	etanercept
Enduron	methyclothiazide
Entex	guaifenesin and phenylephrine
Epifrin	epinephrine bitrate
Epinal	epinephrine bitrate
Epivir	laminudine
Epogen	epoetin alfa (synthetic)
Equanil	meprobamate
Ergonovine	ergonovine
Ergostat	ergotamine tartrate
Eryc	erythromycin
Eryped	erythromycin ethylsuccinate
Esidrix	hydrochlorothiazide (HCTz)
Estrace	estradiol
Estraderm	estradiol
Ethrane	enflurane
Eulexin	flutamide
Eurax	crotimaton
Evista	raloxifene hydrochloride
Ex-Lax	—
Excedrin	acetaminophen, APAP, and caffeine
Excedrin PM	diphenhydramine and APAP
Excedrin IB	ibuprofen
Exelderm	sulconazole nitrate
Exosurf	colfosceril palmitate
Fareston	toremifine
Feen-a-mint	—
Feldene	piroxicam
Femara	letrozole
Feosol	ferrous sulfate
Fergon	ferrous gluconate
Ferosul	ferrous sulfate
Ferralet	ferrous gluconate
Ferro-Sequels	—
Fioricet	caffeine, butalbital, and APAP
Fiorinal	caffeine, butalbital, and ASA
Flagyl	metronidazole
Flarex	fluormetholone ophthalmic
Fleet Preparation	—
Flexeril	cyclobenzaprine hydrochloride
Flonase	fluticasone propionate

Trade Name	Generic
Florinef	fludrocortisone
Flovent	fluticasone propionate
Floxin Otic	ofloxacin
Fludara	fludarabine
Fluex	fluocinonide topical
Fluonid	fluocinolone acetonide
Fluor-Op	fluormetholone ophthalmic
Fluothane	halothane
Flurosyn	fluocinonide topical
FML	fluorometholone ophthalmic
Forane	isoflurane
Fortaz	ceftazidime
Fortovase	saquinavir mesylate
Fosomax	alendronate
Fragmin	dalteparin
Fulvicin P/C	griseofulvin
Furacen	nitrofurazone
Furadantin	nitrofurantoin
Gantrisin	sulfisoxazole
Garamycin	gentamicin sulfate ophthalmic
Gastrocrom	cromolyn sodium
Gaviscon	—
Gemzar	gemcitabine
Genoptic	gentamicin sulfate ophthalmic
Genotropin	somatropin
Gentacidin	gentamicin sulfate
Gentak	gentamicin sulfate ophthalmic
Geodon	ziprasidone
Glatiramer acetate	copaxone
Glaucon	epinephrine bitrate
GlucaGen	glucagon
Glucagon	glucagon
Glucophage	metformin
Glucotrol	glipizide
Glucovance	glyburide/metformin hydrochloride
Glynase	glyburide
Glyset	miglitol
Golytely	—
Grisactin	griseofulvin
Grisfulvin V	griseofulvin
Gyne-Lotrimin	clotrimazole
Halcion	triazolam
Haldol	haloperidol
Halotestin	fluoxymesterone
Haltran	ibuprofen
Herceptin	trastuzumab
Hexadrol	dexamethasone
Hismanal	astemizole
Histerone	testosterone
Hivid	zalcitabine
HMS	medrysone ophthalmic
Humabid	guaifenesin
Humalog	insulin lispro
Humatrope	somatropin
Humulin (L, N, R, or U)	human insulin
Hycamtin	topotecan
Hydrea	hydroxyurea
Hydrocet	hydrocodone and APAP
Hydrocortone	hydrocortisone

Trade Name	Generic
HydroDIURIL	hydrochlorothiazide
Hygroton	chlorthalidone
Hyperstat	diazoxide
Hytakesol	vitamin D preparations
Hytone	hydrocortisone topical
Hytrin	terazosin hydrochloride
Iberet-Folic-500	—
IFEX	ifosfamide
IGIV	immune globulin IV
Ilotycin	erythromycin ophthalmic
Immunex	aminocaproic acid
Imodium	loperamide
Imuran	azathioprine
Incor	amrinone lactate
Inderal	propranolol hydrochloride
Indocin	indomethacin
Intal	cromolyn Na
Intron A	interferon alfa
Intropin	dopamine
Invase	saquinavir mesylate
Ionamin	phentermine
Isoptin	verapamil
Isopto Homatropine	homatropine ophthalmic
Isopto Atropine	atropine ophthalmic
Isopto Carbachol	carbachol
Isopto Carpine	pilocarpine ophthalmic
Isuprel	isoproterenol
K-Tab	potassium chloride
K-Lor	potassium chloride
Kay Ciel	potassium chloride
Kayexalete	sodium polystyrene sulfonate
Keflex	cephalexin
Keftab	cephalexin
Kefzol	cefazolin
Kenalog	triamcinolone acetonide
Ketalar	ketamine hydrochloride
Klonopin	clonazepam
Klor-Con	potassium chloride
Kytril	granisetron
Lactinex	lactobacillus
Lamisil	terbinfine
Lanoxin	digoxin
Lantus	insulin glaring
Lasix	furosemide
Lescol	fluvastatin
Leucovorin Calcium	folinic acid
Leukeran	chlorambucil
Leukine	sargramostim (GM-CSF)
Levbid	hyoscyamine sulfate
Levophed	norepinephrine bitartrate
Levothroid	levothyroxine sodium
Levoxyl	levothyroxine sodium
Levsin	hyoscyamine sulfate
Levsinex	hyoscyamine sulfate
Librax	clidinium and chlordiazepoxide
Librium	chlordiazepoxide
Lidex	fluocinonide topical
Lignocaine	lidocaine
Lioresal	baclofen
Lipitor	atorvastatin

Trade Name	Generic
Lo/Ovral	norgestrel/ethinyl estradiol
Lodine	etodolac
Loestrin	norethindrone acetate and ethinyl estradiol
Lomotil	diphenoxylate with atropine
Loniten	minoxidil
Lopid	gemfibrozil
Lopressor	metoprolol
Loprox	ciclopirox topical
Lopurin	allopurinol
Lorcet	hydrocodone with acetaminophen
Lorelco	probucol
Lortab	hydrocodone and acetaminophen
Lotrimin	clotrimazole topical
Lotrisone	betamethasone and clotrimazole
Lovenox	enoxaparin
Loxitane	loxapine
Lozol	indapamide
Lubath	—
Lugol's Solution	iodine and potassium iodide
Lupron	leuprolide acetate
Lysodren	mitotane
Maalox	—
Macrodantin	nitrofurantoin
Mandol	cefamandole
Mannitol	mannitol
Marcaine	bupivacaine hydrocholoride
Maridex	dexamethasone ophthalmic
Materna 1-60	—
Matulane	procarbazine
Maxidex	dexamethasone
Maxitrol	neomycin, polymyxin, dexamethasone ophthalmic
Maxivate	betamethasone dipropionate
Medrol	methylprednisolone
Megace	megestrol acetate
Mellaril	thioridazine
Menest	esterified estrogen
MESNEX	mesna
Mestinon	pyridostigmine bromide
Metamucil	psyllium preparations
Metaprel	metaproterenol
Methergine	methylergonovine maleate
Methotrexact	methotrexate
Mevacor	lovastatin
Mexate	methotrexate
Mexiletine	mexiletine hydrochloride
Miacalcin	calcitonin salmon
Miacalcin Nasal Spray	calcitonin salmon
Micro-K	potassium chloride
Micronase	glyburide
Midamor	amiloride hydrochloride
Midol	ibuprofen
Milk of Magnesia (MOM)	—
Minipress	prazosin hydrochloride
Minocin	minocycline
Miostat	carbachol
Mircette	—
Mithracin	plicamycin

Trade Name	Generic
Mitrazol	miconazole
Monistat	miconazole
Monistat 7 Vaginal Cream	miconazole nitrate
Monistat-Derm	miconazole
Monocid	cefonicid
Motrin	ibuprofen
Mustargen	mechlorethamine
Mutamycin	mitomycin
Mycelex	clotrimazole topical
Mycelex Troches	clotrimazole
Myciguent	neomycin sulfate
Mycitracin	polymyxin, neomycin, and bacitracin
Mycolog-II	nystatin
Mycostatin	nystatin
Mylanta	—
Myleran	busulfan
Mysoline	primidone
Naftin	naftifine topical
Nalfon	fenoprofen calcium
Naprosyn	naproxen sodium
Nasacort	triamcinolone acetonide
Nasalcrom	cromolyn sodium
Nasalide	flunisolide
Nasarel	flunisolide
Nasonex	mometasone furoate
Natabec Rx	—
Natalins	—
Navane	thiothixene
Navelbine	vinorelbine
Neodecadron	neomycin, dexamethasone
Neoral	cyclosporine
Neosporin ophthalmic	neomycin, polymyxin B, bacitracin
Neosporin G.U. irritant	neomycin, polymyxin B
Neotricin HC	neomycin, polymyxin, hydrocortisone
Nesacaine	chloroprocaine hydrocholoride
Neupogen	filgastim (G-CSF)
Niaspan	nicotinic acid
Nicobid	nicotinic acid
Nicolar	nicotinic acid
Niferex-PN Forte	—
Nilstat	nystatin
Nipride	nitroprusside sodium
Nitrostat	nitroglycerine
Nizoral	ketoconazole
Nolvadex	tamoxifen
Nordette	levonorgestrel/ethinyl estradiol
Norditropin	somatropin
Norinyl	norethindrone/ethinyl estradiol
Norlestrin	—
Noroxin	norfloxacin
Norpace	disopyramide phosphate
Norpramin	desipramine
Norvasc	amlodipine
Norvir	ruonavir
Novantrone	mitoxantrone

Trade Name	Generic
Novocaine	procaine hydrocholoride
Novolin (N, L, or R)	human insulin
Novolog	insulin aspart
Nutracort	hydrocortisone topical
Nutropin	somatropin
Ocu-Cort	neomycin, polymyxin, hydrocortisone
Ocufen	flurbiprofen
Ocuflox	ofloxacin ophthalmic
Ogen	estropipate
Omnipen	ampicillin
Oncovin	vincristine sulfate
Optimine	azatadine maleate
Orapred	prednisoline
Orasone	prednisone
Organidin	iodinated glycerol
Orinase	tolbutamide
Ortho Tri-Cyclen	norgestimate/ethinyl estradiol
Ortho-Novum	norethindrone/mestranol
Ortho-Cyclen	norgestimate/ethinyl estradiol
Ortho-Est	estropipate
Orudis	ketoprofen
Oruvail	ketoprofen
OSCal	oyster shell calcium
Osmoglyn	glycerin
Ovral	norgestral/ethinyl estradiol
Oxistat	oxiconazole topical
Oxsoralen	methoxsalen
OxyContin	oxycodone
P.T.U.	propylthiouracil
Pacerone	amiodarone hydrochloride
Pagitane	cycrimine hydrochloride
Pamelor	nortriptyline
Panadol	acetaminophen and APAP
Pancrease	pancrelipase, pancreatic preparations
Paraplatin	carboplatin
Parisdol	ethopropagine hydrochloride
Parlodel	bromocriptine mesylate
Patanol	olopatadine hydrochloride
Paxil	paroxetine
Pediapred	prednisolone
Pediatric Gentamicin	gentamicin sulfate
Pen-Vee-K	penicillin V and potassium
Penthrane	methoxyflurane
Pentothal Sodium	thiopental sodium
Pepcid	famotidine
Pepto-Bismol	bismuth subsalicylate
Perdiem	—
Pergonal	menotropins
Periactin	cyproheptadine hydrochloride
Peri-Colace	casanthranol and docusate sodium
Peridex	chlorhexidine gluconate
Periogard	chlorhexidine gluconate
Permax	pergolide mesylate
Persantine	dipyridamole
Phenergan	promethazine hydrochloride
Phenobarbital	phenobarbital
Pilocar	pilocarpine ophthalmic

Trade Name	Generic
Pitocin	oxytocin
Pitressin	vasopressin
Platinol	cisplatin
Polocaine	mepivacaine hydrocholoride
Polycillin	ampicillin
Pontocaine	tetracaine
Prandin	repaglinide
Pravachol	pravastatin sodium
Precose	acarbose
Pred Mild	prednisolone acetate ophthalmic
Prelone	prednisolone
Preludin	phenmetrazine
Premarin	conjugated estrogens
Premphase	conjugated estrogens and medroxyprogesterone
Prempro	conjugated estrogen and medroxyprogesterone
Prevacid	lansoprazole
Prevalite	cholestyramine
Prilosec	omeprazole
Primatene	epinephrine
Principen	ampicillin
Prinivil	lisinopril
Pro-Banthine	propantheline bromide
Probalan	probenecid
Procardia	nifedipine
Procrit	epoetin alfa
Profasi HP	chorionic gonadotropin
Prolixin	fluphenazine
Proloid	thyroglobulin
Pronestyl	procainamide hydrochloride
Propine	dipivefrin ophthalmic
Prostigmin	neostigmine bromide
Protonix	pantoprazole
Proventil	albuterol
Provera	medroxyprogesterone acetate
Provil	ibuprofen
Prozac	fluoxetine
Purinethol	6-mercaptopurine
Pyridiate	phenazopyridine hydrochloride
Pyridium	phenazopyridine hydrochloride
Questran	cholestyramine
Quinidex	quinidine
Regitine	phentolamine mesylate
Reglan	metoclopramide
Relafen	nabumetone
Remeron	mirtazapine
Remicade	infliximab
Renacidin Irrigation	citric acid, magnesium carbonate, gluconodelta-lactone
Renova	tretinoin
Rescriptor	delavirdine
Retavase	reteplase
Retin A	tretinoin
Retrovir	zidovudine
Rezine	hydroxyzine
Rheumatrex	methotrexate
Rhinocort	budesonide
Riopan	—
Risperdal	risperidone

Trade Name	Generic
Ritalin	methylphenidate
Rituxan	rituximab
Robaxin	methocarbamol
Robimycin	erythromycin
Robinul	glycopyrrolate
Rocaltrol	calcitriol (man-made vitamin D)
Rocephin	ceftriaxone
Roferon-A	interferon alfa
Rolaids	calcium carbonate and magnesia
Roymicin	erythromycin ophthalmic
Rufen	ibuprofen
Rythmol	propafenone hydrochloride
S.S.K.I.	potassium iodide saturated solution
Sandimmune	cyclosporine
Sandostatin	octreotide acetate
Sansert	methysergide maleate
Seconal	secobarbital
Seldane	terfenadine
Semprex-D	pseudoephedrine and acrivastine
Senokot	—
Sensorcaine	bupivacaine hydrocholoride
Septra	trimethoprim and sulfamethoxazole
Serax	oxazepam
Seroquel	quetiapine fumarate
Serpasil	reserpine
Shohl's solution	sodium citrate, citric acid
Silvadene	silver sulfadiazine
Simron	ferrous gluconate
Sinemet	carbidopa, levodopa
Slo-bid	theophylline
Slo-Niacin	nicotinic acid
Slo-Phyllin	theophylline
Slow-K	potassium chloride
Slow Fe	ferrous sulfate exsiccated
Solu-Cortef	hydrocortisone
Solu-Medrol	methylprednisolone
Soma	carisoprodol
Somnothane	halothane
Spectazole	econazole topical
Sporanox	itraconazole
Starlix	nateglinide
Stelazine	trifluoperazine
Stimate	desmopressin acetate (vasopressin)
Streptase	streptokinase
Sublimaze	fenttanyl citrate
Sudafed	pseudoephedrine
Sufenta	sufentanil citrate
Sulfamylon	mafenide acetate
Sumycin	tetracycline
Suprane	desflurane
Suprax	cefixime
Surfak	docusate calcium
Surmontil	trimipramine
Survanta	beractant
Sustiva	efavirenz
Symmetrel	amantadine
Synalar	fluocinolone acetonide

Trade Name	Generic
Synarel	nafarelin acetate
Synthroid	levothyroxine sodium
Tagamet	cimetidine
Tambocor	flecainide acetate
Tapazole	methimazole
Taxol	paclitaxel
Taxotere	docetaxel
Tegison	etretinate
Tegretol	carbamazepine
Temodal	temozolomide
Temovate	clobetasol topical
Ten-K	potassium chloride
Tenormin	atenolol
Tenuate	diethylpropion
Tequin	gatifloxacin
Terazol Vaginal Cream	terconazole
Testoderm	testosterone
Thalomid	thalidomide
Theo-clear	theophylline
Theo-Dur	theophylline
Thiotepa	thiotepa
Thorazine	chlorpromazine
Thyrogen	thyrotropin
Thyroid U.S.P.	desiccated thyroid
Thyrolar	liotrix
Tigan	trimethobenzamide
Timoptic Ocumeter	timolol maleate ophthalmic
Tobradex	tobramycin, dexamethasone
Tobralcon	tobramycin ophthalmic
Tobramycin	aminoglycosides
Tobrasol	tobramycin ophthalmic
Tobrex	tobramycin ophthalmic
Tofranil	imipramine hydrochloride
Tolectin	tolmetin sodium
Tolinase	tolazamide
Topicort	desoximetasone topical
Toprol XL	metoprolol succinate
Torecan	thiethylperazine maleate
Totacillin	ampicillin
Tranxene	clorazepate dipotassium
Trental	pentoxifylline
Trexall	methotrexate
Tri-Norinyl	ethinyl estradiol/levonorgestrel
Tri-Phasi	ethinyl estradiol/levonorgestrel
Tricor	fenofibrate
Trilafon	perphenazine
Trimox	amoxicillin
Trusopt	dorzolamide
Tylenol with Codeine	acetaminophen with codeine
Tylenol	acetaminophen and APAP
Ultane	sevoflurane
Ultiva	remifentanil hydrochloride
Ultram	tramadol hydrochloride
Ultrase	pancrelipase
Ultravate	halobetasol propionate
Urecholine	bethanechol
Urised (various)	methenamine, phenyl salicylate, atropine, hyoscyamine, benzoic acid, and methylene blue
Urispas	flavoxate

Trade Name	Generic
V-Cillin K	penicillin V potassium
Valisone	betamethasone valerate
Valium	diazepam
Valtrex	valacyclovir
Vancenase	beclomethasone dipropionate
Vanceril	beclomethasone
Vancocin	vancomycin hydrochloride
Vancoled	vancomycin hydrochloride
Vaponephrine	epinephrine
Vasocidin	sulfacetamide, prednisolone
Vasocon-A	naphazoline ophthalmic
Vasotec	enalapril maleate
Velban	vinblastine sulfate
Ventolin	albuterol
VePesid	etoposide
Vermox	mebendazole
Versed	midazolam hydrocholoride
Vexol	rimexolone ophthalmic
Viagra	sildenafil; sildenafil citrate
Vibramycin	doxycycline
Vicodin	hydrocodone with acetaminophen
Videx	didanosine
Vincasar	vincristine sulfate
Vioxx	rofecoxib
Viracept	nelfinavir mesylate
Viramune	neviraprine
Virilon	methyltestosterone
Viroptic	trifluridine ophthalmic
Vistaril	hydroxyzine pamoate
vitamin B12	cyanocobalamin
Vivelle	estradiol

Trade Name	Generic
Voltaren	diclofenac sodium ophthalmic
VoSol Otic	hydrocortisone, acetic acid
Welchol	colesevelam
Wellbutrin	bupropion
Westcort	hydrocortisone valerate
Wycillin	penicillin G and procaine
X-prep	—
Xalatan	latanoprost
Xanax	alprazolam
Xeloda	capecitabine
Xylocaine	lidocaine
Yocon	yohimbine
Yutopar	ritodrine
Zaditor	ketotifen fumarate
Zantac	ranitidine
Zarontin	ethosuximide
Zaroxolyn	metolazone
Zartan	cephalexin
Zenate	—
Zerit	stavudine
Zestril	lisinopril
Zetar	—
Ziagen	abacavir
Zithromax (Z-Pack)	azithromycin
Zocor	simvastatin
Zofran	ondansetron hydrochloride
Zoladex	goserelin
Zoloft	sertraline
Zovirax	acyclovir
Zyloprim	allopurinol
Zyprexa	olanzapine
Zyrtec	cetirizine hydrochloride

Index

Page numbers in boldface indicate references to figures.

681

License Agreement for Delmar Cengage Learning, Educational Software/Data

Audio CD to Accompany *Terminology for Allied Health Professionals*, Fifth Edition

Computer CD Player Instructions

1. Insert the disk into the CD-ROM player of your computer.
2. The media player should automatically start and bring up track 1.
3. Use the media player as directed by the manufacturer.

For Windows: If the media player does not start automatically:

1. From the Start Menu, choose Programs, then Accessories.
2. Choose Entertainment or Multimedia, then a media player such as Windows® Media Player.
3. Browse to your CD-ROM drive and open the audio file you wish to play.

For Macintosh: If the media player does not start automatically:

1. Start the Apple CD Player.
2. Browse to your CD-ROM drive and open the audio file you wish to play.

System Requirements

- Audio CD Player **or**
- Computer with double-spin CD-ROM drive, sound card, speakers or headphones, and media player software.

Tracks

1. Chapter 3 Medical History and Physical Examination (2:03)
2. Chapter 4 Pharmacology (3:02)
3. Chapter 5 The Integumentary System (1:35)
4. Chapter 6 The Musculoskeletal System (3:02)
5. Chapter 7 Surgery (2:08)
6. Chapter 8 The Cardiovascular System (3:08)
7. Chapter 9 The Blood and Lymph Systems (5:38)
8. Chapter 10 Oncology (3:02)
9. Chapter 11 Radiology and Nuclear Medicine (3:02)

Tracks *(continued)*

10. Chapter 12 The Respiratory System (3:18)
11. Chapter 13 The Digestive System (2:57)
12. Chapter 14 Discharge Summaries (3:22)
13. Chapter 15 The Urinary System (2:29)
14. Chapter 16 The Female Reproductive System (3:58)
15. Chapter 17 The Male Reproductive System (3:23)
16. Chapter 18 Pathology and Autopsies (2:47)
17. Chapter 19 The Endocrine System (3:42)
18. Chapter 20 The Nervous System (2:04)
19. Chapter 21 Mental Health (2:44)
20. Chapter 22 The Eye (2:47)
21. Chapter 23 The Ear, Nose, and Throat (1:39)